PHTLS

Prehospital Trauma Life Support

"The fate of the wounded rests in the hands of the one who applies the first dressing."

—**Nicholas Senn, MD (1844-1908)**
American surgeon (Chicago, Illinois)
Founder, Association of Military Surgeons of
the United States

PHTLS

Prehospital Trauma Life Support

SIXTH EDITION

Prehospital Trauma Life Support Committee of The National
Association of Emergency Medical Technicians in Cooperation with
The Committee on Trauma of The American College of Surgeons

MOSBY JEMS

ELSEVIER

Pre HOSPITAL TRAUMA LIFE SUPPORT · NAEMT ·

MOSBY
ELSEVIER

11830 Westline Industrial Drive
St. Louis, Missouri 63146

PHTLS Prehospital Trauma Life Support
**Copyright © 2007, 2003, 1999, 1994 by Mosby, Inc.,
an affiliate of Elsevier Inc.**

ISBN-13: 978-0-323-03331-2
ISBN-10: 0-323-03331-8

Some material was previously published.

Notice

Knowledge and best practice in this field are constantly changing. As new research and experience broaden our knowledge, changes in practice, treatment and drug therapy may become necessary or appropriate. Readers are advised to check the most current information provided (i) on procedures featured or (ii) by the manufacturer of each product to be administered, to verify the recommended dose or formula, the method and duration of administration, and contraindications. It is the responsibility of the practitioner, relying on their own experience and knowledge of the patient, to make diagnoses, to determine dosages and the best treatment for each individual patient, and to take all appropriate safety precautions. To the fullest extent of the law, neither the Publisher nor the [Editors assume any liability for any injury and/or damage to persons or property arising out or related to any use of the material contained in this book.

The Publisher

Previous editions copyrighted 1986, 1990 by Educational Direction, Inc., Akron, Ohio.

ISBN-13: 978-0-323-03331-2
ISBN-10: 0-323-03331-8

Executive Editor: Linda Honeycutt
Senior Developmental Editor: Laura Bayless
Publishing Services Manager: Patricia Tannian
Senior Project Manager: Sarah Wunderly
Design Direction: Julia Dummitt

Printed in Canada

Last digit is the print number: 9 8 7 6 5 4 3 2

IN MEMORIAM

Scott B. Frame, MD, FACS, FCCM	**Richard W. "Rick" Vomacka**	**Joseph D. "Deke" Farrington, MD, FACS**
JANUARY 31, 1952-MARCH 14, 2001	1946-2001	1909-1982

Photo courtesy of Joyce Frame.

Scott was the Associate Medical Director for the PHTLS program. His major emphasis was in the development of the audiovisuals for PHTLS and its promulgation internationally. At the time of his untimely death, he had assumed the responsibility of putting together the fifth edition of the PHTLS course. This included the revision not only of the textbook, but also of the instructor manual and all of the associated teaching materials. He accepted the appointment to become Medical Director of the PHTLS course when the fifth edition was published. He published chapters and articles on EMS and trauma in major textbooks and scientific journals.

The PHTLS program grew immeasurably under Scott's leadership. Its continuation into the future will be because of what Scott did and the part of his life that he lent to PHTLS and to his patients.

Rick was a part of the task force that developed the PHTLS course based on the Advanced Trauma Life Support program of the American College of Surgeons. PHTLS became his passion as the course came together, and he traveled around the country in the early 1980s conducting pilot courses and regional faculty workshops, and worked with Dr. McSwain and the other original task force members to fine-tune the program. Rick was key to the close relationship that developed between PHTLS and the U.S. military, and he also worked on the first international PHTLS course sites. Rick was a big part of PHTLS's beginnings, and we will remember him with gratitude for his hard work and dedication to the cause of trauma patients.

Often referred to as "The Father of EMS," Dr. Farrington penned the article "Death in a Ditch," which many believe signaled the turning point in modern EMS in the United States. In 1958 he convinced the Chicago Fire Department that firefighters should be trained to manage emergency patients. Working with Dr. Sam Banks, Deke started the Trauma Training Program in Chicago. Millions have been trained following the guidelines developed in this landmark program. Deke continued to work at every level of EMS from the field to education to legislation, ensuring that EMS would grow into the profession in which we work today. The principles set forth by Deke's worth form a part of the nucleus of PHTLS, and his are among the shoulders on which we all stand.

Editors

Jeffrey P. Salomone, MD, FACS, NREMT-P
Senior Associate Medical Director, PHTLS
Associate Professor of Surgery
Emory University School of Medicine
Atlanta, Georgia

Peter T. Pons, MD, FACEP
Associate Medical Director, PHTLS
Professor of Emergency Medicine
University of Colorado Health Sciences Center
Denver, Colorado

Editor-in-Chief

Norman E. McSwain, Jr., MD, FACS, NREMT-P
Medical Director, PHTLS
Tulane University Department of Surgery
New Orleans, Louisiana

Associate Editors

Will Chapleau, EMT-P, RN, TNS, CEN
Chairman, PHTLS Executive Council
Chief, Chicago Heights Fire Department
Chicago Heights, Illinois

Gregory Chapman, EMT-P, RRT
Vice Chairman, PHTLS Executive Council
Director, Institute of Prehospital Emergency Medicine
Hudson Valley Community College
Troy, New York

Stephen D. Giebner, MD, MPH
Chairman, Committee on Tactical Combat Casualty Care
CAPT, MC, USN (Ret)
Naval Operational Medicine Institute
San Diego, California

Jeffrey S. Guy, MD, FACS, EMT-P
Associate Medical Director, PHTLS
Associate Professor of Surgery
Director, Regional Burn Center
Vanderbilt University School of Medicine
Nashville, Tennessee

Contributors

Melissa Alexander, MS, NREMT-P
Director, EMS Academy
University of New Mexico
Albuquerque, New Mexico

Jameel Ali, MD, Med, FRCSC, FACS
Professor of Surgery
Division of General Surgery
University of Toronto
Toronto, Ontario, Canada

Brad L. Bennett, PhD
CAPT U.S. Navy
Commanding Officer
Naval School of Health Sciences
Portsmouth, Virginia
Adjunct Faculty
Department of Military and Emergency Medicine
Uniformed University of the Health Sciences School of
Medicine
Bethesda, Maryland
Adjunct Faculty
Emergency Medical Technology
Tidewater Community College
Virginia Beach, Virginia

Matthew Bitner, MD
Chief Resident
Department of Emergency Medicine
Emory University School of Medicine
Atlanta, Georgia

Ernest F. J. Block, MD, FACS, EMT-P
Director of Trauma Services
Orlando Regional Healthcare System
Orlando, Florida

Susan M. Briggs, MD, MPH, FACS
Associate Professor of Surgery
Harvard University, Massachusetts General Hospital
Boston, Massachusetts

Jonnathan Busko, MD, WEMT-P
Medical Director, CDS Outdoor School
Professional Emergency Services
Eastern Maine Medical Center
Bangor, Maine

Christain E. Callsen, Jr., LP
Assistant Director, EMS Operations
Austin-Travis County EMS
Austin, Texas

Howard Champion, MD, FRCS, FACS
Senior Advisory in Trauma
Professor of Surgery and Military and Emergency Medicine
Uniformed Services University of the Health Sciences
Washington, DC

Will Chapleau, EMT-P, RN, TNS, CEN
Chairman, PHTLS Executive Council
Chief, Chicago Heights Fire Department
Chicago Heights, Illinois

Gregory Chapman, RRT, EMT-P
Vice Chairman, PHTLS Executive Council
Director, Institute of Prehospital Emergency Medicine
Hudson Valley Community College
Troy, New York

Hank Christen, MPA
Director, Emergency Response Operations
Unconventional Concepts, Inc.
Battalion Chief (Ret.)
Atlanta Fire Department
Mary Esther, Florida

David L. Ciraulo, DO, FACS, MPH
Associate Clinical Professor of Surgery
University of Vermont College of Medicine
Portland, Maine

Victoria Cleary, RN
EMS Manager
Newport Beach Fire Department
Newport Beach, California

Frederick J. Cole, MD, FACS
Associate Professor of Surgery
Eastern Virginia Medical School
Norfolk, Virginia

Keith Conover, MD, FACEP
Medical Director, Wilderness EMS Institute
Department of Emergency Medicine
Mercy Hospital of Pittsburgh
Clinical Assistant Professor, Department of
Emergency Medicine
University of Pittsburgh
Pittsburgh, Pennsylvania

Arthur Cooper, MD, MS, FACS
Professor of Surgery
Columbia University College of Physicians and Surgeons
Director of Trauma and Pediatric Surgical Services
Harlem Hospital Center
New York, New York

Jel Coward, MD, MBBS, MRCGP
Medical Director, WEMSI-Europe
Pemberton, British Columbia, Canada

Mark Elcock, MBChB, FACEM, FFAEM
Director, Statewide Coordination and Retrieval Services
The Townsville Hospital
Douglas, Queensland, Australia

Mary E. Fallat, MD, FACS
Professor of Surgery
Director, Division of Pediatric Surgery
University of Louisville
Louisville, Kentucky

Jack Grandey, NREMT-P, CCEMT-P
Operations Director
Wilderness EMS Institute
Pemberton, British Columbia, Canada

Jeffrey S. Guy, MD, FACS, EMT-P
Associate Medical Director, PHTLS
Associate Professor of Surgery
Director, Regional Burn Center
Vanderbilt University School of Medicine
Nashville, Tennessee

Nita J. Ham, EMT-P
PHTLS Executive Council
Consultant, EMS Education
Atlanta, Georgia

Mark C. Hodges, BS, NREMT-P, FP-C
PHI Air Medical
Lexington, Kentucky

Alex Isakov, MD
Co-Director, Center for Prehospital and Disaster Medicine
Assistant Professor of Emergency Medicine
Emory University School of Medicine
Atlanta, Georgia

Joseph Pearce, MSN, RN, EMT-P
EMS and Trauma Operations Manager
Orlando Regional Healthcare System
Orlando, Florida

Jon A. King, EMT-P
Performance Improvement Coordinator
WellStar Kennestone Hospital
Marietta, Georgia

Jon R. Krohmer, MD, FACEP
Associate Professor
College of Human Medicine
Michigan State University
Grand Rapids, Michigan

Peter Letarte, MD
Chief of Neurosurgery
Hines VA Hospital
Hines, Illinois

Robert W. Letton, Jr., MD, FACS, FAAP
Director, Pediatric Trauma and Burns
Children's Hospital of Oklahoma
Associate Professor of Pediatric Surgery
Oklahoma University Health Science Center
Oklahoma City, Oklahoma

Gregg C. Lord, BA, NREMT-P
Co-Principal Investigator and
Senior Policy Analyst
Homeland Security Policy Institute
George Washington University
Washington, DC

Paul M. Maniscalco, MPA, PhD(c), EMT-P
Assistant Professor and Senior Research Scientist
George Washington University
Washington, DC
Deputy Chief/Paramedic (Ret.)
Fire Department, New York EMS Command

Merry McSwain, MSN, ACNP, EMT-P
Tulane University Hospital and Clinics
New Orleans, Louisiana

Norman E. McSwain, Jr., MD, FACS, REMT-P
Medical Director, PHTLS
Professor of Surgery
Tulane University School of Medicine
New Orleans, Louisiana

Peter T. Pons, MD, FACEP
Associate Medical Director, PHTLS
Professor of Emergency Medicine
University of Colorado Health Sciences Center
Denver, Colorado

Lou Romig, MD, FAAP, FACEP
Pediatric Emergency Medicine
Miami Children's Hospital
Pediatric Medical Advisor
Miami-Dade Fire Rescue Department
Miami, Florida

Jeffrey P. Salomone, MD, FACS, NREMT-P
Senior Associate Medical Director, PHTLS
Associate Professor of Surgery
Emory University School of Medicine
Atlanta, Georgia

Joseph A. Salomone, MD, FAAEM
Associate Professor of Emergency Medicine
University of Missouri, Kansas City
Kansas City, Missouri

Donald Scelza, BS, EMT-P, WEMT-P
CDS Outdoor School, Inc.
Valencia, Pennsylvania

Brian M. Tibbs, MD
Fellow, Trauma and Surgical Critical Care
Emory University School of Medicine
Atlanta, Georgia

Josh Vayer, EMT-P
Chief, Protective Medicine Branch
Special Operations Division
Federal Protective Service
US Department of Homeland Security
Washington, DC

Carl Werntz, DO, MPH
Assistant Clinical Professor
Institute of Occupational and Environmental Health
West Virginia University
Morgantown, West Virginia

David E. Wesson, MD, FACS
Professor of Pediatric Surgery
Baylor College of Medicine
Houston, Texas

REVIEWERS

Alberto Adduci, MD
Emergency Surgeon
Anesthesiology/Intensive Care Specialist
Piemonte 118 EMS (HEMS/SAR)
Emergency Department–San Giovanni Battista Hospital
("Molinette")
Torino, Italy

Christopher Born, MD, FAAOS, FACS
Director, Orthopedic Trauma Service
Rhode Island Hospital
Professor of Orthopedic Surgery
Brown Medical School
Providence, Rhode Island

Barbara Brennan, EMT-P
Kapiolani Community College
Honolulu, Hawaii

Jeffrey R. Brosius, BS, NREMT-P, FP-C
Banner Health Systems
Phoenix, Arizona

Quirico Manuel Canario, MD, FACS
General Surgery
Assistant Professor, Department of Surgery
University of Puerto Rico School of Medicine
San Juan, Puerto Rico

Lisa K. Cannada, MD
Assistant Professor
University of Texas Southwestern
Dallas, Texas

Jo Ann Cobble, EdD, NREMT-P, RN
Dean, Health Professions
Oklahoma City Community College
Oklahoma City, Oklahoma

Keith Conover, MD, FACEP
Medical Director, Wilderness EMS Institute
Clinical Assistant Professor, Department of
Emergency Medicine
University of Pittsburgh
Pittsburgh, Pennsylvania

Arthur Cooper, MD, MS, FACS
Professor of Surgery
Columbia University College of Physicians and Surgeons
Director of Trauma and Pediatric Surgical Services
Harlem Hospital Center
New York, New York

Orlando J. Dominguez, Jr., REMT-P, MA/MBA
Chief of EMS
Brevard County Fire Rescue
EMS Program Administrator
Health First Training Center
EMS Instructor
Webster University
Space Coast Fire Chief's Association
American Heart Association
Melbourne, Florida

Douglas Fischer, EMT-P
Firefighter/Paramedic
Chicago Heights Fire Department
Chicago Heights, Illinois

Denis J. FitzGerald, MD
Emergency Medicine Physician
Bethesda, Maryland

Greg Friese, MS, NREMT-P, WEMT
President
Emergency Preparedness Systems LLC
Plover, Wisconsin

Rudy Garrett, AS, CCEMT-P, NREMT-P
Flight Paramedic, Training Coordinator
LifeNet Kentucky, Somerset Fire/EMS
Somerset, Kentucky

Ian Greenwald, MD
Assistant Professor of Emergency Medicine
Emory University School of Medicine
Atlanta, Georgia

Jeffrey Hammond MD, MPH
Chief, Trauma/Surgical Critical Care
Professor of Surgery
Robert Wood Johnson Medical School
New Brunswick, New Jersey

Seth C. Hawkins, MD
Physician
Burke County EMS
Morganton, North Carolina

Kevin High, RN, MPH, EMT
Flight Nurse
Vanderbilt LifeFlight
LifeFlight Skyport
Vanderbilt University Medical Center
Nashville, Tennessee

Art Hsieh, MA, NREMT-P
Chief Operating Officer
San Francisco Paramedic Association
San Francisco, California

Andy S. Jagoda
Professor, Emergency Medicine
Mount Sinai School of Medicine
New York, New York

M. Margaret Knudson, MD
Professor of Surgery
University of California San Francisco School of Medicine
San Francisco, California

Peter Letarte, MD
Chief of Neurosurgery
Hines Veterans Hospital
Hines, Illinois

Robert W. Letton, Jr., MD, FACS, FAAP
Director, Pediatric Trauma and Burns
Children's Hospital of Oklahoma
Associate Professor of Pediatric Surgery
Oklahoma University Health Science Center
Oklahoma City, Oklahoma

Mark Lockhart, EMT-P, NREMT-P
Maryland Heights Fire Protection District
Maryland Heights, Missouri

Michelle M. McLean, EMT-P, MD
Emergency Physician
Covenant Hospital
Saginaw, Michigan

Sindre Mellesmo, MD, MHA
Medical Director, PHTLS-Program Norway
Norwegian Air Ambulance
Norway

James B. Miller, NREMT-P
San Antonio, Texas

Fernando da Costa F. Novo, MD
General Surgeon
Hospital das Clínicas
University of São Paulo
São Paulo, São Paulo, Brazil

Gurkan Ozel, BS, NREMT-P
Boulder, Colorado

James Richardson, EMT-P, MBA
EMS Instructor/Field Coordinator
Health One EMS
Englewood, Colorado

Janet Schulte, AS, BS, CCEMT-P, EMT-P
Training Center Coordinator
St. Charles County Ambulance District
St. Peters, Missouri

Henry E. Wang, MD, MPH
Assistant Professor
Department of Emergency Medicine
University of Pittsburgh School of Medicine
Pittsburgh, Pennsylvania

National Association of EMTs Board of Directors

Gregg Lord, EMT-P
Director

Jennifer Frennette, EMT-I
Director

Connie Meyer, EMT-P
Director

PHTLS Executive Council

Will Chapleau, EMT-P, RN, TNS, CEN
Chairman, PHTLS Executive Council
Chief, Chicago Heights Fire Department
Chicago Heights, Illinois

Gregory Chapman, EMT-P, RRT
Vice Chairman, PHTLS Executive Council
Director, Institute of Prehospital Emergency Medicine
Hudson Valley Community College
Troy, New York

Melissa Alexander, MS, NREMT-P
Director, EMS Academy
University of New Mexico
Albuquerque, New Mexico

Augie Bamonti, EMT-P
AFB Consulting
Chicago Heights Fire Department (Ret.)
Chicago Heights, Illinois

Mary-Ann Clarkes, EMT
Director of Administration
Canadian College of Emergency Medical Services
Edmonton, Alberta, Canada

Corine Curd
PHTLS International Office Director
NAEMT Headquarters
Clinton, Mississippi

Jeffrey S. Guy, MD, FACS, EMT-P
Associate Medical Director, PHTLS
Associate Professor of Surgery
Director, Regional Burn Center
Vanderbilt University School of Medicine
Nashville, Tennessee

Nita J. Ham, EMT-P
Consultant, EMS Education
Atlanta, Georgia

Craig H. Jacobus EMT-P, DC
Schuyler, Nebraska

Norman E. McSwain, Jr., MD, FACS, NREMT-P
Medical Director, PHTLS
Professor of Surgery
Tulane University School of Medicine
New Orleans, Louisiana

Steve Mercer, EMT-P, MEd
Iowa Department of Public Health
Des Moines, Iowa

Peter T. Pons, MD, FACEP
Associate Medical Director, PHTLS
Professor of Emergency Medicine
University of Colorado Health Sciences Center
Denver, Colorado

Dennis Rowe, EMT-P
Director, Rural/Metro EMS
Lenoir City, Tennessee

Jeffrey P. Salomone, MD, FACS, NREMT-P
Senior Associate Medical Director, PHTLS
Associate Professor of Surgery
Emory University School of Medicine
Atlanta, Georgia

PHTLS HONOR ROLL

PHTLS continues to prosper and promote high standards of trauma care all over the world. It would not be able to do this without the contributions of many dedicated and inspired individuals over the past two and a half decades. Some of those mentioned below were instrumental in the development of our first textbook. Others were constantly "on the road" spreading the word. Still others "put out fires" and otherwise problem-solved to keep us growing. The PHTLS Executive Council, along with the editors and contributors of this, our sixth edition, would like to express our thanks to all of those listed below. PHTLS lives, breathes, and grows because of the efforts of those who volunteer their time to what they believe in.

Gregory H. Adkisson
Augie Bamonti
J.M. Barnes
Morris L. Beard
Ann Bellows
Chip Boehm
Don E. Boyle
Susan Brown
Frank K. Butler, Jr.
Alexander Butman
H. Jeannie Butman
Steve Carden
Edward A. Casker
Bud Caukin
Philip Coco
Michael D'Auito
Alice "Twink" Dalton
Judith Demarest
Joseph P. Dineen
Leon Dontigney
Blaine L. Endersen

Betsy Ewing
Milton R. Fields, III
Scott B. Frame[†]
Sheryl G.A. Gabram
Bret Gilliam
Vincent A. Greco
Larry Hatfield
Walter Idol
Len Jacobs
Craig Jacobus
Lou Jordan
Richard Judd
Dawn Loehn
Mark Lockhart
Robert Loftus
Fernando
    Magallenes-Negrete
Scott W. Martin
Don Mauger
William McConnell
John Mechtel

Claire Merrick
Bill Metcalf
George Moerkirk
Stephen Murphy
Lawrence D. Newell
Jeanne O'Brien
Joan Drake-Olsen
Dawn Orgeron
Eric Ossmann
James Paturas
Thomas Petrich
Valerie J. Phillips
James Pierce
Brian Plaisier
Mark Reading
Brian Reiselbara
John Sigafoos
Paul Silverston
David Skinner
Dale C. Smith
Richard Sobieray

Sheila Spaid
Michael Spain
Don Stamper
Kenneth G. Swan
Kenneth G. Swan, Jr.
David M. Tauber
Joseph J. Tepas III
Richard Vomacka[†]
Robert K. Waddell, II
Michael Werdmann
Elizabeth Wertz
Keith Wesley
Roger D. White
Kenneth J. Wright
David Wuertz
Al Yellin
Steven Yevich
Doug York
Alida Zamboni

Again, thanks to all of you, and thanks to everyone around the world for making PHTLS work.
PHTLS Executive Council
Editors and Contributors of PHTLS

[†]deceased

ACKNOWLEDGMENTS

In 1624 John Donne wrote that "No man is an island, entire of itself." This describes in many ways the process of the publication of a book. Certainly, no editor is an island. Textbooks such as the PHTLS book and especially courses that involve audiovisual material, instructor manuals, and the textbook cannot be published by editors in isolation. As a matter of fact, much, if not most, of the work in the publishing of a textbook is done not by the editors and the authors whose names appear on the cover and on the inside of the book, but by the editorial staff. The sixth edition of PHTLS is certainly no exception.

Alex Butman and Rick Vomacka worked diligently, and frequently used money out of their own pockets, to bring the first two editions of the PHTLS program to fruition. Without their help and work, PHTLS would never have begun.

From the American College of Surgeons Committee on Trauma, Mary Fallat, MD, FACS, Chairman of the Emergency Services Subcommittee-Prehospital; Steve Parks, MD, FACS, and Christoph Kaufmann, MD, FACS, past and current Chairman of the Advanced Trauma Life Support Subcommittee; and of course, Irvene Hughes, RN, the National-International Coordinator of ATLS, have provided major support of PHTLS generally and the sixth edition specifically. Carol Williams, Executive Secretary of the Committee on Trauma, Wayne Meredith, MD, FACS, the current Chairman of the Committee on Trauma, and David Hoyt, MD, FACS, the ACS Director of Trauma, have provided outstanding support for this edition as well as for PHTLS.

A special thanks is given to the Chicago Heights Fire Department for the use of their facilities and to the crews who participated in the photo shoot for this book.

Within Mosby, Linda Honeycutt has led the effort to bring out this edition out on time, and Joy Knobel has worked hard on the public relations for this book. Jeanne Robertson has created some beautiful new illustrations. The production team, headed by Sarah Wunderly, worked to ensure that our text said what we wanted it to, that the diagrams and tables were accurate, and to get the book to print.

The person to whom we are the most indebted is Laura Bayless. She has worked diligently with the pressures of time, late manuscripts, and difficult illustration issues to get the job done in a superior manner. Laura has been a source of never-ending offers to assist us is all aspects of developing this manuscript and the related items. Without her this sixth edition would not be possible.

The editors and authors whose wives, children, and significant others have tolerated the long hours in the preparation of the material are obviously the backbone of any publication.

Norman McSwain, MD, FACS, NREMT-P
Jeff Salomone, MD, FACS, NREMT-P

FOREWORD

Twenty-five years ago, the American College of Surgeons Committee on Trauma (ACS/COT) and the National Association of Emergency Medical Technicians (NAEMT) joined in an agreement to develop an ATLS-like course for nonphysician prehospital providers. The first courses were presented in 1983, the same year the first PHTLS textbook was published.

Since that time, the course has been delivered in 37 countries to nearly half a million prehospital care providers. The direct benefits to patient care globally are huge but difficult to quantify. The tangential benefit of exporting these invaluable skills worldwide in a culturally competent and language-appropriate manner is equally beneficial for the practice of health diplomacy, which uses the currency of health as a diplomatic tool to achieve health, peace, and security in a challenging world. Many of the global friendships and alliances forged over the years serve to bridge political and ideological differences and signify that our prehospital practices know no geopolitical borders. We serve the world. As the United States Surgeon General and as a Special Forces medic, EMS provider and leader, police officer, registered nurse, and trauma surgeon, I have experienced and continue to appreciate that the world in indeed getting "smaller," and that the broad range of challenges and threats we all face globally do not respect our geopolitical borders. When it comes to prehospital trauma care in the United States and abroad we are one, and PHTLS represents those best practices.

It has been said that we stand on the shoulders of giants in many apparent successes, and PHTLS is no different. With great vision and passion, as well as challenges, a small group of leaders persevered and developed PHTLS over a quarter of a century ago. Its success is heralded by its national and global growth as well as the continued increased demand for this invaluable skill set.

As we move into the sixth edition of PHTLS, we continue to refine our best practices. As with much of EMS and prehospital care, we owe a debt of gratitude to military medicine for many of the concepts we embrace today whose genesis was in wartime combat casualty care. Care at the point of injury by skilled providers, rapid transport to definitive care, and trauma centers are just a few of those best military practices that became institutionalized and now represent the foundation of our emergency medical system. As a nation at war once again, we are learning many new lessons in prehospital trauma care that will ultimately be translated to civilian EMS use. However, the basic science and assessment and management skills serve as the same foundation for both military and civilian prehospital providers. The environment in which each works is unique, and therefore the application of those PHTLS skills will vary according to such issues as geography, weather, and threat level.

To reflect this, the sixth edition civilian and military PHTLS volumes are identical for the first 18 chapters but diverge in the last chapters to reflect the respective "special considerations" unique to the military and civilian prehospital providers. The successful care of the injured patient is a continuum that begins in the prehospital environment. The skill sets necessary to decrease morbidity and mortality and increase survival in the military and civilian prehospital environments are contained in the PHTLS curriculum. Use them wisely, and your community and the world we serve will benefit greatly.

Richard H. Carmona, MD, MPH, FACS, VADM, USPHS
United States Surgeon General

Prehospital care providers should accept the responsibility to provide patient care as close to absolutely perfect as possible. This cannot be achieved with insufficient knowledge of the subject. We must remember that the patient did not choose to be involved in a traumatic situation. The provider, on the other hand, has chosen to be there to take care of the patient. The prehospital care provider is obligated to give 100% of his or her effort during contact with every patient. The patient has had a bad day; the provider cannot also have a bad day. The prehospital care provider must be sharp and capable in the competition between the patient and death and disease.

The patient is the most important person at the scene of an emergency. There is no time to think about the order in which the patient assessment is performed or what treatments should take priority over others. There is no time to practice a skill before using it on a particular patient. There is no time to think about where equipment or supplies are housed within the jump kit. There is no time to think about where to transport the injured patient. All of this information and more must be stored in the mind and all supplies and equipment must be present in the jump kit when the provider arrives on the scene. Without the proper knowledge or equipment, the provider may neglect to do things that could potentially increase the patient's chance of survival. The responsibilities of a provider are too great to make such mistakes.

Those who deliver care in the prehospital setting are integral members of the trauma patient care team, as are the nurses or physicians in the emergency department, operating room, intensive care unit, ward, and rehabilitation unit. Prehospital care providers must be practiced in their skills so that they can move the patient quickly and efficiently out of the environment of the emergency and transport the patient quickly to the closest appropriate hospital.

WHY PHTLS?

Course Education Philosophy

Prehospital Trauma Life Support (PHTLS) focuses on principles, not preferences. By focusing on principles of good trauma care, PHTLS promotes critical thinking. The Executive Committee of the PHTLS Division of the National Association of Emergency Medical Technicians (NAEMT) believes that, given a good fund of knowledge, prehospital care providers are capable of making reasoned decisions regarding patient care. Rote memorization of mnemonics is discouraged. Furthermore, there is no one "PHTLS way" of performing a specific skill. The principle of the skill is taught, and then one acceptable method of performing the skill that meets the principle is presented. The authors realize that no one method can apply to the myriad of unique situations encountered in the prehospital setting.

Up-to-Date Information

Development of the PHTLS program began in 1981, immediately on the heels of the inception of the Advanced Trauma Life Support (ATLS) program for physicians. As the ATLS course is revised every 4 to 5 years, pertinent changes are incorporated into the next edition of PHTLS. This sixth edition of the PHTLS program has been significantly revised based on the 2005 ATLS course. While still following the ATLS principles, PHTLS is specifically designed for the unique requirements of caring for trauma patients in the prehospital setting. Many new chapters have been added, while others have been extensively revised. New chapters include information on scene assessment and management, environmental emergencies, disaster management, weapons of mass destruction, civilian tactical EMS, and trauma care in the wilderness. We have also included a CD-ROM with video clips of skills and practice questions. Note that throughout the book, the ⊙ symbol references where more information can be found on the CD-ROM.

Scientific Base

The authors and editors have adopted an "evidence-based" approach that includes references from the medical literature supporting the key principles and additional position papers published by the national organizations are cited where applicable. Many references have been added, allowing those providers with an inquisitive mind to read the scientific data supporting our recommendations.

Support for NAEMT

The NAEMT provides the administrative structure for the PHTLS program. No proceeds from the PHTLS program (surcharges or royalties from the text and audiovisuals) go to the editors or authors of this work, nor to the American College of Surgeons Committee on Trauma or any other physician-oriented organization. All profits from the PHTLS program are channeled back into NAEMT to provide funding for issues and programs that are of prime importance to EMS professionals, such as educational conferences and lobbying of legislators on behalf of prehospital care providers.

PHTLS Is a World Leader

Because of the unprecedented success of the fifth edition of PHTLS, the program has continued to grow by leaps and bounds. PHTLS courses continue to proliferate across the United States, and the U.S. military has adopted it, teaching the program to U.S. Armed Forces personnel at over 100 training sites worldwide. PHTLS has been exported to more than 32 nations, and many others are expressing interest in bringing PHTLS to their countries in efforts to improve prehospital trauma care levels.

Prehospital care providers have the responsibility to assimilate this knowledge and these skills in order to use them for the benefit of the patients for whom the providers are responsible. The editors and authors of this material and the Executive Committee of the PHTLS Division of the NAEMT hope that you will incorporate this information into your practice and daily rededicate yourself to the care of those persons who cannot care for themselves—the trauma patients.

Jeffrey P. Salomone, MD, FACS, NREMT-P
Peter T. Pons, MD, FACEP
Editors

Norman E. McSwain, Jr., MD, FACS, NREMT-P
Editor-in-Chief, PHTLS

Will Chapleau, EMT-P, RN, TNS, CEN
Gregory Chapman, EMT-P, RRT
Jeffrey S. Guy, MD, FACS, EMT-P
Associate Editors

CONTENTS

As happens so often in life, a personal experience brought about the changes in emergency care that resulted in the birth of the ATLS course. My own personal part in the role of ATLS started 29 years ago when a plane crashed in a rural area of Nebraska. The ATLS course was born out of that mangled mass of metal, the injured, and the dead. This is what I remember.

On February 17, 1976, my family left Los Angeles to return to Lincoln, Nebraska, after a wedding. I flew a 6-seat Beach Barron twin-engine plane. My wife, Charlene, sat in the copilot's seat. Our eldest son, Christopher, age 10, sat behind me facing the oxygen bottle that was strapped to the back of the pilot's seat. Kimberly, his 3-year-old sister, sat on his lap, strapped in with the lap seat belt around both of them. The two middle boys sat next to the rear luggage door; 7-year-old Randy was on the right, with 8-year-old Richard beside him. The temperature was 29° F (−1.66° C) that night.

Five hours into the flight (6:00 PM), trying to stay below a layer of clouds, I became disoriented and lost altitude. We flew into a row of trees at 163 miles per hour (311 km/hour). The wings of the plane were ripped off, the fuel tanks emptied, and a large hole was torn in the right side of the aircraft. We dropped into a thicket that cushioned the landing and then rocketed us onto a field. A piece of the propeller came through my pilot's window, missed me, and hit Charlene's head. She died instantly. At impact, Charlene was ejected. The plane traveled another 294 feet (89.6 meters), rotating 180 degrees, but it stayed upright.

What seemed like an eternity actually took 2$^1/_2$ seconds. There was a tremendous noise. I waited to die. Then I remember silence.

My face had hit the dash. I sustained fractured ribs over the spleen. My forehead and face were lacerated. My left eye was closed, and I had difficulty seeing out of the right one. The right zygomatic arch had an open fracture. I had a frozen shoulder from a fall 2 months earlier. Kimberly's head hit the oxygen bottle. She sustained a blow-out fracture of the orbit and a forehead laceration. Richard had lacerations to his forehead and the right supraorbital nerve. He and Kimberly were unconscious for 7 days. Chris crashed into Kimberly's back and was spared a head injury but had a fractured right forearm and a severe laceration of the dorsum of the right hand. Randy sustained an open depressed skull fracture. His right leg came out of the luggage door and was

impaled at the knee by a piece of metal, under the aircraft. He remained in a coma for 3 days.

I don't know how long I sat after the world became silent. The first thing I thought was *fire*, and I exited through the opening, running straight into barbed wire that entangled the aircraft. This got my attention. Then I realized *the kids are still in the plane!* I saw Randy and started to pull him free when I realized he was pinned under the fuselage. Chris passed Kim to me. I set her away from the aircraft and removed Richard next. Chris was able to extract himself. I returned to Randy and used my hands to dig his leg out. I don't know how hard the ground was, but there were no marks on my hands. His leg fell off the impalement, and I waited for the bleeding that never started.

Once we all were away from the aircraft and fire was not a problem, I realized the potential for hypothermia. We gathered clothing from scattered suitcases, and made a bed in the back compartment where I placed the kids and piled more clothes over them. Chris and I sat in the front and waited, but help never came. The overcast from earlier in the evening dissipated into a clear night sky with a near-full moon. I went looking for my wife and found her on the third try. I checked her, and confirmed she was gone. I would go back three more times to be sure she was really gone.

We could see a road some distance away from the plane. After waiting until approximately 2:00 AM, I decided to go for help. I instructed Chris to stay with the children. I walked $^5/_8$ of a mile along a dirt road to a highway and flagged down a car after two trucks didn't stop. The occupants' names were Rick and David. I told them what had happened, and we drove to the accident site and loaded the kids in the car.

I cannot recall how we assembled seven people in the car or how much protection we gave their necks.

I felt no pain while I was digging out my son's leg and lifting the kids. After help arrived, I was unable to lift because of chest and shoulder pain. I don't recall any facial pain either. Adrenaline is amazing.

At the crash site, I had to worry about fire and hypothermia. The wounds were possible bleeding problems. We protected the children's necks as best we could. I did most of the lifting because of Chris's fractured arm. He acted as my eyes. Without him the task would have been nearly impossible. We splinted his arm, I said goodbye to my wife, and we drove to Hebron Hospital, a few miles south of the crash site.

We arrived as a motley crew and approached the locked emergency room door of this rural hospital. We knocked and the night nurse opened the door. We explained our predicament and asked if we could get the kids inside. She told us that we would have to wait until the doctors arrived. I cannot remember our response, but we got in. A little later Drs. Pembry and Bunting, the two general practitioners in this small farming community, arrived. I remember standing at a mirror picking dried blood off my face and trying to help. Richard was becoming agitated. A doctor picked him up by the shoulders and the knees and took him into the x-ray room. Picture the motion of his head and neck with this maneuver. Later he returned with Richard and announced there was no skull fracture. The cervical spine had not been considered. He then began suturing the laceration. An IV was placed in Richard and he was given Valium. I don't remember anyone else receiving IVs. I called my partner, Bruce Miller, and told him what had happened and that we would get to Lincoln as soon as we could; he notified the hospital.

The doctors and staff in Hebron had little or no preparation for this type of situation. There was an obvious lack of training for triage and proper treatment.

A sheriff's department helicopter piloted by Larry Russell was assigned to the search (12:00 AM). An aircraft called *Looking Glass* came from South Dakota, picked up our emergency locator beacon, and directed the helicopter to the crash site. He landed about half an hour after we had vacated the scene and proceeded to the hospital after being notified of our arrival.

The civil air patrol was now also searching for us. They arrived at the crash site hours later. The FAA rule at that time was that all airports had to be checked first, then a search and rescue could begin, which took about 6 hours!

The helicopter pilot assessed the situation and suggested we ask the Lincoln Air National Guard for transport. They arrived with a transport helicopter and we were loaded for the 110-mile flight to Lincoln. There was a crew of three, Dr. Pembry, a nurse, and the five of us. Rick and David disappeared, and I never saw them again. We departed, and I noted that Richard's IV had been discontinued.

This was the first air evacuation by the National Guard. The CAP (civil air patrol) from its formation in the 1950s to 1976 responded to its first crash that had survivors.

We landed at Lincoln Airport and an ambulance transported us to Lincoln General Hospital. The emergency department and the operating rooms were ready for us. We arrived at 8:00 AM, 14 hours after the crash. Waiting for us were the emergency doctor, Ron Craig, my partner, Bruce Miller, and a plastic surgeon, Larry Ruth. This experience was like coming out of a hostile dark hell into civilization. So ended the longest night of my life.

ATLS Is Born

For the next year or so we tried to heal our physical and emotional scars.

Folks got tired of my criticism of the treatment we received before our arrival in Lincoln. I wasn't complaining about care at any particular facility, but the general lack of a delivery system to treat the acute trauma patient in the rural setting. The statement, "When I can provide better care in the field with limited resources than my children and I received at the primary facility, there is something wrong with the system and the system has to be changed," emphasizes this observation. Simply, you have to *train* them before you can blame them. Ron Craig and I started talking about how to prevent a recurrence of my experience. He probably said something like, "Quit your griping and put your money where your mouth is." We decided we wanted to educate rural physicians in a systematic way to treat trauma patients, so we connected with Jodie Bechtel (now Upright), a nurse with the Lincoln Area Mobile heart team, now a paramedic group. The three of us decided to do a training course for Nebraska. Jodie had worked with Steve Carvith (also from Lincoln) when he created the ACLS course. We decided to use a similar format and call it ATLS.

A syllabus was created and organized into a logical approach to trauma. Eventually we got the idea of seeing and fixing a problem before attacking the next one, rather than looking at every system involved and then going back to treat. Among those who joined was a Mobile heart team nurse with unending energy, Irvene Hughes, who is now the ATLS program manager. Paul (Skip) Collicott, a peripheral vascular surgeon, was also with us from the beginning. He had the political know-how and took the lead. Several doctors joined our efforts, and we each wrote chapters in our specialties for the syllabus. The ABCs of trauma were developed to prioritize the order of assessment and treatment. The prototype was field tested in Auburn, Nebraska, in 1978 with the help of many. Skip presented the course to the University of Nebraska, who helped with the surgical skill lab using live, anesthetized dogs. Skip got the American College of Surgeons Committee on Trauma involved. We presented the finished course to the College's 13 regions. It was arborized in each region.

Since that first course in Auburn, 28 years have passed and ATLS keeps spreading and growing. What was originally intended as a course for rural Nebraska became a course for the whole world in all types of trauma settings—500,000 students have trained in 46 countries with 25,000 courses, and 24,000 trained physicians graduate each year. We're definitely on a roll! Everyone involved with the trauma victim speaks the same ATLS "language." This ability to communicate and anticipate at all levels decreases morbidity and mortality in that precious "golden hour."

ATLS Today

Compared with the recent tsunami, 9-11 at the twin towers in New York, the Gulf Coast hurricanes, and other natural and manmade disasters over the past 20 years, our experience was minor. Our hope is that the ATLS family has played a part in saving lives since that night so many years ago when my own family's lives were in peril.

People often wonder or ask about how we have fared since the crash. The kids have all done well. Kim graduated with a degree in psychology from college, then went on to get a master's in human resources, and now heads that department in a small company. Chris started college, but never finished. He and his wife work in real estate and are doing well. Randy graduated with a degree in biological science and works for Orange County, California, in waste management. Richard has a master's degree in education from Brown University and teaches computers, biological science, and astronomy at San Leandro High School south of Oakland, California.

James K. Styner, MD, FACS
Retired Orthopedic Surgeon

In 1979, care of trauma patients took a giant step forward with the inauguration of the Advanced Trauma Life Support (ATLS) course. The first chairman of the ATLS ad hoc committee for the American College of Surgeons and Chairman of the Prehospital Care Subcommittee on Trauma for the American College of Surgeons, Dr. Norman E. McSwain, Jr., FACS, knew that what they had begun would have a profound effect on the outcome of trauma patients. Moreover, he had a strong sense that an even greater effect could come from bringing this type of critical training to prehospital care providers.

Dr. McSwain, a founding member of the board of directors of the National Association of Emergency Medical Technicians (NAEMT), gained the support of the Association's president, Gary Labeau, and began to lay plans for a prehospital version of ATLS. President Labeau directed Dr. McSwain and Robert Nelson, NREMT-P, to determine the feasibility of an ATLS-type program for prehospital care providers.

As a professor of surgery at Tulane University School of Medicine in New Orleans, Louisiana, Dr. McSwain gained the university's support in putting together the draft curriculum of what was to become Prehospital Trauma Life Support (PHTLS). With this draft in place, a PHTLS committee was established in 1983. This committee continued to refine the curriculum, and later that same year, pilot courses were conducted in Lafayette and New Orleans, Louisiana, and at Marian Health Center, Sioux City, Iowa, Yale University School of Medicine, New Haven, Connecticut, and Norwalk Hospital, Norwalk, Connecticut.

National dissemination began with three intensive workshops, taught in Denver, Colorado, Bethesda, Maryland, and Orlando, Florida, between September 1984 and February 1985. The graduates of these early courses formed what would be the "Barnstormers," PHTLS national and regional faculty members who traveled the country training additional faculty members, spreading the word that PHTLS had arrived.

Early courses focused on advanced life support (ALS). In 1986, a course that encompassed basic life support (BLS) was developed. The course grew exponentially. Beginning with those first few enthusiastic faculty members, first dozens, then hundreds, and now thousands of providers annually participate in PHTLS courses all over the world.

As the course grew, the PHTLS committee became a division of the NAEMT. Course demand and the need to maintain course continuity and quality necessitated the building of networks of affiliate, state, regional, and national faculty members. There are national coordinators for every country, and in each country there are regional and state coordinators along with affiliate faculty members to make sure that information is disseminated and courses are consistent whether a provider participates in a program in Chicago Heights, Illinois, or Buenos Aires, Argentina.

Throughout the growth process, medical oversight has been provided through the American College of Surgeons Committee on Trauma. For nearly 20 years the partnership between the American College of Surgeons and the NAEMT has ensured that course participants receive the opportunity to give trauma patients everywhere their best chance at survival.

PHTLS in the Military

Beginning in 1988, the U.S. military aggressively set out to train its medics in PHTLS. Coordinated by DMRT, the Defense Medical Readiness Training Institute at Fort Sam Houston in Texas, PHTLS is taught all over the United States, Europe, and Asia, and anywhere the flags of the U.S. military fly. In 2001, the Army's 91WB program standardized the training of over 58,000 Army medics to include PHTLS. A military chapter was added in the fourth edition. After the fifth edition was initially published, a strong relationship was forged between the PHTLS organization and the newly established Committee on Tactical Combat Casualty Care. The initial fruit born of this relationship was an extensively revised military chapter in the fifth edition (revised), and a military version of the book was published in 2004. This collaboration has now led to the creation of multiple military chapters for the sixth edition military PHTLS text. PHTLS has been taught numerous times "in theater" during the Afghanistan and Iraq wars and has contributed to the lowest mortality rate from any armed conflict in U.S. history.

International PHTLS

The sound principles of prehospital trauma management emphasized in the PHTLS course have led prehospital care providers and physicians outside the United States to request the importation of the program to their various countries. ATLS faculty members presenting ATLS courses worldwide have assisted in this. This network provides medical direction and course continuity.

As PHTLS has moved across the United States and around the globe, we have been struck by the differences in our cultures and climates and also by the similarities of the people who devote their lives to caring for the sick and injured. All of us who have been blessed with the opportunity to teach overseas have experienced the fellowship with our international partners and know that we are all one people in pursuit of caring for those who need care the most.

The nations in the growing PHTLS family include Argentina, Australia, Barbados, Bolivia, Brazil, Canada, Chile, China, Colombia, Denmark, England, France, Greece, Grenada, Holland, Ireland, Israel, Italy, Luxembourg, Mexico, New Zealand, Norway, Panama, Peru, Portugal, Saudi Arabia, Scotland, Spain, Sweden, Switzerland, Trinidad, United Arab Emirates, the United States, Uruguay, and Venezuela. Demonstration courses have been run in Bulgaria, Macedonia, and soon, Croatia, with hopes to establish faculty members there soon. Japan, Korea, South Africa, Germany, Ecuador, Paraguay, Lithuania, Poland, and Nigeria all hope to join the family in the near future.

Translations

Our growing international family has spawned translations of the text. The text is currently available in English, Spanish, Greek, Portuguese, French, Dutch, and Italian. Negotiations are ongoing to have the text published in a number of additional languages. Toward that end, there are subtitles in several languages on the DVD that accompanies this book.

Vision for the Future

The vision for the future of PHTLS is family. The father of PHTLS, Dr. McSwain, is the root of the growing family that provides vital training and contributes knowledge and experience to the world. The inaugural international PHTLS Trauma Symposium was held near Chicago, Illinois, in the year 2000. This first program pitted the controversies facing trauma care against the will and energy of prehospital trauma providers. These programs will bring the work of practitioners and researchers around the globe together to determine the standards of trauma care for the new millennium.

The support of the PHTLS family worldwide, all volunteering countless hours of their lives, allows the PHTLS leadership to keep PHTLS growing. This leadership consists of the following:

PHTLS Executive Council
Medical Director of PHTLS International

| Norman E. McSwain, Jr., MD, FACS, NREMT-P | 1983-present |

Associate PHTLS Medical Directors

Scott B. Frame, MC, FACS, FCCM	1994-2001
Jeffrey Salomone, MD, FACS, NREMT-P	1996-present
Peter T. Pons, MD, FACEP	2000-present
Jeffrey S. Guy, MD, FACS, EMT-P	2001-present

International PHTLS Chairs

Richard Vomacka, REMT-P	1983-1985
James L. Paturas	1985-1988
David Wuertz, EMT-P	1988-1990
John Sinclair, EMT-P	1990-1991
James L. Paturas	1991-1992
Elizabeth M. Wertz, RN, BSN, MPM	1992-1996
Will Chapleau, EMT-P, RN, TNS	1996-present

As we continue to pursue the potential of the PHTLS course and the worldwide community of prehospital care providers, we must remember our commitment to the following:

- Rapid and accurate assessment
- Identification of shock and hypoxemia
- Initiation of the right interventions at the right time
- Timely transport to the right place

It is also fitting to reprise our mission statement, which was written in a marathon session at the NAEMT conference in 1997. The PHTLS mission continues to be to provide the highest quality prehospital trauma education to all who wish to avail themselves of this opportunity. The PHTLS mission also enhances the achievement of the NAEMT mission. The PHTLS program is committed to quality and performance improvement. As such, PHTLS is always attentive to changes in technology and methods of delivering prehospital trauma care that may be used to enhance the clinical and service quality of this program.

National Association of Emergency Medical Technicians

The NAEMT represents the interests of prehospital care providers all over the world.

NAEMT was founded with the help of the National Registry of EMTs (NREMT) in 1975. Since its inception, the association has worked to promote professional status for prehospital care providers from the first responder to the administrator. Its educational programs began as a way of providing meaningful continuing education to providers at every level and have become the standard of prehospital continuing education all over the world.

NAEMT has reciprocal relationships with dozens of United States and international federal and private agencies that influence every aspect of prehospital care. The NAEMT's participation ensures that the voice of prehospital care is heard in determining the future of our practice.

NAEMT MISSION

The mission of the National Association of Emergency Medical Technicians, Inc., is to be a professional representative organization that will receive and represent the views and opinions of prehospital care personnel and to influence the future advancement of EMS as an allied health profession. NAEMT will serve its professional membership through educational programs, liaison activity, development of national standards and reciprocity, and development of programs to benefit prehospital care personnel.

With this mission clearly defined and passionately pursued, NAEMT will continue to provide leadership in this developing specialty of prehospital care into the future.

CHAPTER 1

Introduction to PHTLS

Our patients did not choose us. Rather, they present to us because of some traumatic occurrence that has resulted in injury requiring our assistance. We, however, have chosen to treat them. We could have chosen another profession, but we did not. We have accepted the responsibility for patient care in some of the worst situations: when patients are at their most stressed and anxious, when we are tired or cold, when it is rainy and dark, and often when conditions are unpredictable. We must either accept this responsibility or surrender it. We must give our patients the very best care that we can—not with unchecked equipment, not with incomplete supplies, not with yesterday's knowledge, and not with indifference. We cannot know what medical information is current, and we cannot claim to be ready to care for our patients, without reading and learning each day. The Prehospital Trauma Life Support (PHTLS) course contributes to the knowledge of a prehospital care provider and, more importantly, ultimately benefits the patient. At the end of each run, we should feel that the patient received nothing short of our very best.

Trauma Care in the Twenty-First Century

The opportunity for a prehospital care provider to help another person is greater in the management of trauma patients than in any other patient encounter. The number of trauma patients we will encounter is higher than most other patient populations, and the chance for survival of the trauma patient who receives excellent trauma care, both in the prehospital and the hospital setting, is probably greater than that of any other patient. The prehospital care provider can lengthen the life span and productive years of the trauma patient and benefit society by virtue of the care provided. The prehospital care provider, through effective management of the trauma patient, has a significant influence on society.

Understanding, learning, and practicing the principles of PHTLS is more beneficial to patients than any other educational program. The following facts have led to the revised and expanded Chapter 2 on injury prevention in this edition of *Prehospital Trauma Life Support.*

Trauma is the leading cause of death in persons between 1 and 44 years of age. About 80% of teenage deaths and 60% of childhood deaths are secondary to trauma. Trauma continues to be the seventh leading cause of death in elderly persons. Three times more Americans die of trauma each year than died in the Vietnam War. Every 10 years, more Americans die of trauma than have died in all U.S. military conflicts combined. Only in the fifth decade of life do cancer and heart disease compete with trauma as a leading cause of death. About 80 times as many patients die yearly from blunt and penetrating trauma than died in the first 3 years of the Iraqi conflict.

Prehospital care providers can do little to increase the survival of a cancer patient. For the trauma patient, however, prehospital care providers can often make the difference between life and death; between temporary disablement and serious or permanent disability; or between a life of productivity and a life of destitution and welfare. In the United States, about 60 million injuries occur each year, 30 million will require medical care, and 9 million of these are disabling. About 8.7 million trauma patients will be temporarily disabled, and 300,000 will be permanently disabled.

The cost for care of trauma patients is staggering. Billions of dollars are spent on the management of trauma patients, not including the dollars lost in wages, insurance administration costs, property damage, and employer costs. Lost productivity from disabled trauma patients is the equivalent of 5.1 million years at a cost of more than $65 billion. For patients who die, 5.3 million years of life are lost (34 years per person) at a cost of more than $50 billion. Comparatively, the costs (measured in dollars and in years lost) for cancer and heart disease are much less, as illustrated in Figure 1-1. For example, proper protection of the

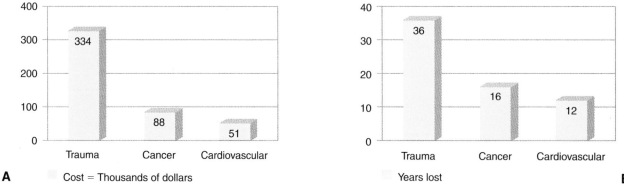

FIGURE 1-1   A, Comparative costs in thousands of dollars to United States victims of trauma, cancer, and cardiovascular disease each year. **B,** Comparative number of years lost as a result of trauma, cancer, and cardiovascular disease.

fractured cervical spine by a prehospital care provider may make the difference between lifelong quadriplegia and a productive healthy life of unrestricted activity. Prehospital care providers encounter many more examples almost every day.

Trauma care is divided into three phases: preevent, event, and postevent. The prehospital care provider has responsibilities in each phase.

Preevent Phase

Trauma is no accident, even though it is often referred to as such. An *accident* is defined as either "an event occurring by chance or arising from unknown causes" or "an unfortunate occurrence resulting from carelessness, unawareness, ignorance." Most trauma deaths and injuries fit the second definition and are preventable. Traumatic incidents fall into two categories: *intentional* and *unintentional.*

The preevent phase involves circumstances leading up to an injury. Efforts in this phase are primarily focused on injury prevention. In working toward preventing injuries, the public must be educated to increase the use of vehicle occupant restraint systems, promote methods to reduce the use of weapons in criminal activities, and promote nonviolent conflict resolution. In addition to caring for the trauma patient, all members of the health care delivery team have a responsibility to reduce the number of victims. Currently, violence and unintentional trauma cause more deaths annually in the United States than all diseases combined. Violence accounts for more than one third of these deaths (Figure 1-2). Motor vehicles and firearms are involved in more than one half of all trauma deaths, most of which are preventable (Figure 1-3).

Motorcycle helmet usage laws are one example of legislation that has affected injury prevention. In 1966 the U.S. Congress gave the Department of Transportation the authority to mandate that states pass legislation requiring the use of motorcycle helmets. The use of helmets subsequently increased to almost 100%, and the fatality rate decreased dramatically. Congress rescinded this authority in 1975. More than half the states repealed or modified the existing legislation, leading to an increase in related fatalities. As some states reinstate or repeal these laws, the rates have changed. Recently, more states have repealed rather than instituted such laws, resulting in increased death rates in 1998 and 1999 (Figure 1-4).

Another example of preventable trauma deaths involves drunk driving. As a result of pressure to change state laws for the level of intoxication while driving and through the educational activities of such organizations as Mothers Against Drunk Drivers (MADD), the number of drunk drivers involved in fatal crashes has been consistently decreasing since 1989.

Another way to prevent trauma is through the use of child safety seats. Many trauma centers, law enforcement organizations, and emergency medical services (EMS) conduct programs to educate parents in the correct installation and use of child safety seats.

FIGURE 1-3 Motor vehicle trauma and firearms account for more than half the deaths that result from trauma and violence.

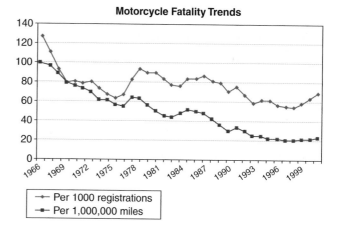

FIGURE 1-4 Motorcycle helmet legislation and therefore the mandated use of helmets significantly reduce the motorcycle fatality rate. Repeal of this law in 1975 produced a marked increase in the number of fatalities. Many states have reinstated their own laws, reducing the number of fatalities for registered motorcyclists to as low as it was before the repeal of this law.

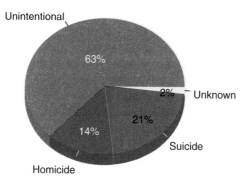

FIGURE 1-2 Unintentional trauma and violence account for more deaths than all other causes of death combined.

Event Phase

This phase is the moment of the actual trauma. Steps performed in the preevent phase can influence the outcome of the event phase. This applies not only to our patients, but also to ourselves. Whether driving a personal vehicle or an emergency vehicle, prehospital care providers need to protect themselves and teach by example. It is important that they always drive safely, follow traffic laws, and use the protective devices available, such as vehicle restraints, in the driving compartment and in the passenger or patient care compartment.

Postevent Phase

Donald Trunkey, MD, has described a trimodal categorization of trauma deaths.[1] The *first phase* of deaths occurs within the first few minutes of and up to an hour after an incident. These deaths would likely occur even with prompt medical attention. The best way to combat these deaths is through injury prevention and safety strategies. The *second phase* of deaths occurs within the first few hours of an incident. These deaths can be prevented by good prehospital care and good hospital care. The *third phase* of deaths occurs several days to several weeks after the incident. These deaths are generally caused by multiple organ failure. Much more needs to be learned about managing and preventing multiple organ failure; however, early and aggressive management of shock in the prehospital setting can prevent some of these deaths (Figure 1-5).

R. Adams Cowley, MD, founder of the Maryland Institute of Emergency Medical Services (MIEMS), one of the first trauma centers in the United States, described and defined what he called the "Golden Hour." Based on his research, Cowley believed that patients who received definitive care soon after an injury had a much higher survival rate than those whose care was delayed. One reason for this improvement

When Casualties Die from Trauma

■	Immediate (50%) Minutes to 1 hour
□	Early (30%) First 4 hours
■	Late (20%) 2 to 5 weeks

FIGURE 1-5 Immediate deaths can be prevented only by injury prevention education because some patients' only chance is for the incident not to have occurred. Early deaths can be prevented through timely, appropriate prehospital care to reduce mortality and morbidity. Late deaths can be prevented only through prompt transport to a hospital appropriately staffed for trauma care.

in survival is preservation of the body's ability to produce energy to maintain organ function. For the prehospital care provider, this translates into maintaining oxygenation and perfusion and providing rapid transportation to a facility set up to continue that process.

An average urban EMS system has a *response time* (from the time the incident occurs until arrival on the scene) of 6 to 8 minutes. A typical transport time to the receiving facility is another 8 to 10 minutes. Between 15 and 20 minutes of the magic "Golden Hour" are used just to arrive at the scene and transport the patient. If prehospital care at the scene is not efficient and well organized, an additional 30 to 40 minutes can be spent on the scene. With this time on the scene added to the transport time, the "Golden Hour" has already passed before a physician has an opportunity to treat the patient. Research data are starting to support this concept.[2,3] One of these studies showed that critically injured patients had a significantly lower mortality rate (17.9% vs. 28.2%) when transported by a private vehicle rather than an ambulance. This unexpected finding was most likely the result of prehospital care providers spending too much time on the scene. One trauma center documented that EMS scene times averaged 23 minutes for patients injured in motor vehicle crashes (MVCs) and 22 minutes for victims of penetrating trauma. This begs the questions that all prehospital providers need to ask: "Is what I'm doing going to benefit the patient? Does that benefit outweigh the risk of delaying transport?" One of the most important responsibilities of a prehospital care provider is to spend as little time on the scene as possible. In the first precious minutes a prehospital care provider rapidly assesses the patient, performs lifesaving maneuvers, and prepares the patient for transportation.

A second responsibility is actually transporting the patient to an appropriate facility. The factor most critical to any patient's survival is the length of time that elapses between the incident and definitive care. For a cardiac arrest patient, definitive care is the restoration of normal heart rhythm and adequate perfusion. Cardiopulmonary resuscitation (CPR) is merely a holding pattern. For a patient whose airway is compromised, definitive care is the management of the airway and restoration of adequate ventilation. The reestablishment of either ventilation or normal cardiac rhythm by defibrillation is usually easily achieved in the field; therefore, transportation time is not as critical for the cardiac patient.

The management of trauma patients is different. Definitive care is usually hemorrhage control and restoration of adequate perfusion. Hemostasis (hemorrhage control) cannot always be achieved in the field or in the emergency department (ED); it must often be achieved in the operating room (OR). Therefore, in determining an appropriate facility, it is important that the prehospital care provider consider the transport time to a given facility and the capabilities of that facility.

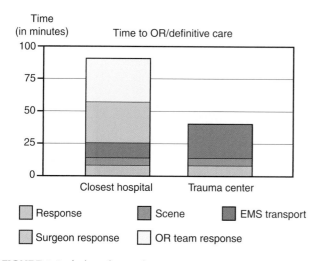

FIGURE 1-6 In locations where trauma centers are available, bypassing hospitals not committed to the care of trauma patients can significantly improve patient care. In severely injured trauma patients, definitive patient care generally occurs in the operating room (OR). An extra 10 to 20 minutes spent en route to a hospital with an in-house surgeon and in-house OR staff will significantly reduce the time to definitive care in the OR. *Blue,* EMS response time. *Purple,* On-scene time. *Red,* EMS transport time. *Orange,* Surgical response from out of hospital. *Yellow,* OR team response from out of hospital.

A trauma center that has an in-house surgeon and an OR team can often have a trauma patient with life-threatening hemorrhage in the OR within 10 to 15 minutes of the patient's arrival. On the other hand, a hospital without in-house surgical capabilities must await the arrival of the surgeon and the surgical team before transporting the patient from the ED to the OR. Additional time may then elapse before the hemorrhage can be controlled, resulting in an associated increase in mortality rate (Figure 1-6).

History of Emergency Medical Services

This text, the PHTLS course, and care of the trauma patient are based on the objectives developed and taught by the early pioneers of prehospital care. The list of these innovators is long; however, a few especially deserve our recognition.

As early as the late 1700s, Baron Dominick Jean Larrey, Napoleon's chief military physician, recognized the need for prompt prehospital care. He developed the horse-drawn "flying ambulance" for timely retrieval of men injured on the battlefield and introduced the premise that individuals working in these "flying ambulances" should be trained in medical care to provide on-scene and en route care for patients.

J.D. "Deke" Farrington, MD, the father of modern EMS, stimulated the development of improved prehospital care with his landmark article, "Death in a Ditch."[4] His work as chairman on three of the initial documents establishing the basis of EMS—the essential equipment list for ambulances of the American College of Surgeons (ACS), the KKK ambulance design specifications of the U.S. Department of Transportation, and the first emergency medical technician (EMT) basic training program—also propelled the idea and development of prehospital care. Robert Kennedy, MD, was the author of "Early Care of the Sick and Injured Patient."[5] Sam Banks, MD, who with Dr. Farrington taught the first prehospital training course to the Chicago Fire Department in 1957, initiated proper care of the trauma patient. Minimal change occurred between the 1700s and the time that Farrington and the early leaders, such as Oscar Hampton, MD, and Curtis Arts, MD, brought the United States into the modern era of EMS and prehospital care.[6,7]

A 1965 text edited and compiled by George J. Curry, MD, a leader of the ACS and its Committee on Trauma, states the following:

Injuries sustained in accidents affect every part of the human body. They range from simple abrasions and contusions to multiple complex injuries involving many body tissues. This demands efficient and intelligent primary appraisal and care, on an individual basis, before transport. It is obvious that the services of trained ambulance attendants are essential. If we are to expect maximum efficiency from ambulance attendants, a special training program must be arranged.

Although prehospital care was rudimentary when Curry wrote this passage, the words still hold true as prehospital care providers address the specific area of *prehospital trauma* care rather than the broad field of general EMS.

Curry's call for specialized training of "ambulance attendants" has been answered *for trauma* during the past 25 years by this text and by the landmark "white paper" *Accidental Death and Disability: the Neglected Disease of Modern Society.* The National Academy of Sciences/National Research Council issued this paper just 1 year after Curry's call. The first training efforts were primitive but have greatly progressed in a brief time. However, despite the continual rush of new developments, procedures, equipment, provider levels, and standards, a need exists to go back and rethink issues to fill in the spaces left by the "march of progress" through the field of EMS.[7,8]

All these innovators taught the following basic principles, which have been expanded on and refined over time:

■ Rapidly respond to the patient.
■ Provide efficient but prompt care to reestablish adequate ventilation, provide sufficient oxygenation, and preserve adequate perfusion to maintain the needed energy production for organ preservation.

■ Rapidly transport the patient to the most appropriate facility.[7]

Rapid access to the patient depends on a prehospital care system that offers easy access for the system. This access can be aided by a single emergency phone number (e.g., 9-1-1 in the United States, other numbers in other countries), a good communication system to dispatch the unit, and well-prepared and well-trained prehospital care providers. Many people have heard that early access and early CPR save the lives of those experiencing cardiac arrest. Trauma can be approached the same way. The three principles just listed can save lives.

Efficient on-scene medical care requires prehospital care providers who are well trained in rapid identification of the patient's condition and skilled in airway management, shock management, and proper immobilization procedures. The prehospital care provider needs to exercise good judgment to decide what action to take on the scene, how to perform it efficiently, and which steps to carry out en route to the receiving facility.

It is important for the prehospital care provider to ensure that the patient is transported to an appropriate facility. This facility is the one that can most promptly and most appropriately provide definitive care to the patient. The prehospital care provider often has no choice in a rural area with only one hospital available in the community. The next hospital may be miles away, and the trauma center could be even farther. In this situation the prehospital provider needs to decide whether helicopter transport from the scene is warranted. This is a fairly simple calculation. The approximate time of ground transportation is on one side of the equation. On the other side is the time necessary for helicopter alert and lift off, travel to the scene, management on the scene, and travel back to the hospital. The prehospital care provider determines the means of transportation based on which time is shorter.

PHTLS is designed to assess patients rapidly and begin lifesaving therapy early and appropriately. Two studies conducted by Dr. Jameel Ali in Trinidad and Tobago demonstrated an improved process in patient care resulting in a decreased mortality rate from trauma after teaching PHTLS to all prehospital care providers[9,10] (Figure 1-7). This text and the PHTLS course provide the necessary tools to save lives. Prehospital care works.

Reading the EMS Literature

A major goal of PHTLS has been to ensure that the practice recommendations presented in this text accurately represent the best medical evidence available at the time

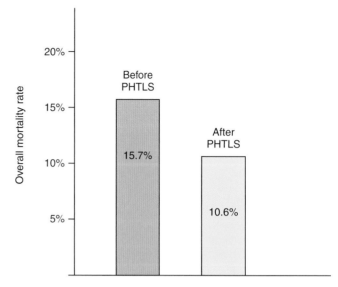

FIGURE 1-7 Trauma deaths decreased by about one-third after the introduction of PHTLS to the nation of Trinidad and Tobago.
(Modified from Ali J, Adam RU, Gana TJ, et al: *J Trauma* 42:1018, 1997.)

of publication in support of these recommendations. To that end, we have begun the process of adding, as References and Suggested Readings, those manuscripts, sources, and resources that are fundamental components of each chapter and recommendation. (See Suggested Readings at the end of this chapter for further information on evaluating the EMS literature.) It is our hope that every practitioner and health care provider obtain, read, and critically evaluate the publications and sources that make up the foundation and basis for all the components of our daily practice.

To accomplish this, it is important to have an understanding of exactly what constitutes the medical literature and of how to interpret the various sources of information. In many cases the first place that is accessed for information about a particular topic is a medical textbook. As our level of interest and sophistication grows, a search is undertaken to find the specific references that are referred to in those book chapters or to find what, if any, primary research studies have been performed and published. Then, after reviewing and analyzing the various sources, a decision can be made about the quality and strength of the evidence that will guide our decision making and patient care interventions.

Types of Evidence

There are a number of different systems for rating the quality and strength of medical evidence. Regardless of the exact rating system used, several common assessments can be found among them. The highest-quality source that leads to the strongest recommendation about the treatment being studied is the randomized, double-blind controlled study. Studies of this type are usually referred to as *Class I evidence.* This type of study is considered to be the best type of study because all patients entered into the study are *randomized* (meaning each patient has an equal chance of being assigned to whatever type of treatment is being studied); the researchers as well as the patients do not know which type of treatment the subject is receiving *(double blinding)*; and investigators are controlling for as many other aspects of the study as possible. These factors minimize the chances of any bias entering into the study or affecting the results or interpretation of the results.

Class II evidence generally includes the other types of studies that can be found in the medical literature, including nonrandomized nonblinded studies, retrospective case-control series, and cohort studies.

Finally, *Class III evidence* consists of case studies, case reports, consensus documents, textbook material, and medical opinion. Class III evidence is the weakest source of evidence, although often the easiest to obtain.

Unfortunately, if the literature related to prehospital care is critically reviewed, the majority qualifies as Class III evidence. There has been remarkably little research that would qualify as Class I. Much of the practice of medicine that has been applied to the prehospital setting has been adopted from and adapted to the out-of-hospital environment from the in-hospital delivery of emergency care. The result is that most of the prehospital care provided today is based on Class III evidence. Specifically, with few exceptions, the medical practice of prehospital care is based on "expert" opinion usually found in textbook chapters, the credentials and qualifications of the individual offering that opinion, and the forcefulness and "volume" of the delivery of that opinion.

Steps in Evaluation

It is important that every medical practitioner read the medical literature and critically evaluate every study published that might alter his or her treatment decisions, in order to be able to distinguish useful information and therapy from that which is useless or potentially even harmful. How, then, does one go about reading and critically evaluating the medical literature?

The first step in this process is to develop a list of journals, which will form the foundation of a regular literature review. This list should comprise not only those journals with the desired specialty in their name, but also those publications that address related specialties or topics and have a high likelihood of also publishing applicable studies (Box 1-1).

An alternative to reviewing multiple journals is to perform a computerized literature search when there is a particular topic of interest. The use of computerized search engines such as Medline or Ovid allows the computer to search a massive database of multiple medical journals and automatically develop a list of suggested studies and publications (Box 1-2).

> ### BOX 1-1   Suggested Journals for Review
>
> Academic Emergency Medicine
> American Journal of Emergency Medicine
> Annals of Emergency Medicine
> Journal of Emergency Medicine
> Journal of Trauma
> Prehospital Emergency Care

> ### BOX 1-2   Performing a Computerized Literature Search
>
> Medline can be accessed through the National Library of Medicine website at the following website address: www.ncbi.nlm.nih.gov/pubmed.
>
> To perform a journal search for articles and studies, it is necessary to enter search terms into Medline that will be used as key words to find appropriate articles. The more specific that you can be with the terms, the more likely you are to find articles that will meet your needs. However, being too specific can occasionally exclude articles that might also apply. Therefore, a good strategy to follow is to first conduct a search using very specific terms and then do a follow-up search with more generic terms. For example, if you are interested in finding articles about cricothyroidotomy in the prehospital setting, the initial search you perform might be done using the terms "Cricothyroidotomy" and "Prehospital." The next search might be performed using the terms "Airway management" and "Emergency Medical Services," recognizing that "airway management" may well yield articles that include not only cricothyroidotomy but other forms of airway management as well.

The next step is to review the title of every article in the table of contents of each of the selected journals to narrow down the article choices to those that clearly relate to the topic of interest. It would be impossible to read each of the selected journals from cover to cover, nor is it necessary. By reviewing the table of contents, articles that are of no interest can be immediately dismissed.

Once the selection has been narrowed, there are still a number of preliminary actions to take before reading the text of the article. Look at the authors listed on the articles to see if any are already known for their work in this area. Next, read the summary or abstract of the article to see if this overview of the article fulfills the expectations generated when the title was first reviewed. Then, review the site where the study was conducted to assess the similarities, differences, and applicability to the setting in which the results of the study may be subsequently applied. It must be stressed that reading the abstract alone is not enough. It serves only as the "teaser" to determine whether the full article should be reviewed. Medical practice should never be changed based on the abstract.

Once these initial points have been evaluated, the full text of the article is now read and critically assessed. In doing so, several specific issues are important to determine. The first issue is to *evaluate the study and the randomization of the patients* entered into the study. Every patient included should have had the same probability of receiving one or the other treatments or interventions being compared in the study, and that probability should be known beforehand. The method for assigning patients to their treatment should be described and should be similar to the flip of a coin.

Next, the *patient population* entered into the study is assessed to determine the similarities or differences with the target population where the study conclusions will be implemented. To do so, adequate information must be provided in the text describing the clinical and sociodemographic makeup of the study population.

The next issue for consideration is the *outcome measure* selected by the authors. All outcomes that are clinically relevant should be considered and reported in the study. For example, cardiac arrest studies may describe such endpoints or outcomes as cardiac rhythm conversion, return of spontaneous circulation, survival to hospital admission, or survival to discharge from the hospital.

Analysis of the *results* section also requires critical review. Just as it is important to evaluate the study population and entry criteria, it is equally important to see if all patients entered into the study at the beginning are accounted for at the end of the study. Specifically, the authors should describe any criteria used to exclude patients from the study analysis. Simple addition by the reader of the various treatment groups or subgroups will quickly confirm if all patients were accounted for. The authors should also describe occurrences that might introduce bias into the results. For example, the authors should report mishaps such as control patients accidentally receiving the treatment or study patients receiving other diagnostics or interventions.

In addition, the clinical, as well as the statistical, significance of the results are important to consider. Although the *statistical* analyses may be difficult to understand, a basic comprehension of statistical test selection and utilization will validate the statistical tests performed. Equally and perhaps more important than the statistical significance of a result is the *clinical* significance of the reported result. For example, in evaluating the effect of a new antihypertensive medication, the statistical analysis may show that the new drug causes a statistically significant decrease in blood pressure of 4 mm Hg. Clinically, however, the reported decrease is insignificant. Thus, the health care provider must assess not only the statistical significance of the result but also the clinical significance.

If all the prior issues have been answered satisfactorily, the last issue relates to the *implementation* of the study results and conclusion in the reader's health care system. To determine the practicality of applying the therapy, the authors needed to describe the treatment in sufficient detail, the intervention or therapy must be available for use, and it must be clinically sensible in the planned setting.

Some differences exist in the evaluation of consensus statements, overviews, and textbook chapters. Ideally, the statement or overview should address a specific focused question. The authors should describe the criteria used to select the articles included as references, and the reader will determine the appropriateness of these criteria. This in turn will help determine the likelihood that important studies were included and not missed. In addition, the reference list should be reviewed for known studies that should have been included.

A high-quality overview or consensus statement will include a discussion of the process by which the *validity* of the included studies was appraised. The validity assessment should be reproducible regardless of who actually performed the appraisal. Also, multiple studies with similar results help support the conclusions and ultimate decision about whether or not to change current practice.

Similar to the review of individual studies, the review and assessment of consensus statements, overviews, and textbook chapters include a determination of whether all clinically relevant outcomes were considered and discussed and whether the results can be applied to the reader's patient care setting. This also includes an analysis of the benefits versus the potential risks and harm.

The final step in evaluation is to determine when a publication should cause a *change in daily medical practice.* Ideally, any change in medical practice will result from a study of the highest quality, specifically a randomized, controlled, double-blind study. The conclusion of that study will be based on results that have been critically evaluated, have both statistical and clinical significance, and have been reviewed and judged to be valid. The study should be the best information currently available on the issue. In addition, the change in practice must be "doable" in the system planning to make the change, and the benefit of making the change must outweigh the risks.

All the medical practice in the out-of-hospital setting should be based on high-quality, Class I evidence that supports practice. As noted, however, most of the EMS literature qualifies as Class III evidence.

References

1. Trunkey DD: Trauma, *Sci Am* 249:28, 1983.
2. Demetriades D, Chan L, Cornwell EE, et al: Paramedic vs. private transportation of trauma patients: effect on outcome, *Arch Surg* 131:133, 1996.

3. Cornwell EE, Belzberg H, Hennigan K, et al: Emergency medical services (EMS) vs. non-EMS transport of critically injured patients: a prospective evaluation, *Arch Surg* 135(3):315, 2000.

4. Farrington JD: Death in a ditch, *Bull Am Coll Surg* 52:121, 1967.

5. Kennedy R: *Early care of the sick and injured patient*, Chicago, 1964, American College of Surgeons.

6. Rockwood CA, Mann CM, Farrington JD, et al: History of emergency medical services in the United States, *J Trauma* 16:299, 1976.

7. McSwain NE: Prehospital care from Napoleon to Mars: the surgeon's role, *J Am Coll Surg* 200:487, 2005.

8. National Academy of Sciences/National Research Council: *Accidental death and disability: the neglected disease of modern society*, Washington, DC, 1966, NAS/NRC.

9. Ali J, Adam RU, Gana TJ, et al: Effect of the prehospital trauma life support program (PHTLS) on prehospital trauma care, *J Trauma* 42:786, 1997.

10. Ali J, Adam RU, Gana TJ, et al: Trauma patient outcome after the prehospital trauma life support program, *J Trauma* 42: 1018, 1997.

Suggested Readings

Callaham M: Quantifying the scanty science of prehospital emergency care, *Ann Emerg Med* 30:785, 1997.

Cone DC, Lewis RJ: Should this study change my practice? *Acad Emerg Med* 10:417, 2003.

Haynes RB, McKibbon KA, Fitzgerald D, et al: How to keep up with the medical literature. II. Deciding which journals to read regularly, *Ann Intern Med* 105:309, 1986.

Keim SM, Spaite DW, Maio RF, et al: Establishing the scope and methodological approach to out-of-hospital outcomes and effectiveness research, *Acad Emerg Med* 11:1067, 2004.

Lewis RJ, Bessen HA: Statistical concepts and methods for the reader of clinical studies in emergency medicine, *J Emerg Med* 9:221, 1991.

MacAvley D: Critical appraisal of medical literature: an aid to rational decision making, *Fam Pract* 12:98, 1995.

Reed JF III, Salen P, Bagher P: Methodological and statistical techniques: what do residents really need to know about statistics? *J Med Syst* 27:233, 2003.

Sackett DL: How to read clinical journals. V. To distinguish useful from useless or even harmful therapy, *Can Med Assoc J* 124:1156, 1981.

Chapter Objectives

*At the completion of this chapter, the reader
will be able to do the following:*

✓ Describe the concept of energy as a cause of injury.

✓ Build a Haddon Matrix for a type of injury of interest.

✓ Relate the importance of accurate, attentive scene observations
and documentation of data by emergency medical services (EMS)
providers to the success of injury prevention initiatives.

✓ Assist in the development, implementation, and evaluation of injury
prevention programs in his or her community or EMS organization.

✓ Advocate the role of EMS providers in injury prevention.

✓ Identify strategies that prehospital care providers can implement that
will reduce the risk of injury.

CHAPTER 2

Injury Prevention

SCENARIO

The "guys" were sitting around the station after the monthly meeting of the Lanier County Volunteer Ambulance Squad. As is often the case, conversation turned to "war stories." This session became particularly animated because there were three new members inducted tonight. Steve, Bill, and Marilyn had just gotten their state certification as emergency medical technicians (EMTs) and were bona fide active members in good standing. Everyone was taking turns telling about their most spectacular save or closest brush with death. The stories were becoming more exaggerated than ever before. Mike, a 10-year veteran of the squad, had the "newbies" wide-eyed as he told how he had old Medic 1 on two wheels going around the sharp curve on Highway 138. Of course, his years of experience were the only thing that saved him. "But you have to drive like a maniac on 138 because it's a long way to the hospital at the other end of the county." He went on to say he thought about putting his seat belt on after that but remembered how it always got tangled up with his lapel mic when he exited the ambulance, and anyway, he was already through the worst part of the highway. His partner on that call, Belinda, had the group in stitches when she added that she ended up kissing the old guy on the stretcher when she got thrown around in the back. "But, that's the risk you have to take to work in this business."

Steve and Marilyn were talking just 2 weeks later about how they were thinking of "hanging it up because it's just not worth it." Bill's funeral had taken the strength out of them. He was driving Medic 1 that rainy night when he took the curve on Highway 138 too fast. If he'd had his seat belt on, he might have survived. The consensus is that the patient he was transporting will never wake up or come off the ventilator, and the patient's family will probably sue.

What factors contributed to these injuries? How could this tragedy have been prevented? What can Steve and Marilyn do as EMTs to reduce the incidence of injury in the community they serve as well as in their own service? How do you think EMS providers' perceptions about their jobs affect their actions as medical providers? ■

A major impetus in the development of modern emergency medical services (EMS) systems was the publication of the 1966 "white paper" by the National Academy of Sciences/National Research Council (NAS/NRC), *Accidental Death and Disability: the Neglected Disease of Modern Society*. The paper spotlighted shortcomings in injury management in the United States, which helped launch a formal system of on-scene care and rapid transport for patients injured as a result of "accidents." This educational initiative was instrumental in the creation of a more efficient system to deliver prehospital care to sick and injured patients.[1]

Death and disability from injury in the United States have fallen since the publication of the white paper.[2] Despite this progress, however, injury remains a major public health problem. More than 152,000 Americans die from injuries annually, and millions more are adversely affected to some degree.[3] However, injury is a global problem as well. Approximately 5.2 million people worldwide died from injuries in 2002. Injuries remain a leading cause of death for all age groups.[4] For some age groups, particularly children, teenagers, and young adults, injury is *the* leading cause of death.

The desire to care for patients stricken by injury draws many into the field of EMS. The Prehospital Trauma Life Support (PHTLS) course teaches prehospital providers to be efficient and effective in injury management. The need for well-trained prehospital providers to care for injured

patients will always exist. However, the *most* efficient and effective method to combat injury is to prevent it from happening in the first place. Health care providers at all levels play an active role in injury prevention to achieve the best results for not only the community at large but for themselves as well.

Even in 1966, the authors of the NAS/NRC white paper recognized the importance of injury prevention when they wrote:

The long-term solution to the injury problem is prevention .... Prevention of accidents involves training in the home, in the school, and at work, augmented by frequent pleas for safety in the news media; first aid courses and public meetings; and inspection and surveillance by regulatory agencies.[1]

Prehospital personnel can easily play an active role in most, if not all, of the current recommendations for injury prevention.

Prevention of some diseases, such as rabies, has been so effective that the occurrence of a single case makes front-page news. Public health officials recognize that prevention results in the greatest reward toward the amelioration of disease. Emergency medical technician (EMT) curricula have long included formal instruction in scene safety and personal protective equipment as a means of self-injury prevention for the EMT. To spur EMS systems to take a more active role in community prevention strategies, the

EMS Agenda for the Future, developed by and for the EMS community, lists prevention as one of 14 attributes to develop further in order to "improve community health and result in more appropriate use of acute health resources."[5] To this end, the U.S. Department of Transportation (DOT) paramedic curriculum has included community injury prevention training.

EMS systems are transforming themselves from a solely reactionary discipline to a broader, more effective discipline that includes more emphasis on prevention. This chapter introduces key concepts of injury prevention to the prehospital care provider.

Scope of the Problem

Death from injuries is a major health problem worldwide, resulting in more than 14,000 deaths *daily* (Box 2-1). In most countries, regardless of their level of development, injuries appear among the five leading causes of death.[4] Although causes of injury deaths vary little between countries, wide variability does exist between which causes have the greatest impact on specific age groups. Because of economic, social, and developmental issues, the cause of injury-related death varies from country to country and even region to region within the same country.

For example, in low-income and middle-income countries of the Western Pacific, the leading injury-related causes of death are road traffic injuries, drowning, and suicide, whereas in Africa the leading causes are road traffic injuries, war, and interpersonal violence. In high-income countries of the Americas, the leading cause of death among people between 15 and 29 years of age is road traffic injuries. In low-income and middle-income countries of the Americas,

the leading cause is interpersonal violence for the same age group.[4] Figure 2-1 demonstrates that injury plays a leading role in the global burden of disease.

In the United States, injuries are the third leading cause of death after cardiovascular disease and cancer, accounting for more than 152,000 deaths annually[3] (Figure 2-2). Injury is an especially serious problem for the youth of America as well as most industrialized nations of the world. In the United States, injury kills more children and young adults than all diseases combined (almost 19,000 in 1997).[6]

Unfortunately, deaths from injury are only the tip of the iceberg. The "injury triangle" provides a more complete picture of the *public health impact* of injury (Figure 2-3). In the United States in 2002, just over 161,000 people died from injury, but another 2.8 million were hospitalized because of nonfatal injuries. Injury also resulted in more than 40 million emergency department visits.[3]

The impact can be further realized by examining the number of *years of potential life lost* (YPLL) as a result of injury. YPLL is calculated by subtracting age-at-death from a fixed age of the group being examined, usually 65 or 70 years or the life expectancy of the group. Injury unnecessarily kills or disables people of all ages, but it disproportionately affects children, youth, and young adults, especially in industrialized nations. Because injury is the leading killer of Americans between 1 and 44 years of age, it is responsible for more YPLL than any other cause. In 1995, injury stole an estimated 3.5 million years from its victims compared with 2 million years for cancer, even though cancer claims more lives than injury.[7]

A third measure of injury severity can be demonstrated financially. The *economics of injury* are felt far beyond the patient and the immediate family. The cost of injury is spread across a wide spectrum. All members of society feel the effect because the costs of injury are borne by federal

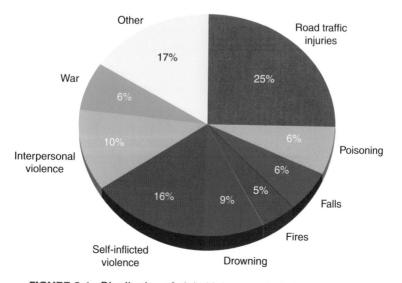

FIGURE 2-1   Distribution of global injury mortality by cause, 2000.
(From World Health Organization: *The injury chart book*, Geneva, 2002, WHO.)

BOX 2-1   Worldwide Injury-Related Statistics, 2000

INJURY OVERALL
- The top eight injury-related causes of mortality in order were:
  1. Road traffic injuries
  2. Self-inflicted violence
  3. Interpersonal violence
  4. Drowning
  5. Poisoning
  6. War
  7. Falls
  8. Fires
- An estimated 5.2 million people died worldwide from injuries.
- Injuries accounted for 9% of the world's deaths.
- The burden of disease related to injuries, particularly road traffic injuries, interpersonal violence, war, and self-inflicted injuries, is expected to rise dramatically by the year 2020.
- Twice as many men die from injury as women; fire-related deaths are the notable exception.
- Males in Africa have the highest injury-related mortality rates.
- Southeast Asia and the Western Pacific account for approximately one half of the total number of injury-related deaths worldwide.
- Injury accounts for 12% of "total lost years of life" either from premature death or from disability.

ROAD TRAFFIC INJURY
- An estimated 1.2 million people died as a result of road traffic injuries.
- 90% of road traffic injuries occurred in low- and middle-income countries.
- Road traffic mortality for males is almost three times higher than for females.
- Southeast Asia accounts for the highest percentage of road traffic injury deaths.
- More than 50% of global mortality caused by road traffic injuries occurs in the 15-44 age group.

FIRE-RELATED BURNS
- Females in Southeast Asia have the highest fire-related burn mortality rates.
- Children under age 5 years and elderly persons have the highest fire-related mortality rates.
- Southeast Asia alone accounts for just over one half of fire-related burn deaths.

DROWNING
- 450,000 persons drowned in 2000.
- 97% of drowning deaths occurred in low- and middle-income countries.
- Among the various age groups, children under age 5 years have the highest drowning mortality rates, accounting for more than 50%.
- Males in Africa and the Western Pacific have the highest drowning mortality rates.

FALLS
- 283,000 people died as a result of falls in 2000.
- A quarter of all fatal falls occurred in high-income countries.
- In all regions of the world, adults over age 70, particularly women, have the highest fall mortality rate.
- Europe and the Western Pacific combined account for almost 60% of the total number of fall-related deaths.

POISONING
- An estimated 315,000 people died from poisoning worldwide.
- More than 94% of fatal poisonings occurred in low- and middle-income countries.
- The overall poisoning rate among males in Europe is approximately three times higher than the rate in either gender in any other world region.
- The European region accounts for more than one third of all poisoning deaths worldwide.

INTERPERSONAL VIOLENCE
- An estimated 520,000 people died worldwide as a result of interpersonal violence.
- 95% of homicides occurred in low- and middle-income countries.
- The highest interpersonal violence rates are found in the Americas among males age 15 to 29 years.
- Among females, Africa has the highest mortality rate from interpersonal violence.

SUICIDE
- 815,000 people worldwide committed suicide.
- 86% of all suicides occurred in low- and middle-income countries.
- Women in China have a suicide rate that is approximately twice that of women in other parts of the world.
- More than 50% of suicides occur in persons age 15 to 44 years.

All figures compiled from World Health Organization data.

Rank	<1	1-4	5-9	10-14	15-24	25-34	35-44	45-54	55-64	65+	All Ages
					Age Groups						
1	Congenital Anomalies 5,623	Unintentional Injury 1,641	Unintentional Injury 1,176	Unintentional Injury 1,542	Unintentional Injury 15,412	Unintentional Injury 12,569	Unintentional Injury 16,710	Malignant Neoplasms 49,637	Malignant Neoplasms 93,391	Heart Disease 576,301	Heart Disease 696,947
2	Short Gestation 4,637	Congenital Anomalies 530	Malignant Neoplasms 537	Malignant Neoplasms 535	Homicide 5,219	Suicide 5,046	Malignant Neoplasms 16,085	Heart Disease 37,570	Heart Disease 64,234	Malignant Neoplasms 391,001	Malignant Neoplasms 557,271
3	SIDS 2,295	Homicide 423	Congenital Anomalies 199	Suicide 260	Suicide 4,010	Homicide 4,489	Heart Disease 13,688	Unintentional Injury 14,675	Chronic Low. Respiratory Disease 11,280	Cerebro-vascular 143,293	Cerebro-vascular 162,672
4	Maternal Pregnancy Comp. 1,708	Malignant Neoplasms 402	Homicide 140	Congenital Anomalies 218	Malignant Neoplasms 1,730	Malignant Neoplasms 3,872	Suicide 6,851	Liver Disease 7,216	Diabetes Mellitus 10,022	Chronic Low. Respiratory Disease 108,313	Chronic Low Respiratory Disease 124,816
5	Placenta Cord Membranes 1,028	Heart Disease 165	Heart Disease 92	Homicide 216	Heart Disease 1,022	Heart Disease 3,165	HIV 5,707	Suicide 6,308	Cerebro-vascular 9,897	Influenza & Pneumonia 58,826	Unintentional Injury 106,742
6	Unintentional Injury 946	Influenza & Pneumonia 110	Benign Neoplasms 44	Heart Disease 163	Congenital Anomalies 492	HIV 1,839	Homicide 3,239	Cerebro-vascular 6,055	Unintentional Injury 8,345	Alzheimer's Disease 58,289	Diabetes Mellitus 73,249
7	Respiratory Distress 943	Septicemia 79	Septicemia 42	Chronic Low. Respiratory Disease 95	Chronic Low. Respiratory Disease 192	Diabetes Mellitus 642	Liver Disease 3,145	Diabetes Mellitus 5,496	Liver Disease 6,097	Diabetes Mellitus 54,715	Influenza & Pneumonia 65,681
8	Bacterial Sepsis 749	Chronic Low. Respiratory Disease 65	Chronic Low. Respiratory Disease 41	Cerebro-vascular 58	HIV 178	Cerebro-vascular 567	Cerebro-vascular 2,425	HIV 4,474	Suicide 3,618	Nephritis 34,316	Alzheimer's Disease 58,866
9	Circulatory System Disease 667	Perinatal Period 65	Influenza & Pneumonia 38	Influenza & Pneumonia 53	Cerebro-vascular 171	Congenital Anomalies 475	Diabetes Mellitus 2,164	Chronic Low. Respiratory Disease 3,475	Nephritis 3,455	Unintentional Injury 33,641	Nephritis 40,974
10	Intrauterine Hypoxia 583	Benign Neoplasms 60	Cerebro-vascular 33	Septicemia 53	Diabetes Mellitus 171	Liver Disease 374	Chronic Low. Respiratory Disease 1,008	Viral Hepatitis 2,331	Septicemia 3,360	Septicemia 26,670	Septicemia 33,865
11	Atelectasis 400	Cerebro-vascular 53	Anemias 29	Benign Neoplasms 45	Influenza & Pneumonia 167	Influenza & Pneumonia 345	Influenza & Pneumonia 971	Septicemia 2,074	Influenza & Pneumonia 2,987	Hypertension 17,345	Suicide 31,655
12	Neonatal Hemorrhage 387	Acute Bronchitis 23	Perinatal Period 15	Diabetes Mellitus 29	Septicemia 118	Septicemia 314	Septicemia 856	Influenza & Pneumonia 1,918	Hypertension 1,526	Parkinson's Disease 16,577	Liver Disease 27,257
13	Necrotizing Enterocolitis 352	Anemias 21	Meningitis 10	Anemias 24	Anemias 111	Chronic Low. Respiratory Disease 301	Nephritis 749	Homicide 1,915	Aortic Aneurysm 1,460	Pneumonitis 16,236	Hypertension 20,261
14	Birth Trauma 345	Meningitis 19	Nephritis 9	HIV 21	Complicated Pregnancy 89	Nephritis 269	Viral Hepatitis 740	Nephritis 1,893	HIV 1,347	Athero-sclerosis 13,085	Homicide 17,638
15	Chronic Respiratory Disease 314	Nephritis 14	Two Tied 7	Meningitis 21	Benign Neoplasms 87	Anemias 180	Congenital Anomalies 572	Hypertension 923	Benign Neoplasms 1,193	Aortic Aneurysm 12,187	Pneumonitis 17,593

FIGURE 2-2   Leading causes of death in the United States by age group, 2002. *Blue,* Death from unintentional injury. *Red,* Death from intentional injury committed by others. *Green,* Death from intentional injury committed by self. (Produced by the Office of Statistics and Programming, National Center for Injury Prevention and Control, CDC. Data source: National Center for Health Statistics [NCHS] Vital Statistics System.)

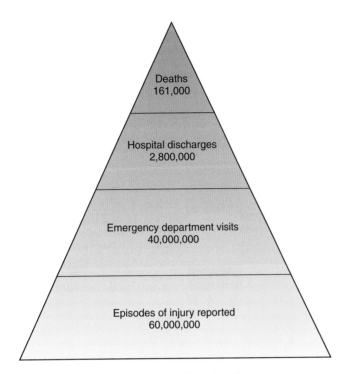

FIGURE 2-3   Injury triangle.

and other agencies, private insurance programs that pass the expense on to other subscribers, and employers as well as the patient. As a result, everyone pays when an individual is seriously injured. Cost estimates for injury run as high as $325 billion annually, which includes the direct cost of medical care and indirect costs such as lost earnings.[8]

The toll of injury in terms of morbidity, mortality, and economic stress is excessive:

Injuries have always been a threat to the public's well-being, but until the mid-twentieth century, infectious diseases overshadowed the terrible contribution injury made to human morbidity and mortality. Public health's success in other areas has left injury as a major public health concern, one that has been termed "the neglected epidemic."[8]

Society is calling on all segments of the medical community to increase its prevention activities. With more than 600,000 prehospital providers in the United States alone, EMS systems can make a tremendous contribution to community-based injury prevention efforts.

Injury in EMS

Obtaining a clear picture of the impact of injury on the EMS provider is difficult because no single national data-gathering process deals with our industry. Even determining how many providers are in the United States is only an estimate of 600,000 to 832,000. However, several studies and publications have sought to answer this question.

EMS personnel are undoubtedly exposed to a wide variety of situations that can result in worker injury. We go where people are hurt and sick. Sometimes those scenes are unsecured despite our best efforts and those of law enforcement because we are dealing with people in emotional and physical crisis. Even the very nature of the work presents opportunities for injury. Just driving to the scene can be hazardous. Lifting, exposure to environmental hazards and infectious disease, and stress of the job also present opportunities for injury.

For the years 1992 through 1997, an estimated 12.7 fatalities occurred per 100,000 workers per year in EMS.[9] This compares with a national average fatality rate of 5.0 per 100,000 over the same period. More than 58% of those fatalities involved ambulance crashes; 9% involved assault or homicide. As with fatalities, estimating nonfatal injury can be difficult as well. However, one serious, disabling injury requiring hospitalization per 31,616 dispatches has been documented among urban providers.[10]

These numbers reveal a disturbing truth. "The most dangerous times for EMS personnel are when they are inside their truck when it is moving or when they are working at a crash scene near other moving vehicles."[11] It is critical that EMS personnel know and understand the concepts of injury and injury prevention so that the risks inherent in EMS can be identified and corrected. From almost the first day of EMT education, it is taught that no one is more important at the scene than the EMT, so his or her safety must come first. Seat belt use is the first step of safety.

Concepts of Injury

Definition of Injury

A discussion of injury prevention should begin with a definition of the term *injury*. The wide variability of the causes of injury initially represented a major hurdle in its study and prevention. For example, what does a fractured hip caused by a fall in an elderly person have in common with a self-inflicted gunshot wound to the head of a young adult? All possible causes of injury, from vehicle crashes, to stabbings, to suicides, to drownings, have one factor in common: energy transfer. *Injury* is now commonly defined as a harmful event that arises from the release of specific forms of physical energy or barriers to normal flow of energy.[12]

Typically, energy exists in five physical forms: mechanical, chemical, thermal, radiation, or electrical. *Mechanical energy,* the most common cause of injury, is expended when an unrestrained driver collides with the windshield during a vehicle crash. Injury from *chemical energy* occurs when a curious child drinks ammonia found in an unlocked cabinet in the kitchen. *Thermal energy* causes injury when a cook sprays lighter fluid on actively burning charcoal in an outdoor grill, which then flashes in his face. *Radiation energy* produces sunburn to the teenager searching for a golden tan for the summer. *Electrical energy* damages the skin, nerves, and blood vessels of a prehospital care provider who fails to do a proper scene assessment before touching a vehicle that hit a power pole.

The body requires basic elements such as oxygen and heat to produce the internal energy needed to function properly. If conditions arise that prevent the body from using these necessary elements, injury can result. Suffocation and hypothermia are physical injuries that result from an interruption of the body's normal energy flow.

Any form of physical energy in sufficient quantity can cause tissue damage. The body can tolerate energy transfer within certain limits. If this threshold is breached, an injury results. A bullet fired from a pistol at point-blank range easily passes through skin and soft tissue, causing massive injury. If the intended victim is far enough away, theoretically the potential victim can simply stick out a hand, and the bullet would hit his palm and fall harmlessly to the ground. As the bullet's energy dissipates in the air on its flight, it does not have enough energy on impact to exceed the body's tolerance level. Such a situation rarely happens.

Energy Out of Control

People harness and use all five forms of energy in many productive endeavors every day. In these situations, energy is under control and is not allowed to affect the body adversely. A person's ability to maintain control of energy depends on two factors: task performance and task demand.[13] As long as a person's ability to perform a task exceeds the demands of a task, energy is released in a controlled, usable manner.

In the following three situations, however, demand may exceed performance, leading to an uncontrolled release of energy:

1. *When the difficulty of the task suddenly exceeds the individual's performance ability.* For example, a prehospital care provider may operate an ambulance safely during normal driving conditions but loses control when the vehicle hits a sheet of black ice. The sudden increase in the demands of the task exceeds the prehospital care provider's performance capabilities, leading to a crash.
2. *When the individual's performance level falls below the demands of the task.* Falling asleep at the wheel of a vehicle while driving down a country road causes a sudden drop in performance with no change in task demand, leading to a crash.
3. *When both factors change simultaneously.* Talking on a cellular phone while driving may reduce a driver's concentration on the road. If an animal darts in front of the vehicle, task demand suddenly rises. Under normal circumstances, the driver may be able to handle the

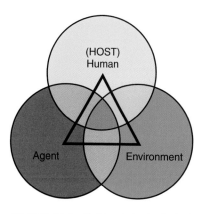

FIGURE 2-4 Epidemiological triad.

increased demands of the task. A drop in concentration at the very moment when additional skill is required may lead to a crash.

Injury as a Disease

The disease process has been studied for years. It is now understood that three factors must be present and interact simultaneously for an illness to occur: (1) an agent that causes the illness, (2) a host in which the agent can reside, and (3) a suitable environment in which the agent and host can come together. Once public health professionals recognized this "epidemiological triad," they discovered how to combat the disease (Figure 2-4). Eradication of certain diseases has been possible by vaccinating the host, destroying the agent with antibiotics, reducing environmental transmission through improved sanitation, or a combination of all three.

Only since the late 1940s has significant exploration of the *injury process* occurred. Pioneers in the study of injury demonstrated that despite the obviously different results, illness and injury behave similarly. Both require the presence of the three elements of the epidemiological triad, and therefore both are treated as a disease:

1. For an injury to occur, a host (i.e., the human) must exist. As with illness, *susceptibility* of the host does not remain constant from individual to individual; it varies as a result of internal and external factors. *Internal* factors include intelligence, gender, and reaction time. *External* factors include intoxication, anger, and social beliefs. Susceptibility also varies over time within the same person.
2. As described previously, the agent of injury is *energy*. Velocity, shape, material, and time of exposure to the object that releases the energy all play a role in whether the host's tolerance level is overwhelmed.
3. The host and agent must come together in an environment that allows the two to interact. Typically, the environment is divided into physical and social components. *Physical* environmental factors can

be seen and touched. *Social* environmental factors include attitudes, beliefs, and judgments. For example, teenagers are more likely to participate in risk-taking behavior (the physical component) because they have more of a sense of invincibility (the social component) than other age groups.

The characteristics of the host, agent, and environment change with time and circumstance:

To illustrate, think of the components of the Epidemiological Triad as constantly turning wheels. Inside each wheel are pie-shaped sections, one for each possible circumstantial variable—good and bad. The three wheels turn at different rates, so different characteristics interact (meet) at different times and in different combinations. Some combinations predict that no injury will occur; some predict disaster.[14]

In the case of injury, the host might be a curious, mobile 2-year-old child; the agent of injury might be a swimming pool filled with water with a beach ball floating just beyond the edge; the environment might be a pool gate left open while the babysitter runs inside to answer the telephone. With the host, agent, and environment all coming together at the same time, an unintentional injury—in this case, drowning—can occur.

Haddon Matrix

Dr. William J. Haddon, Jr., is considered the father of the science of injury prevention. Working within the concept of the epidemiological triad, in the mid-1960s he recognized that an injury can be broken down into the following three temporal phases:

1. *Preevent:* Before the injury.
2. *Event:* The point when harmful energy is released.
3. *Postevent:* The aftermath of the injury.

By examining the three factors of the epidemiological triad during each temporal phase, Haddon created a nine-cell "phase-factor" matrix (Table 2-1). This grid has become known as the *Haddon Matrix.* It provides a means to depict graphically the events or actions that increase or decrease the odds that an injury will occur. It can also be used to identify prevention strategies. The Haddon Matrix demonstrates that *multiple* factors can lead to an injury, and therefore multiple opportunities exist to prevent or reduce its severity. The matrix played a major role in dispelling the myth that injury is the result of a single cause, bad luck, or fate.

Table 2-1 depicts a Haddon Matrix for an ambulance crash. The components in each cell of the matrix are different depending on the injury being examined. The *preevent phase* includes factors that can contribute to the likelihood

of a crash; however, energy is still under control. This phase may last from a few seconds to several years. The *event phase* depicts the factors that influence the severity of the injury. During this time, uncontrolled energy is released and injury occurs if energy transfer exceeds the body's tolerance. The event phase is typically very brief; it may last only a fraction of a second but rarely lasts more than a few minutes. Factors in the *postevent phase* affect the outcome once an injury has occurred. Depending on the type of event, it may last from a few seconds to the remaining life span of the host. (See also Chapter 1.)

Classification of Injury

A common method to subclassify injuries is based on *intent.* Injury may result from either intentional or unintentional causes. Although this is a logical way to view injuries, it underscores the difficulty of injury prevention efforts.

Intentional injury is typically associated with an act of interpersonal or self-directed violence. Problems such as homicide, suicide, spousal abuse, and war fall into this category. Previously, prevention of intentional injury was thought to be the sole responsibility of the criminal justice and mental health systems. Although these agencies are integral to reducing violent deaths, intentional injuries can best be prevented through a broad multidisciplinary approach, which includes the medical profession.

In the past, *unintentional injuries* were called "accidents." The authors of the NAS/NRC white paper appropriately referred to "accidental" death and disability; this was the vocabulary of the time.[1] Because it is now understood that very specific factors must come together for an injury to occur, health care providers now realize that the term *accidental* does not describe unintentional injury resulting from events such as vehicle crashes, drownings, falls, and electrocutions. EMS systems have embraced this concept by using the term *motor vehicle crashes* (MVCs) rather than "motor vehicle accidents" (MVAs). However, public perception has changed much more slowly. News reporters still describe persons injured in "automobile accidents" or "accidental shootings." The term *accident* suggests that a person was injured as a result of fate, divine intervention, or bad luck. It implies that the injury was random and therefore unavoidable. As long as this misperception exists, implementation of corrective measures will be impeded.

Prevention as the Solution

Preventing injury is even more important than treating injury. When injury is prevented, it spares the patient and family from suffering and economic hardship. The National Center for Injury Prevention and Control (NCIPC) of the

TABLE 2-1   Haddon Matrix for an Ambulance Crash

Time phases (Epidemiological Triad)	Host	Agent	Environment
Preevent	Driver's visual acuity Experience and judgment Amount of time in the ambulance per shift Level of fatigue Proper nutrition Stress level Adherence to company and community driving laws Quality of driver education courses	Maintenance of brakes, tires, etc. Defective equipment Ambulance's high center of gravity Speed Ease of control	Visibility hazards Road curvature and gradient Surface coefficient of friction Narrow road shoulder Traffic signals Speed limits
Event	Safety belt use Physical conditioning Injury threshold Ejection	Speed capability Ambulance size Automatic restraints Hardness and sharpness of contact surfaces Hardness and sharpness of loose items (e.g., clipboards, flashlights) Steering column Practice of safe driving habits: speed, use of lights/siren, passing, intersections, backing Practice of good partner habits en route: watching road, clearing intersections Park safely	Lack of guardrails Median barriers Distance between roadway and immovable objects Speed limits Other traffic Attitudes about safety belt use Maintain an escape route Make no assumptions about an environment being safe (e.g., "nice part of town," high-income home) Weather
Postevent	Age Physical condition Type or extent of injury	Fuel system integrity Entrapment	Emergency communication capability Distance to and quality of responding EMS Training of EMS personnel Availability of extrication equipment Trauma care system of the community Rehabilitation programs in the community

Centers for Disease Control and Prevention (CDC) estimates the following[6]:

- $1 spent on smoke detectors saves $69.
- $1 spent on bicycle helmets saves $29.
- $1 spent on child safety seats saves $32.
- $1 spent on center and edge lines on roads saves $3 in medical costs alone.

- $1 spent on counseling by pediatricians to prevent injuries saves $10.
- $1 spent on poison control center services saves $7 in medical expenses.
- A CDC-funded evaluation study of a regional trauma care system in Portland, Oregon, found a 35% decrease in the risk of dying for severely injured patients who were treated in the system.

■ A smoke detector distribution program in Oklahoma reduced burn-related injuries by 83%.

Because of the variability among the host, agent, and environment at any given time, health care providers cannot always predict or prevent every individual injury. However, it is possible to identify high-risk populations (which include EMS providers), high-risk products, and high-risk environments. Prevention efforts centered on high-risk groups or settings influence as wide a range of society as possible. Health care providers can pursue prevention in multiple ways. Some strategies have proven successful across the United States and around the world. However, other strategies work in one region but not in another. Before implementing an injury prevention strategy, efforts must center on determining if it will work. Although it is not necessary to "reinvent the wheel," health care providers may need to modify a prevention strategy to improve its chances of success. Methods for doing this are examined in the following section.

Concepts of Injury Prevention

Goal

The goal of injury prevention programs is to bring about a change in knowledge, attitude, and behavior on the part of a preidentified segment of society. Simply providing information to potential victims is not enough to prevent injury. A program must be implemented in a manner that will influence society's attitude and, most importantly, change behavior. The hope is that any change in behavior will be long term. This task is monumental but not insurmountable.

Opportunities for Intervention

Prevention strategies can be arranged according to their effect on the injury event. They coincide with the temporal phases of the Haddon Matrix. Preevent interventions, known as *primary interventions,* strive to prevent the injury from occurring. Actions intended to keep intoxicated drivers off the road, lower speed limits, and install traffic lights are designed to prevent crashes from occurring. Event-phase interventions are intended to reduce injury severity by softening the blow of injuries that occur. Wearing safety belts, installing cushioned dashboards in vehicles, and enforcing child safety seat laws are means to reduce the severity of injury sustained in crashes. Postevent interventions provide a means to improve the likelihood of survival for those who are injured. Encouraging physical fitness, designing

fuel systems for vehicles that do not explode on impact, and implementing high-quality EMS systems are intended to reduce the recovery time for persons who are injured.

Prehospital systems have traditionally limited their community involvement to the postevent phase. Countless lives have been saved as a result. However, because of the limitations inherent in waiting until injury has occurred, the best results have not been achieved. EMS systems must look at entering the injury cycle earlier. Using the Haddon Matrix, EMS systems can identify opportunities to collaborate with other public health and public safety organizations to prevent injuries from occurring or to soften their blow.

Potential Strategies

No single strategy provides the best approach to injury prevention. The most effective option or options depends on the type of injury being studied. However, Haddon developed a list of 10 generic strategies designed to break the chain of injury-producing events at numerous points (Table 2-2). These strategies represent ways that the release of uncontrolled energy can be prevented or at least reduced to amounts the body can better tolerate. Table 2-2 also presents countermeasures that can be taken in the preevent, event, and postevent phases and that are directed toward the host, agent, or environment. This list is not complete and merely serves as a starting point to help determine the most effective options for the particular problem under study.

Most injury prevention strategies are either active or passive. *Passive strategies* require little or no action on the part of the individual; sprinkler systems and vehicle air bags are examples. *Active strategies* require the cooperation of the person being protected; examples include manual seat belts and choosing to wear a motorcycle or bicycle helmet. Passive measures are generally more effective because people do not need to do anything consciously to take advantage of the protection. Nonetheless, passive strategies are usually more difficult to implement because they can be expensive or require legislative or regulatory action. Sometimes a combination of active and passive strategies is the best option.

Strategy Implementation

Three common approaches to implementing an injury prevention strategy have become known as the "Three Es of Injury Prevention": *E*ducation, *E*nforcement, and *E*ngineering.

Education

Educational strategies are meant to impart information. To be effective, the target audience must embrace the new-found knowledge with enough enthusiasm to alter behavior in the manner prescribed by the program. Because the

TABLE 2-2 Basic Strategies for Injury Countermeasures*

Strategy	Possible countermeasures
Prevent initial creation of the hazard	Do not produce firecrackers, three-wheeled all-terrain vehicles, or various poisons Eliminate spearing in high school football
Reduce amount of energy contained in the hazard	Limit the horsepower of motor vehicle engines Package toxic drugs in smaller, safer amounts Reduce speed limits Mandate public transportation to reduce the number of vehicles on the road Limit temperature of tap water in homes through regulators at the water heater Limit the muzzle velocity of guns Limit the amount of gunpowder in firecrackers
Prevent release of a hazard that already exists	Store firearms in locked containers Close pools and beaches when no lifeguard is on duty Make bathtubs less slippery Childproof containers for all hazardous household drugs and chemicals Limit cell phone use in vehicles to hands-free models Require safety shields on rotating farm machinery Improve vehicle handling
Modify rate or spatial distribution of the hazard	Use seat belts Provide antilock brakes Use short cleats on football shoes so feet rotate rather than transmit sudden force to the knees Require vehicle air bags Provide hydraulic bumpers on vehicles Provide safety nets to protect workers from falls Wear flame-retardant pajamas
Separate in time or space the hazard from that which is to be protected	Provide pedestrian overpasses at high-volume crossings Keep roadsides clear of poles and trees Do not have play areas near unguarded bodies of water Install bike paths Spray pesticides at a time when people are not present Install sidewalks Route trucks carrying hazardous material along low-density roads
Separate the hazard from that which is to be protected by a material barrier	Install fencing around all sides of swimming pools Provide protective eyewear for racquet sports Build highway medians Build protective shields around hazardous machinery Install guardrails between sidewalks and roads Install reinforced panels in vehicle doors Require EMS personnel to place used needles directly into a sharps container
Modify basic nature of the hazard	Provide air bags in motor vehicles Provide collapsible steering columns Provide breakaway poles Make crib slats too narrow to strangle a baby Adopt breakaway baseball bases Install nonslip surfaces in bathtubs Round the corners of cabinetry in the patient compartment of ambulances

Continued

TABLE 2-2   Basic Strategies for Injury Countermeasures*—cont'd

Strategy	Possible countermeasures
Make what is to protected more resistant to the hazard	Encourage calcium intake to reduce osteoporosis Encourage musculoskeletal conditioning in athletes Prohibit alcohol sales and consumption near recreational water areas Treat medical conditions such as epilepsy to prevent episodes that can result in burns, drownings, and falls Check earthquake-resistant building codes in susceptible areas
Begin to counter the damage already done by the hazard	Provide emergency medical care Employ system to route injured persons to appropriately trained prehospital care providers Develop school protocols for responding to injury emergencies Provide first-aid training to residents Install automatic sprinkler systems
Stabilize, repair, and rehabilitate the object of the damage	Develop rehabilitation plans at an early stage of injury treatment Make use of occupational rehabilitation for paraplegic patients

*The examples listed are for illustrative purposes only and are not necessarily the official recommendations of PHTLS, the National Association of EMTs, or the American College of Surgeons.

audience is required to do something, education is an active countermeasure. The target audience may be individuals who engage in high-risk activities, policymakers who have then the authority to enact further prevention legislation or regulation, or prehospital care providers learning to become active participants in injury prevention. The NAS/NRC white paper is an example of an education initiative.

Education once was the primary means of implementing prevention programs because society believed that most injuries were simply the result of human error. Although this is true to a certain extent, many failed to recognize the role that energy and the environment play in causing injury. Education is still often used, however, and is probably the easiest of the three strategies to implement.

Experience has demonstrated that education strategies have not met with overwhelming success for several reasons. The target audience may never hear the message. If the message is heard, some may reject it outright or not embrace it enough to alter behavior. Those who embrace it may do so sporadically or with declining enthusiasm over time.[15] However, education still can be particularly useful in reducing injury in the following four areas[9]:

1. *Teaching young children basic safety behaviors and skills that stay with them later in life.* Examples include what to do when a smoke detector sounds an alarm, calling 9-1-1 for help in an emergency, or fastening seat belts.
2. *Teaching about certain types and causes of injury for certain age groups.* Education may be the only strategy available for these groups.
3. *Altering the public's perception of risk and acceptable risk to change social norms and attitudes.* This was

used regarding drinking and driving and occurs now regarding wearing a helmet when riding a bicycle, scooter, skateboard, or rollerblades.
4. *Promoting policy change and educating consumers to demand safer products.*

As a singular approach to injury prevention, educational programs have had disappointing results. However, when coupled with other forms of implementation strategies, education can be a valuable tool. Education often serves as a starting point to pave the way for enforcement and engineering strategies.

Enforcement

Enforcement seeks to tap the persuasive power of law to compel adherence to simple but effective prevention strategies. Certain government entities have the power to enact statutes, regulations, and laws in an effort to promote public health, safety, and general welfare even when such actions restrict individual autonomy to a limited degree. Generally, courts tend to uphold injury prevention laws that pose a minimal burden on individuals if they are fairly enforced and the public health benefit is substantial.

Statutory commands can either *require* or *prohibit*, and they can be directed at individual behavior (people), products (things), or environmental conditions (places), as follows[8]:

- Legal requirements that apply to people are mandatory seat belt, child restraint, and helmet use laws.
- Prohibitions that apply to people are drunk-driving laws, speed limits, and making assaultive behavior a crime.

- Legal requirements that apply to products include design and performance standards, such as the federal Motor Vehicle Safety Standards.
- Prohibitions that apply to products include restrictions on dangerous animals and flammable fabrics.
- Legal requirements that apply to places include the installation of breakaway signposts along highways and fencing around swimming pools.
- Prohibitions that apply to places include the outlawing of rigid structures along highways and firearms in airport terminals.

Enforcement is also an *active* countermeasure because people must obey the law to benefit from it. Enforcement typically has wide application because laws apply to all members of society within a given jurisdiction. The effectiveness of enforcement initiatives depends on the willingness of society to obey and the feasibility and visibility of its enforcement. The target audience may be less likely to comply if they believe that the directive infringes on personal freedom, they have little chance of getting caught, or they will not face consequences of violating the law.

Because society as a whole tends to obey laws or at least stay within narrow limits around them, enforcement is often more effective than education. Enforcement in tandem with education appears to produce better results than either initiative alone.

Engineering

Often the most effective means of injury prevention are those in which destructive energy release is permanently separated from the host. Passive countermeasures accomplish this goal with little or no effort on the part of the individual. Engineering strategies strive to build injury prevention into products or environments so that the host does not have to act differently to be protected. Engineering strategies help the people who actually need them, and they do so every time. Measures such as automatic sprinkler systems in buildings, flotation hulls in boats, and backup alarms on ambulances have all been proven to save lives with little or no effort on the part of the host.

Engineering seems to be the perfect answer to injury prevention. It is passive, effective, and usually the least disruptive of the "Three Es." Unfortunately, it is often the most expensive to implement. Designing safety into a product usually makes it more expensive and may require legislative or regulatory initiation. The price may be more than the manufacturer is willing to absorb or the customer is willing to pay. Society dictates how much safety it wants built into a product and how much it is willing to support the endeavor financially.

Enforcement and engineering strategies should be preceded with education initiatives. The most effective countermeasures may be those that incorporate all three implementation strategies.

Public Health Approach

Much has been learned about injury and injury prevention. Unfortunately, a wide discrepancy exists between what is known about injury and what is being done about it.[8] EMS systems are critical to help close that gap. Injury is a complex problem in all societies of the world. A single person or single agency unfortunately will usually have little impact. A public health approach has demonstrated success in dealing with other diseases and is making progress with injury prevention as well. EMS agencies that have joined forces with other public and private organizations have been able to accomplish as much or more than they could on their own. Partnerships bring together a community's expertise to tackle a complex and perplexing issue.

A public health approach creates a community-based coalition to combat a community-based disease through a four-step process, as follows:

1. Surveillance
2. Risk factor identification
3. Intervention evaluation
4. Implementation

The coalition is composed of experts from such diverse fields as epidemiology, the medical community, schools of public health, public health agencies, community advocacy programs, economics, sociology, and criminal justice. EMS systems have an important place in a public health approach to injury prevention. Being part of a coalition to improve playground safety may not have the immediate effect of providing care at the scene of a horrific vehicle crash, but the results will be much more widespread.

Surveillance

Surveillance is the process of collecting data within a community. Collection of population-based data aids in discovery of an injury's true magnitude and effect on the community. A community can be a neighborhood, city, county, state, or even the ambulance service itself. Support for the program, proper allocation of resources, and even knowing who to include on the interdisciplinary team depends on understanding the scope of the problem.

Sources of information available within a community include the following:

- Mortality data
- Hospital admission and discharge statistics
- Medical records
- Trauma registries
- Police reports
- EMS run sheets
- Insurance reports
- Unique surveillance data collected solely for the study at hand

Risk Factor Identification

After a problem is identified and researched, it is necessary to know who is at risk to direct a prevention strategy at the correct population. "Shotgun" approaches to injury prevention are less successful than targeted ones. Identification of causes and risk factors determines who is injured; what types of injuries are sustained; and where, when, and why those injuries occur.[16] Sometimes a risk factor is an obvious cause, such as the presence of alcohol in fatal vehicles crashes. At other times, research is required to discover the true risk factors involved in injury events. EMS systems can serve as the "eyes and ears" of public health at the scene of injuries to identify actual risk factors that no one else may be able to uncover. Risk factors can then be charted on a Haddon Matrix as they are properly identified.

Intervention Evaluation

As risk factors become clear, intervention strategies begin to emerge. Haddon's list of 10 injury prevention strategies serves as a starting point (see Table 2-2). Even though communities have different characteristics, with modification an injury prevention initiative from one community may work in another. Once a potential intervention has been selected, a pilot program using one or more of the "Three Es" may give indications of the success of full-scale implementation.

Implementation

The final step in the public health approach is implementation and evaluation of the intervention. Detailed implementation procedures are prepared so others interested in implementation of similar programs will have a guide to follow. Collection of evaluation data measures the effectiveness of a program. Answering the following three questions may help determine the success of a program[12]:

1. Have attitudes, skills, or judgment changed?
2. Has behavior changed?
3. Does behavioral change lead to a favorable outcome?

The public health approach provides a proven means to combat a disease such as injury. Through a multidisciplinary, community-based effort, it is possible to identify the "who, what, where, when, and why" of an injury problem and develop a plan of action. EMS systems need to play a much more substantial role to help close the gap between what is known about injury and what is being done about it.

Evolving Role of EMS

Traditionally, the prehospital care provider's role in health care focuses almost exclusively on postevent, one-on-one

treatment of the individual. Little emphasis is placed on understanding the causes of the injuries or what a prehospital care provider could do to prevent them. As a result, patients may return to the same environment only to be injured again. In addition, information that could aid in the development of a community-wide prevention program to keep others from being injured in the first place may not be documented and therefore may remain unavailable to other sectors of public health.

The public health approach to injury is more proactive. It works to determine how to alter the host, agent, and environment to prevent injuries. Through coalitions that conduct surveillance and implement interventions, public health works to develop community-wide prevention programs. The *Emergency Medical Services Agenda for the Future* envisions closer ties between EMS systems and public health that would make both sectors of health care more effective.[5]

Prehospital care providers can take a more active role in development of community-wide injury prevention programs. EMS systems enjoy a unique position in the community. With more than 600,000 providers in the United States alone, basic and advanced prehospital care providers are widely distributed at the community level. Prehospital care providers enjoy a credible reputation in the community, making them high-profile role models. In addition, they are readily welcomed into homes and businesses. All phases of the public health approach to injury prevention will benefit from an EMS presence.

One-on-One Interventions

EMS systems do not have to give up their one-on-one approach to patient care to conduct valuable injury prevention interventions. The one-on-one approach makes EMS systems uniquely able to conduct injury prevention initiatives. Prehospital care providers can bring injury prevention messages directly to high-risk individuals. One indicator of a successful educational program is that the information is received with enough enthusiasm to change behavior. Prehospital care providers can use their role model status to deliver important prevention messages. Implicitly, people look up to role models, listen to what they have to say, and emulate what they do.

On-scene prevention counseling takes advantage of a "teachable moment." A teachable moment is the time when the patient who does not require critical medical interventions or the family members may be in a state that makes them more susceptible to what a role model says. The prehospital care provider may think of the on-scene time as wasted when it becomes apparent that little or no medical interventions are necessary. However, this may be the best time to deliver primary prevention.[17]

Not every call allows for injury prevention counseling. Serious and life-threatening calls require concentration on acute care. However, as many as 95% of ambulance calls are non–life threatening. A significant proportion require minor, if any, treatment. One-on-one prevention counseling may be appropriate during these noncritical calls.

Patient interactions are typically short encounters, especially those that require little or no treatment. However, they provide enough time to discuss and demonstrate to patients and family members practices that may prevent an injury in the future. A role model who discusses the importance of replacing a burned-out light bulb and removing a slippery throw rug in a dimly lit hallway may prevent a fall by an elderly resident. Prehospital care providers have an attentive audience during the ride to a hospital. Prevention is a more valuable topic to discuss than the weather or the local sports team. Teachable moments take 1 to 2 minutes to complete and do not interfere with treatment or transport.

Educational programs have been developed to train prehospital care providers to administer on-scene injury prevention counseling.[17,18] These types of programs must be further developed and evaluated to discover which are the most valuable and therefore worthy of inclusion in the primary education of a prehospital care provider.

Community-Wide Interventions

The public health approach to injury prevention is community based and involves a multidisciplinary team. EMS personnel have the expertise to be a valuable member of that team. Community-wide prevention strategies depend on data to address properly the "who, what, when, where, and why" of an injury problem. Multiple sources of information, as described previously, provide the needed data. Prehospital care providers, perhaps more than any other team member, have the opportunity to examine patient interaction with the environment at the time of the injury. This may allow identification of a high-risk individual, high-risk attitude, or high-risk behavior that is not present by the time the patient arrives at the emergency department.

The prehospital care provider can use documentation acquired en route to a medical facility in the following two ways:

1. Data can be used immediately by emergency personnel who receive the patient. Emergency room physicians and nurses are also being called on to improve and increase their role in injury prevention. Their "teachable moment" can reinforce and supplement the prehospital care provider's on-scene counseling if they know what has already been discussed or demonstrated.
2. Others in public health can use injury data provided by prehospital care providers retrospectively to help develop a comprehensive, community-wide injury prevention program.

Prehospital care providers usually do not practice documentation to help support a community-wide prevention program. Knowing what to acquire and when to document information beneficial to the development of community-wide prevention programs requires opening a dialogue with other members of the public health team. Leaders in the EMS system need to build a coalition with others in public health to develop documentation policies that promote complete documentation of injuries.

EMS can be the spearhead for workable, effective injury prevention programs that make a profound impact in a community. Programs have been created out of the desire of a small group of EMS professionals to prevent childhood fatalities.[19] Services in Louisiana, Florida, Washington state, Oregon, and Hawaii have been recognized for their efforts in designing, coordinating, and conducting injury prevention programs through the Nicholas Rosecrans Award for best practices in injury prevention in EMS.[20,21]

Injury Prevention for EMS Providers

"Who's the most important person at an incident scene?" EMT students are always asked this question early in their training to make them think about their own safety. Invariably, one or two students will say "the patient," which is what the instructor wanted to hear. This provides a teachable moment for the instructor to begin the course-long directive to reinforce the point that self-injury prevention is the most valuable service an EMT can provide.

Hostile environments resulting from terrorist activities or hazardous materials spills unfortunately make the news too often. However, the everyday activities of prehospital providers provide sufficient opportunity to end an EMT's career or life because of injury. The Bureau of Labor Statistics paints an accurate picture of the "normal" dangers in EMS:

EMTs and paramedics work both indoors and outdoors, in all types of weather. They are required to do considerable kneeling, bending, and heavy lifting. These workers risk noise-induced hearing loss from sirens and back injuries from lifting patients. In addition, EMTs and paramedics may be exposed to diseases such as hepatitis-B and AIDS, as well as violence from drug overdose victims or mentally unstable patients. The work is not only physically strenuous, but also stressful, involving life-or-death situations and suffering patients.[22]

Providers can become complacent to the everyday dangers of the job. *Complacency* is a feeling of security or safety in the unacknowledged face of potential danger. Compounding the situation is the idealism and invincibility of youth typical to some EMS personnel.[23] Management is needed to create a culture of injury prevention by instituting prevention policy, maintaining adherence to procedure, and rewarding positive performance. It is necessary that the providers themselves be equally committed to the principles of injury prevention. Failure of either management or providers can have potentially devastating effects.

In a prehospital service, employees are not only the most valuable asset but also the most expensive. The service, community, and most importantly the EMT benefit when the employee remains uninjured. An in-house injury prevention program is worthwhile on its own merits. When conducted through a public health approach, however, it provides valuable experience for involvement in community injury prevention initiatives as well. The community (e.g., the ambulance service) is small; there is 100% access to it; and surveillance is easier because the ambulance service has access to many of the data sources it may need. Identification of risk factors is simplified because the target audience consists of fellow employees. Gaining evaluation information should be almost immediate. Outcome data collection should be readily available as well.

Kinnane and colleagues[18] mention in-house prevention programs that utilize education, enforcement, and engineering implementation strategies. The wide variability of the programs demonstrates the dangers involved in EMS systems and the need for prevention initiatives. It also demonstrates the variability among EMS communities. Even though all EMS services are similar, individual services (communities) have different risk factors and different prevention priorities.

As described previously, education programs enhance wellness, prevent back injury, and increase awareness of the potential for violent patients. Enforcement programs introduced mandatory fitness programs and established protocols to deal with violent patients. Engineering initiatives addressed increasing seat belt use in the back of the ambulance by evaluating the position of equipment and location of the seat and reduced back injury through preemployment screening and physical strengthening.

A small-scale, in-house injury prevention program may reap rewards beyond the most important outcome of improved employee health. Small successes lay the groundwork for participation in larger, more complicated endeavors. They provide a valuable on-the-job learning tool about injury prevention for all employees. In addition, in-house prevention programs provide an introduction of the EMS service to other public health agencies in the community that assist in in-house program implementation and evaluation.

SUMMARY

Trauma is the most neglected current epidemic. Although EMS systems have progressed dramatically in the management of injuries since the 1966 publication of the NAS/NRC "white paper," the health care industry has failed to measurably decrease the incidence of injuries. More than 161,000 people die as a result of injuries each year in the United States alone despite the development of highly evolved EMS systems. EMS providers are in a unique position to influence injury morbidity and mortality rates through prevention. This position has been recognized, and the role of EMS personnel in illness and injury prevention is evolving.

It is necessary that EMS personnel integrate knowledge, skills, and tools used in public health into the practice of the EMS profession. This is an opportunity for EMS systems to have a significant effect on the health of all individuals. The advancement of EMS systems in injury prevention depends on the adoption of this new role by each individual prehospital care provider. Prehospital care providers need to have knowledge and skills in injury prevention, believe in its importance, commit to the effort, and serve as an advocate to their peers.

SCENARIO SOLUTION

After much soul searching, Steve and Marilyn decided not to quit the volunteer ambulance squad. They determined that they could do more than simply run ambulance calls. They approached the staff officers with an idea to create a safety committee so that another tragedy could be avoided. The leadership liked their ideas and appointed them co-chairs.

One year later, Marilyn and Steve had spearheaded the creation of a set of safety policies for the squad, worked with a local engineering firm to create lockdown devices for all the equipment previously loose in the patient compartment, and conducted the safety orientation for the latest group of "newbies" to be inducted. They discovered the wealth of injury prevention information available on the internet, in safety texts and journal articles geared specifically to EMS, and by talking to other ambulance services and community businesses with injury prevention programs in place. Next month, another member will attend her first meeting as the Lanier County Rescue Squad representative at the Safe Communities coalition of Lanier County. ■

References

1. National Academy of Sciences/National Research Council: *Accidental death and disability: the neglected disease of modern society,* Washington, DC, 1966, NAS/NRC.
2. National Center for Health Statistics: *Health, United States, 2000, with adolescent health chartbook,* Hyattsville, Md, 2000, NCHS.
3. National Center for Health Statistics: *Fastats A to Z,* http://www.cdc.gov/nchs/fastats/injury.htm (accessed April 2006).
4. Peden M, McGee K, Sharma G: *The injury chart book: a graphical overview of the global burden of injuries,* Geneva, 2002, World Health Organization.
5. National Highway Traffic Safety Administration, US Department of Health and Human Services, Health Resources and Services Administration, Maternal and Child Health Bureau: *Emergency medical services agenda for the future,* Washington, DC, 1999, NHTSA.
6. National Center for Injury Prevention and Control: *Fact book for the year 2000: working to prevent and control injury in the United States,* 2000, http://www.cdc.gov/ncipc/pub-res/FactBook/default.htm (accessed May 2001).
7. National Committee for Injury Prevention and Control: *Injury prevention: meeting the challenge,* New York, Oxford University Press, *Am J Prev Med* 5(suppl):4, 1989.
8. Christoffel T, Gallagher SS: *Injury prevention and public health: practical knowledge, skills, and strategies,* Gaithersburg, Md, 1999, Aspen.
9. Maguire BJ, Huntington KL, Smith GS, Levick NR: Occupational fatalities in emergency medical services: a hidden crisis, *Ann Emerg Med* 40:6, 2002.
10. Tortella BJ, Lavery RF: Disabling job injuries among EMS providers, *Prehosp Disaster Med* 9, 1994.
11. Garrison HG: Keeping rescuers safe, *Ann Emerg Med* 40:6, 2002.
12. Martinez R: Injury control: a primer for physicians, *Ann Emerg Med* 19:1, 1990.
13. Waller JA: *Injury control: a guide to the causes and prevention of trauma,* Lexington, Mass, 1985, Lexington Books.
14. PIER: Public Information, Education, and Relations for EMS injury prevention modules, DOT HS 809 520, Washington, DC, 2002, US Department of Transportation, National Highway Traffic Safety Administration.
15. Kellerman AL, Hutson HR: Injury control. In Schwartz GR: *Principles and practice of emergency medicine,* Philadelphia, 1992, Lea & Febiger.
16. Kellerman AL, Todd KH: Injury control. In Tintinelli JE, Kelen GD, Stapczynski JS, editors: *Emergency medicine: a comprehensive study guide,* New York, 1999, McGraw-Hill.
17. Todd KH: *Accident's aren't: proposal for evaluation of an injury prevention curriculum for EMS providers: a grant proposal to the National Association of State EMS Directors,* Atlanta, 1998, Department of Emergency Medicine, Emory University School of Medicine.
18. Kinnane JM, Garrison HG, Coben JH, Alonzo-Serra HM: Injury prevention: is there a role for out-of-hospital emergency medical services? *Acad Emerg Med* 4:306, 1997.
19. EPIC Medics: http://www.epicmedics.ord (accessed July 2004).
20. Griffiths K: Best practices in injury prevention, *J Emerg Med Serv* 27:8, 2002.
21. Krimston J, Griffiths K: Best practices in injury prevention, *J Emerg Med Serv* 28:9, 2003.
22. Emergency Medical Technicians and Paramedics. In *Occupational Outlook Handbook, 2004-2005 Edition,* US Department of Labor, Bureau of Labor Statistics, http://stats.bls.gov/oco/ocos101.htm (accessed July 2004).
23. Federal Emergency Management Agency, US Fire Administration: EMS safety: techniques and applications, International Association of Fire Fighters, FEMA contract EMW-91-C-3592.

Suggested Reading

American College of Surgeons Committee on Trauma: *Advanced trauma life support for doctors, student course manual,* ed 7, Chicago, 2004, ACS.

Chapter Objectives

At the completion of this chapter, the reader will be able to do the following:

✓ Define energy in the context of production of injury.

✓ Describe the association between the laws of motion energy and the kinematics of trauma.

✓ Describe the relationship of injury and energy exchange to speed.

✓ Discuss energy exchange and the production of cavitation.

✓ Given the description of a motor vehicle crash, use kinematics to predict the likely injury pattern for an unrestrained occupant.

✓ Associate the principles of energy exchange with the pathophysiology of the head, spine, thorax, abdomen, and extremities resulting from that exchange.

✓ Describe the specific injuries and their causes as related to interior and exterior vehicle damage.

✓ Describe the function of restraint systems for vehicle occupants.

✓ Relate the laws of motion and energy to mechanisms other than motor vehicle crashes (e.g., blasts, falls).

✓ Describe the five phases of blasts and the injuries produced in each phase.

✓ Describe the differences in the production of injury with low-, medium-, and high-energy weapons.

✓ Discuss the relationship of the frontal surface of an impacting object to energy exchange and injury production.

✓ Integrate principles of the kinematics of trauma into patient assessment.

CHAPTER 3

Kinematics of Trauma

SCENARIO

At 1750 on a rainy cool Sunday, you are dispatched to a crash scene at the intersection of a busy noninterstate highway. Dispatch tells you and your partner that two cars are involved with an unknown number of patients and that law enforcement is en route.

On arrival at the scene, you note that one vehicle has frontal damage and the second has lateral damage. Air bags are deployed on both vehicles. The first car has moderate front-end damage, steam coming from under the hood, and the fenders pushed back on the tires. The unbelted occupant is still in the car. The second car has about 18 inches (45 cm) of intrusion into the passenger compartment on the driver's side. The driver is still in the vehicle, slumped over the steering wheel.

Based on this information, what injuries would you expect with the two drivers? As the senior emergency medical technician–paramedic (EMT-P) on the scene, which patient will you access, and which will you send to your partner, who finished EMT-P school only 3 months ago? ◼

Unexpected traumatic injuries are responsible for more than 161,000 deaths in the United States each year. Vehicle collisions accounted for 44,000 deaths and more than 3 million injured persons in 2002. This problem is not limited to the United States; other countries have an equal frequency of vehicular trauma, although the vehicles may be different. Penetrating trauma from guns is very high in the United States. Blast injuries are a growing cause of injuries in many countries because of terrorism. Successful management of trauma patients depends on identification of injuries or potential injuries and good assessment skills.

When the provider, at any level of care, does not understand the principles of kinematics or the mechanisms involved, injuries may be missed. An understanding of these principles will increase the level of suspicion based on the pattern of injuries likely associated with the survey of the scene on arrival. The appropriate information and the suspected injuries can be transmitted to the physicians and nurses in the emergency department (ED). At the scene and en route, these suspected injuries can be managed to provide the most appropriate patient care, and "do no further harm."

Injuries that are not obvious but still severe can be fatal because they are not managed at the scene and en route to the trauma center or appropriate hospital. Knowing where to look and how to assess for injuries is as important as knowing what to do after finding injuries. A complete, accurate history of a traumatic incident and proper interpretation of this information can provide such information. Most of a patient's injuries can be predicted by a proper survey of the scene, before examining the patient.

This chapter discusses the general principles and mechanical principles involved in the kinematics of trauma; sections on the regional effects of blunt and penetrating trauma address local injury pathophysiology. The general principles are the physics laws that govern energy exchange and the general effects of the energy exchange. Mechanical principles address the interaction with the human body and the components of the crash for blunt trauma (e.g., motor vehicles, three- and two-wheeled vehicles, falls), penetrating trauma, and blasts. A crash is the energy exchange that occurs when an energy force, usually a solid object, impacts the human body. It is not only the collision of a motor vehicle, but also the crash of a falling body into the pavement, the impact of a bullet on the internal tissues of the body, and the overpressure and debris of a blast. All these involve energy exchange. All involve injury. All involve potentially life-threatening conditions. All require the correct management by the knowledgeable and insightful prehospital care provider.

General Principles

The conditions of assessment and management of the injured patient are divided into three phases: precrash, crash, and postcrash. Again, the term *crash* does not necessarily mean a vehicular crash. The crash of a vehicle into a pedestrian, a missile (bullet) into the abdomen, and a construction worker striking the asphalt after a fall are all crashes. In each case, energy is exchanged between a moving object and the tissue of the human body or between the moving human body and a stationary object.

The *precrash phase* includes all the events that precede the incident, such as the ingestion of alcohol or drugs. Conditions that are present before the incident, but important in the management of the patient's injuries, are assessed as part of the precrash history, such as a patient's acute or preexisting medical conditions (and medications to treat those conditions), ingestion of recreational substances (illegal and prescription drugs, alcohol), and a patient's state of mind. Typically, young trauma patients do not have chronic illnesses. With older patients, however, medical conditions that are present before the trauma event can cause serious complications in the prehospital assessment and management of the patient and can significantly influence the outcome. For example, the elderly driver of a vehicle that has struck a utility pole may have chest pain indicative of a myocardial infarction (heart attack). Did the driver hit the utility pole and have a heart attack, or did he have a heart attack and then strike the utility pole? Does the patient take medication (e.g., beta blocker) that will prevent elevation of the pulse in shock? Most of these conditions directly influence the assessment and management strategies discussed in Chapters 4 and 5 but are important in overall patient care as well, even if they do not necessarily influence the kinematics of the crash.

The *crash phase* begins at the time of impact between one moving object and a second object. The second object can be moving or stationary and can be either an object or a person. Three impacts occur in most vehicular crashes: (1) the impact of the two objects, (2) the impact of the occupants into the vehicle, and (3) the impact of the vital organs inside the occupants. For example, when a vehicle strikes a tree, the first impact is the collision of the vehicle into the tree. The second impact is the occupant of the vehicle striking the steering wheel or windshield. If the patient is restrained, an impact occurs between the occupant and the seat belt. The third impact is between the patient's internal organs and his or her chest wall or abdominal wall.

In a fall, only the second and third impacts are involved.

The direction in which the energy exchange occurs, the amount of energy that is exchanged, and the effect that these forces have on the patient are all important considerations as assessment begins.

During the *postcrash phase* the information gathered about the crash and precrash phases is used to manage a patient. This phase begins as soon as the energy from the crash is absorbed. The onset of the complications of life-threatening trauma can be slow or fast (or these complications can be prevented or significantly reduced), depending in part on the care provided at the scene and en route to the hospital. In the postcrash phase the understanding of the kinematics of trauma, the index of suspicion regarding injuries, and strong assessment skills all become crucial to the patient outcome.

To understand the effects of the forces that produce bodily injury, the prehospital care provider needs first to understand two components—energy and anatomy.

Energy

The first step in obtaining a history is to evaluate the events that occurred at the time of the crash (Figure 3-1). For example, in a motor vehicle crash (MVC), what does the

FIGURE 3-1 Evaluating the scene of an incident is critical. Such information as direction of impact, passenger compartment intrusion, and amount of energy exchange provides insight into the possible injuries of the occupants. This photograph was in the first edition of this text and, although an older-model vehicle, continues to show the concept of mechanism of injury.

scene look like? Who hit what and at what speed? How long was the stopping time? Were the victims restrained by seat belts? Did the air bag deploy? Were the children restrained properly in seats, or were they unrestrained and thrown about the vehicle? Were occupants thrown from the vehicle? Did they strike objects? If so, how many objects? These and many other questions must be answered if the prehospital care provider is to understand the exchange of forces that took place and translate this information into a prediction of injuries and appropriate patient care.

The process of surveying the scene to determine what injuries might have resulted from the forces and motion involved is called *kinematics.* Because kinematics is based on fundamental principles of physics, an understanding of the pertinent laws of physics is necessary.

Laws of Energy and Motion

Newton's first law of motion states that a body at rest will remain at rest and a body in motion will remain in motion unless acted on by an outside force. The motorcycle in Figure 3-2 was stationary until the energy from the engine moved it along the dirt track. Once in motion, although it leaves the ground, the motorcycle remains in motion until it hits something or returns to the ground and the brakes are applied. The same is true of the person sitting in the front seat of a vehicle. Even if the vehicle hits a tree and stops, the unrestrained person continues in motion and at the same rate of speed until he or she hits the steering column, dashboard, and windshield. The impact with these objects stops the forward motion of the torso or head. The internal organs of the person remain in motion until they hit the chest wall or abdominal wall, halting the forward motion.

Why does the sudden starting or stopping of motion result in trauma and injury to an individual? The *law of*

FIGURE 3-2 A motorcycle going over a jump does not suddenly stop when it loses contact with the ground. The momentum of the motorcycle and the previously existing energy carry the motorcycle and rider forward unless something obstructs the motion.

conservation of energy states that energy cannot be created or destroyed but can be changed in form. The motion of the vehicle is a form of energy. To start the vehicle, the engine explodes the energy in gasoline, which moves the pistons. Motion of the pistons is transferred by set of gears to the wheels, which grasp the road as they turn and impart motion to the vehicle. To stop the vehicle, the energy of its motion must be changed to another form, such as heating up the brakes or crashing into an object and bending the frame. When a driver brakes, the energy of motion is converted into the heat of friction (thermal energy) by the brake pads on the brake drums and by the tires on the roadway. The vehicle decelerates. Similarly, the mechanical energy of a vehicle crashing into a wall is dissipated by the bending of the frame or other parts of the vehicle. The energy remaining is transferred to the occupants and their internal organs.

Kinetic energy is a function of an object's weight and speed. A victim's weight and mass are the same thing. Likewise, speed and velocity are the same. The relationship between weight and speed as it affects kinetic energy is as follows:

Kinetic energy = One-half the mass times the velocity squared

$$KE = \tfrac{1}{2}mv^2$$

Thus the kinetic energy involved when a 150-lb (68-kg) person travels at 30 mph (48 km/hr) is calculated as follows:

$$KE = \frac{150}{2} \times 30^2$$

KE = 67,500 units

For the purpose of this discussion, no specific physical unit of measure (e.g., foot-pounds, joules) is used. The units are used merely to illustrate how this formula affects the change in energy. As just shown, a 150-lb (68-kg) person traveling at 30 mph (48 km/hr) would have 67,500 units

of energy converted to another form when he or she stops. This change takes the form of damage to the vehicle and injury to the person in it, unless the energy dissipation can take some less harmful form, such as on a seat belt or into an air bag.

Which factor, however, has the greatest effect on the amount of kinetic energy produced: mass or velocity? Consider a 160-lb (72-kg) person traveling at 30 mph (48 km/hr):

$$KE = \frac{160}{2} \times 30^2$$

KE = 72,000 units

Returning to the previous example of a 150-lb (68-kg) person and increasing the speed by 10 mph (16 km/hr), the kinetic energy is as follows:

$$KE = \frac{150}{2} \times 40^2$$

KE = 120,000 units

These calculations demonstrate that increasing the velocity (speed) increases the rate of production of kinetic energy much more than increasing the mass. Much more energy exchange will occur (and therefore produce injury to either the occupant or the vehicle or both) in a high-speed crash than in a crash at a slower speed.

Although the velocity is exponential and the mass is linear, this can be critical when there is a great mass disparity between two objects. In a collision between a small car and a semitrailer truck or between a car and a pedestrian, the advantage goes to the vehicle with the most momentum (force).

Mass × acceleration = force = mass × deceleration

Another important factor in a crash is the *stopping distance.* A vehicle that stops against a brick wall or when

FIGURE 3-3 The energy exchange from a moving vehicle to a pedestrian crushes tissue and imparts speed and energy to the pedestrian to knock the victim away from the point of impact. Injury to the patient can occur at the point of impact as the pedestrian is hit by the vehicle and as the pedestrian is thrown to the ground or into another vehicle.

the brakes are applied dissipates the same amount of energy, just in a different manner and over a different distance. In the first instance, the energy is absorbed by the bending of the frame of the vehicle. In the latter case, the energy is absorbed by the heat of the brakes. The forward motion of the occupant of the vehicle (energy) is absorbed in the first instance by damage to the soft tissue and bones of the occupant. In the latter case, the energy is dissipated along with the energy of the vehicle into the brakes.

This inverse relationship between stopping distance and injury also applies to falls. A person has a better chance of surviving a fall if he or she lands on a compressible surface, such as deep powder snow. The same fall terminating on a hard surface, such as concrete, can produce more severe injuries. The compressible material (i.e., the snow) increases the stopping distance and absorbs at least some of the energy rather than allowing all the energy to be absorbed by the body. The result is decreased injury and damage to the body. This principle also applies to other types of crashes. In addition, an unrestrained driver will be more severely injured than a restrained driver. The restraint system, rather than the body, will absorb a significant portion of the damage energy.

Therefore, once an object is in motion and has a specific energy of motion, to come to a complete rest, the object must lose all its energy by converting the energy to another form or transferring it to another object. For example, if a vehicle strikes a pedestrian, the pedestrian is knocked away from it (Figure 3-3). Although the vehicle is somewhat slowed by the impact, the greater force of the vehicle imparts much

more acceleration to the lighter-weight pedestrian than it loses in speed.

$$\text{Mass} \times \text{deceleration} = \text{force} = \text{mass} \times \text{acceleration}$$

The energy in terms of acceleration imparted to the pedestrian is much more than the vehicle is slowed. The softer body parts of the pedestrian versus the harder body parts of the vehicle also means more damage to the pedestrian than to the vehicle.

Energy Exchange between a Solid Object and the Human Body

As the human body collides with a solid object, or vice versa, the number of body tissue particles that are impacted by the solid object determines the amount of energy exchange that takes place and therefore the amount of damage (injury) that occurs to the patient. The number of tissue particles affected is determined by (1) the density (particles per volume) of the tissue and (2) the size of the contact area of the impact.

Density

The more dense a tissue (measured in particles per volume), the greater is the number of particles that will be hit by a moving object. Driving a fist into a feather pillow and driving a fist at the same speed into a brick wall will produce different effects on the hand. The fist absorbs more energy colliding with the dense brick wall than with the less dense feather pillow.

Simplistically, the body has three different types of tissue densities: *air density* (much of the lung and some portions of the intestine), *water density* (muscle and most solid organs, e.g., liver, spleen), and *solid density* (bone). Therefore, amount of energy exchange (with resultant injury) will depend on which type of organ is impacted.

Contact Area

Wind exerts pressure on a hand when it is extended out of the window of a moving vehicle. When the palm of the hand is horizontal and parallel to the direction of the flow through the wind, some backward pressure is exerted on the front of the hand (fingers) as the particles of air strike the hand. Rotating the hand 90 degrees to a vertical position places a larger surface area into the wind; thus more air particles make contact with the hand, increasing the amount of force on it. The surface area can be modified by the size of the object, its motion within the body, and fragmentation. Examples of this variation on the human body could include the front of an automobile, a baseball bat, and a bullet. The automobile's front surface would contact a large portion of the victim. A baseball bat would contact a smaller area and a bullet a very small area. The amount of energy exchange that would produce damage to the patient depends then on the energy of the object and the density of the tissue in the pathway of the energy exchange.

Cavitation

The basic mechanics of energy exchange are relatively simple. The impact of the object on the tissue particles accelerates the tissue particles away from the point of impact. These tissues then become moving objects themselves and crash into other tissue particles, producing a "falling domino" effect. A common game that provides a visual effect of cavitation is pool.

The cue ball is driven down the length of a pool table by the force of the muscles in the arm. The cue ball crashes into the racked balls at the other end of the table. The energy from the arm into the cue ball is transferred onto each of the racked balls (Figure 3-4). The cue ball gives up its energy and slows or even stops. The other balls take on this energy as motion and move away from the impact point. The same kind of energy exchange occurs when a bowling ball rolls down the alley, hitting the set of pins at the other end. The pool balls and bowling pins are knocked out of their positions.

Similarly, when a solid object strikes the human body or when the human body is in motion and strikes a stationary object, the tissue particles of the human body are knocked out of their normal position, creating a hole or cavity. Thus this process is called *cavitation*.

Two types of cavities are created. A temporary cavity forms at the time of impact; some or all of the cavity returns to its previous position. The amount returning depends on the crush of the tissue particles at the site of the impact and the elasticity of the tissue. This cavity may not be visible when the prehospital or hospital provider examines the patient later. The temporary cavity causes stretching of the tissues. A permanent cavity also forms at the time of impact and is caused by compression or tearing of tissue. It is also caused partly by stretch, but because it does not necessarily rebound to its original shape, it can be seen later (Figure 3-5).

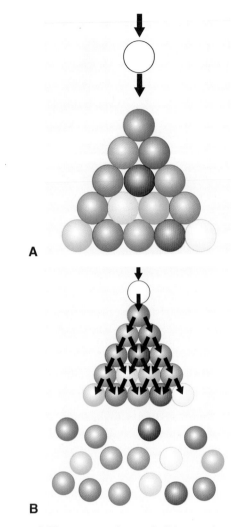

FIGURE 3-4 **A,** The energy of a cue ball is transferred to each of the other balls. **B,** The energy exchange pushes the balls apart, or creates a cavity.

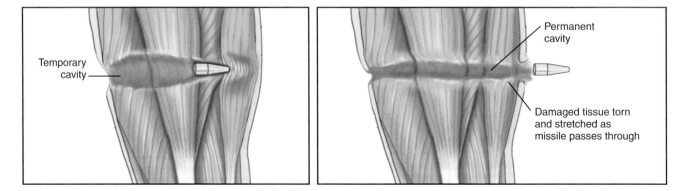

FIGURE 3-5 Damage to tissue is greater than the permanent cavity that remains from a missile injury. The faster or heavier the missile, the larger the temporary cavity and the greater the zone of tissue damage.

The amount of temporary cavity that remains as a permanent cavity is related to the elasticity of the tissue involved. For example, forcefully swinging a baseball bat into a steel drum leaves a dent, or cavity, in its side. Swinging the same baseball bat with the same force into a similarly sized and shaped mass of foam rubber will leave no dent once the bat is removed (Figure 3-6). The difference is *elasticity;* the foam rubber is more elastic than the steel drum. The human body is more like the foam rubber than the steel drum. If a person punches a fist into another person's abdomen, he or she would feel it go in. However, when the person pulls the fist away, a dent is not left. Similarly, a baseball bat swung

FIGURE 3-6 A, Swinging a baseball bat into a steel drum leaves a dent, or cavity, in its side. **B,** Swinging a baseball bat into a piece of foam leaves no visible cavity.

into the chest will leave no obvious cavity in the thoracic wall, but it would cause damage, both from direct contact and the cavity created by the energy exchange. The history of the incident and its interpretation will provide the information needed to determine the potential size of the cavity at the time of impact and accurately predict injuries.

When the trigger of a loaded gun is pulled, the firing pin strikes the cap and produces an explosion in the cartridge. The energy created by this explosion is exchanged onto the bullet, which speeds from the muzzle of the weapon. The bullet now has energy, or force (acceleration × mass = force).

Once such force is imparted, the bullet cannot slow down until acted on by an outside force (Newton's first law of motion). In order for the bullet to stop inside the human body, an explosion equivalent to the explosion in the weapon must occur within the tissues (acceleration × mass = force = mass × deceleration) (Figure 3-7). This explosion is the result of energy exchange accelerating the tissue particles out of their normal position, creating a cavity.

Blunt and Penetrating Trauma

Trauma is generally classified as either blunt or penetrating. However, the energy exchange and the injury produced are similar in both types of trauma. The only real difference is penetration of the skin. If an object's entire energy is concentrated on one small area of skin, the skin likely will tear, and the object will enter the body and create a more concentrated energy exchange. This can result in greater destructive power to one area. A larger object whose energy is dispersed over a much larger area of skin may not penetrate the skin. The damage will be distributed over a larger area of the body, and the injury pattern will be less localized.

Energy exchange is directly related to the density and size of the frontal area at the point of contact between the object and the victim's body. In blunt trauma, injuries are produced as the tissues are compressed, decelerated, or accelerated. In penetrating trauma, injuries are produced as the tissues are crushed and separated along the path of the penetrating object. Both types create a cavity, forcing the tissues out of their normal position.

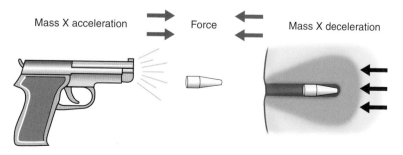

FIGURE 3-7 As a bullet travels through tissue, its kinetic energy is transferred to the tissue that it comes in contact with, accelerating it away from the bullet.

Blunt trauma creates both shear tears and cavitation. The cavitation is frequently only a temporary cavity and is directed away from the point of impact. Penetrating trauma creates both a permanent and a temporary cavity. The energy of a rapidly moving object with a small frontal surface area will be concentrated in one area and may exceed the tensile strength of the tissue and penetrate it. The temporary cavity that is created will spread away from the pathway of this missile in both frontal and lateral directions.

Mechanical Principles

Blunt Trauma

The observations in a crash during blunt trauma that provide clues as to the patterns of injury, the severity of these injuries, and the potential organs involved are (1) direction of the impact, (2) external damage to the vehicle (type and severity), and (3) internal damage (e.g., occupant compartment intrusion, steering wheel/column bending, windshield bull's-eye fractures, mirror damage, dashboard knee impacts).

In blunt trauma, two forces are involved in the impact: shear and compression. *Shear* is the result of one organ or structure (or part of an organ or structure) changing speed faster than another organ or structure (or part of an organ or structure). *Compression* is the result of an organ or structure (or part of an organ or structure) being directly squeezed between other organs or structures. Injury can result from any type of impact, such as MVCs (vehicle or motorcycle), pedestrian collisions with vehicles, falls, sports injuries, or blast injuries. All these mechanisms are discussed separately, followed by the results of this energy exchange on the specific anatomy in each of the body regions.

Motor Vehicle Crashes

Many forms of blunt trauma occur, but MVCs (including motorcycle crashes) are the most common. In 1999, 86% of fatalities were vehicle occupants. The remaining 14% were pedestrians, cyclists, and other nonoccupants, as reported by the National Highway Traffic Safety Administration (NHTSA). MVCs can be divided into the following five types:

1. Frontal impact
2. Rear impact
3. Lateral impact
4. Rotational impact
5. Rollover

Although each pattern has variations, accurate identification of the five patterns will provide insight into other, similar types of crashes.

FIGURE 3-8   As a vehicle impacts a utility pole, the front of the car stops but the rear portion of the vehicle continues traveling forward, causing deformation of the vehicle.

In MVCs and other rapid-deceleration mechanisms, such as snowmobile, motorcycle, and boating crashes and falls from heights, three collisions occur: (1) the vehicle collides with an object or with another vehicle, (2) the unrestrained occupant collides with the inside of the vehicle, and (3) the occupant's internal organs collide with one another or with the wall of the cavity that contains them.

An example is a vehicle hitting a tree. The first collision occurs when the vehicle strikes the tree. Although the vehicle stops, the unrestrained driver keeps moving forward (consistent with Newton's first law of motion). The second collision occurs when the driver hits the steering wheel and windshield. Although the driver stops moving forward, many internal organs keep moving (Newton's first law again) until they strike another organ or cavity wall or are suddenly stopped by a ligament, fascia, vessel, or muscle. This is the third collision.

One easy way to estimate the injury pattern to the occupant is to look at the vehicle and determine which of the five types of collisions occurred. The occupant receives the same type of force as the vehicle and from the same direction. The amount is reduced by absorption of energy onto the vehicle. The energy exchange will be similar and will take place in a similar direction. In Figure 3-8, for example, the vehicle has hit a utility pole in the center of the car. The impact point stopped its forward motion, but the rest of the car continued forward until the energy was absorbed by the bending of the car. The same type of injury occurs to the driver if the steering column impacts the center of the sternum. The car continued in forward motion, significantly deforming it; the driver's chest does the same.

In Figure 3-9 the front of the car stopped against a dirt embankment, but the rear did not stop until the energy was absorbed by the bending of the frame. This pattern is similar to that occurring to the chest. As the sternum stops forward motion against the dash, the posterior thoracic wall

FIGURE 3-9   Vehicle stops suddenly against a dirt embankment.

FIGURE 3-10   Configuration of the seat and position of the occupant can direct the initial force on the upper torso, with the head as the lead point.

continues until the energy is absorbed by the bending and possible fracture of the ribs.

Frontal Impact.   In a frontal impact (or "head-on" collision) involving a motor vehicle, such as a vehicle hitting a brick wall, the first collision occurs when the vehicle hits the wall, resulting in damage to the front of the vehicle. The amount of damage to the vehicle indicates the approximate speed of the vehicle at the time of impact. The greater the intrusion into the body of the vehicle, the greater is the speed at the time of impact. The greater the vehicle speed, the greater the energy exchange and the more likely the occupants are to be injured.

Although the vehicle suddenly ceases to move forward in a frontal impact, the occupant continues to move and will follow one of two possible paths: either up-and-over or down-and-under. The use of a seat belt and the deployment of an airbag will absorb some or most of the energy, thus reducing the injury to the victim.

Up-and-Over Path.   In this sequence the body's forward motion carries it up and over the steering wheel (Figure 3-10). The head is usually the lead body portion striking the windshield or windshield frame or roof. The head stops its forward motion. The torso continues in motion until its energy/force is absorbed along the spine. The cervical spine is the least protected segment of the spine. The chest or abdomen then collides with the steering column, depending on the position of the torso. Impact of the chest into the steering column produces thoracic cage, cardiac, lung, and aortic injuries (see Regional Effects of Blunt Trauma). Impact of the abdomen into the steering column can compress and crush the solid organs, produce overpressure injuries, especially to the diaphragm, and rupture of the hollow organs. The kidneys, spleen, and liver are also subject to shear injury as the abdomen strikes the steering wheel

and abruptly stops. An organ may be torn from its normal anatomic restraints and supporting tissues. For example, the continued forward motion of the kidneys after the vertebral column has stopped moving produces shear along the attachment of the organs at their blood supply. These great vessels adhere tightly to the posterior abdominal wall and vertebral column. The continued forward motion of the kidneys can stretch the renal vessels to the point of rupture. A similar action may tear the aorta as the unattached arch becomes the tightly adhered descending aorta.

Down-and-Under Path.   In a down-and-under path the occupant moves downward and out of the seat forward into the dashboard (Figure 3-11). The importance of understanding kinematics is illustrated by injuries produced to the lower extremity in this pathway. Many of the injuries are difficult to identify if not suspected because of the mechanism.

The foot, if planted on the floor panel or on the brake pedal with a straight knee, can twist as the continued torso motion angulates and fractures the ankle joint. More often, however, the knees are already bent, and the force is not directed to the ankle. Therefore the knees strike the dashboard.

The knee has two possible impact points against the dashboard, the tibia and the femur (Figure 3-12). If the tibia hits the dashboard and stops first, the femur remains in motion and overrides it. A dislocated knee, with torn ligaments, tendons, and other supporting structures, can result. Because the popliteal artery lies close to the knee joint, dislocation of the joint is frequently associated with injury to the vessel. The artery can be completely disrupted

FIGURE 3-11   The occupant and the vehicle travel forward together. The vehicle stops, and the unrestrained occupant continues forward until something stops that motion.

FIGURE 3-12   The knee has two possible impact points in a motor vehicle crash: the femur and the tibia.

or the lining alone (intima) may be damaged (Figure 3-13). In either case, a blood clot may form in the injured vessel, resulting in significantly decreased blood flow to the leg tissues below the knee. Early recognition of the potential of vascular injury will alert the physicians to the need for assessment of the vessel in this area.

Early identification and treatment of such a popliteal artery injury significantly decreases the complications of distal limb ischemia. Perfusion to this tissue needs to be reestablished within about 6 hours. Delays could occur because the prehospital care provider failed to consider the kinematics of the injury or overlooked important clues during assessment of the patient.

Although most of these patients have evidence of injury to the knee, an imprint on the dashboard where the knee impacted is a key indicator that significant energy was focused on this joint and adjacent structures (Figure 3-14).

When the femur is the point of impact, the energy is absorbed on the bone shaft, which can then break (Figure 3-15). The continued forward motion of the pelvis onto the femur that remains intact can override the femoral head, resulting in a posterior dislocation of the acetabular joint (Figure 3-16).

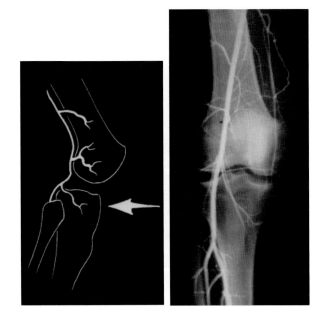

FIGURE 3-13   The popliteal artery lies close to the joint, tightly tied to the femur above and tibia below. Separation of these two bones stretches, kinks, and tears the artery.

FIGURE 3-14   The impact point of the knee on the dashboard indicates both a down-and-under pathway and a significant absorption of energy along the lower extremity.

After the knees and legs stop forward motion, the upper body will rotate forward into the steering column or dashboard. The victim may then sustain many of the same injuries described previously for the up-and-over pathway.

Recognizing these potential injuries and relaying the information to the ED physicians can result in long-term benefits to the patient.

Rear Impact.   Rear-impact collisions occur when a slower-moving vehicle or stationary object is struck from behind by a vehicle moving at a faster rate of speed. For ease of understanding, the more rapidly moving vehicle is called

FIGURE 3-15 When the femur is the point of impact, the energy is absorbed on the bone shaft, which can then break.

FIGURE 3-16 The continued forward motion of the pelvis onto the femur can override the femur's head, resulting in a posterior dislocation of the acetabular joint.

FIGURE 3-17 A rear-impact collision forces the torso forward. If the headrest is improperly positioned, the head is hyperextended over the top of the headrest.

FIGURE 3-18 If the headrest is up, the head moves with the torso, and neck injury is prevented.

> If it can be proved that the victim's headrest was not properly positioned when the neck injury occurred, some courts consider reducing the liability of the party at fault in the crash on the grounds that the victim's negligence contributed to the injuries *(contributory negligence)*. Similar measures have been considered in cases of failure to use occupant restraints.

the "bullet vehicle," and the slower or stopped object is called the "target vehicle." In such collisions the energy of the bullet vehicle at impact is converted to damage to both vehicles and acceleration of the target vehicle. The greater the difference in the momentum of the two vehicles, the greater the force of the initial impact and the more energy is available to create damage and acceleration.

With rear impact the target vehicle in front is accelerated forward. Everything that is attached to the frame will also move forward and at the same rate of speed. The unattached objects in the vehicle, including the occupants, will begin forward motion only after something in contact with the frame begins to transmit the energy of the frame motion to these objects or occupants. As an example, the torso is accelerated by the seat after some of the energy has been

absorbed by the springs in the seats. If the headrest is positioned behind and below the occiput of the head, the head will begin forward motion after the torso as it comes into contact with the headrest. This may result in hyperextension of the neck. Shear and stretching of the ligaments and other support structures, especially in the anterior part of the neck, can result in injury (Figure 3-17). If the headrest is properly positioned, the head moves at approximately the same time as the torso with hyperextension (Figure 3-18).

If the vehicle is allowed to move forward without interference until it slows to a stop, the occupant will probably not be injured because most of the body's motion is supported by the seat, similar to the astronaut launching into orbit. However, if the vehicle strikes another vehicle or object or if the driver slams on the brakes and stops suddenly, the occupants will continue forward, following the characteristic pattern of a frontal-impact collision. The collision then involves two impacts, rear and frontal. The double impact increases the likelihood of injury.

Lateral Impact. Lateral-impact mechanisms come into play when the vehicle is involved in an intersection ("T-bone") collision or when the vehicle veers off the road and impacts a utility pole, tree, or other obstacle on the roadside. If the collision is at an intersection, the target vehicle is accelerated from the impact in the direction away from the force created by the bullet vehicle. The side of the vehicle or the door is thrust against the side of the occupant. The occupants may then be injured as they are accelerated laterally (Figure 3-19) or as the passenger compartment is bent inward by the door's projection (Figure 3-20). Injury caused by the vehicle's

movement is less severe if the occupant is restrained and moves with the initial motion of the vehicle.

Four body regions can sustain injury in a lateral impact, as follows:

1. *Chest.* Compression of the thoracic wall inward can result in fractured ribs, pulmonary contusion, or compression injury to solid organs inside the rib cage but below the diaphragm, as well as overpressure injuries (e.g., pneumothorax) (Figure 3-21). Shear injuries to the aorta can result from the lateral acceleration (25% of aortic shear injuries occur in lateral-impact collisions). The clavicle can be compressed and fractured if the force is against the shoulder (Figure 3-22).
2. *Abdomen and pelvis.* The intrusion compresses and fractures the pelvis and pushes the head of the femur

FIGURE 3-19 Lateral impact of the vehicle pushes the entire vehicle into the unrestrained passenger. A restrained passenger moves laterally with the vehicle.

FIGURE 3-21 Compression against the lateral chest and abdominal wall can fracture ribs and injure the underlying spleen, liver, and kidney.

FIGURE 3-20 Intrusion of the side panels into the passenger compartment provides another source of injury.

FIGURE 3-22 Compression of the shoulder against the clavicle produces midshaft fractures of this bone.

through the acetabulum (Figure 3-23). Occupants on the driver's side are vulnerable to splenic injuries because the spleen is on the left side of the body, whereas those on the passenger side are more likely to receive an injury to the liver.

3. *Neck.* The torso can move out from under the head in lateral collisions as well as in rear impacts. The attachment point of the head is posterior and inferior to the center of gravity of the head. Therefore the motion of the head in relationship to the neck is lateral flexion and rotation. This can fracture the vertebrae or more likely produce jumped facets and possible dislocation (Figure 3-24).
4. *Head.* The head can impact the frame of the door.

Near-side impacts produce more injuries than far-side impacts.

FIGURE 3-23 Lateral impact on the femur pushes the head through the acetabulum or fractures the pelvis.

Rotational Impact. Rotational-impact collisions occur when one corner of a vehicle strikes an immovable object, the corner of another vehicle, or a vehicle moving slower or in the opposite direction of the first vehicle. Following Newton's first law of motion, this corner of the vehicle will stop while the rest of the vehicle continues its forward motion until all its energy is completely transformed.

Rotational-impact collisions result in injuries that are a combination of those seen in frontal impacts and lateral collisions. The victim continues to move forward and then is hit by the side of the vehicle (as in a lateral collision) as the vehicle rotates around the point of impact. *More severe injuries are seen in the victim closest to the point of impact.*

Rollover. During a rollover, a vehicle may undergo several impacts at many different angles, as may the unrestrained occupant's body and internal organs (Figure 3-25). Injury and damage can occur with each of these impacts. In rollover collisions a restrained patient often sustains shearing-type injuries because of the significant forces created by a rolling vehicle. The forces are similar to the forces of a spinning carnival ride. Although the occupants are held securely by restraints, the internal organs still move and can tear at the connecting tissue areas. More serious injuries result from being unrestrained. In most cases the occupants are ejected from the vehicle as it rolls and are either crushed as the vehicle rolls over them or sustain injuries from the impact with the ground. If the occupants are ejected onto the roadway, they can be struck by oncoming traffic.

Vehicle Incompatibility. The type of vehicles involved in the crash plays a significant role in the potential for injury and death to the occupants. For example, in a lateral impact between two cars that lack air bags, the occupants of the car struck on its lateral aspect are 5.6 times more likely to die than the occupants in the vehicle striking that car. This

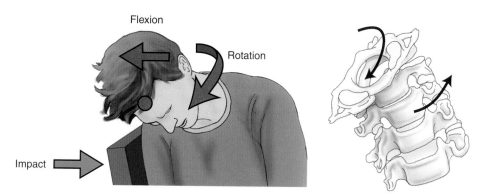

FIGURE 3-24 The center of gravity of the skull is anterior and superior to its pivot point between the skull and cervical spine. During a lateral impact, when the torso is rapidly accelerated out from under the head, the head turns toward the point of impact, in both lateral and anterior-posterior angles. Such motion separates the vertebral bodies from the side of opposite impact and rotates them apart. Jumped facets, ligaments, tears, and lateral compression fractures result.

FIGURE 3-25 During a rollover, the unrestrained occupant can be wholly or partially ejected out of the vehicle or can bounce around inside the vehicle. This action produces multiple and somewhat unpredictable injuries that are usually severe.

FIGURE 3-26 A properly positioned seat belt is located below the anterior superior iliac spine on each side, above the femur, and is tight enough to remain in this position. The bowl-shaped pelvis protects the soft intraabdominal organs.

can be largely explained by the relative lack of protection on the side of a car compared with the large amount of deformation that can occur to the front end of a vehicle before there is intrusion into the passenger compartment. However, when the vehicle that is struck in a lateral collision (by a car) is a sport utility vehicle (SUV), van, or pickup truck rather than a car, the risk of death to occupants is almost the same for all vehicles involved. Thus, SUVs, vans, and pickup trucks provide additional protection to their occupants because the passenger compartment sits higher off the ground than that of a car, and the occupants sustain less of a direct blow in a lateral impact.

More serious injuries and a greatly increased risk of death to vehicle occupants have been documented when a car is struck on its lateral aspect by a van, SUV, or pickup. In a lateral-impact collision between a van and a car, the occupants of the car struck broadside are 13 times more likely to die than those in the van. If the striking vehicle is a pickup truck or SUV, the occupants of the car struck broadside are 25 to 30 times more likely to die than those in the pickup truck or SUV. This tremendous disparity results from the higher center of gravity and increased mass of the van, SUV, or pickup truck. Knowledge of vehicle types where occupants were located in a crash may lead the prehospital care provider to have a higher index of suspicion for serious injury.

Seat Belts. In the injury patterns described previously, the victims were assumed to be unrestrained, as are most vehicle occupants in the United States (67% in a 1999 NHTSA report). Ejection from vehicles accounted for approximately 25% of the 44,000 vehicular deaths in 2002. About 75% of passenger vehicle occupants who were totally ejected were killed; 1 in 13 ejection victims sustained a spine fracture. After ejection from a vehicle, the body is subjected to a

second impact as the body strikes the ground (or another object) outside the vehicle. This second impact can result in injuries that are even more severe than the initial impact. The risk of death for ejected victims is six times greater than for those who are not ejected. Clearly, seat belts save lives.

The NHTSA reports that 49 states and the District of Columbia have safety belt legislation. In 1999, more than 11,000 lives were saved by the use of these restraining devices. Over 123,000 lives have been saved since 1975. If all occupants wore restraints, the total lives saved for 1999 would have been more than 20,000.

What occurs when the victims are restrained? If a seat belt is positioned properly, the pressure of the impact is absorbed by the pelvis and the chest, resulting in few, if any, serious injuries (Figure 3-26). The proper use of restraints transfers the force of the impact from the patient's body to the restraint belts and restraint system. With restraints, the chance of receiving life-threatening injuries is greatly reduced.

Seat belts must be worn properly to be effective. An improperly worn belt may not protect against injury in the event of a crash, and it may even cause injury. When lap belts are worn loosely or are strapped above the anterior iliac crests, compression injuries of the soft abdominal organs can occur. Compression injuries of the soft intraabdominal organs (spleen, liver, and pancreas) result from compression between the seat belt and the posterior abdominal wall (Figure 3-27). Increased intraabdominal pressure can cause diaphragmatic rupture and herniation of abdominal organs. Anterior compression fractures of the lumbar spine can also

FIGURE 3-27   A seat belt that is incorrectly positioned above the brim of the pelvis allows the abdominal organs to be trapped between the moving posterior wall and the belt. Injuries to the pancreas and other retroperitoneal organs result, as well as blowout ruptures of the small intestine and colon.

FIGURE 3-28   Abrasions of the forearm are secondary to rapid expansion of the air bag when the hands are tight against the steering wheel.
(From McSwain NE Jr, Paturas JL: *The basic EMT: comprehensive prehospital patient care,* ed 2, St Louis, 2001, Mosby.)

occur as the upper and lower parts of the torso pivot over the restrained twelfth thoracic (T12), first lumbar (L1), and second lumbar (L2) vertebrae. Lap belts should also not be worn alone. Many occupants of vehicles still place the diagonal strap under the arm and not over the shoulder.

As mandatory laws on seat belt use are passed and enforced, the overall severity of injuries decreases, and the number of fatal crashes is significantly reduced.

Air Bags.   Air bags (in addition to seat belts) provide supplemental protection. Originally, front-seat driver and passenger air bag systems were designed to cushion the forward motion of only the front-seat occupant. They absorbed energy slowly by increasing the body's stopping distance. They are extremely effective in the first collision of frontal and near-frontal impacts (the 65% to 70% of crashes that occur within 30 degrees of the headlights). Air bags deflate immediately after the impact and therefore are not effective in multiple-impact or rear-impact collisions. An air bag deploys and deflates within 0.5 second. As the vehicle veers into the path of an oncoming vehicle or off the road into a tree after the initial impact, no air bag protection is left. Side air bags are adding to the protection of occupants.

When air bags deploy, they can produce minor but noticeable injuries that the prehospital care provider needs to manage. These include abrasions of the arms, chest, and face (Figure 3-28); foreign bodies to the face and eyes; and injuries caused by the occupant's eyeglasses (Figure 3-29). Air bags that do not deploy can still be dangerous to both the patient and the prehospital care provider. Air bags can be deactivated by an extrication specialist trained to do so properly and safely. Such deactivation should *not* delay patient care or extrication of the critical patient.

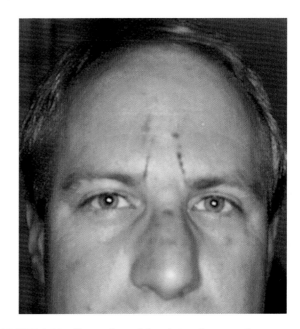

FIGURE 3-29   Expansion of the air bag into eyeglasses produces abrasions.
(From McSwain NE Jr, Paturas JL: *The basic EMT: comprehensive prehospital patient care,* ed 2, St Louis, 2001, Mosby.)

Motorcycle Crashes

Motorcycle crashes account for a significant number of the motor vehicle deaths each year. The laws of physics are the same, but the mechanism of injury varies slightly

Front-seat passenger air bags have been shown to be dangerous to children and small adults, especially when children are placed in incorrect positions in the front seat or with incorrectly installed child car seats. Children 12 years of age and younger should always be in the proper restraint device for their size and should be in the back seat.

Drivers should always be at least 10 inches (25 cm) from the air bag cover, and front-seat passengers should be at least 18 inches (45 cm) away. In most cases, when the proper seating arrangements and distances are used, air bag injuries are limited to simple abrasions.

FIGURE 3-31   The body travels forward and over the motorcycle, impacting the thighs and the femurs into the handlebars. The driver can also be ejected.

Bilateral femur fractures

FIGURE 3-30   The position of a motorcycle driver is above the pivot point of the front wheel as the motorcycle impacts an object head-on.

from automobile and truck crashes. This variance occurs in each of the following types of impacts: head-on, angular, and ejection.

Head-on Impact.   A head-on collision into a solid object stops the forward motion of a motorcycle (Figure 3-30) because the motorcycle's center of gravity is above and behind the front axle, which is the pivot point in such a collision. The motorcycle will tip forward, and the rider will crash into the handlebars. The rider may receive injuries to the head, chest, abdomen, or pelvis depending on which part of the anatomy strikes the handlebars. If the rider's feet remain on the pegs of the motorcycle and the thighs hit the handlebars, the forward motion will be absorbed by the midshaft femur, usually resulting in bilateral femoral fractures (Figure 3-31).

Angular Impact.   In an angular-impact collision, the motorcycle hits an object at an angle. The motorcycle will then collapse on the rider or cause the rider to be crushed between the motorcycle and the object struck. Injuries to the upper

or lower extremities can occur, resulting in fractures and extensive soft tissue injury (Figure 3-32). Injuries can also occur to organs of the abdominal cavity as a result of energy exchange.

Ejection Impact.   Because of lack of restraint, the rider is susceptible to being ejected. The rider will continue in flight until the head, arms, chest, abdomen, or legs strike another object, such as a motor vehicle, a telephone pole, or the road. Many riders do not use proper protection (e.g., helmets). Injury will occur at the point of impact and will radiate to the rest of the body as the energy is absorbed.

Injury Prevention.   Protection for motorcyclists includes boots, leather clothing, and helmets. Of the three, the *helmet* affords the best protection. It is built similar to the skull: strong and supportive externally and energy-absorbent internally. The helmet's structure absorbs much of the impact, thereby decreasing injury to the face, skull, and brain. The helmet provides only minimal protection for the neck but does not cause neck injuries. Failure to use helmets has been shown to increase head injuries by more than 300%. Mandatory helmet laws work. For example, Louisiana had a 60% reduction in head injuries in the first 6 years after passing a helmet law. Most states that have passed mandatory helmet legislation have found an associated reduction in motorcycle incidents.

"Laying the bike down" is a protective maneuver used by bikers to separate them from the motorcycle in an impending crash (Figure 3-33). The rider turns the motorcycle sideways and drags the inside leg on the ground. This action slows the rider more than the motorcycle so that the motorcycle will move out from under the rider. The rider will then slide along on the pavement but will not be trapped between the motorcycle and the object it hits. These riders usually

FIGURE 3-33 To prevent being trapped between two pieces of steel (motorcycle and vehicle), the rider "lays the bike down" to dissipate the injury. This often causes abrasions ("road rash") as the rider's speed is slowed on the asphalt.

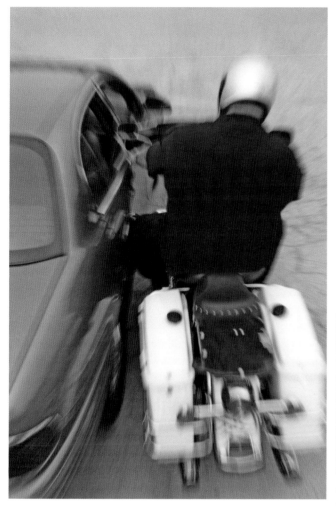

FIGURE 3-32 If the motorcycle does not hit an object head-on, it collapses like a pair of scissors, trapping the rider's lower extremity between the object impacted and the motorcycle.

FIGURE 3-34 Road burns after a motorcycle crash without protective clothing.
(From McSwain NE Jr, Paturas JL: *The basic EMT: comprehensive prehospital patient care,* ed 2, St Louis, 2001, Mosby.)

receive abrasions ("road rash") and minor fractures but avoid the severe injuries associated with the other types of impact (Figure 3-34).

Pedestrian Injuries

Pedestrian crashes versus MVCs have three separate phases, each with its own injury pattern, as follows:

1. The initial impact is to the legs and sometimes the hips (Figure 3-35, *A*).
2. The torso rolls onto the hood of the vehicle (Figure 3-35, *B*).
3. The victim falls off the vehicle and onto the ground, usually headfirst, with possible cervical spine trauma (Figure 3-35, *C*).

The injuries produced in pedestrian crashes vary according to the height of the victim. Visualize the impact points

on a child and an adult standing in front of a car. Because they are shorter, children are initially struck higher on the body than adults (Figure 3-36, *A*). The first impact generally occurs when the bumper strikes the child's legs (above the knees) or pelvis, damaging the femur or pelvic girdle. The second impact occurs almost instantly afterward when the front of the vehicle's hood continues forward and strikes the child's thorax. The head and face strike the front or top of the vehicle's hood (Figure 3-36, *B*). Because of the child's smaller size and weight, the child may not be thrown clear of the vehicle, as usually occurs with an adult. Instead, the child can be dragged by the vehicle while partially under the vehicle's front end (Figure 3-36, *C*). If the child falls to the side, the lower limbs may also be run over by a front

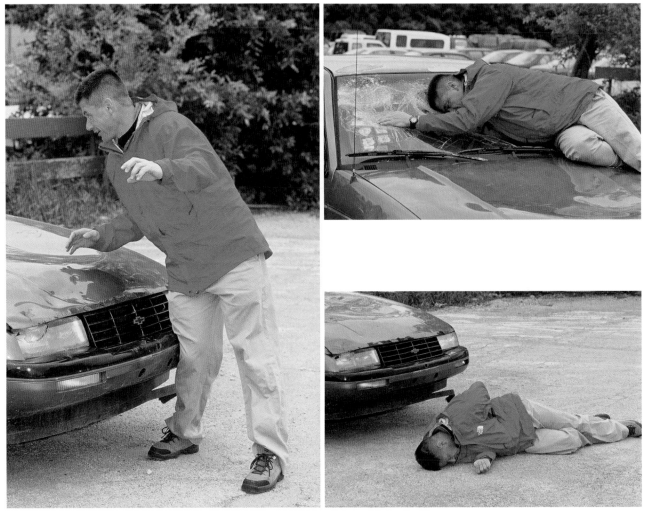

FIGURE 3-35 **A,** *Phase 1.* When a pedestrian is struck by a vehicle, the initial impact is to the legs and sometimes to the hips. **B,** *Phase 2.* The torso of the pedestrian rolls onto the hood of the vehicle. **C,** *Phase 3.* The pedestrian falls off the vehicle and hits the ground.

wheel. If the child falls backward, ending up completely under the vehicle, almost any injury can occur (e.g., being dragged, struck by projections, or run over by a wheel).

If the foot is planted on the ground at the time of impact, the child will receive energy exchange at the upper leg, hip, and abdomen. This will force the hips and abdomen away from the impact. The upper part of the torso will come along later, as will the planted foot. The severe angulation at the point of impact can produce fractures of the spine and femur.

To complicate these injuries further, the child will likely turn toward the car out of curiosity, exposing the anterior body and face to injuries, whereas the adult will attempt to escape and will be hit in the back or the side.

Adults are usually struck first by the vehicle's bumper in the lower legs, fracturing the tibia and fibula and driving the legs out from under the pelvis and torso. As the victim folds forward, the pelvis and upper femur are struck by the front of the vehicle's hood. As the abdomen and thorax fall forward, they strike the top of the hood. This substantial second strike can result in fractures of the upper femur, pelvis, ribs, and spine and produce serious intraabdominal or intrathoracic damage. Injury to the head and face at this point depends on the victim's ability to protect them with the arms. If the victim's head strikes the hood or if the victim continues to move up the hood so that the head strikes the windshield, injury to the face, head, and spine can occur.

The third impact occurs as the victim falls off the vehicle and strikes the pavement. The victim can receive a significant blow on one side of the body to the hip, shoulder, and head. Head injury often occurs when the victim strikes either the vehicle or the pavement and must always be considered. Similarly, because all three impacts produce sudden, violent movement of the torso, neck, and head, the prehospital care provider always assumes the patient

Knowing the specific sequence of multiple impacts in pedestrian versus motor vehicle crashes and understanding the multiple underlying injuries that they can produce are key to making an initial assessment and determining the appropriate management of a patient.

Falls

Victims of falls can also sustain injury from multiple impacts. An estimation of the height of the fall, the surface on which the victim landed, and part of the body struck first is part of the kinematics assessment of falls. Victims who fall from greater heights have a higher incidence of injury because their velocity increases as they fall. Falls from greater than three times the height of the victim are frequently severe. The type of surface on which the victim lands, and particularly its degree of *compressibility* (ability to be deformed by the transfer of energy), also has an effect on stopping distance.

The pattern of falls occurring feetfirst is called *Don Juan syndrome.* However, only in the movies can the character Don Juan jump from a balcony, land on his feet, and walk painlessly away. In real life, bilateral fractures of the calcaneus (heel bone), fractures of the ankles, and distal tibial or fibular fractures are often associated with this syndrome. After the feet land and stop moving, the legs are the next body part to absorb energy. Knee fractures, long-bone fractures, and hip fractures can result. The body is compressed by the weight of the head and torso, which are still moving, and can cause compression fractures of the spinal column in the thoracic and lumbar areas. Hyperflexion occurs at each concave bend of the S-shaped spine, producing compression injuries on the concave side and distraction injuries on the convex side. This victim is often described as breaking his or her "S" (Figure 3-37).

If a victim falls forward onto the outstretched hands, the result can be bilateral Colles' fractures of the wrists. If the victim did not land on the feet, the prehospital care provider will assess the part of the body that struck first, evaluate the pathway of energy displacement, and determine the injury pattern.

If the falling victim lands on the head with the body almost in-line, as often occurs in shallow-water diving injuries, the entire weight and force of the moving torso, pelvis, and legs compress the head and cervical spine. A fracture of the cervical spine can result, as with the up-and-over pathway of the frontal-impact collision.

Sports Injuries

Severe injury can occur during many sports or recreational activities, such as skiing, diving, baseball, and football. These injuries can be caused by sudden deceleration forces or by excessive compression, twisting, hyperextension, or hyperflexion. In recent years, various sports activities have become available to a wide spectrum of occasional, recreational participants who often lack the necessary

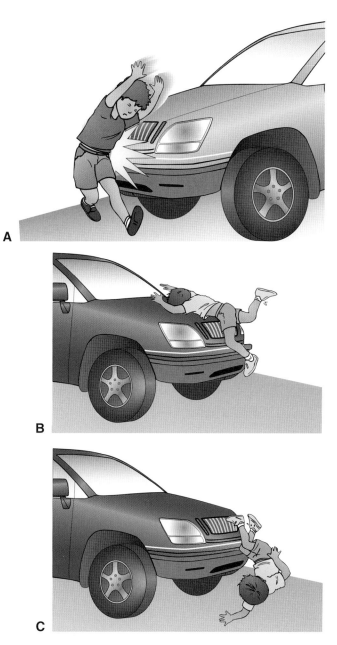

FIGURE 3-36 A, The initial impact on a child occurs when the vehicle strikes the child's upper leg or pelvis. **B,** The second impact occurs when the child's head and face strike the front or top of the vehicle's hood. **C,** A child may not be thrown clear of a vehicle but may be trapped and dragged by the vehicle.

has an unstable spine. An evaluation of the mechanism of injury should also include a determination if the victim, after hitting the roadway, was struck again by a second vehicle traveling next to or behind the first.

As with an adult, any child struck by a vehicle can receive some type of head injury. Because of the sudden, violent forces acting on the head, neck, and torso, cervical spine injuries are high on the suspicion list.

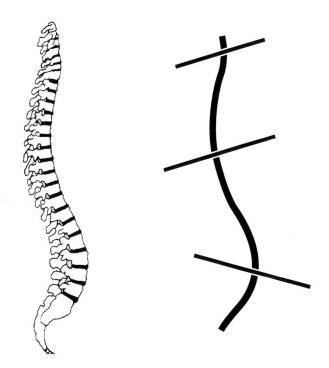

FIGURE 3-37 As the lower part of the spine stops its forward motion, the continued motion of the upper torso and head compresses the spine. This motion tends to produce compression injuries on the side of the concavity and distraction injuries on the side of the convexity.

training and conditioning or the proper protective equipment. Recreational sports and activities include participants of all ages. Sports such as downhill skiing, water-skiing, bicycling, and skateboarding are potentially high-velocity activities. Other sports, such as trail biking, all-terrain vehicle (ATV) riding, and snowmobiling, can produce velocity deceleration, collisions, and impacts similar to motorcycle crashes or MVCs.

The potential injuries of a victim who is in a high-speed collision and is then ejected from a skateboard, snowmobile, or bicycle are similar to those sustained when a person is ejected from a vehicle at the same speed because the amount of energy is the same. The specific mechanisms of MVCs and motorcycle crashes are described earlier.

The potential mechanisms associated with each sport are too numerous to list in detail. However, the general principles are the same as for MVCs. While assessing the mechanism of injury, the prehospital care provider considers the following:

■ What forces acted on the victim, and how?
■ What are the apparent injuries?
■ To what object or part of the body was the energy transmitted?
■ What other injuries are likely to have been produced by this energy transfer?
■ Was protective gear being worn?

■ Was there sudden compression, deceleration, or acceleration?
■ What injury-producing movements occurred (e.g., hyperflexion, hyperextension, compression, excessive lateral bending)?

When the mechanism of injury involves a high-speed collision between two participants, as in a crash between two skiers, reconstruction of the exact sequence of events from eyewitness accounts is often difficult. In such crashes the injuries sustained by one skier are often guidelines for examination of the other. In general, the prehospital care provider needs to know which part struck what, and what injury resulted from the energy transfer. For example, if one victim sustains an impact fracture of the hip, a part of the other skier's body must have struck with substantial force and therefore must have sustained a similar high-impact injury. If the second skier's head struck the first skier's hip, the prehospital care provider will suspect potentially serious head injury and an unstable spine for the second skier.

Broken or damaged equipment is also an important indicator of injury and must be included in the evaluation of the mechanism of injury. A broken sports helmet is evidence of the force with which it struck. Because skis are made of highly durable material, a broken ski indicates that extreme localized force came to bear, even when the mechanism of injury may appear unimpressive. A snowmobile with a severely dented front can indicate the force with which it struck a tree. The presence of a broken stick after an ice hockey skirmish raises the question of whose body broke it, how, and specifically what part of the victim's body was struck by the stick or fell on it.

Significant crashes with no apparent injuries must be assessed as if severe injuries exist. The steps are as follows:

1. Evaluate the patient for life-threatening injury.
2. Evaluate the patient for mechanism of injury. (What happened, and exactly how?)
3. Determine how the forces that produced injury in one victim may have affected any other person.
4. Determine whether protective gear was worn (it may have already been removed).
5. Assess damage to equipment. (What are the implications of this damage relative to the patient's body?)
6. Assess patient for possible associated injuries.

High-speed falls, collisions, and falls from heights without serious injury are common in many contact sports. The ability of athletes to experience incredible collisions and falls while sustaining only minor injury, largely a result of impact-absorbing equipment, may be confusing. The potential for injury in sports injury victims may be overlooked. The principles of kinematics and carefully

FIGURE 3-38 Three initial phases of injury that occur during a blast. In the first phase *(1)* the pressure wave first reaches the victim. This is followed by the second phase *(2),* in which flying debris can become missiles that produce injury. In the third phase *(3)* the victim becomes a missile and can be thrown into other objects or the ground.

considering the exact sequence and mechanism of injury will provide insight into sports collisions in which greater forces than usual came to bear. Kinematics is an essential tool in identifying possible underlying injuries and determining which patients require further evaluation and treatment at a medical facility.

Blast Injuries

The incidence of blast injuries increases during warfare, but these injuries are also becoming more common in the civilian world as terrorist activities and hazardous material incidents increase. Blasts may injure 70% of the people in the vicinity, whereas an automatic weapon used against the same-size group may injure only 30%. Mines, shipyards, chemical plants, refineries, fireworks firms, factories, and grain elevators are areas in which explosions are a particular hazard. However, because many volatile materials are transported by truck or rail, and domestic and bottled gas are common household items, an explosion can occur almost anywhere. The most insidious threat of blast injury, however, comes from the huge upsurge of terrorist bombings throughout the world in recent years. These occur on an almost daily basis, and military as well as civilian emergency medical services (EMS) personnel are routinely called on to treat injuries from explosions. Blast injuries have unique kinematics that distinguish them from other types of trauma.

Explosions can be divided into three initial phases—primary, secondary, and tertiary (Figure 3-38)—and two subsequent phases (quaternary and quinary). Different mechanisms create different types of injuries during each of these phases.

Primary Injuries. The pressure wave of the blast travels at speeds up to 10,000 feet per second and can cause a wide variety of injuries, including dismemberment. Most survivable injuries usually occur at the interface between tissues of different densities, primarily affecting those in the gas-containing organs, such as the eardrum, lungs, and bowel. Primary injuries include pulmonary bleeding, pneumothorax, air emboli, and perforation of the gastrointestinal organs. Pressure waves rupture and tear the small vessels and membranes of the gas-containing organs (cavitation) and may also injure the central nervous system; a classic sign of primary blast injury is tympanic rupture. These waves may cause severe damage or death without external signs of injury. Cardiopulmonary arrest and pulmonary injury are typical, with the latter (known as "blast lung") being the most common cause of death associated with primary blast. Clinical presentation may be immediate or delayed; therefore, EMS care for patients with a high index of suspicion for primary blast injury should include the following:

- Continual screening for respiratory distress and characteristic frothy secretions from the mouth.
- Periodic measurement of oxygen (O_2) saturation.
- Oxygen administration.

Land mines, because of their proximity to the body when detonated, produce devastating damage from blast overpressure, with stress waves extending from the foot to the thigh.

Underwater explosions also produce primary blast injuries, with the increased density and reduced compressibility of water greatly increasing risk of injury.

Secondary Injuries. Secondary, or *fragmentation,* injuries occur when the victim is struck by primary fragments (parts of the explosive device itself), secondary fragments (vehicle parts, flying glass, falling mortar, other debris generated by blast), or both. Secondary injuries include penetrating wounds, lacerations, and fractures. Triage of casualties with such injuries is guided by the location and severity of injury. Many superficial wounds to the skin and extremities often result, but thoracic and ocular injuries have higher associated morbidity and thus higher priority. Injuries to the eye from flying shards of glass or metal are a significant cause of morbidity associated with secondary fragments.

Tertiary Injuries. Tertiary injuries occur when the victim is (1) thrown against an object or hit with a large object or objects propelled by the explosion *(translational injury)* or (2) crushed during structural collapse induced by the blast wind (not the overpressure blast wave). Injury occurs at the point of impact, and the force of the blast is transferred to other organs of the body as the energy from the impact is absorbed. Tertiary injuries are usually apparent, but the prehospital care provider needs to look for associated injuries according to the type of impact that occurred. The injuries that occur in the tertiary phase (e.g., rib and vertebral fractures) are similar to those sustained in ejections from vehicles and falls from significant heights.

Quaternary and Quinary Injuries. Two additional categories of injury can result from explosions. Quaternary injuries are those imposed by heat or fumes created by the explosion, which may result in burns, inhalation injury, or even asphyxiation. The newest category, quinary injuries, includes the myriad of health effects that may be caused by additives to bombs, such as bacteria, radiation, and chemicals. A recent addition to the category of quinary injury associated with suicide bomb attacks in Israel is fragments of human remains (e.g., pieces of bone belonging to the suicide bomber) that become embedded in the bodies of victims; in addition to the injuries caused, this has devastating psychological and potentially infectious disease consequences.

Treatment. Secondary and tertiary injuries are the most obvious and are usually the most aggressively treated. Primary injuries may be the most severe, but they are often overlooked and sometimes never suspected. Adequate assessment of the various types of injuries is vital if the prehospital care provider is to manage the patient properly. Blast injuries often cause severe complications that may result in death if they are overlooked or ignored. For this reason, individuals who were close to the source of the explosion who do not have any obvious injuries should be monitored carefully for frothy secretions and respiratory distress, with sequential O_2 saturation measurements taken and oxygen administered as needed. Decreased O_2 saturation is an early warning sign of "blast lung" injury in the absence of other symptoms.

FIGURE 3-39   A bull's-eye fracture of the windshield is a major indication of skull impact and energy exchange to both the skull and the cervical spine.

Although each wound should be treated individually, bomb explosions usually generate a large number of victims that can reduce the capability to provide individualized treatment. The limited mass-casualty scenario typically created by explosions is typically managed using the "minimal acceptable care" model, developed in Israel, in which resources and personnel are focused on as many salvageable patients as possible.

Regional Effects of Blunt Trauma

The body can be divided into several regions: head, neck, thorax, abdomen, pelvis, and extremities. Each body region is subdivided into (1) the external part of the body, usually composed of skin, bone, soft tissue, vessels, and nerves, and (2) the internal part of the body, usually vital internal organs. The injuries produced as a result of shear, cavitation, and compression forces are used to provide an overview in each component and region for potential injuries.

Head

The only indication that compression and shear injuries have occurred to the patient's head may be a soft tissue injury to the scalp, a contusion of the scalp, or a bull's-eye fracture of the windshield (Figure 3-39).

Compression. When the body is traveling forward with the head leading the way, as in a frontal vehicular crash or a headfirst fall, the head is the first structure to receive the impact and the energy exchange. The continued momentum of the torso then compresses the head. The initial energy exchange occurs on the scalp and the skull. The skull can be compressed and fractured, pushing the broken bony segments of the skull into the brain (Figure 3-40).

Shear. After the skull stops its forward motion, the brain continues to move forward, becoming compressed against the intact or fractured skull with resultant concussion, contusions, or lacerations. The brain is soft and compressible;

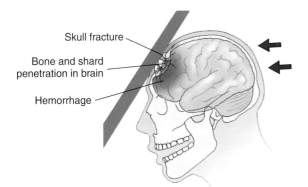

FIGURE 3-40 As the skull impacts a movable object, pieces of bone are fractured and are pushed into the brain substance.

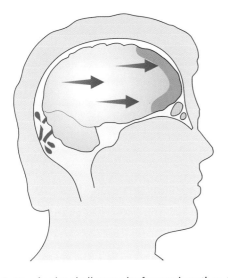

FIGURE 3-41 As the skull stops its forward motion, the brain continues to move forward. The part of the brain nearest the impact is compressed, bruised, and perhaps even lacerated. The portion farthest from the impact is separated from the skull, with tearing and lacerations of the vessels involved.

FIGURE 3-42 The skull frequently stops its forward motion, but the torso does not. Just as the brain compresses within the skull, the torso continues its forward motion until its energy is absorbed. The weakest point of this forward motion is the cervical spine.

FIGURE 3-43 The spine can be compressed directly along its own axis or angled in hyperextension or hyperflexion.

therefore its length is shortened. The posterior part of the brain can continue forward, pulling away from the skull, which has already stopped moving. Therefore the brain separates from the skull, stretching or breaking (shearing) any vessels in the area (Figure 3-41). Hemorrhage into the epidural, subdural, or subarachnoid space can then result. If the brain separates from the spinal cord, it will most likely occur at the brain stem.

Neck

Compression. The dome of the skull is fairly strong and can absorb the impact of a collision; however, the cervical spine is much more flexible. The continued pressure from the momentum of the torso toward the stationary skull produces angulation or compression (Figure 3-42). Hyperextension or hyperflexion of the neck often results in fracture or

dislocation of the vertebrae and injury to the spinal cord (Figure 3-43). Direct inline compression crushes the bony vertebral bodies. Both angulation and inline compression can result in an unstable spine.

Shear. The skull's center of gravity is anterior and cephalad to the point at which the skull attaches to the bony spine. Therefore a lateral impact on the torso when the neck is unrestrained will produce lateral flexion and rotation of the neck (see Figure 3-24). Extreme flexion or hyperextension may also cause stretching injuries to the soft tissues of the neck.

Thorax

Compression. If the impact of a collision is centered on the anterior part of the chest, the sternum will receive the initial energy exchange. When the sternum stops moving, the posterior thoracic wall (muscles and thoracic spine) and

FIGURE 3-44 Ribs forced into the thoracic cavity by external compression usually fracture in multiple places, producing the clinical condition known as *flail chest.*

FIGURE 3-45 Compression of the lung against a closed glottis, by impact on either the anterior or the lateral chest wall, produces an effect similar to compressing a paper bag when the opening is closed tightly by the hands. The paper bag ruptures, as does the lung.

the organs in the thoracic cavity continue to move forward until they compress against the sternum.

The continued forward motion of the posterior thorax bends the ribs until their tensile strength is exceeded. Fractured ribs and a flail chest can develop (Figure 3-44). This is similar to what happens when a vehicle stops suddenly against a dirt embankment (see Figure 3-9). The frame of the vehicle bends, which absorbs some of the energy. The rear of the vehicle continues to move forward until the bending of the frame absorbs all the energy. In the same way, the posterior thoracic wall continues to move until the ribs absorb all the energy.

Compression of the chest wall is common with frontal and lateral impacts and produces an interesting phenomenon called the *paper bag effect,* which may result in a pneumothorax. A victim instinctively takes a deep breath and holds it just before impact. This closes the glottis, effectively sealing off the lungs. With a significant energy exchange on impact, the lungs may then burst like a paper bag full of air that is popped (Figure 3-45). The lungs can also become compressed and contused, compromising ventilation.

Compression injuries to the internal structures of the thorax may also include a cardiac contusion, which occurs as the heart is compressed between the sternum and the spine and can result in significant dysrhythmias.

Shear. The heart, ascending aorta, and aortic arch are relatively unrestrained within the thorax. The descending aorta tightly adheres to the posterior thoracic wall and the vertebral column. The resultant motion is analogous to holding the flexible tubes of a stethoscope just below where the rigid tubes from the earpiece end and swinging the acoustic head of the stethoscope from side to side. As the skeletal frame stops abruptly in a collision, the heart and the initial segment of the aorta continue their forward

motion. The shear forces produced can tear off the aorta at the junction of the portion of free motion and the tightly bound portion (Figure 3-46).

An aortic tear may result in an immediate, complete transection of the aorta. More often, aortic tears are only partial, and one or more layers of tissue remain intact. However, the remaining layers are under great pressure, and a traumatic aneurysm often develops, similar to the bubble that can form on a weak part of a tire. The aneurysm can eventually rupture within minutes, hours, or days after the original injury. Approximately 80% of these patients die on the scene at the time of the initial impact. Of the remaining 20%, one third will die within 6 hours, one third will die within 24 hours, and one third will live 3 days or longer. It is important that the prehospital care provider recognize the potential for such injuries and relay this information to the hospital personnel.

Abdomen

Compression. Internal organs pressed by the vertebral column into the steering wheel or dashboard during a frontal collision may rupture. The effect of this pressure is similar to the effect of placing the internal organ on an anvil and striking it with a hammer. Solid organs frequently injured in this manner include the pancreas, spleen, liver, and kidneys.

Injury may also result from a buildup of pressure in the abdomen. The *diaphragm* is a 1/4-inch thick (5-mm) muscle located across the top of the abdomen and separating the abdominal cavity from the thoracic cavity. Its contraction causes the pleural cavity to expand for ventilation. The anterior abdominal wall comprises two layers of fascia and one very strong muscle. Three lateral muscle layers have

A

B

FIGURE 3-46 A, The descending aorta is a fixed structure that moves with the thoracic spine. The arch, aorta, and heart are freely movable. Acceleration of the torso in a lateral-impact collision or rapid deceleration of the torso in a frontal-impact collision produces a different rate of motion between the arch-heart complex and the descending aorta. **B,** Tears at the junction of the arch and descending aorta.
(**A** from McSwain NE Jr, Paturas JL: *The basic EMT: comprehensive prehospital patient care,* ed 2, St Louis, 2001, Mosby.)

associated fascia, and the lumbar spine and its associated muscles provide strength to the posterior abdominal wall. The multilayered perineum lies inferior to the diaphragm. The diaphragm is the weakest of all the walls and structures surrounding the abdominal cavity. It may be torn or ruptured as the intraabdominal pressure increases (Figure 3-47). This injury has four common consequences, as follows:

1. The "bellows" effect that is usually created by the diaphragm is lost.

FIGURE 3-47 With increased pressure inside the abdomen, the diaphragm can rupture.

2. The abdominal organs can enter the thoracic cavity and reduce the space available for lung expansion.
3. The displaced organs can become ischemic from compression of their blood supply.
4. If intraabdominal hemorrhage is present, the blood can also cause a hemothorax.

Another injury caused by increased abdominal pressure is a rupture of the aortic valve as a result of retrograde blood flow (Figure 3-48). This injury is rare but does exist. It occurs when a collision with the steering wheel or involvement in another type of incident (e.g., ditch or tunnel cave-in) has produced a rapid increase in intraabdominal pressure. This rapid pressure increase results in a sudden increase of aortic blood pressure. Blood is pushed back (retrograde) against the aortic valve with enough pressure to cause rupture of the valve cusps.

Shear. Injury to the abdominal organs occurs at their points of attachment to the mesentery. During a collision, the forward motion of the body stops, but the organs continue to move forward, causing tears at the points of attachment of organs to the abdominal wall. If the organ is attached by a pedicle (a stalk of tissue), the tear can occur where the pedicle attaches to the organ, where it attaches to the abdominal wall, or anywhere along the length of the pedicle (Figure 3-49). Organs that can shear this way are the kidneys, small intestine, large intestine, and spleen.

Another type of injury that often occurs during deceleration is laceration of the liver caused by its impact with the ligamentum teres. The liver is suspended from the diaphragm but is only minimally attached to the posterior abdomen near the lumbar vertebrae. The ligamentum teres attaches to the anterior abdominal wall at the umbilicus and to the left lobe of the liver in the midline of the body.

FIGURE 3-48 Increased intraabdominal pressure can force blood in a retrograde fashion up the aorta and against the aortic valve. The aortic valve may then tear.

FIGURE 3-49 Organs can tear away from their point of attachment to the abdominal wall. The spleen, kidney, and small intestine are particularly susceptible to these types of shear forces.

(The liver is not a midline structure; it lies more on the right than on the left.) A down-and-under pathway in a frontal impact or a feet first fall causes the liver to bring the diaphragm with it as it descends into the ligamentum teres (Figure 3-50). The ligamentum teres will fracture or transect the liver, analogous to a cheese slicer cutting cheese.

Pelvic fractures are the result of damage to the external abdomen and may cause injury to the bladder or lacerations of the blood vessels in the pelvic cavity. Approximately 10%

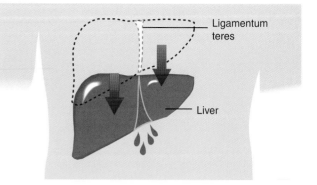

FIGURE 3-50 The liver is not supported by any fixed structure. Its major support is by the diaphragm, which is freely movable. As the body travels in the down-and-under pathway, so does the liver. When the torso stops but the liver does not, the liver continues downward onto the ligamentum teres, tearing the liver. This is much like pushing a cheese-cutting wire into a block of cheese.

of patients with pelvic fractures also have a genitourinary injury.

Penetrating Trauma
Physics of Penetrating Trauma

The principles of physics discussed earlier are equally important when dealing with penetrating injuries. Again, the kinetic energy that a striking object transfers to body tissue is represented by the following formula:

$$KE = \tfrac{1}{2}mv^2$$

Energy cannot be created or destroyed, but it can be changed in form. This principle is important in understanding penetrating trauma. For example, although a lead bullet is in the brass cartridge casing that is filled with explosive powder, the bullet has no force. However, when the primer explodes, the powder burns, producing rapidly expanding gases that are transformed into force. The bullet then moves out of the gun and toward its target.

According to Newton's first law of motion, after this force has acted on the missile, the bullet will remain at that speed and force until it is acted on by an outside force. When the bullet hits something, such as a human body, it strikes the individual tissue cells. The energy (speed and mass) of the bullet's motion is exchanged for the energy that crushes these cells and moves them away (cavitation) from the path of the bullet.

Factors That Affect the Size of the Frontal Area
The larger the frontal area of the moving missile, the greater is the number of particles that will be hit; therefore the greater the energy exchange that occurs and the larger

the cavity that is created. The size of the frontal surface area of a projectile is influenced by three factors: profile, tumble, and fragmentation. Energy exchange or potential energy exchange can be analyzed based on these factors.

Profile. *Profile* describes an object's initial size and whether that size changes at the time of impact. The profile, or frontal area, of an ice pick is much smaller than that of a baseball bat, which in turn is much smaller than that of a truck. A hollow-pointed missile, if crushed and deformed as a result of striking a body, will have a much larger frontal area than before its shape was changed. A hollow-point bullet flattens and spreads on impact (Box 3-1). This change enlarges the frontal area so that it hits more tissue particles and produces greater energy exchange. A larger cavity forms, and more injury results (Figure 3-51).

In general, as a bullet travels through the air after being discharged from a weapon, it will strike fewer air particles and will maintain most of its speed if its frontal area is kept small and is streamlined by its conical shape. If that missile strikes the skin and becomes deformed, covering a larger area, a much greater energy exchange will occur than if its frontal surface area did not expand. Therefore, the ideal bullet keeps its shape while in the air and only deforms on impact.

Tumble. *Tumble* describes whether the object tumbles and assumes a different angle inside the body than the angle assumed as it entered the body. A wedge-shaped bullet's center of gravity is located nearer to the base than to the nose of the bullet. When the nose of the bullet strikes something, it slows rapidly. Momentum continues to carry the base of the bullet forward, with the center of gravity seeking to become the leading point of the bullet. This movement causes an end-over-end motion, or tumble. As the bullet tumbles, the normally horizontal sides of the bullet become its leading edges, thus striking far more particles than when the nose was the leading edge (Figure 3-52). More energy exchange is produced, and therefore greater tissue damage occurs.

FIGURE 3-51 Changes in the profile or trauma projection increase the particles hit and therefore the amount of energy dispersal.
(From McSwain NE Jr: Pulmonary chest trauma. In Moylan JA, editor: *Principles of trauma,* New York, 1992, Gower.)

FIGURE 3-52 Tumble motion of a missile maximizes its damage at 90 degrees.

Fragmentation. *Fragmentation* describes whether the object breaks up after it enters the body. Bullets with soft noses or vertical cuts in the nose and safety slugs that contain many small fragments increase body damage by breaking apart on impact. The resulting mass of fragments creates a larger frontal area than a single solid bullet, and energy is dispersed rapidly into the tissue. If the missile shatters, it will spread out over a wider area, with two results: (1) more tissue particles will be struck by the larger frontal projection, and (2) the injuries will be distributed over a larger portion of the body because more organs will be struck (Figure 3-53). The multiple pieces of shot from a shotgun blast produce similar results. Shotgun wounds are an excellent example of the fragmentation injury pattern (Figure 3-54).

FIGURE 3-53 **A,** Missile made of soft lead or another component that breaks up will cause damage over a wider area and create maximum absorption of the energy because many more tissue particles are impacted than with a hard missile. **B,** When the missile breaks up into smaller particles, this fragmentation increases its frontal area and increases the energy distribution.
(**B** from McSwain NE Jr: Pulmonary chest trauma. In Moylan JA, editor: *Principles of trauma,* New York, 1992, Gower.)

FIGURE 3-54 Maximum fragmentation damage is caused by a shotgun.

Damage and Energy Levels

The damage caused in a penetrating injury can be estimated by classifying penetrating objects into three categories according to their energy capacity: low-, medium-, and high-energy weapons. Penetrating trauma can result from impaled objects such as fence posts and street signs in vehicle crashes, ski poles in snow sports, and handlebar injuries in bicycling.

Low-Energy Weapons. Low-energy weapons include hand-driven weapons such as a knife or ice pick. These missiles produce damage only with their sharp points or cutting edges. Because these are low-velocity injuries, they are usually associated with less secondary trauma (i.e., less cavitation will occur). Injury in these victims can be pre-

dicted by tracing the path of the weapon into the body. If the weapon has been removed, the prehospital care provider should try to identify the type of weapon used and the gender of the attacker whenever possible. Men tend to stab with the blade on the thumb side of the hand and with an upward or inward thrust, whereas women tend to hold the blade on the little finger side and stab downward.

An attacker may stab a victim and then move the knife around inside the body. A simple entrance wound may produce a false sense of security. The entrance wound may be small, but the damage inside may be extensive. The potential scope of the movement of the inserted blade is an area of possible damage (Figure 3-55).

Evaluation of the patient for associated injury is important. For example, the diaphragm can reach as high as the nipple line on deep expiration. A stab wound to the lower chest can injure intrathoracic as well as intraabdominal structures.

Medium-Energy and High-Energy Weapons. Firearms fall into two groups, medium energy and high energy. Medium-energy weapons include handguns and some rifles. As the amount of gunpowder in the cartridge increases, the

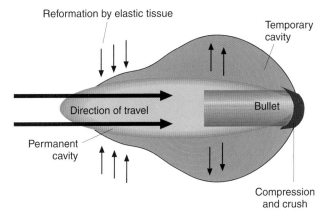

FIGURE 3-57   A bullet crushes tissues directly in its path. A cavity is created in the wake of the bullet. The crushed part is permanent. The temporary expansion can also produce injury.

FIGURE 3-55   Damage produced by a knife depends on the movement of the blade inside the victim.

FIGURE 3-56   Medium-energy weapons are usually guns that have short barrels and contain cartridges with less power.
(From McSwain NE Jr, Paturas JL: *The basic EMT: comprehensive prehospital patient care,* ed 2, St Louis, 2001, Mosby.)

speed of the bullet and therefore its kinetic energy increase (Figure 3-56).

In general, medium-energy and high-energy weapons damage not only the tissue directly in the path of the missile, but also the tissue on each side of the missile's path. The variables of profile, tumble, and fragmentation influence the extent and direction of the injury. The pressure on tissue particles, which are moved out of the direct path of the missile, compresses and stretches the surrounding tissue. A temporary cavity is always associated with weapons in the medium- or high-energy classification. This cavity is usually three to six times the size of the missile's frontal surface area (Figure 3-57).

High-energy weapons include assault weapons, hunting rifles, and other weapons that discharge high-velocity

missiles (Figure 3-58). These missiles not only create a permanent track but also produce a much larger temporary cavity than lower-velocity missiles. This temporary cavity expands well beyond the limits of the actual bullet track and damages a wider area than is apparent during the initial assessment. Tissue damage is much more extensive with a high-energy penetrating object than with one of medium energy. The vacuum created by this cavity pulls clothing, bacteria, and other debris from the surrounding area into the wound.

A consideration in predicting the damage from a gunshot wound is the range or *distance* from which the gun (either medium or high energy) is fired. Air resistance slows the bullet; therefore, increasing the distance will decrease the velocity at the time of impact and will result in less injury. Most shootings are done at close range with handguns, so the probability of serious injury is high.

Entrance and Exit Wounds

Tissue damage will occur at the site of entry into the body, in the path of the weapon's entrance, and on exit from the body. Knowledge of the victim's position, the attacker's position, and the weapon used is essential in determining the path of injury.

Evaluating wound sites provides valuable information to direct the management of the patient and to relay to the receiving facility. Do two holes in the victim's abdomen indicate that a single missile entered and exited, or that two missiles are both still inside the patient? Did the missile cross the midline (usually causing more severe injury) or remain on the same side? In what direction did the missile travel? What internal organs are likely to have been in its path?

Entrance and exit wounds usually produce identifiable injury patterns to soft tissue. An entrance wound from a gunshot lies against the underlying tissue, but an exit wound has no support. The former is a round or oval

FIGURE 3-58 A, High-energy weapons. **B,** Graze wound to the scalp created by a projectile from a high-velocity weapon. The skull was not fractured. **C,** High-velocity gunshot wound to the leg demonstrating the large, permanent cavity.
(**A** from McSwain NE Jr, Paturas JL: *The basic EMT: comprehensive prehospital patient care,* ed 2, St Louis, 2001, Mosby.)

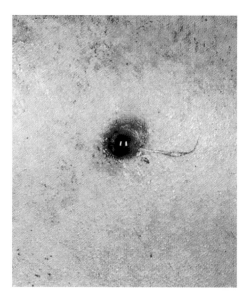

FIGURE 3-59 Entrance wound is round or oval in shape, and exit wound is stellate or linear.
(From McSwain NE Jr, Paturas JL: *The basic EMT: comprehensive prehospital patient care,* ed 2, St Louis, 2001, Mosby.)

FIGURE 3-60 The abraded edge indicates that the bullet traveled from top right to bottom left.

wound depending on the entry path, and the latter is a *stellate* (starburst) wound (Figure 3-59). Because the missile is spinning as it enters the skin, it leaves a small area of abrasion (1-2 mm in size) that is pink (Figure 3-60). Abrasion is not present on the exit side. If the muzzle was placed directly against the skin at the time of discharge, the expanding gases will enter the tissue and produce crepitus on examination (Figure 3-61). Within 2 to 3 inches (5-7 cm) the burning gases will burn the skin, at 2 to 6 inches (5-15 cm) the smoke will adhere to the skin, and inside 10 inches (25 cm) the burning cordite particles will tattoo the skin with small (1-2 mm) burned areas (Figure 3-62).

Regional Effects of Penetrating Trauma

This section discusses the injuries sustained by various parts of the body during penetrating trauma.

Head. After a missile penetrates the skull, its energy is distributed within a closed space. Particles accelerating away from the missile are forced against the unyielding

FIGURE 3-61   Hot gases coming from the end of a muzzle held in proximity to the skin produce partial-thickness and full-thickness burns on the skin.

FIGURE 3-63   The bullet may follow the curvature of the skull. (From McSwain NE Jr, Paturas JL: *The basic EMT: comprehensive prehospital patient care,* ed 2, St Louis, 2001, Mosby.)

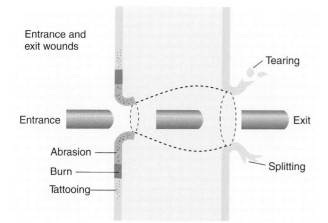

FIGURE 3-62   Spin and compression of the bullet on entrance produce round or oval holes. On exit the wound is pressed open.

FIGURE 3-64   Lung damage produced by the cavity at a distance from the point of impact.

skull, which cannot expand as skin can. Thus the brain tissue is compressed against the inside of the skull, producing more injury than if it could expand freely. If the forces are strong enough, the skull may explode from the inside out.

A bullet may follow the curvature of the interior of the skull if it enters at an angle and has insufficient force to exit the skull. This path can produce significant damage (Figure 3-63). Because of this characteristic, medium-velocity weapons, such as the 0.22-caliber or 0.25-caliber pistol, have been called the "assassin's weapon."

Thorax. Three major groups of structures are inside the thoracic cavity: the pulmonary system, vascular system, and gastrointestinal tract.

Pulmonary System. Lung tissue is less dense than blood, solid organs, or bone; therefore a penetrating object does less damage to lung tissue than to other thoracic tissues. Much of the area traversed by the missile is air, fewer particles are hit, and less energy is transferred, so less damage is produced. However, damage to the lungs can be clinically significant (Figure 3-64).

Vascular System. Smaller vessels that are not attached to the chest wall may be pushed aside without significant damage. However, if larger vessels, such as the aorta and vena cava, are hit, they cannot move aside easily and are more susceptible to damage.

The myocardium stretches as the bullet passes through and then contracts, leaving a smaller defect. The thickness of the muscle may control a low-energy penetration, such as by a knife or 0.22-caliber bullet, preventing immediate exsanguination and allowing time to transport the victim to an appropriate facility.

Gastrointestinal Tract. The *esophagus*, the part of the gastrointestinal tract that traverses the thoracic cavity, can be penetrated and can leak its contents into the thoracic cavity. The signs and symptoms of such an injury may be delayed for several hours or several days.

Abdomen. The abdomen contains structures of three types: air filled, solid, and bony. Penetration by a low-energy missile may not cause significant damage; only 30% of knife wounds penetrating the abdominal cavity require surgical exploration to repair damage. A medium-energy injury (e.g., handgun wound) is more damaging; 85% to 95% require surgical repair. However, even with injuries caused by medium-energy missiles, the damage to solid and vascular structures may not produce immediate exsanguination. Temporary control of the hemorrhage can be provided indirectly in the abdomen with a compression bandage or air splint or by using a *pneumatic antishock garment* (PASG). This enables prehospital care providers to transport the patient to an appropriate facility in time for effective surgical intervention.

Extremities. Penetrating injuries to the extremities can include damage to bones, muscles, or vessels. When bones are hit, bony fragments become secondary missiles, lacerating surrounding tissue (Figure 3-65). Muscles often expand away from the path of the missile, causing hemorrhage. The missile may penetrate blood vessels, or a near-miss may damage the lining of a blood vessel, causing clotting and obstruction of the vessel within minutes or hours.

Shotgun Wounds

Although shotguns are not high-velocity weapons by most definitions, at close range they can be more lethal than some of the most high-energy rifles. Handguns and rifles predominantly use *rifling* (grooves) on the inside of the barrel to spin a single missile in a flight pattern toward the target. In contrast, most shotguns possess a smooth, cylindrical tube barrel that directs a load of missiles in the direction of the target. Devices known as *chokes* and *diverters* can be attached to the end of a shotgun barrel to shape and form the column of missiles into specific patterns (e.g., cylindrical or rectangular). Regardless, when a shotgun is fired, a large number of missiles are ejected in a *spread,* or *spray,* pattern. The barrels may be shortened ("sawed off") to widen prematurely the trajectory of the missiles.

Although shotguns may use various types of ammunition, the structure of most shotgun shells is similar. A typical shotgun shell contains gunpowder, wadding, and projectiles. When discharged, all these individual components are

FIGURE 3-65 Bone fragments become secondary missiles themselves, producing damage by the same mechanism as the original penetrating object.

propelled from the muzzle and can inflict injury on the victim. Certain types of gunpowder can *stipple* ("tattoo") the skin in close-range injuries. Wadding, which is usually lubricated paper, fibers, or plastic used to separate the shot (missiles) from the charge of gunpowder, can introduce another source of infection into the wound if not removed. The missiles can vary in size, weight, and composition. A wide variety of missiles are available, from compressed metal powders to *birdshot* (small metal pellets), *buckshot* (larger metal pellets), *slugs* (a single metal missile), and more recently, plastic and rubber alternatives. The average shell is loaded with 1 to 1 1/2 ounces of shot. Fillers that are placed with the shot (polyethylene or polypropylene granules) can become embedded in the superficial layers of the skin.

An average birdshot shell may contain 200 to 2000 pellets, whereas a buckshot shell may contain only 6 to 20 pellets. It is important to note that as the size of the buckshot pellets increases, they approach the wounding characteristics of 0.22-caliber missiles, in regard to effective range and energy transfer characteristics. Larger or "magnum" shells are also available. These shells may contain more shot and a larger charge of gunpowder, or only the larger powder charge, to boost the muzzle velocity of the shot.

The type of ammunition used is important in gauging injuries, but the *range* (distance) at which the patient was shot provides the most important variable when evaluating the shotgun injury victim. Shotguns eject a large number of missiles, most of which are spherical. These projectiles are especially susceptible to the effects of air resistance,

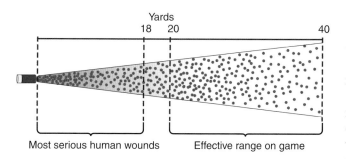

FIGURE 3-66 The diameter of the spread of a shot column expands as range increases.
(From DeMuth WE: The mechanism of gunshot wounds, *J Trauma* 11:219, 1971.)

thereby quickly slowing the shot that exits the muzzle at its peak velocity (Figure 3-66). The effect of air resistance on the projectiles decreases the effective range of the weapon and changes the basic characteristics of wounds that it generates. Consequently, shotgun wounds have been classified into four major categories: contact, close-range, intermediate-range, and long-range wounds (Table 3-1).

Contact wounds occur when the muzzle is touching the patient at the time the weapon is discharged. This typically results in circular entrance wounds, which may or may not have soot or an imprint of the muzzle. Searing or burning of the wound edges is common, secondary to the high temperatures and the expansion of hot gases as the missiles exit the muzzle. Some contact wounds may be more stellate (star shaped) in appearance, caused by the superheated gases from the barrel escaping from the tissue. Contact wounds usually result in widespread tissue damage

and are associated with high mortality. The length of a standard shotgun barrel makes it difficult to commit suicide with this weapon, since it is difficult to pull the trigger. Such attempts usually result in a split face without the shot reaching the brain.

Close-range wounds, although still typically characterized by circular entrance wounds, will likely have more evidence of soot, gunpowder, or filler stippling around the wound margins than contact wounds. Additionally, abrasions and markings from the impact of the wadding that coincide with the wounds from the missiles may be found. Close-range wounds also create significant damage in the patient; missiles fired from this range still retain sufficient energy to penetrate deep structures and exhibit a slightly wider spread pattern. This increases the extent of injury as missiles travel through soft tissue.

Intermediate-range wounds are characterized by the appearance of satellite pellet holes emerging from the border around a central entrance wound. This pattern is a result of individual pellets spreading from the main column of shot. These injuries are a mixture of deep penetrating wounds and superficial wounds and abrasions. Because of the deep penetrating components of this injury, however, victims may still have a relatively high mortality rate.

Long-range wounds are rarely lethal. These wounds are typically characterized by the classic spread of scattered pellet wounds. However, even at these slower velocities, the pellets can cause significant damage to certain sensitive tissues (e.g., eyes). In addition, larger buckshot pellets can retain sufficient velocity to inflict damage to deep structures, even at long range. The prehospital care provider also needs to consider the cumulative effects of many small

TABLE 3-1 Patterns of Shotgun Injury

Type	Wound appearance	Injury	Mortality
Contact		Widespread tissue damage	85%-90%
Close		Penetrates beyond deep fascia	15%-20%
Intermediate		Penetrates SQ tissue and deep fascia	0-5%
Long Range		Superficial skin penetration	0%

Modified from Sherman RT, Parrish RA: Management of shotgun injuries: a review of 152 cases, *J Trauma* 18:236, 1978.

missile wounds and their locations, focusing on sensitive tissues. *Adequate exposure* is key to examining all patients involved in trauma, and shotgun injuries are no exception.

These varying characteristics need to be taken into account when evaluating injury patterns in patients with shotgun injuries. For example, a single circular shotgun wound could represent a contact or close-range injury with birdshot or buckshot in which the missiles have retained a tight column or grouping. Conversely, this may also represent an intermediate-range to long-range injury with a slug or solitary missile. Only detailed examination of the wound will allow differentiation of these injuries that will likely involve significant damage to internal structures despite strikingly different missile characteristics.

Contact and close-range wounds to the chest may result in an impressive open pneumothorax, and bowel may eviscerate from such wounds to the abdomen. On occasion, a single pellet from an intermediate-range wound may penetrate deep enough to perforate the bowel, leading eventually to peritonitis, or may damage a major artery, resulting in vascular compromise to an extremity. Alternatively, a patient who presents with multiple small wounds in a spread pattern may have dozens of entrance wounds. However, none of the missiles may have retained enough energy to penetrate through fascia, let alone produce significant damage to internal structures.

Although immediate patient care must always remain paramount, any information (shell type, suspected range of patient from weapon, number of shots fired) that prehospital care providers can gather from the scene and relay to the receiving facility can assist with appropriate diagnostic evaluation and treatment of the shotgun-injured patient. Furthermore, recognition of various wound types can aid providers in maintaining a high index of suspicion for internal injury regardless of the initial impression of the injury.

Using Kinematics in Assessment

The assessment of a trauma patient must involve knowledge of kinematics. For example, a driver who hits the steering wheel (blunt trauma) will have a large cavity in the anterior chest at the time of impact; however, the chest rapidly returns to, or near to, its original shape as the driver rebounds from the steering wheel. If two prehospital care providers examine the patient separately—one who understands kinematics and another who does not—the one without knowledge of kinematics will be concerned only with the bruise visible on the patient's chest. The prehospital care provider who understands kinematics will recognize that a large cavity was present at the time of impact; that the ribs had to bend in for the cavity to form; and that the heart, lungs, and great vessels were compressed by the formation of the cavity. Therefore the knowledgeable provider will suspect injuries to the heart, lungs, great vessels, and chest wall. The other prehospital care provider will not even be aware of these possibilities.

The knowledgeable prehospital care provider will assess the injuries, manage the patient, and initiate transport more aggressively, suspecting serious intrathoracic injuries, rather than reacting to what otherwise appears to be only a minor closed, soft tissue injury. Early identification, adequate understanding, and appropriate treatment of underlying injury will significantly influence whether a patient lives or dies.

SUMMARY

Integrating the principles of the kinematics of trauma into assessment of the trauma patient is the key to discovering otherwise unnoticed and unsuspected injuries. Left unsuspected, undetected, and therefore untreated, these injuries contribute significantly to morbidity and mortality resulting from trauma. A thorough comprehension of the kinematics of trauma is also significant in the prehospital care provider's emerging role in injury prevention. To apply the kinematics of trauma, the provider needs to consider both the physics of energy and the effect of the energy of motion on the structures of the body.

Energy cannot be created or destroyed, only changed in form. The kinetic energy of an object, expressed as a function of velocity (speed) and mass (weight), is transferred to another object on contact. Damage to the object or body tissue impacted is not only a function of the amount of kinetic energy applied to it, but also a function of its ability to tolerate the forces applied to it. The prehospital care provider's knowledge of body structure, combined with clues about the types of forces and amount of energy involved, has a significant predictive value for injuries sustained.

In applying a critical thinking process to relate kinetic energy to the potential for injury, the following questions can be asked and answered:

- What mechanism of trauma is involved?
- Is it an impact, blast, fall, or penetrating trauma?

Blunt trauma
- What type of vehicle impact occurred: frontal, lateral, rear, rotational, rollover, or angular?
- Was the victim ejected?
- How many impacts occurred? For example, was an ejected victim then struck by another vehicle? Was the victim of an assault struck multiple times?
- What speeds were involved?
- What was the stopping distance (or time)?
- Was the victim using appropriate protective devices and using them correctly (e.g., seat belts, air bags, helmets, body armor)?
- In field triage, which victims are most likely to have been more severely injured?
- Which part or parts of the body impacted another object? For example, was there an up-and-over path that caused the head or chest to impact the vehicle interior? Was the victim of an assault struck with a club, pipe, fists, or other weapon?

- Is the victim an adult or child? How will the pattern of injury vary?

Falls
- How far did the victim fall? How does that distance relate to the patient's height?
- On what type of surface did the victim land?
- Did the victim sustain multiple impacts caused by objects in the path of the fall?
- Which part of the victim's body made the initial impact on landing?

Blasts
- How close was the victim to the explosion?
- What primary-, secondary-, and tertiary-phase injuries should be suspected?

Penetrating trauma
- What was the size and gender of the assailant?
- What type of weapon was used?
- What was the angle of injury?
- If a gun was used, is there an indication of the velocity and type of projectile?
- What was the range?
- What is the pattern of injury that is likely to have occurred?

Through the use of this knowledge, the incidence, morbidity, and mortality rates caused by injuries can be significantly improved.

SCENARIO SOLUTION

The driver of the lateral-impact vehicle is moaning and has a decreased level of consciousness. He is breathing about 10 times a minute. Based on the mechanism of injury and the findings of the primary survey (initial assessment), the paramedics call a trauma alert, requesting a helicopter for transport, and decide to perform a rapid extrication. If the transport time by ground to the trauma center is significantly longer than flight time of a helicopter plus the added time to access the scene, a helicopter can be requested. The paramedics administer oxygen at 15 L/min via a nonrebreathing mask and secure the patient to a longboard with a cervical collar and head blocks in place.

Two large-bore intravenous (IV) lines of normal saline should be started en route. Depending on local protocol, these IV lines should be at a "keep vein open" (KVO) rate or full flow. The potential injuries are severely damaged spleen and left kidney, lateral flail chest, pulmonary contusion, pneumothorax, aortic shear injury, pelvic fracture, and clavicular fracture. The potential injuries for the frontal-impact patient would be cervical (C-spine) fracture; head injury; aortic shear injury; compression of the spleen, liver, and pancreas; overpressure tear of the diaphragm; pneumothorax; and cardiac contusion. ■

Suggested Reading

Alderman B, Anderson A: Possible effect of airbag inflation on a standing child. In Proceedings of 18th American Association of Automotive Medicine, September 1974.

American College of Surgeons (ACS) Committee on Trauma: *Advanced trauma life support course,* Chicago, 2002, ACS.

Anderson PA, Henley MB, Rivara P, Maier RV: Flexion distraction and chance injuries to the thoracolumbar spine, *J Orthop Trauma* 5(2):153, 1991.

Anderson PA, Rivara FP, Maier RV, Drake C: The epidemiology of seatbelt-associated injuries, *J Trauma* 31(1):60, 1991.

Bartlett CS. Gunshot wound ballistics, *Clin Orthop* 408:28, 2003.

DePalma RG, Burris DG, Champion HR, Hodgson MJ: Current concepts: blast injuries, *N Engl J Med* 352:1335, 2005.

Di Maio VJM: *Gunshot wounds: practical aspects of firearms, ballistics and forensic techniques,* Boca Raton, Fla, 1999, CRC Press.

Fackler ML, Surinchak JS, Malinowski JA, Bowen RE: Bullet fragmentation: a major cause of tissue disruption, *J Trauma* 24:35, 1984.

Fackler ML, Surinchak JS, Malinowski JA, Bowen RE: Wounding potential of the Russian AK-47 assault rife, *J Trauma* 24:263, 1984.

Garrett JW, Braunstein PW: The seat belt syndrome, *J Trauma* 2:220, 1962.

Huelke DF, Mackay GM, Morris A: Vertebral column injuries and lap-shoulder belts, *J Trauma* 38:547, 1995.

Huelke DF, Moore JL, Ostrom M: Air bag injuries and occupant protection, *J Trauma* 33(6):894, 1992.

Joksch H, Massie D, Pichler R: Vehicle aggressivity: fleet characterization using traffic collision data, Washington, DC, 1998, NHTSA/Department of Transportation.

McSwain NE Jr: Kinematics. In Mattox KL, Feliciano DV, Moore EE, editors: *Trauma,* ed 4, New York, 1999, McGraw-Hill.

McSwain NE Jr, Brent CR: Trauma rounds: lipstick sign, *Emerg Med* 21:46, 1898.

National Safety Council (NSC): *Accident facts 1994,* Chicago, 1994, NSC.

Ordog GJ, Wasserberger JN, Balasubramaniam S: Shotgun wound ballistics, *J Trauma* 28:624, 1988.

Oreskovich MR, Howard JD, Compass MK, et al: Geriatric trauma: injury patterns and outcome, *J Trauma* 24:565, 1984.

Rutledge R, Thomason M, Oller D, et al: The spectrum of abdominal injuries associated with the use of seat belts, *J Trauma* 31(6):820, 1991.

States JD, Annechiarico RP, Good RG, et al: A time comparison study of the New York State Safety Belt Use Law utilizing hospital admission and police accident report information, *Accid Anal Prev* 22(6):509, 1990.

Swierzewski MJ, Feliciano DV, Lillis RP, et al: Deaths from motor vehicle crashes: patterns of injury in restrained and unrestrained victims, *J Trauma* 37(3):404, 1994.

Sykes LN, Champion HR, Fouty WJ: Dum dums, hollowpoints, and devastators: techniques designed to increase wounding potential of bullets, *J Trauma* 28:618, 1988.

Chapter Objectives

*At the completion of this chapter, the reader
will be able to do the following:*

✓ Identify potential threats to the safety of the patient, bystanders, and emergency personnel that are common to all emergency scenes.

✓ Identify potential threats that are unique to a given scenario, such as a motor vehicle crash (MVC).

✓ Integrate analysis of scene safety, scene situation, and kinematics into assessment of the trauma patient to make patient care decisions.

✓ Describe appropriate steps to take to mitigate potential threats to safety.

✓ Given a mass-casualty incident (MCI) scenario (hazardous material incident, weapon of mass destruction), make triage decisions based on assessment findings.

CHAPTER 4

Scene

SCENARIO

You are awakened at 0400 on a Saturday to respond to the scene of a person struck by a vehicle. As you go to the ambulance, you notice that it is raining; the temperature is 50° F (10° C). Dispatch provides the additional information that after hitting the pedestrian, the vehicle crashed into a utility pole. Fluid from the vehicle is leaking onto the street, leaving a sheet on the rainwater. According to dispatch, bystanders report that the patient lost consciousness. On arrival, you detect no additional threats to safety in your scene assessment.

What are your concerns about the scene? ■

The prehospital care provider has the following three priorities on arrival to a scene:

1. The first priority for everyone involved at a trauma incident is assessment of the scene. *Scene assessment* involves establishing that the scene is safe and carefully considering the exact nature of the situation. Assessment of the scene safety and situation can be initiated enroute to the scene based on information from the dispatcher, as the emergency medical services (EMS) unit arrives on the scene, and as the providers approach the patient; however, the issues identified in this evaluation must be addressed before beginning assessment of individual patients. In some situations, such as combat or tactical situations, this becomes even more critical and can alter the methods of how the principles of patient care are accomplished

2. After performing the scene assessment, attention can be turned to evaluating individual patients; Chapter 5 discusses this in detail. Scene assessment includes an abbreviated form of triage so that the most severely injured patients are assessed first. The emphasis in order of priority is (a) conditions that may result in the loss of life, (b) conditions that may result in the loss of limb, and (c) all other conditions that do not threaten life or limb.

3. If the scene involves more than one patient, the situation is classified as either a multiple-patient incident or a mass-casualty incident (MCI). In an MCI the priority shifts from focusing all resources on the most injured patient to saving the maximum number of patients, that is, providing the greatest good to the greatest number. Triage is discussed in the final section of this chapter.

Scene Assessment

Patient assessment starts long before the prehospital care provider arrives at the patient's side. Dispatch begins the process by providing the initial information about the incident and the patient, based on bystander reports or information provided by other prehospital care units first on the scene. The on-scene information-gathering process begins immediately on arrival at the incident. Before making contact with the patient, the prehospital care provider can evaluate the scene by (1) observing family members and bystanders, (2) looking for the outcome of the incident, and (3) obtaining a general impression of the situation. A majority of patient injuries can be predicted based on an understanding of the kinematics and the effects on the patients.

Taking the time to prepare mentally for a call and practicing basic communication between partners may be the difference between a well-managed scene and a hostile confrontation (or a physical assault). Good observation, perception, and communication skills are the best tools.

The scene's appearance creates an impression that influences the entire assessment; therefore, correct evaluation of the scene is crucial. A wealth of information is gathered by simply watching, listening, and cataloging as much information as possible, including the mechanisms of injury, the present situation, and the overall degree of safety.

Just as the patient's condition can improve or deteriorate, so can the condition of the scene. Evaluating the scene initially, then failing to reassess how the scene may be changing, can result in serious consequences to the care providers and the patient.

Scene assessment includes the following two major components:

1. *Safety.* The primary consideration when approaching any scene is the safety of the medical and rescue personnel. Rescue attempts should not be done by those untrained in the techniques required. When medical personnel become victims, they will no longer be able to assist other injured people and will add to the number of patients and decrease the number of care

providers. Patient care needs to wait until the scene is secured.

Scene safety involves not only rescuer safety but also patient safety. In general, patients in a hazardous situation should be moved to a safe area before assessment and treatment begin. Threatening conditions to patient or rescuer safety include fire, downed electrical lines, explosives, hazardous materials, including blood or body fluid, traffic, floodwater, weapons (e.g., guns, knives), and environmental conditions. Also, an assailant may still be on the scene and may intervene to harm the patient, rescuers, or others.

2. *Situation.* Assessment of the situation follows the safety assessment. What really happened at the scene? Why was help summoned? What was the mechanism of injury (kinematics), and what forces and energies led to the victims' injuries? (See Chapter 3.) How many people are involved, and what are their ages? Are additional EMS units needed for treatment or transport? Is mutual aid needed? Are any other personnel or resources needed (e.g., law enforcement, fire department, power company)? Is special extrication or rescue equipment needed? Is helicopter transport necessary? Is a physician needed to assist with triage? Could a medical problem be the instigating factor that led to the trauma (e.g., a vehicle crash that resulted from the driver's heart attack)?

Issues related to both safety and situation have significant overlap; many safety topics are also specific to certain situations, and certain situations pose serious safety hazards. These issues are discussed in further detail in the following sections.

Safety Issues

Traffic Safety

The majority of EMS responders who are killed or injured each year are involved in motor vehicle–related incidents.[1] Although most of these are related to direct ambulance collisions during the response phase, a subset of these fatalities and injuries occurs while working on the scene of a motor vehicle crash (MVC). In the United States, MVCs resulted in more than 1.9 million EMS responses in 2003.[2] Many factors can result in prehospital care providers being injured or killed on the scene of an MVC (Figure 4-1). Some factors, such as weather conditions (e.g., snow, ice, rain, fog) and road design (e.g., limited-access or rural roads), cannot be changed; however, the responder can be aware that these conditions exist and can act appropriately to mitigate these situations.[3]

FIGURE 4-1 A significant number of prehospital care providers who are injured or killed are working at the scene of a motor vehicle crash.
(From McSwain N, Paturas J: *The basic EMT,* ed 2, St Louis, 2003, Mosby.)

Weather/Light Conditions

Many prehospital care responses to MVCs take place in adverse weather conditions and at night. These weather conditions vary by geographic location and time of the year. Many areas need to deal with ice and snow during the winter months, whereas coastal and mountainous areas confront fog. Rainstorms are common in most geographic areas, and sandstorms affect other regions. Incoming traffic may not see or be able to stop in time to avoid emergency vehicles or personnel parked on the scene.

Highway Design

High-speed, limited-access highways have made moving large amounts of traffic efficient in urban areas, but when a crash occurs, the resulting traffic backup and "rubber necking" by drivers create dangerous situations for responders. Law enforcement is usually reluctant to shut down a limited-access highway and strives to keep the flow of traffic moving. Although this may seem to produce further danger to responders, it may prevent additional rear-end collisions caused by the backup of vehicles.

Rural roads present other problems. Although the volume of traffic is much less than on urban roadways, the windy, narrow, and hilly nature of these roads creates short sight distances for drivers as they approach the scene of an MVC. Rural roads may not be as well maintained as those in urban areas, resulting in slippery conditions long after a storm has passed and catching unsuspecting drivers off guard. Isolated areas of snow, ice, or fog that caused the original MVC may still be present before EMS arrival and may result in suboptimal conditions for oncoming drivers.

Mitigation Strategies

It would be safest to respond to MVCs only during daylight hours on clear days; unfortunately, prehospital care providers need to respond at all times of day and in any weather condition. However, steps can be taken to reduce the risks of becoming a victim while working at an MVC. The best way is not to be there, particularly on limited-access highways. The number of people on the scene at any given time should be the number needed to accomplish the tasks at hand. Having three ambulances and a supervisor's vehicle at a scene that has only one patient dramatically increases the risk of a provider being hit by a passing vehicle. Although many dispatch protocols require multiple-ambulance response to limited-access highways, all but the initial ambulance should be staged at an on ramp nearby unless immediately needed.

The location of equipment on the ambulance also plays a role in safety. Equipment should be placed so that it can be gathered without stepping into the traffic flow. The passenger's side of the ambulance is usually toward the guardrails, and placing the equipment most often used at MVCs in these compartments will keep responders out of the traffic flow.

Reflective Clothing. In most cases of prehospital care responders being hit by oncoming vehicles, the drivers stated that they did not see the responder in the road. Both the National Fire Protection Association and the Occupational Safety and Health Administration (OSHA) have standards for reflective warning garments used on highways. OSHA has three levels of protection for workers on highways, with the highest level (level 3) being used at night on a high-speed roadway. Although it is not the purpose of this text to set standards for appropriate clothing (e.g., safety vest) at an MVC, common sense indicates that prehospital care providers need to be as well or better protected than workers flagging traffic at construction sites. It is recommended that outerwear used by responders should at least meet American National Standards Institute (ANSI) class 2 or 3 standards. These standards can be met either by affixing reflective material to the outer jacket or by wearing an approved reflective vest.

Vehicle Positioning and Warning Devices. Vehicle positioning at the scene of an MVC is of the utmost importance. The incident commander or the safety officer should ensure that the responding vehicles are placed in the best positions to protect prehospital care providers. It is important for the first arriving emergency vehicles to "take the lane" of the accident (Figure 4-2). Placement of the ambulance behind the scene will not facilitate loading of the patient, but it will protect the responders and patients from oncoming traffic. As additional emergency vehicles arrive, they should generally be placed on the same side of the road as the incident. These vehicles should be placed farther away from the incident to give increased warning time to oncoming drivers.

Headlights, especially high beams, should be turned off so as not to blind oncoming drivers, except if the beams are

FIGURE 4-2 Correct positioning of emergency vehicle. (From McSwain N, Paturas J: *The basic EMT,* ed 2, St Louis, 2003, Mosby.)

being used to illuminate the scene. The number of warning lights at the scene should be evaluated; too many lights will only serve to confuse oncoming drivers. Many departments use warning signs stating "accident ahead" to give ample warning time for drivers. Flares may be arranged to warn and direct traffic flow; however, care should be used in dry conditions so as not to start grass fires. Reflective cones serve as good devices to direct traffic flow away from the lane taken up by the emergency (Figure 4-3).

If traffic needs to be directed, this should be done by law enforcement or those with special training in traffic behavior. Confusing or contradicting instructions given to drivers only create further safety risks. The best situations are created when traffic is not impeded and normal flow can be maintained around the emergency. Construction sites provide an example of traffic flow around obstructions. These traffic issues can be handled in much the same way; prehospital care providers can observe construction sites to gain insight into how traffic flow may work better at an MVC.

Violence

Prehospital care providers need to remember that each call has the potential to take them into an emotionally charged

FIGURE 4-3 Placement of traffic delineation devices.
(From Henry M, Stapleton E: *EMT prehospital care,* ed 3, St Louis, 2004, Mosby.)

demonstrating respect and concern is important in gaining the patient's trust and achieving control of the scene.

It is important that EMS personnel train themselves to "observe" the scene and not just "look" at it. Learn to notice numbers and locations of individuals when arriving on the scene, movement of bystanders into or out of the scene, indicators of stress or tension, unexpected or unusual reactions to EMS presence, or other "gut" feelings that may be developing. Watch the hands; look for unusual bulges in waistbands or oversized clothing that could easily hide a weapon.

If a developing threat is perceived, immediately begin preparing to leave the scene. An assessment or a procedure may need to be finished in the ambulance. The safety of the prehospital care providers takes priority.

Safety Scenario

You and your partner are in the living room of your patient's home. While your partner is checking the patient's blood pressure, an apparently intoxicated individual enters the room from the back of the house. He looks angry, and you notice what appears to be the butt of a gun sticking out of the waistband of his pants. Your partner does not see or hear this person enter the room because he is focused on the patient. The suspicious person begins to question your presence and is extremely agitated about your uniform and your badge. His hands repeatedly move toward, then away from, his waist. He begins to pace and mumble. What do you do?

Safety Suggestions

Partners can use a hands-on/hands-off approach, as well as predetermined code words and hand signals, for emergencies. The role of the *hands-on* prehospital care provider is to take charge of the patient assessment, giving necessary attention to the patient. The *hands-off* provider stands back (until needed) to observe the scene, interact with family or bystanders, collect necessary information, and create better access and egress. In essence, the hands-off provider is monitoring the scene and "covering" his partner's back. A predetermined *code word* and *hand signals* allow partners to communicate a threat without alerting others of their concerns.

In many situations, tension and anxiety are immediately reduced when an attentive prehospital care provider begins interacting with and assessing the patient. However, if both providers have all their attention centered on the patient, the scene can quickly become threatening, and early clues (as well as opportunities to retreat) may be missed.

Violent Scene Safety Rules

1. **Don't be there.** When responding to a known violent scene, stage at a safe location until the scene has been rendered safe by law enforcement and clearance to respond has been given.

environment. The patient, family, or bystanders on the scene may not be able to perceive the situation rationally. These individuals may think that the response time was too long, may be oversensitive to words or actions, and may misunderstand the "usual" approach to patient assessment. Maintaining a confident and professional manner while

2. **Retreat.** If threats are presented when approaching the scene, tactfully retreat to the vehicle and leave the scene. Stage at a safe location and notify appropriate personnel.

3. **Diffuse.** If a scene becomes threatening during patient care, use verbal diffusion skills to reduce tension and aggression (while preparing to leave the scene).

4. **Defend.** *As a last resort,* the prehospital care provider may find it necessary to defend himself. It is important that such efforts are to "disengage and get away." Do not attempt to chase or subdue an aggressive party. Ensure that law enforcement personnel have been notified and are en route. Again, the safety of the providers is the priority.

Bloodborne Pathogens

Before the recognition of acquired immunodeficiency syndrome (AIDS) in the early 1980s, health care workers (HCWs) showed little concern over exposure to blood and body fluids. Despite knowledge that blood was known to transmit certain hepatitis viruses, prehospital care providers and others involved in emergency medical care often viewed contact with a patient's blood as an annoyance rather than an occupational hazard. Because of the high mortality rate associated with contracting AIDS, and the identification that human immunodeficiency virus (HIV), the causative agent of AIDS, could be transmitted in blood, HCWs became much more concerned about the patient as a vector of disease. Federal agencies, such as the Centers for Disease Control and Prevention (CDC) and OSHA, developed guidelines and mandates for HCWs to minimize exposure to bloodborne illness, including HIV and hepatitis.

Epidemiologic data demonstrate that HCWs are much more likely to contract bloodborne illness from their patients than their patients are to contract disease from health professionals. Exposures to blood are typically characterized as either percutaneous or mucocutaneous. *Percutaneous exposures* occur when an individual sustains a puncture wound from a contaminated sharp object, such as a needle or scalpel, with the risk of transmission being directly related to both the contaminating agent and the volume of infected blood introduced by the injury. *Mucocutaneous exposures* typically are less likely to result in transmission and include exposure of blood to nonintact skin, such as a soft tissue wound (e.g., abrasion, superficial laceration) or a skin condition (e.g., acne), or to mucous membranes (e.g., conjunctiva of eye). The primary infections transmitted through blood include both hepatitis B (HBV) and hepatitis C (HCV) viruses and HIV.

Viral Hepatitis

Although a number of hepatitis viruses have been identified, HBV and HCV are of most concern to HCWs experiencing a blood exposure. Viral hepatitis causes acute inflammation of the liver, often resulting in right upper quadrant pain, fatigue, loss of appetite, nausea, vomiting, and alteration in liver function. Jaundice, a yellowish coloration of the skin, results from an increased level of bilirubin in the bloodstream. The incubation period, from exposure to manifestation of symptoms, is generally 60 to 90 days. Up to 30% of those infected with HBV may have an asymptomatic course. Although most individuals with hepatitis recover without serious problems, a small percentage develop *acute fulminant hepatic failure* and may die. A significant number of those who recover will develop a carrier state, in which their blood can transmit the virus.

As in HBV, infection with HCV can range from a mild, asymptomatic course to liver failure and death. The incubation period for HCV is somewhat shorter than for HBV, typically 6 to 9 weeks. Chronic infections with HCV are much more common than with HBV, and about 80% to 85% of those who contract HCV will develop persistently abnormal liver function, predisposing them to *hepatocellular carcinoma*. Hepatitis C is primarily transmitted through blood, whereas hepatitis B can be transmitted through blood or sexual contact. About two thirds of intravenous drug abusers have been infected with HCV. Before routine testing of donated blood for presence of HBV and HCV, blood transfusion was the primary reason patients contracted hepatitis. Hepatitis can be transmitted to HCWs through needlesticks and mucocutaneous exposures on nonintact skin.

A vaccine derived from the hepatitis B surface antigen (HBsAg) can immunize individuals against HBV.[4] Before the development of this vaccine, more than 10,000 HCWs became infected with HBV annually, and several hundred would die each year from either severe hepatitis or complications of chronic HBV infection. OSHA now requires employers to offer HBV vaccine to those workers in high-risk environments. All prehospital care providers should be immunized against HBV. Almost all those who complete the series of three vaccines will develop antibody (Ab) to HBsAg, and immunity can be determined by testing blood for the presence of HBsAb. If an HCW is exposed to blood potentially infected with HBV before developing immunity (i.e., before completing the vaccine series), passive protection from HBV can be conferred with the administration of hepatitis B immune globulin (HBIG).

At present, no immune globulin or vaccine is available to protect HCWs from exposure to HCV, emphasizing the need for using Standard Precautions.

Human Immunodeficiency Virus

After infection, HIV targets the immune system of its new host. Over time the number of certain types of white blood cells falls dramatically, leaving the individual prone to developing unusual infections or cancers. When patients develop one of these opportunistic infections or cancers, they transition from being *HIV positive* to having AIDS.

In the last decade, significant advances have been made in the treatment of HIV disease, primarily in developing new drugs to combat its effects. This has resulted in many individuals with HIV infection being able to lead fairly normal lives because the progression of the disease is slowed dramatically.

Although HCWs typically are more concerned about contracting HIV because of its uniformly fatal prognosis, they are at greater risk of contracting HBV or HCV. Only about 0.3% (about 1 in 300) of needlestick exposures to HIV-positive blood lead to infection, compared to infection rates of 23% to 62% (1 in 4 to 1 in 2) with exposure to HBV-infected needles. Infection with HCV falls between these two rates (1.8%; 1 in 50). The probable explanation for the varying rates of infection is the relative concentration of virus particles found in infected blood. In general, HBV-positive blood contains 100 million to 1 billion virus particles/mL, whereas HCV-positive and HIV-positive blood contains 1 million and 100 to 10,000 particles/mL, respectively. The risk of infection appears higher with exposure to a larger quantity of blood, exposure to blood from a patient with a more advanced stage of disease, a deep percutaneous injury, or an injury from a hollow-bore, blood-filled needle. Since 2001, the risk of contracting HIV, HBV, or HCV from a blood transfusion has been estimated at about 1 in 1 million transfusions.

Two serotypes of HIV have been identified. *HIV-1* accounts for virtually all AIDS in the United States and equatorial Africa, and *HIV-2* is found almost exclusively in Western Africa. Although early victims of HIV were male homosexuals, intravenous drug users, or hemophiliacs, HIV disease is now found in many teenage and adult heterosexual populations, with the fastest-growing numbers in minority communities. The screening test for HIV is very sensitive, and false-positive tests occasionally occur. All positive screening tests should be confirmed with a more specific technique (e.g., Western blot electrophoresis).

HIV is primarily transmitted through infected blood or semen, but vaginal secretions and pericardial, peritoneal, pleural amniotic, and cerebrospinal fluids are all considered potentially infected. Unless obvious blood is present, tears, urine, sweat, feces, and saliva are generally considered noninfectious.

Standard Precautions

Because clinical examination cannot reliably identify all patients who pose a potential threat to HCWs, Standard Precautions were developed to prevent HCWs from coming into direct contact with a patient's blood or body fluid (e.g., saliva, vomit). OSHA has developed regulations that mandate employers and their employees to follow Standard Precautions in the workplace. Standard Precautions consist of both physical barriers to blood and body fluid and exposure as well as safe handling practices for needles and other "sharps." Because trauma patients often have external

FIGURE 4-4 At a minimum, personal protective equipment for prehospital care providers should consist of gloves, mask, and eye protection.
(From Chapleau W: *Emergency first responder,* St Louis, 2004, Mosby.)

hemorrhage and because blood is an extremely high-risk body fluid, protective devices should be worn while caring for patients.

Physical Barriers

Gloves. Gloves should be worn when touching nonintact skin, mucous membranes, or areas contaminated by gross blood or other body fluids. Because perforations may readily occur in gloves while caring for a patient, gloves should be examined regularly for defects and changed immediately if a problem is noted (Figure 4-4).

Masks and Face Shields. Masks serve to protect the HCW's oral mucous membranes from exposure to infectious agents. Masks and face shields should be changed immediately if they become wet or soiled.

Eye Protection. Eye protection must be worn in circumstances where droplets of infected fluid may be splattered, such as while providing airway management to a patient with blood in the oropharynx. Standard eyeglasses are not considered adequate because they lack side shields.

Gowns. Disposable gowns with impervious plastic liners offer the best protection, but they may be extremely uncomfortable and impractical in the prehospital environment. Gowns or clothing should be changed immediately if significant soilage occurs.

Resuscitation Equipment. HCWs should have access to bag-valve-mask devices or mouthpieces to protect them from direct contact with a patient's saliva, blood, and vomit.

Handwashing. Handwashing is a fundamental principle of infection control. Hands should be washed with soap and

BOX 4-1   **Preventing Sharps Injury**

Prehospital care providers are at significant risk for injury from needles and other sharps. Strategies for reducing sharps injuries include the following:

- Use safety devices, such as shielded or retracting needles and scalpels and automatically retracting lancets.
- Use "needleless" systems that allow injection of medication at ports without needles.
- Refrain from recapping needles and other sharps.
- Immediately dispose of contaminated needles into rigid sharps containers rather than setting them down.
- Use prefilled medication syringes rather than drawing medication from an ampule.
- Provide a written exposure control plan, and ensure that all employees are aware of the plan.
- Maintain a sharps injury log.

running water if gross contamination with blood or body fluid occurs. Alcohol-based hand antiseptics are useful at preventing transmission of many infectious agents but are not appropriate for situations where obvious soiling has occurred; however, they can provide some cleansing and protective effect in situations where running water and soap are not available. After removal of gloves, hands should be cleansed with either soap and water or an alcohol-based antiseptic.

Preventing Sharps Injury. As noted earlier, percutaneous exposure to a patient's blood or body fluid constitutes a significant manner in which viral infections could be transmitted to HCWs. Many percutaneous exposures are caused by injuries from needlesticks with contaminated needles or other sharps. Attempt to eliminate unnecessary needles and sharps, never try to recap a used needle, and implement safety devices when possible (Box 4-1).

Management of Occupational Exposure. In the United States, OSHA mandates that every organization providing health care have a control plan for managing occupational exposures of its employees to blood and body fluids. Each exposure should be thoroughly documented, including the type of injury and estimation of the volume of inoculate. If an HCW has mucocutaneous or percutaneous exposure to blood or sustains an injury from a contaminated sharp, efforts are taken to prevent bacterial infection, including tetanus, and HBV and HIV infection. No prophylactic therapy to prevent HCV infection is currently approved or available. Box 4-2 describes a typical blood and body fluid exposure protocol.

Hazardous Materials

Understanding the prehospital care provider's risk of exposure to hazardous materials is not as simple as recognizing environments that have obvious potential for hazardous material exposure. Hazardous materials are widespread in the modern world; vehicles, buildings, and even homes have hazardous material potential. For this reason, all prehospital care providers require training to a minimum of the awareness level.

Awareness is the first of four levels of training available to responders. The next level is *operations;* these responders are trained to set up perimeters and safety zones, limiting the spread of the event. Whereas awareness represents the minimum level of training, the operations level would be helpful for all responders, as well as providing the training to help control the event. The next level is *technician.* Technicians are trained to stop the release of hazardous materials. The highest level of training is *specialist.* This advanced level allows the responder to provide command and support skills to a hazardous materials ("hazmat," HazMat) event.

Prehospital care providers accept that scene safety is the first part of the approach to every patient and every scene. An important part of determining the safety of the scene is to evaluate for the potential of hazmat exposure. Assessment of potential hazards should begin with dispatch. The information given by dispatch may establish a high index of suspicion. Additional information can be requested while en route if prehospital care providers have any concerns or questions that could be relayed to the scene.

Once a scene has been determined to have hazmat involvement, the focus must shift to securing the scene and summoning help to safely isolate the scene and remove and decontaminate the patients. The general simple rule is, "If the scene is not safe, make it safe." If the provider cannot make the scene safe, help should be summoned. The *Emergency Response Guidebook* (ERG), produced by the U.S. Department of Transportation, can be used to identify potential hazards (Figure 4-5). The book uses a simple system that allows identification of a material by its name or placard number. The text then refers the reader to a guide page that provides basic information about safe distances for rescuers, life and fire hazards, and the patient's likely complaints. Binoculars should be used to read labels; if labels can be read without the use of viewing devices, the provider is likely to be exposed.

At a hazmat scene, security must be ensured: "nobody in, nobody out." The staging area should be established upwind and upgrade at a safe distance from the hazard. Entry into and exit from the scene should be denied until the arrival of hazmat specialists. In most cases, patient care will begin when the decontaminated patient is delivered to the prehospital care provider.

It is important for the prehospital care provider to understand the command system and structure of the work

---

BOX 4-2 Sample Exposure Protocol

After a percutaneous or mucocutaneous exposure to blood or other potentially infected body fluids, the following actions constitute appropriate postexposure prophylaxis (PEP):

1. Prevention of bacterial infection.
   - Cleanse exposed skin thoroughly with germicidal soap and water; exposed mucous membranes (mouth, eyes) should be irrigated with copious amounts of water.
   - Administer tetanus toxoid booster, if not received in previous 5 years.
2. Baseline laboratory studies are performed on both the exposed health care worker (HCW) and the source patient, if known.
   - *HCW:* Hepatitis B surface antibody (HBsAb), hepatitis C virus (HCV), and human immunodeficiency virus (HIV) tests.
   - *Source patient:* Hepatitis B and C serology and HIV test.
3. Prevention of hepatitis B virus (HBV) infection.
   - If the HCW has not been immunized against hepatitis B, the first dose of HBV vaccine is administered along with hepatitis B immune globulin (HBIG).
   - If the HCW has begun but not yet completed the HBV vaccine series, or if the HCW has completed all HBV immunizations, HBIG is given if the HBsAb test fails to show the presence of protective antibodies and the source patient's tests demonstrate active infection with HBV. HBIG may be administered up to 7 days after an exposure and still be effective.
4. Prevention of HIV infection.
   - For percutaneous injuries:
     — If the source patient is HIV negative, no PEP is warranted.

   — If the source patient is of unknown HIV status or has asymptomatic HIV and the exposure is superficial, a 28-day course of two medications is typically prescribed.*
   — If the exposure is more severe (deep, obvious blood on device) or if the source patient has symptomatic HIV (AIDS), a three-drug regimen is typically prescribed for 28 days.†
   - For mucocutaneous exposures:
     — If the source patient is HIV negative, no PEP is warranted.
     — If the source patient is of unknown HIV status, generally no PEP is warranted, unless there are significant HIV risk factors. In the latter case, a 28-day course of two medications is typically prescribed.*
     — If the source patient has asymptomatic HIV infection, or if the exposure was a small amount (few drops) of blood from a patient with symptomatic HIV, a 28-day course of two medications is typically prescribed.*
     — If the exposure involves a large volume of blood from a patient with symptomatic HIV, a three-drug regimen is typically prescribed for 28 days.†
   - Follow-up laboratory tests:
     — If PEP is prescribed for HIV, a complete blood count (CBC) and blood chemistries are performed at 14 days to check for adverse effects.
     — If the source patient is HIV negative, the HCW needs no further HIV testing.
     — If source patient has HIV, or if the HIV status is unknown, the HCW should undergo follow-up HIV testing at 6 weeks, 3 months, 6 months, and 12 months after the exposure.

*Two-drug PEP regimen typically consists of zidovudine and lamivudine (medications are discontinued if an HIV test on the source patient is negative).
†Three-drug PEP regimen typically consists of zidovudine, lamivudine, and a protease inhibitor.

---

zones in a hazmat operation. Hazmat control operations are set up in zones. The "hot" zone is the area of highest contamination, and only specially trained and protected workers may enter this area. If patients are in this area, the hazmat team will bring them out. A contamination reduction corridor runs through the next zone, called the "warm" zone, to the "cold" zone, where the patients will be decontaminated by the hazmat team. They are then delivered to the prehospital care provider outside the cold zone. The command post, treatment, and triage areas will be outside the cold zone. (See Weapons of Mass Destruction for further hazmat considerations.)

Situation Issues

Crime Scenes

Unfortunately, a sizable percentage of trauma patients encountered by many prehospital care providers, especially in urban settings, are intentionally injured. In addition to shootings and stabbings, patients may be victims of other types of violent crimes, including assaults with fists or blunt objects and attempted strangulation. In other cases, victims may have been intentionally struck by a vehicle

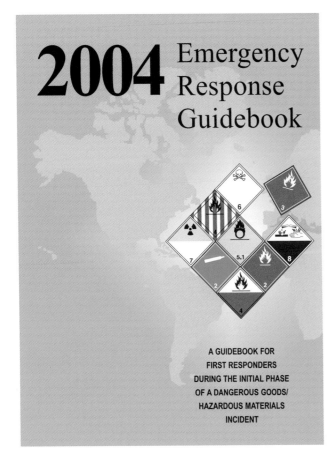

FIGURE 4-5 The *Emergency Response Guidebook* produced by the U.S. Department of Transportation provides critical information at the scene of a potential hazardous material ("hazmat") incident.

FIGURE 4-6 Prehospital care providers often have to manage patients at the scene of a crime and need to collaborate with law enforcement to preserve evidence. (From McSwain N, Paturas J: The *basic EMT,* ed 2, St Louis, 2003, Mosby.)

or pushed from a structure, resulting in a significant fall. Even an MVC can be considered a crime scene, if one of the drivers is thought to be legally intoxicated, driving recklessly, or speeding (Figure 4-6).

When managing these types of patients, prehospital care personnel will interact with law enforcement personnel. Although both EMS and law enforcement share the goal of preserving life, prehospital care providers and law enforcement personnel occasionally find that their duties at a crime scene come into conflict. EMS personnel may focus on the need to assess a victim for signs of life and viability, whereas law enforcement personnel are concerned with preserving evidence at a crime scene or bringing a perpetrator to justice. By being aware of the general approach taken by law enforcement personnel at a crime scene, prehospital care providers not only may aid their patient, but also may better cooperate with law enforcement personnel, leading to the arrest of their patient's assailant.

At the scene of a major crime (homicide, suspicious death, rape, traffic death), most law enforcement agencies will collect and process evidence. Officers will typically perform the following duties:

- Initially canvass the scene to identify all evidence, including weapons and shell casings.
- Photograph the scene.
- Sketch the scene.
- Create a log of everyone who has entered the scene.
- Conduct a more thorough search of the entire scene, looking for all potential evidence.
- Look for and collect trace evidence, ranging from fingerprints to items that may contain DNA evidence (e.g., cigarette butts, strands of hair, fibers).

Police investigators believe that everyone who enters a crime scene brings some type of evidence to the scene and may unknowingly remove some evidence from the scene. To solve the crime, a detective's goal is to identify the evidence deposited and removed by the perpetrator. To accomplish this, the investigators have to account for any evidence left or removed by other law enforcement officers, EMS personnel, and citizens who may have entered the scene. Careless behavior by prehospital care personnel at a crime scene may disrupt, destroy, or contaminate vital evidence, hampering a criminal investigation.

On occasion, prehospital care providers may arrive at a potential crime scene before any law enforcement officers. If the victim is obviously dead, providers can carefully back out of the location without touching any items and await the arrival of officers. Although they would prefer that a crime scene not be disturbed, investigators realize that in some circumstances, prehospital care providers need to turn a body or move objects at a crime scene to access a victim and determine viability. If providers needed to transport a patient or move a body or other objects in the area before the arrival of law enforcement, investigators will typically ascertain the following:

- When were the alterations made to the scene?
- What was the purpose of the movement?
- Who made the alterations?
- At what time was the person's death identified by EMS personnel?

If prehospital care providers entered a crime scene before law enforcement personnel, investigators may want to interview and formally take a statement from the providers regarding their actions or observations. Prehospital care providers should never be alarmed or concerned about such a request. The purpose of the interview is not to critique the actions of the providers but to learn information that may prove helpful to the investigator in solving the case. Investigators may also request to take fingerprints of the prehospital care personnel if items in the crime scene were touched or handled by the crew without gloves.

Proper handling of a patient's clothing may preserve valuable evidence. If a patient's clothing needs to be removed, law enforcement officers and medical examiners prefer that prehospital care providers refrain from cutting through bullet or knife holes in the clothing. If the clothing is cut, investigators may ask what alterations were made to the clothing, who made the alterations, and the reason for alterations. Any clothing that is removed should be placed in a paper (not plastic) bag and turned over to investigators.

One final important issue involving victims of violent crimes is the value of any statements made by the patient while under the care of prehospital care providers. Some patients, realizing the critical nature of their injuries, may tell providers who inflicted their injuries. This information should be documented and passed on to investigators. If possible, prehospital care personnel should inform officers of the critical nature of a patient's injuries so that a sworn officer can be present if the patient is capable of providing any information regarding the perpetrator: a "dying declaration."

Weapons of Mass Destruction

The response to a scene involving hazardous materials, as discussed earlier, includes similar safety and other concerns as the response to the scene involving a weapon of mass destruction (WMD).

Every scene that involves multiple victims or that was reported to have resulted from an explosion should trigger the question of whether a WMD was involved. In particular, when many victims complain of similar symptoms or present with similar findings, a WMD should be considered.

The prehospital care provider needs to approach such scenes with extreme caution and resist the urge to rush in to care for the sickest victim.[5] This natural response of providers only serves to increase the victim count. Instead, the provider can approach the scene from an upwind position and take a moment to stop, look, and listen for clues that will alert the team to the possible presence of a WMD. Obvious spills of wet or dry material, visible vapors, and smoke should be avoided until the nature of the material has been ascertained. Enclosed or confined spaces should never be entered without appropriate personal protective equipment (PPE).

Once a WMD has been included as a possible cause, the prehospital care provider needs to take all appropriate steps for self-protection. These steps include the use of PPE appropriate to the function of the individual provider. Information that this may be a WMD incident should be relayed back to dispatch to alert incoming responders from all services. Staging areas for additional equipment, responders, and helicopters should be established upwind and at a safe distance from the site.

If possible, the scene should be secured and zones indicating hot, warm, and cold areas designated. Sites for decontamination should also be determined. Once the nature of the agent has been determined (chemical, biologic, or radiologic), specific requests for the antidote or antibiotics should be made.

Scene Control Zones

To limit the spread of a hazardous material or WMD, the National Institute of Occupational Safety and Health (NIOSH) and the Environmental Protection Agency (EPA) have developed and advocated the use of control zones. The objective of this concept is to perform specific activities in specific zones. Adherence to such principles reduces the likelihood of spread of contamination and injury to rescue personnel and bystanders.

The zones are three concentric circles (Figure 4-7). The innermost zone, the *hot zone,* is the region immediately adjacent to the hazmat or WMD incident. The task of rescuers in this region is to evacuate the contaminated, injured patient, with no provision of patient care. The next zone, the *warm zone,* is where decontamination of victims, personnel, and equipment occurs. In this zone the only patient care administered is primary assessment and spinal immobilization. The outermost zone, the *cold zone,* is where equipment and personnel are staged. Once the patient is evacuated to the cold zone, providers can deliver definitive

FIGURE 4-7   The scene of a WMD or hazmat incident is generally divided into hot, warm, and cold zones. (From Chapleau W: *Emergency first responder*, St Louis, 2004, Mosby.)

patient care. Table 4-1 lists safe evacuation distances for bomb threats.

If a patient is delivered to the hospital or aid station from a hazmat or WMD scene, it is most prudent to reevaluate if that patient has been decontaminated and to mimic the concepts of these zones.

Decontamination

Whether the incident involves a hazmat situation or a WMD, decontamination of an exposed individual often may be required. *Decontamination* is the reduction or removal of hazardous chemical, biologic, or radiologic agents. The highest priority in the care of an exposed patient, as in any emergency, is personal and scene safety. If there is any question of a continued exposure hazard, assurance of personal safety is the first priority. Failure to do so will only produce an additional victim (the provider) and deprive those already injured of the provider's skills. Decontamination of the patient is the next priority. This will minimize the exposure risk to the provider during assessment and treatment of the patient and will prevent contamination of equipment, thereby avoiding the risk of exposure of other individuals from contaminated equipment and vehicles.

OSHA provides regulatory guidelines for PPE used by prehospital care providers during the emergency care of victims in a potentially hazardous environment. Individuals providing medical care in environments of an unknown

hazard must have a minimum of appropriate training and be supplied and trained with level B protection. Level B protection consists of splash-protective, chemical-resistant clothing and self-contained breathing sources.

If the patient is conscious and able to assist, it is best to enlist their cooperation to have them perform as much of the decontamination as possible to reduce the likelihood of cross-contamination to providers. Carefully remove the patient's clothes as well as jewelry and place these in plastic bags. Transfer the removed clothing carefully so as not to spread any particulate matter or splash any liquid onto noncontaminated personnel or surfaces. Brush any particulate matter off the patient, then irrigate copiously with water. Lavage with water will dilute the concentration of the potentially hazardous material and wash away any remaining agent. A common axiom is, "The solution to pollution is dilution." Successful decontamination will use large amounts of water. A common mistake made by the inexperienced prehospital care provider is to irrigate the patient with water only until the irrigant begins to spill onto the floor, which usually occurs after 1 or 2 L of irrigation. This practice has two problems: the area of body contamination is increased, and the offending agent is not diluted sufficiently to render the agent harmless. Failure to provide adequate runoff and drainage of lavage fluid may cause injury to previously unexposed areas of the body as the contaminated lavage accumulates. One simple way of promoting runoff in a prehospital setting for nonambulatory

TABLE 4-1   Bomb Threats: Safe Evacuation Distances

Threat description	Explosives capacity (TNT capacity) (pounds)	Building evacuation distance (feet)	Outdoor evacuation distance (feet)
Pipe bomb	5	70	850
Briefcase/suitcase bomb	50	150	1850
Compact sedan	500	320	1500
Full-size sedan	1000	400	1750
Passenger/cargo van	4000	650	2750
Small moving van, delivery truck	10,000	860	3750
Moving van, small tank truck	30,000	1240	6500
Semitrailer	60,000	1570	7000

Modified from Messier DM: Explosive Prospects: terrorist bombings present multifaceted response challenge, *Homeland Response* 2(1), 2004.

patients is to place the patient on a backboard and then tilt the backboard with cribbing or other means to elevate an end of the board. Ideally, the contaminated runoff would be collected and disposed of; however, with mass decontamination and large amounts of runoff, it is acceptable to dilute the runoff further and let it run into the sewer system.

Neutralizing agents for chemical burns are typically avoided. Often in the neutralizing process the agents give off heat in an exothermic reaction. Therefore a well-meaning provider may create a thermal burn in addition to the chemical burn. Most commercially available decontamination solutions are made for the purpose of decontaminating equipment, not people.

Decontamination after exposure of chemical warfare agents deserves special consideration. Decontamination of chemical agents can usually be accomplished by copious irrigation and showering with water. Household bleach diluted with water can also be used on intact skin, but decontamination should not be delayed to find bleach. A simple solution of 0.5% hypochlorite solution can be rapidly prepared for decontamination of chemical warfare agents by mixing one part household bleach with nine parts water. This solution can be applied to skin. After irrigation with the 0.5% hypochlorite solution, rinse the area with large amounts of saline or water. Do not use this solution on open head, chest, or abdominal wounds. Also, this solution is contraindicated for use on the eye. M291 is a dry resin used on pads that removes the agent by physical absorption. M291 is useful in decontamination of small, spot areas of skin contaminated with chemical weapon agents.

Secondary Devices

Within months after the bombing at the 1996 Atlanta Summer Olympics, the metropolitan Atlanta area experienced two additional bombings. These bombings, at an abortion clinic and a nightclub, represented the first time in 17 years in the United States that secondary bombs had been planted, presumably to kill or injure rescuers responding to the scene of the first blast. Luckily, in both situations, the secondary devices were identified before their detonation, and no additional injuries occurred. However, all prehospital care personnel need to be mindful of the potential presence of a secondary device. After these incidents, the Georgia Emergency Management Agency developed the following guidelines for rescuers and prehospital care personnel responding to the scene of a bombing where a secondary bomb might be planted[6]:

1. *Refrain from use of electronic devices.* Sound waves from cell phones and radios may cause a secondary device to detonate, especially if used close to the bomb. Equipment used by the news media may also trigger a detonation.

2. *Ensure sufficient boundaries for the scene.* The potential zone of danger (hot zone) should extend 1000 feet in all directions (including vertically) from the original blast site. As more powerful bombs are created, shrapnel may travel further. The initial bomb blast may damage infrastructure, including gas lines and power lines, which may jeopardize the safety of

rescuers. Access to and exit from the hot zone should be carefully controlled.

3. *Provide rapid evacuation of victims from the scene and hot zone.* Because the scene of a bomb blast is considered unsafe, triage of victims should not occur in the hot zone. An EMS command post (or triage area) should be established 2000 to 4000 feet from the scene of the initial bombing. Rescuers can rapidly evacuate victims from the bombing site, with minimal interventions, until victims and rescuers are out of the hot zone.

4. *Collaborate with law enforcement personnel on preserving and recovering evidence.* Bombing sites constitute a crime scene, and rescuers may disrupt the scene only as necessary to evacuate victims. Any potential evidence that is inadvertently removed from the scene with a victim should be documented and turned over to law enforcement personnel to ensure proper chain of custody. Prehospital care personnel can document exactly where they were in the scene and which items they touched.

Command Structure

All hazmat and WMD incidents are assessed using an incident command system, whether formalized or not. An EMT ambulance responding to a call will usually have one person in charge (the incident commander) and another person assisting in a rudimentary incident command structure. As an incident grows larger and more responders from various public safety and other agencies respond to the scene, the need for a formal system and structure to oversee and control the response becomes increasingly important.

Incident Command

The *incident command system* (ICS) has developed over the years as an outgrowth of planning systems used by firefighting services for multiple-service responses to major fire situations. The program gained acceptance particularly from the experience of wildland firefighters battling expansive firefronts, with deployment of dozens of diverse agencies. The collective wisdom of their efforts resulted in FIRESCOPE, or Firefighting Resources of California Organized for Potential Emergencies. Meanwhile, the Phoenix Fire Department developed the Fire Ground Command System (FGC). Although many similarities existed between these two approaches, there were also differences, and attempts were made to combine the two systems into one comprehensive command structure.

In 1987 the National Fire Protection Association (NFPA) published NFPA Standard 1561, the Standard on Fire Department Incident Command Management System. NFPA 1561 was later revised and titled the Standard on Emergency Services Incident Management. This version can be implemented and adjusted to any type or size of event by

any agency managing an incident. In the 1990s the National Fire Incident Management System (IMS) was created, which further refined the single-incident management approach.

Dealing with any incident, large or small, is enhanced by the precise command structure afforded by the ICS. At the core of ICS is the establishment of centralized command at the scene and the subsequent buildup of divisional responsibilities. The first arriving unit establishes the command center, and communications are established through command for the buildup of the response. The five key elements of incident command are as follows:

1. *Command* provides overall control of the event and the communications that will coordinate the movement of resources in and patients out of the incident scene.
2. *Operations* include divisions to handle the tactical needs of the event. Fire suppression, EMS, and rescue are examples of operational divisions.
3. *Planning* is a continuous process of evaluating immediate and potential needs of the incident and planning the response. Throughout the event, this element will be used to evaluate the effectiveness of operations and to make suggested alterations in the response and tactical approach.
4. *Logistics* handles the task of acquiring resources and moving them where needed; these include personnel, shelter, vehicles, and equipment.
5. *Finance* tracks the money. Contractors, personnel, and vendors brought into service in the incident will be tracked so that the cost of the event can be determined and these groups can be paid for goods, supplies, equipment, and services.

Unified Command

An expansion of the ICS is the *unified command system.* This expansion takes into account the needs of coordinating agencies from across jurisdictional boundaries. The technical aspects of bringing resources to bear from multiple communities, counties, and states are covered by this additional coordinating structure.

National Incident Management System

On February 28, 2003, President George W. Bush directed the Secretary of Homeland Security through Presidential Directive HSPD-5 to produce a National Incident Management System (NIMS). This would establish a consistent, nationwide approach for federal, state, and local governments to work effectively together to prepare for, respond to, and recover from domestic incidents regardless of cause, size, or complexity. The Department of Homeland Security authorized NIMS on March 1, 2004, after collaborating with detailed working groups consisting of state and local government officials and representatives of the National Association of Emergency Medical Technicians (NAEMT), Fraternal Order of Police (FOP), International Association of Fire Chiefs (IAFC), and International Association of Emergency Managers (IAEM), as well as a wide range of other public safety organizations.

NIMS focuses on the following incident management characteristics:

- Common terminology
- Modular organization
- Management by objectives
- Reliance on an incident action plan
- Manageable span of control
- Predesignated "incident mobilization center" locations and facilities
- Comprehensive resource management
- Integrated communications
- Establishment of transfer of command
- Chain of command and unity of command
- Unified command
- Accountability of resources and personnel
- Deployment
- Information and intelligence management

The key elements of NIMS are as follows:

1. ICS
2. Communications and information management
3. Preparedness
4. Joint information systems (consistent public information)
5. National Incident Management Integration Center (NIC)

Command

Command comprises the *incident commander* (IC) and command staff. Command staff positions are made as appropriate to the size and nature of the event and may include public information officer (PIO), safety officer (SO), and liaison officer. Other positions can be created as deemed necessary by the IC.

As described earlier, unified command is an enhancement to incident command in situations involving multiple jurisdictions. In a single-command situation, the IC is solely responsible for the incident management. In a unified command structure, individuals representing various jurisdictions jointly determine objectives, plans, and priorities. The unified command system seeks to solve problems involving differences in communications and operational standards (Figure 4-8).

One element not included in ICS that is added with unified command and NIMS is *intelligence.* Based on the size of the event, intelligence and information gathering related to national security may also include risk management assessment, medical intelligence, weather information, structural design of buildings, and information on toxic containment. Although these functions are typically handled in the planning section, in certain situations the IC may separate information gathering from planning.

In NIMS the IC can assign intelligence and information as follows:

- Within the command staff
- As a unit of the planning section
- As a branch of operations
- As a separate general staff function

Incident Action Plans

Incident action plans (IAPs) include overall incident objectives and strategies established by the IC or unified command. The planning section develops and documents the IAP. The IAP also addresses the tactical objectives and support activities for the operational period, which is generally 12 to 24 hours. The planning section also provides an ongoing critique, or "lessons learned" process, to ensure the response meets the needs of the event.

In very large incidents, multiple ICS organizations may be established. Area command may be established to manage multiple ICS organizations. Area command does not have operational responsibilities but will perform the following duties:

1. Set overall incident-related priorities for the agency
2. Allocate critical resources according to established priorities
3. Ensure that incidents are managed properly
4. Ensure effective communications
5. Ensure that incident management objectives are met and do not conflict with each other or with agency policies
6. Identify critical resource needs and report to the Emergency Operations Center(s)
7. Ensure that short-term emergency recovery is coordinated to assist in the transition to full recovery operations
8. Provide for personnel accountability and safe operating environments

Patient Assessment and Triage

Once all the preceding issues have been addressed, the actual process of assessing and treating patients can begin. The greatest challenge occurs when the prehospital care provider is faced with multiple victims.

Mass-casualty incidents (MCIs) occur in many sizes. Most rescuers have responded to incidents with more than one victim, but large-scale events with hundreds to thousands of victims are rarely encountered. *Triage* is a French word meaning "to sort."

In the prehospital environment, triage is used in two different contexts, as follows:

1. **Sufficient resources are available to manage all patients.**
   In this triage situation, the most severely injured patients

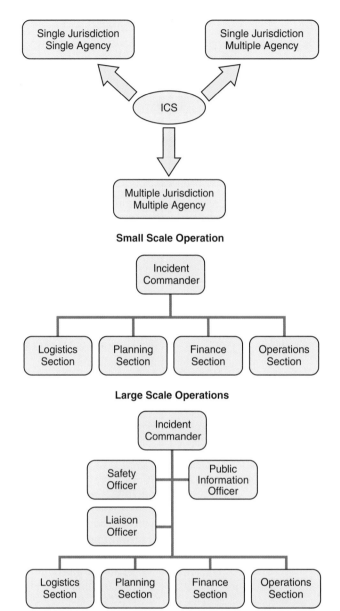

FIGURE 4-8 The incident command structure is flexible and can be expanded or decreased based on the number of patients and the complexity of the event. The operational functions of each of the sections under incident command are the branches. The Medical Services Branch is the operational component that is responsible for coordinating and providing medical services needed to meet the tactical objectives of the incident. This would include martialling equipment and personnel, triage, communications with medical facilities, and transport. *Continued*

are treated and transported first, and those with lesser injuries are treated and transported later.

2. **Triage is primarily used to deal with MCIs in which the number of patients exceeds the immediate capacity of on-scene resources.** The objective in such triage is to ensure survival of the largest possible number of injured patients. Patients are sorted into categories for patient care. In an MCI, patient care must be rationed because the number of patients exceeds the available resources. Relatively few prehospital care providers ever experience an MCI with 80 to 120 simultaneously injured persons, but many will be involved in MCIs with 10 to 20 patients, and most prehospital veterans have managed an incident with 2 to 10 patients.

Incidents that involve sufficient rescuers and medical resources allow for treatment and transport of the most severely injured patients first. In a large-scale MCI, limited

Larger Scale Operation

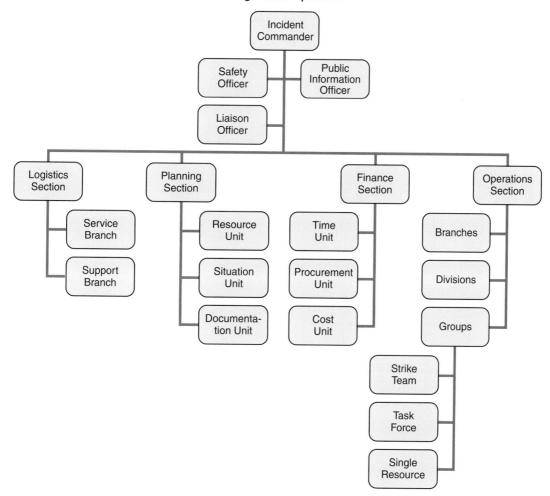

FIGURE 4-8   Cont'd

resources will require that patient treatment and transport be prioritized to salvage the victims with the greatest chance of survival (Figure 4-9). These victims would be prioritized for transport.

The goal of patient management at the MCI scene is to do the most good for the most patients with the resources available. It is the responsibility of the prehospital care provider to make decisions about who is to be managed first. The usual rules about saving lives are different in MCIs. The decision is always to save the most lives; however, when the available resources are not sufficient for the needs of all the injured patients present, these resources should be used for the patients who have the best chance of surviving. In a choice between a patient with a catastrophic injury such as severe brain trauma and a patient with acute intra-abdominal hemorrhage, the proper course of action in an MCI is to manage first the salvageable patient—the victim with the abdominal hemorrhage. Treating the patient with severe head trauma first will probably result in the loss of both patients; the head trauma patient may die because he or she may not be salvageable, and the abdominal hemorrhage patient may die because time, equipment, and personnel spent managing the unsalvageable patient kept this salvageable patient from receiving the simple care needed to survive until definitive surgical care was available.

In a triage MCI situation, the catastrophically injured patient may need to be considered "lower priority," with treatment delayed until more help and equipment become available. These are difficult circumstances, but a prehospital care provider must respond quickly and properly. A medical care team should not make efforts to resuscitate a traumatic cardiac arrest patient with little or no chance of survival while three other patients die because of airway compromise or external hemorrhage. The "sorting scheme" most often used divides patients into five categories based on need of care and chance of survival, as follows:

1. *Immediate.* Patients whose injuries are critical but who will require only minimal time or equipment to manage and who have a good prognosis for survival.

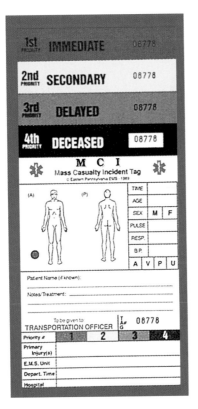

FIGURE 4-9 Example of a triage tag.
(From McSwain N, Paturas J: *The basic EMT,* ed 2, St Louis, 2003, Mosby.)

An example is the patient with a compromised airway or massive external hemorrhage.

2. *Delayed.* Patients whose injuries are debilitating but who do not require immediate management to salvage life or limb. An example is the patient with a long-bone fracture.

3. *Minor.* Patients, often called the "walking wounded," who have minor injuries that can wait for treatment or who may even assist in the interim by comforting other patients or helping as litter bearers.

4. *Expectant.* Patients whose injuries are so severe that they have only a minimal chance of survival. An example is the patient with a 90% full-thickness burn and thermal pulmonary injury.

5. *Dead.* Patients who are unresponsive, pulseless, and breathless. In a disaster, resources rarely allow for attempted resuscitation of cardiac arrest patients.

Box 4-3 describes the accepted triage scheme known as START, which uses only four categories: Immediate, Delayed, Minor, and Dead.

BOX 4-3   START Triage

Triage is the basic tool used to manage victims at a multicasualty incident. It helps prehospital care providers and other rescuers efficiently use the available resources. Precious time can be wasted if providers do not have a simple triage tool to identify those patients most at risk for early death. Failure to perform triage will prolong time at the incident and delay definitive treatment.

In 1983, medical personnel from Hoag Memorial Hospital and firefighter paramedics from the Newport Beach Fire Department created a triage process for first responders, *Simple Triage and Rapid Treatment* (START) (Figure 4-10). This triage process was designed to identify critically injured patients easily and quickly. START does not establish a medical diagnosis but instead provides a rapid and simple sorting process.

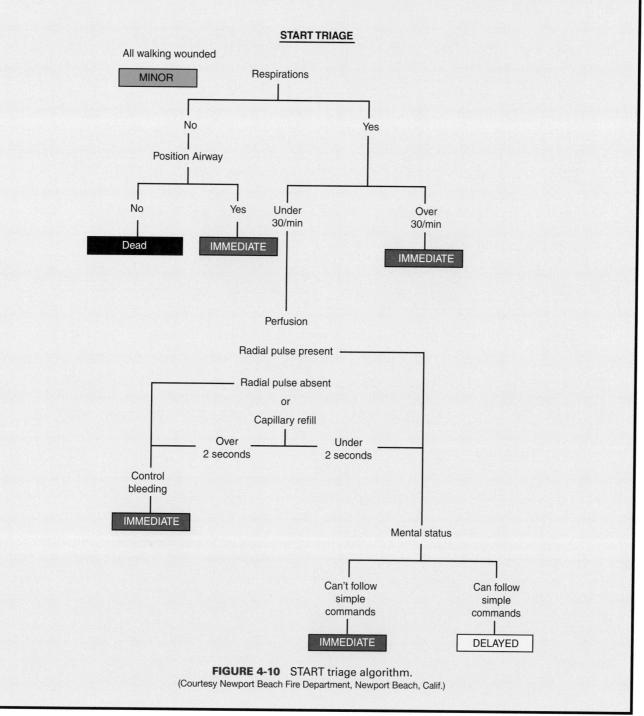

FIGURE 4-10   START triage algorithm.
(Courtesy Newport Beach Fire Department, Newport Beach, Calif.)

Continued

BOX 4-3 START Triage—cont'd

START uses three simple assessments to identify those victims most at risk to die from their injuries. Typically, the process takes 30 to 60 seconds per victim. START requires no tools, specialized medical equipment, or special knowledge.

HOW DOES IT WORK?

The first step is to direct anyone who can walk to a designated safe area. If the victims can walk and follow commands, their condition is categorized as "minor," and they will be further triaged and tagged when more rescuers arrive. This now leads to a smaller group of injured victims remaining for rescuers to triage. The mnemonic "30-2-can-do" is used as the START triage prompt. The "30" refers to the patient's respiratory rate, the "2" refers to capillary refill, and the "can-do" refers to the ability of the patient to follow commands. Any victim with respirations fewer than 30 per minute, capillary refill of less than 2 seconds, and the ability to follow verbal commands and who can walk is categorized as a "minor" patient. When victims meet these criteria but cannot walk, they are categorized as "delayed." Victims who are unconscious or have rapid breathing or who have delayed capillary refill or absent radial pulse are categorized as "immediate." Any of these physiologic abnormalities can be caused by serious injuries. While at the victim's side, two basic lifesaving measures can be performed: opening the airway and controlling external hemorrhage. Bystanders or the "walking wounded"

Respirations	**30**
Perfusion	**2**
Mental status	**CAN DO**

can be directed by the rescuer to maintain these simple interventions. For those victims who are not breathing, the rescuer should open the airway, and if breathing resumes, the victim is categorized as "immediate." No cardiopulmonary resuscitation (CPR) should be attempted. If the victim does not resume breathing, the victim is categorized as "dead."

Retriage is also needed if lack of transportation prolongs the time the victims remain at the scene. Using START criteria, significantly injured victims may be categorized as "delayed." The longer they remain without treatment, the greater the chance their condition will deteriorate. Therefore, repeat evaluation and triage are appropriate over time.

SUMMARY

To do the most good for the most people, to make sure that provider personnel and equipment are not compromised and unavailable for others, and to ensure that other health care professionals are protected from hazards that are not identified, isolated, or removed, it is important that prehospital care providers assess for hazards as a part of assessing for scene safety with each patient situation. Sometimes hazards will be ruled out quickly, but if they are not looked for, they won't be seen, and this is what can cause harm.

SCENARIO SOLUTION

Providing emergency medical care along roadsides ranks as one of the most dangerous situations encountered by prehospital care providers. Assessment of the scene reveals many potential hazards, the most apparent being the environmental conditions. Rain not only obscures vision, but also makes the roadway slippery and increases stopping distances. Lying on the ground in the rain, combined with nighttime temperatures, may predispose the patient to hypothermia. The darkness adds to the risk and makes it imperative that personnel wear reflective clothing. Law enforcement personnel are essential for traffic control along the scene. A damaged utility pole creates the risk of downed power lines, and the electrical company should be notified to respond. Fuel spills and other vehicle fluids may create a hazardous material situation. Fire department personnel can isolate or neutralize the fluids while monitoring the scene for fires that may erupt. In addition, a bloody patient exposes prehospital care personnel to the risks of bloodborne infections, and the caregivers should wear physical barriers, including gloves, masks, and eye protection. ■

Note: Now that the scene has been assessed, this scenario is continued in Chapter 5.

References

1. Maguire BJ, Hunting KL, Smith GS, Levick NR: Occupational fatalities in emergency medical services, *Ann Emerg Med* 40(6):625, 2002.
2. National Highway Traffic and Safety Administration: Traffic safety facts, 2003, http://www-nrd.nhtsa.dot.gov/pdf/nrd-30/NCSA/TSFAAnn/2003/cov2.htm.
3. Schaeffer J: Prevent run downs: best practices for roadside incident management, 2002, http://www.jems.com/jems/news02/0903a.html (accessed September 2002).
4. Poland GA, Jacobson RM: Prevention of hepatitis B with the hepatitis B vaccine, *N Engl J Med* 351:2832, 2004.
5. Georgia Emergency Management Agency: Surviving weapons of mass destruction, www.ojp.usdoj.gov/odp/docs/video.htm.
6. Georgia Emergency Management Agency, Department of Justice Bureau of Justice Assistance: Surviving the secondary device: the rules have changed, www.ojp.usdoj.gov/odp/docs/video.htm.

Rinnert KJ: A review of infection control practices, risk reduction, and legislative regulations for blood-borne disease: applications for emergency medical services, *Prehosp Emerg Care* 2(1):70, 1998.

Rinnert KJ, O'Connor RE, Delbridge T: Risk reduction for exposure to blood-borne pathogens in EMS: National Association of EMS Physicians, *Prehosp Emerg Care* 2(1):62, 1998.

Suggested Reading

Centers for Disease Control and Prevention: See website for information on Standard Precautions and postexposure prophylaxis, www.cdc.gov.

Training Resoures

Federal Emergency Management Agency (FEMA): Incident command system (ICS) training:

ICS-100, Introduction to ICS

ICS-200, Basic ICS

ICS-300, Intermediate ICS

ICS-400, Advanced ICS

National Incident Management System (NIMS) and FEMA training: Contact your state Emergency Management Agency or Emergency Management Institute and National Fire Academy, Emmitsburg, Md. A variety of online correspondence and on-site courses are available.

For more information on NIMS, contact the NIMS Integrations Center: www.dhs.gov.

Chapter Objectives

At the completion of this chapter, the reader will be able to do the following:

✓ Provide an illustration of the significance of patient assessment in the context of overall management of the trauma patient.

✓ Systematize the discrete steps involved in assessing and managing the trauma patient into an organized and rational process.

✓ Given a scenario, adapt the 15-second global survey and primary survey to the particulars of the situation.

✓ Employ a process of critical questioning to associate examination and scene findings with their likely causes and consequences.

CHAPTER 5

Patient

SCENARIO

You are awakened at 0400 on a Saturday to respond to the scene of a person struck by a vehicle. As you go to the ambulance, you notice that it is raining; the temperature is 50° F (10° C). Dispatch provides the additional information that after hitting the pedestrian, the vehicle crashed into a utility pole. Fluid from the vehicle is leaking onto the street, leaving a sheet on the rainwater. According to dispatch, bystanders report that the patient lost consciousness. On arrival, you detect no additional threats to safety in your scene assessment. Bystanders confirm that they witnessed the patient's loss of consciousness for a period of "several minutes." Approaching the patient, a young adult female, you kneel at her head, observing that she is conscious and her clothes are wet, and you position your hands to provide cervical spine stabilization. In response to your questioning, you discover that the patient's chief complaint is leg pain. Your questioning serves the dual purpose of obtaining the patient's complaint and assessing her ventilatory effort by noting that speech is difficult only because of her chattering teeth. Detecting no shortness of breath, you proceed with further questioning as your partner obtains the patient's vital signs. The patient answers your questions appropriately to establish that she is oriented to person, place, and event.

Based on kinematics as they relate to pedestrian versus motor vehicle injuries, what are the problems for which you should maintain a high index of suspicion in your assessment? What are your next priorities? How will you proceed with this patient? ■

Assessment is the cornerstone of excellent patient care. For the trauma patient, as for other critically ill patients, assessment is the foundation on which all management and transportation decisions are based. The first goal in assessment is to determine a patient's current condition. In doing so, the prehospital care provider can develop an overall impression of a patient's condition and establish baseline values for the status of the patient's respiratory, circulatory, and neurologic systems. The provider then rapidly assesses life-threatening conditions and initiates urgent intervention and resuscitation. The prehospital care provider identifies and addresses any conditions that require attention before a patient is moved. If time allows, the provider conducts a secondary survey of non–life-or-limb-threatening injuries. Often this occurs during transportation of the patient.

The prehospital care provider performs all these steps quickly and efficiently, with a goal of minimizing time spent on the scene. Critical patients cannot remain in the field for care other than that needed to stabilize them for transport, unless they are trapped or other complications exist that prevent early transportation. By applying the principles learned in this course, a prehospital care provider can minimize on-scene delay and rapidly move patients to an appropriate medical facility. Successful assessment and intervention require a strong knowledge base of trauma physiology and a well-thought-out plan of management that is carried out quickly and effectively.

The trauma management literature frequently mentions the need to transport the trauma patient to definitive surgical care within an absolute minimum amount of time after the onset of the injury. This is because a critical trauma patient who does not respond to initial therapy is most likely bleeding internally. This blood loss will continue until the hemorrhage can be controlled. Except for the most basic external bleeding, this hemorrhage control can be accomplished only in the operating room (OR).

The primary concerns for assessment and management of the trauma patient, in order of importance, are (1) airway, (2) ventilation, (3) oxygenation, (4) hemorrhage control, (5) perfusion, and (6) neurologic function. This sequence protects the ability of the body to oxygenate and the ability of the red blood cells (RBCs) to deliver oxygen to the tissues. Hemorrhage control, which is only temporary in the field but permanent in the OR, depends on rapid transportation by the prehospital care providers and the presence of a trauma team who is immediately available on arrival at the medical facility.

R. Adams Cowley, MD, developed the concept of the "Golden Hour" of trauma. He believed that the time between injury occurrence and definitive care was critical. During this period, when bleeding is uncontrolled and inadequate tissue oxygenation is occurring because of decreased perfusion, damage occurs throughout the body. If bleeding is not controlled and tissue oxygenation is not restored within 1 hour of the injury, the patient's chances of survival plummet.

The Golden Hour is now referred to as the "Golden Period" because some patients have less than an hour to receive care whereas others have more time. A prehospital care provider is responsible for transporting a patient as quickly as possible to a facility where definitive care can be accomplished. To deliver the trauma patient to definitive care, the prehospital care provider quickly identifies the seriousness of the patient's life-threatening injuries; provides only essential, lifesaving care at the scene; and provides for rapid transportation to an appropriate medical facility. In many urban prehospital systems, the average time between injury and arrival on the scene is 8 to 9 minutes. The prehospital care providers spend another 8 to 9 minutes transporting the patient. If the providers spend only 10 minutes on the scene, 30 minutes of the Golden Period will have passed by the time a patient arrives at the receiving facility. Every additional minute spent on the scene is additional time that the patient is bleeding, and valuable time is taken away from the Golden Period. To address this critical trauma management issue, quick, efficient evaluation and management of the patient is the ultimate objective. Scene time should not exceed 10 minutes; the shorter the scene time, the better. The longer the patient is kept on scene, the greater the potential for blood loss and death. These time parameters change as delayed extrication, delayed transportation, and other unexpected circumstances arise.

This chapter covers the essentials of patient assessment and initial management in the field and is based on the approach taught to physicians in the Advanced Trauma Life Support (ATLS) program.[1] The principles described are identical to those learned in initial basic or advanced provider training programs, although different terminology may occasionally be used. For example, the phrase "primary survey" is used in the ATLS and Prehospital Trauma Life Support (PHTLS) programs to describe the patient assessment activity known as "initial assessment" in a U.S. Department of Transportation (DOT) Emergency Medical Technician (EMT) course. What the PHTLS course refers to as the "secondary survey" is essentially the same activity that the basic provider learns as either the "detailed history and physical examination" or the "focused history and physical examination" of the trauma patient. For the most part, the activities performed in each phase are exactly the same; the various courses simply use different terminology. Similarly, activities of monitoring and reassessing the patient are called the "ongoing assessment" in the DOT system (Table 5-1).

TABLE 5-1   Assessment Terminology

PHTLS	EMT National Standard Curricula
Scene assessment	Scene size-up
Primary survey	Initial assessment
Secondary survey	Detailed or focused history and physical examination
Monitoring and reassessment	Ongoing assessment

Establishing Priorities

The prehospital care provider has three priorities on arrival to a scene, as follows:

1. The first priority for everyone involved at a trauma incident is assessment of the scene. Chapter 4 discusses this in detail.
2. The prehospital care provider needs to recognize the existence of multiple-patient incidents and mass-casualty incidents (MCIs). In an MCI the priority shifts from focusing all resources on the most injured patient to saving the maximum number of patients (providing the greatest good to the greatest number). Chapter 4 also discusses triage.
3. Once the prehospital care providers have performed a brief scene assessment, they should turn their attention to evaluating individual patients. They begin the assessment and management process by focusing on the patient or patients who have been identified as most critical, as resources allow. Emphasis is placed on the following, in this order: (a) conditions that may result in the loss of life, (b) conditions that may result in the loss of limb, and (c) all other conditions that do not threaten life or limb. Depending on the severity of the injury, the number of injured patients, and the proximity to the receiving facility, the prehospital care provider may never address the conditions that do not threaten life or limb.

Most of this chapter focuses on the *critical thinking* skills required for prehospital care providers to learn to conduct a proper assessment, interpret the findings, and set priorities for proper patient care.

Primary Survey (Initial Assessment)

In the critical multisystem trauma patient, the priority for the prehospital care provider is the rapid identification and management of life-threatening conditions (Box 5-1). More than 90% of trauma patients have simple injuries that involve only one system (e.g., an isolated limb fracture). For these single-system trauma patients, the prehospital care provider has time to be thorough in both the primary and the secondary survey. For the critically injured patient, the provider may never conduct more than a primary survey. The emphasis is on rapid evaluation, initiation of resuscitation, and transportation to an appropriate medical facility. This does not eliminate the need for prehospital management; it means that the prehospital care provider

---

BOX 5-1 Multisystem versus Single-System Trauma Patient

- A *multisystem trauma patient* has injuries involving more than one body system, including the pulmonary, circulatory, neurologic, gastrointestinal, musculoskeletal, and integumentary systems. An example would be a patient involved in a motor vehicle crash who has a traumatic brain injury, pulmonary contusions, a splenic injury with shock, and a femur fracture.
- A *single-system trauma patient* has injury to only one body system. An example would be a patient with a simple ankle fracture and no evidence of blood loss or shock.

---

needs to *do it faster, do it more efficiently, and do it en route to the receiving facility.*

Quick establishment of priorities and the initial evaluation of life-threatening injuries must be routine. Therefore the prehospital care provider needs to memorize the components of the primary and secondary surveys by understanding the logical progression of priority-based assessment and treatment. A prehospital care provider has to think about the pathophysiology of a patient's injuries and conditions; the provider cannot waste time trying to remember which priorities are the most important.

The most common basis of life-threatening injuries is lack of adequate tissue oxygenation, which leads to anaerobic (without oxygen) metabolism (energy production). Decreased energy production that occurs with anaerobic metabolism is termed *shock*. Three components are necessary for normal metabolism: (1) oxygenation of RBCs in the lungs, (2) delivery of RBCs to the cells throughout the body, and (3) offloading of oxygen to these cells. The activities involved in the primary survey are aimed at identifying and correcting problems with the first two components.

General Impression

The primary survey begins with a simultaneous, or *global,* overview of the status of a patient's respiratory, circulatory, and neurologic systems to identify obvious significant external problems with oxygenation, circulation, hemorrhage, or gross deformities. When approaching a patient, the prehospital care provider observes whether the patient appears to be moving air effectively, is awake or unresponsive, is holding himself or herself up, and is moving spontaneously. Once at the patient's side, a reasonable starting point is to ask the patient, "What happened to you?" If the patient answers with a coherent explanation in complete sentences, the prehospital care provider can conclude that the patient has a patent airway, sufficient respiratory function to support speech, adequate cerebral perfusion, and reasonable neurologic functioning; that is, there are probably no immediate threats to this patient's life.

If a patient is unable to provide such an answer, the prehospital care provider begins a detailed primary survey to identify life-threatening problems. While asking follow-up questions (e.g., "Where do you hurt?"), respiratory function is observed and airway patency is further assessed. A quick check of the radial pulse allows the prehospital care provider to evaluate the presence, quality, and rate (very fast, very slow, or generally normal) of circulatory activity. The provider can simultaneously feel the temperature and moistness of the skin while noting skin color and capillary refill. The patient's level of consciousness and mentation are determined by the appropriateness of verbal responses. The prehospital care provider then scans the patient from head to foot, looking for signs of hemorrhage while gathering all the preliminary data for the primary survey. During this time, the provider has taken a quick, overall look at the patient, making the first few seconds with the patient a global survey of overall condition and an evaluation of life-threatening possibilities. The provider can classify the information according to priorities, categorize the severity of the patient's injuries and conditions, and identify which injury or condition needs to be managed first. Within 15 to 30 seconds, the prehospital care provider has gained a general impression of the patient's overall condition.

The general impression establishes whether the patient is presently or imminently in a critical condition and rapidly evaluates the patient's overall systemic condition. The general impression often provides all the information necessary to determine whether additional resources, such as advanced life support (ALS), are required. If helicopter transportation to a trauma facility is appropriate, this is often when the prehospital care provider decides to request the helicopter. Delay in deciding that additional resources are necessary will only extend on-scene time. Early decision making will ultimately shorten scene time. Once the prehospital care provider gains a general impression of the patient's condition, he or she can rapidly complete the primary survey unless a complication requires more care or evaluation.

The primary survey must proceed rapidly. The following discussion addresses the specific components of the primary survey and the order of priority for optimal patient management.

The following are the five steps involved in the primary survey, in order of priority:

A—Airway management and cervical spine stabilization
B—Breathing (ventilation)
C—Circulation and bleeding
D—Disability
E—Expose/environment

Step A—Airway Management and Cervical Spine Stabilization
Airway

The prehospital care provider should check the patient's airway quickly to ensure that it is *patent* (open and clear) and that no danger of obstruction exists. If the airway is compromised, the prehospital care provider will have to open it initially using manual methods (trauma chin lift or trauma jaw thrust) and clear blood and body substances if necessary (Figure 5-1). Eventually, as equipment and time become available, airway management can advance to mechanical means (oral airway, nasal airway, or endotracheal intubation) or to transtracheal methods (percutaneous transtracheal ventilation) (see Chapter 6).

Cervical Spine Stabilization

As a prehospital care provider learns in an initial training program, every trauma patient with a significant mechanism of injury is suspected of spinal injury until spinal injury is conclusively ruled out. (See Chapter 9 for a complete list of indications for spinal immobilization.) Therefore, when establishing an open airway, the prehospital care provider needs to remember that a possibility of cervical spine injury exists. Excessive movement could either aggravate or produce neurologic damage because bony compression may occur in the presence of a fractured spine. The solution is to ensure that the patient's neck is manually maintained in the neutral position during the opening of the airway and the administration of necessary ventilation. This does not mean that the prehospital care provider cannot or should not apply the necessary airway maintenance procedures just described. Instead, it means that the provider will perform the procedures while protecting the patient's spine from unnecessary movement. After initiating precautions for cervical injury, the prehospital care provider immobilizes the patient's entire spine. Therefore the patient's entire body must be in line and secured.

Step B—Breathing (Ventilation)

The prehospital care provider will first effectively deliver oxygen to a patient's lungs to fuel the metabolic process. Hypoxia can result from inadequate ventilation of the lungs and leads to lack of oxygenation to the patient's tissues. Once the patient's airway is open, the quality and quantity of the patient's breathing (ventilation) can be evaluated, as follows:

1. Check to see if the patient is breathing.
2. If the patient is not breathing (apneic), immediately begin assisting ventilations with a bag-valve-mask (BVM) device with supplemental oxygen before continuing the assessment.
3. Ensure that the patient's airway is patent, continue assisted ventilation and prepare to insert an oral or nasal airway, intubate, or provide other means of mechanical airway protection.
4. If the patient is breathing, estimate the adequacy of the ventilatory rate and depth to determine whether the patient is moving enough air, and assess oxygenation. Ensure that the inspired oxygen concentration is 85% or greater.
5. Quickly observe the patient's chest rise, and if the patient is conscious, listen to the patient talk to assess whether he or she can speak a full sentence without difficulty.

The ventilatory rate can be divided into the following five levels:

1. *Apneic.* The patient is not breathing.
2. *Slow.* A very low ventilatory rate may indicate ischemia (decreased supply of oxygen) of the brain. If the ventilatory rate has dropped to 12 breaths/min or less (*bradypnea*), the prehospital care provider either assists or completely takes over the patient's breathing with a BVM device. Assisted or total ventilatory support with the BVM device should include supplemental oxygen that achieves an oxygen concentration of 85% or greater, or a fraction of inspired oxygen (Fio_2) of 0.85 or greater (Table 5-2).

FIGURE 5-1   If the airway appears compromised, it must be opened while continuing to protect the spine.

Although commonly referred to as the "respiratory rate," a more correct term is *ventilatory rate. Ventilation* refers to the process of inhalation and exhalation, whereas *respiration* best describes the physiologic process of gas exchange between the arteries and the alveoli. This text uses the term *ventilatory rate* rather than *respiratory rate.*

TABLE 5-2   Airway Management Based on Spontaneous Ventilation Rate

Ventilatory rate (breaths/min)	Management
Slow (<12)	Assisted or total ventilation with ≥85% oxygen (Fio$_2$ ≥0.85)
Normal (12-20)	Observation; consider supplemental oxygen
Too fast (20-30)	Administration of ≥85% oxygen (Fio$_2$ ≥0.85)
Abnormally fast (>30)	Assisted ventilation (Fio$_2$ ≥0.85)

Fio$_2$, Fraction of inspired oxygen concentration.

3. *Normal.* If the ventilatory rate is between 12 and 20 breaths/min (*eupnea,* a normal rate for an adult), the prehospital care provider watches the patient closely. Although the patient may appear stable, supplemental oxygen should be considered.

4. *Fast.* If the ventilatory rate is between 20 and 30 breaths/min *(tachypnea),* the prehospital care provider again watches the patient closely. The provider determines whether the patient is improving or deteriorating. The drive for increasing the ventilatory rate is increased accumulation of carbon dioxide (CO_2) in the blood or a decreased level of blood oxygen (O_2). When a patient displays an abnormal ventilatory rate, the provider investigates why. A rapid rate indicates that not enough oxygen is reaching the body tissue. This lack of oxygen initiates anaerobic metabolism (see Chapter 7) and ultimately an increase in CO_2. The body's detection system recognizes an increased level of CO_2 and tells the ventilatory system to speed up to exhale this excess. Therefore an increased ventilatory rate may indicate that the patient needs better perfusion or oxygenation, or both. Administration of supplemental oxygen to achieve an oxygen concentration of 85% or greater (Fio$_2$ ≥0.85) is indicated for this patient, at least until the patient's overall status is determined. The provider will be suspicious of the patient's ability to maintain adequate ventilation and remains alert for any deterioration in overall condition.

5. *Abnormally fast.* A ventilatory rate greater than 30 breaths/min *(severe tachypnea)* indicates hypoxia, anaerobic metabolism, or both, with a resultant acidosis. The prehospital care provider immediately begins assisted ventilation with a BVM device with supplemental oxygen that achieves an oxygen concentration of 85% or greater (Fio$_2$ ≥0.85). A search for the cause of the rapid ventilatory rate should begin

at once. Is this an oxygenation problem or an RBC delivery problem? Once the cause is identified, the prehospital care provider will intervene immediately.

In the patient with abnormal ventilation, the prehospital care provider exposes, observes, and palpates the chest rapidly. The provider auscultates the lungs to identify abnormal, diminished, or absent breath sounds. Injuries that may impede ventilation include tension pneumothorax, spinal cord injuries, and traumatic brain injuries. These injuries should be identified during the primary survey and require that ventilatory support be initiated at once.

When assessing the trauma patient's ventilatory status, the prehospital care provider assesses the ventilatory *depth* as well as the *rate.* A patient can be breathing at a normal ventilatory rate of 16 breaths/min but have a greatly decreased ventilatory depth. Conversely, a patient can have a normal ventilatory depth but an increased or decreased ventilatory rate. The ventilatory depth and rate combine to produce the *total minute ventilation* of the patient (see Chapter 6).

Step C—Circulation (Hemorrhage and Perfusion)

Assessing for circulatory system compromise or failure is the next step in caring for the trauma patient. Oxygenation of the RBCs without delivery to the tissue cells is of no benefit to the patient. In the primary survey of a trauma patient, the prehospital care provider needs to identify and control external hemorrhage. The provider can then obtain an adequate overall estimate of the patient's cardiac output and perfusion status.

Hemorrhage Control

The prehospital care provider identifies and controls external hemorrhage in the primary survey. Hemorrhage control is included in circulation because if gross bleeding is not controlled as soon as possible, the potential for the patient's death increases dramatically. The three types of external hemorrhage are as follows:

1. *Capillary bleeding* is caused by abrasions that have scraped open the tiny capillaries just below the skin's surface. Usually capillary bleeding will have slowed or even stopped before the arrival of prehospital care.

2. *Venous bleeding* is from deeper areas within the tissue and is usually controlled with a small amount of direct pressure. Venous bleeding is usually not life threatening unless the injury is severe or blood loss is not controlled.

3. *Arterial bleeding* is caused by an injury that has lacerated an artery. This is the most important and most difficult type of blood loss to control. It is characterized by spurting blood that is bright red in

color. Even a small, deep arterial puncture wound can produce life-threatening arterial blood loss.

Hemorrhage control is a priority because every red blood cell counts. Rapid control of blood loss is one of the most important goals in the care of a trauma patient. The primary survey cannot advance unless hemorrhage is controlled.

In cases of external hemorrhage, application of direct pressure will control most major hemorrhage until the prehospital care provider can move the patient to a location where an OR and adequate equipment are available. The prehospital care provider needs to initiate hemorrhage control and maintain it throughout transport. The provider may require assistance to accomplish both ventilation and bleeding control.

The prehospital care provider can control hemorrhage in the following ways:

1. *Direct pressure.* Direct pressure is exactly what the name implies—applying pressure to the site of bleeding. The prehospital care provider accomplishes this by placing a dressing (e.g., 4 × 4–inch gauze) or abdominal pads directly over the site and applying pressure. Applying direct pressure will require all of one provider's attention, preventing the provider from continuing patient care. However, if assistance is limited, a pressure dressing can be fashioned out of gauze pads and an elastic bandage. If bleeding is not controlled, it will not matter how much oxygen or fluid the patient receives; perfusion will not improve in the face of ongoing hemorrhage.
2. *Tourniquets.* In the previous edition of this text, tourniquets were described as the technique of "last resort." Military experience in Afghanistan and Iraq, plus the routine and safe use of tourniquets by surgeons, has led to reconsideration of this approach. The use of "elevation" and pressure on "pressure points" is no longer recommended because of insufficient data supporting their effectiveness.[2] Tourniquets are very effective in controlling severe hemorrhage and should be used if direct pressure or a pressure dressing fails to control hemorrhage from an extremity.

If internal hemorrhage is suspected, the prehospital care provider quickly exposes the patient's abdomen to inspect and palpate for signs of injury. The provider also palpates the pelvis because a pelvic fracture is a major source of intraabdominal bleeding. Pelvic fractures are managed with rapid transport, use of a pneumatic antishock garment (PASG), and rapid, warm intravenous (IV) fluid replacement.

Many causes of hemorrhage are not easy to control outside the hospital. The prehospital treatment is rapid delivery of the patient to a facility equipped and staffed for rapid control of hemorrhage in the OR (e.g., trauma center, if available).

Perfusion

The prehospital care provider can obtain the patient's overall circulatory status by checking the pulse; skin color, temperature, and moisture; and capillary refilling time.

Pulse. The prehospital care provider evaluates the pulse for presence, quality, and regularity. The presence of a palpable peripheral pulse also provides an estimate of blood pressure. A quick check of the pulse reveals whether the patient has tachycardia, bradycardia, or an irregular rhythm. It can also reveal information about the systolic blood pressure. If a radial pulse is not palpable in an uninjured extremity, the patient has likely entered the *decompensated phase* of shock, a late sign of the patient's critical condition. In the primary survey, determination of an exact pulse rate is not necessary. Instead, a gross estimate is rapidly obtained, and assessment moves on to other gross evaluations. The actual pulse rate is obtained later in the process. If the patient lacks a palpable carotid or femoral pulse, he or she is in cardiopulmonary arrest (see later discussion).

Skin

Color. Adequate perfusion produces a pinkish hue to the skin. Skin becomes pale when blood is shunted away from an area. Bluish coloration indicates incomplete oxygenation. Pale coloration is associated with poor perfusion. The bluish color is caused by lack of blood or oxygen to that region of the body. Skin pigmentation can often make this determination difficult. Examination of the color of nail beds and mucous membranes serves to overcome this challenge because these changes in color usually first appear in the lips, gums, or fingertips.

Temperature. As with overall skin evaluation, skin temperature is influenced by environmental conditions. Cool skin indicates decreased perfusion, regardless of the cause. The prehospital care provider usually assesses skin temperature by touching the patient with the back of the hand; therefore an accurate determination can be difficult with gloves donned. Normal skin temperature is warm to touch, neither cool nor hot. Normally the blood vessels are not dilated and do not bring the heat of the body to the surface of the skin.

Moisture. Dry skin indicates good perfusion. Moist skin is associated with shock and decreased perfusion. This decrease in perfusion is caused by blood being shunted to the core organs of the body through the vasoconstriction of peripheral vessels.

Capillary Refilling Time. The prehospital care provider checks capillary refilling time by pressing over the nail beds. This removes the blood from the visible capillary bed. The rate of return of blood to the beds (refilling time) is a tool in estimating blood flow through this most distal part of circulation. A capillary refilling time of greater than 2 seconds indicates that the capillary beds are not receiving adequate perfusion. However, capillary refilling time by itself is a poor indicator of shock because it is influenced by so many other factors. For example, peripheral vascular disease (arteriosclerosis), cold temperatures, the use of pharmacologic vasodilators or constrictors, or the presence of neurogenic shock can skew the result. Refilling becomes a less useful check of cardiovascular function in these cases. Capillary refilling time has a place in the evaluation of circulatory adequacy, but it should always be used in conjunction with other physical examination findings, just as the prehospital care provider uses other indicators (e.g., blood pressure).

Step D—Disability

Having evaluated and corrected, to the extent possible, the factors involved in delivering oxygen to the lungs and circulating it throughout the body, the next step in the primary survey is assessment of cerebral function, which is an indirect measurement of cerebral oxygenation. The goal is to determine the patient's level of consciousness (LOC) and ascertain the potential for hypoxia.

The prehospital care provider can infer that a belligerent, combative, or uncooperative patient is hypoxic until proved otherwise. Most patients want help when their lives are medically threatened. If a patient refuses help, the reason must be questioned. Why does the patient feel threatened by the presence of a prehospital care provider on the scene? If the patient appears threatened by the situation, the provider needs to establish rapport and gain the patient's trust. If nothing in the situation seems to be threatening, the provider can assume that the source is physiologic and identify and treat reversible conditions. During the assessment, the provider determines from the history whether the patient lost consciousness at any time since the injury occurred, what toxic substances might be involved, and whether the patient has any preexisting conditions that may produce a decreased LOC or aberrant behavior.

A decreased LOC alerts a prehospital care provider to the following four possibilities:

1. Decreased cerebral oxygenation (caused by hypoxia/hypoperfusion)
2. Central nervous system (CNS) injury
3. Drug or alcohol overdose
4. Metabolic derangement (diabetes, seizure, cardiac arrest)

The Glasgow Coma Scale (GCS) score is a tool used for determining LOC.[3] It is a quick, simple method for determining cerebral function and is predictive of patient

Eye Opening	Points
Spontaneous eye opening	4
Eye opening on command	3
Eye opening to painful stimulus	2
No eye opening	1
Best Verbal Response	
Answers appropriately (oriented)	5
Gives confused answers	4
Inappropriate response	3
Makes unintelligible noises	2
Makes no verbal response	1
Best Motor Response	
Follows command	6
Localizes painful stimuli	5
Withdrawal to pain	4
Responds with abnormal flexion to painful stimuli (decorticate)	3
Responds with abnormal extension to pain (decerebrate)	2
Gives no motor response	1
Total	

FIGURE 5-2 Glasgow Coma Scale (GCS).

outcome, especially the best motor response. It also provides a baseline of cerebral function for serial neurologic evaluations. The GCS score is divided into three sections: (1) *eye* opening, (2) best *verbal* response, and (3) best *motor* response (EVM). The prehospital care provider assigns the patient a score according to the *best* response to each component of the EVM (Figure 5-2). For example, if a patient's right eye is so severely swollen that the patient cannot open it, but the left eye opens spontaneously, the patient receives a "4" for the best eye movement. If a patient lacks spontaneous eye opening, the provider should use a verbal command ("Open your eyes"). If the patient does not respond to a verbal stimulus, a painful stimulus, such as nail bed pressure with a pen or squeezing of the axillary tissue, can be applied.

The prehospital care provider can examine the patient's verbal response using a question such as, "What happened to you?" If fully oriented, the patient will supply a coherent answer. Otherwise, the patient's verbal response is scored as confused, inappropriate, unintelligible, or absent. If a patient is intubated, the GCS score contains only the eye and motor scales, and a "T" is added to note the inability to assess the verbal response (e.g., "8T").

The third component of the GCS is the motor score. The prehospital care provider can give the patient a simple, unambiguous command such as, "Hold up two fingers," or "Show me a hitchhiker's sign." A patient who squeezes or grasps the finger of a provider may simply be demonstrating a grasping reflex and not purposefully following a command. If the patient fails to follow a command, a painful stimulus, as noted previously, should be used, and the patient's *best* motor response should be scored. A patient who attempts to push away a painful stimulus is considered to be "localizing." Other possible responses to pain include withdrawal from the stimulus, abnormal flexion *(decorticate posturing)* or extension *(decerebrate posturing)* of the upper extremities, and absence of motor function. Recent evidence suggests that the motor component of the GCS alone is essentially as good in evaluating a patient as the entire score.[4]

The maximum GCS score is 15, indicating a patient with no disability, whereas the lowest score of 3 is generally an ominous sign. A score of less than 8 indicates a major injury, 9 to 12 a moderate injury, and 13 to 15 a minor injury. A GCS score of 8 is an indication for intubating a patient. The prehospital care provider can easily calculate the score and will include it in the verbal report to the receiving facility as well as in the patient care record.

If a patient is not awake, oriented, or able to follow commands, the prehospital care provider can assess the pupils quickly. Are the pupils equal and round, reactive to light (PEARRL)? Are the pupils equal to each other? Is each pupil round and of normal appearance, and does it appropriately react to light by constricting, or is it unresponsive and dilated? A GCS score of less than 14 in combination with an abnormal pupil examination can indicate the presence of a life-threatening traumatic brain injury (see Chapter 8).

Previous editions of this text used the acronym AVPU to describe the patient's LOC. In this system, *A* stands for *alert*, *V* for responds to *verbal* stimulus, *P* for responds to *painful* stimulus, and *U* for *unresponsive*. This approach, although very simple, fails to provide *how* the patient responds to verbal or painful stimuli. In other words, if the patient responds to verbal questioning, is the patient oriented, confused, or mumbling incomprehensibly? Likewise, when the patient responds to painful stimulus, does the patient withdraw, or demonstrate decorticate or decerebrate posturing? Because of its lack of precision, the use of AVPU should be abandoned. Although the GCS is more complicated to remember than AVPU, repeated practice will make this crucial assessment second nature.

Step E—Expose/Environment

An early step in the assessment process is to remove a patient's clothes because exposure of the trauma patient is critical to finding all injuries (Figure 5-3). The saying, "The one part of the body that is not exposed will be the most severely injured part," may not always be true, but it is true often enough to warrant a total body examination. Also, blood can collect in and be absorbed by clothing and thereby go unnoticed. After seeing the patient's entire body, the prehospital care provider covers the patient again to conserve body heat. Although it is important to expose a trauma patient's body to complete an effective assessment,

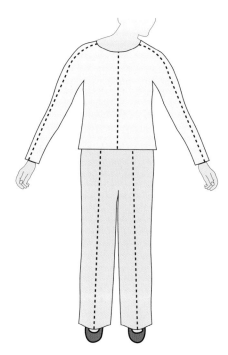

FIGURE 5-3 Clothing can be quickly removed by cutting, as indicated by the dotted lines.

hypothermia is a serious problem in the management of a trauma patient. Only what is necessary should be exposed to the outside environment. Once inside the warm emergency medical services (EMS) unit, the provider can complete the examination and then cover the patient again as quickly as possible.

The amount of the patient's clothing that should be removed during an assessment varies depending on the conditions or injuries found. A general rule is to remove as much clothing as necessary to determine the presence or absence of a condition or injury. The prehospital care provider need not be afraid to remove clothing if it is the only way to complete assessment and treatment properly. On occasion, patients can sustain multiple mechanisms of injury, such as experiencing a motor vehicle crash after being shot. Potentially life-threatening injuries may be missed if the patient is inadequately examined. Injuries cannot be treated if they are not first identified. Special care should be taken when cutting and removing clothing from a victim of a crime (Box 5-2).

Resuscitation

Resuscitation describes treatment steps taken to correct life-threatening problems as identified in the primary survey. PHTLS assessment is based on a "treat as you go" philosophy, in which treatment is initiated as each threat to life is identified, or at the earliest possible moment.

Simultaneous Evaluation

In discussing the process of patient assessment, management, and decision making, the information must be presented in a linear format (i.e., step A followed by step B followed by step C, etc.). Although presentation of information in this manner makes explanation easier and perhaps makes the concepts easier for a student to understand, that is not how the real world functions. The prehospital care provider's brain is similar to a computer that can receive input from several sources at once (cerebral multitasking). The brain can assess data received simultaneously. The brain is also capable of prioritizing the information from all input sources, sorting them in such a way that orderly decision making follows.

The brain can gather most data in about 15 seconds. Simultaneous processing of these data and appropriate prioritization of the information by the prehospital care provider can identify the component that the provider must manage first. Although the ABCDE approach described in this chapter may not necessarily be the order in which the prehospital care provider collects or receives the information, it does serve to establish priorities for management.

The primary survey addresses life-threatening conditions. The secondary survey of the patient identifies possible limb-threatening injuries as well as other, less significant problems.

BOX 5-2   Forensic Evidence

Unfortunately, some trauma patients are victims of violent crimes. In these situations, prehospital care providers have a duty to help preserve evidence for law enforcement personnel. When cutting clothing from a crime victim, care should be taken *not* to cut through holes in the clothing made by bullets (projectiles), knives, or other objects because this can compromise valuable forensic evidence. If clothing is removed from a victim of a potential crime, it should be placed in a paper (not plastic) bag and turned over to law enforcement personnel on scene before patient transport. Any weapons, drugs, or personal belongings found during patient assessment should also be turned over to law enforcement personnel, as well as thoroughly documented on the prehospital care report (PCR). If the patient's condition warrants transport before the arrival of law enforcement, these items are brought with the patient to the hospital, and the law enforcement agency is contacted and appraised of the destination facility.

Limited Scene Intervention

The prehospital care provider manages airway problems as the top priority. If the airway is open but the patient is not breathing, the provider initiates ventilatory support. Ventilatory support should include administration of high concentrations of oxygen (≥85%; Fio$_2$ ≥0.85) as early as possible. If the patient is exhibiting signs of ventilatory distress and lowered levels of air exchange, ventilatory assistance is needed by way of a BVM. The provider identifies cardiac arrest during the assessment of circulation and initiates chest compressions, if appropriate. The provider also controls exsanguinating hemorrhage. In a patient with adequate airway and breathing, the prehospital care provider can rapidly correct hypoxia and shock (anaerobic metabolism), if present.

Transport

If life-threatening conditions are identified during the primary survey, the patient should be rapidly "packaged" after initiating limited field intervention. Transport of critically injured trauma patients to the closest appropriate facility should be initiated as soon as possible (Box 5-3). Unless extenuating circumstances exist, the prehospital care provider limits the scene time to 10 minutes or less for these patients. The provider needs to realize that limiting scene time and initiation of rapid transport to the closest appropriate facility, preferably a trauma center, are fundamental aspects of prehospital trauma resuscitation.

Fluid Therapy

Another important step in resuscitation is the restoration of the cardiovascular system to an adequate perfusing volume as quickly as possible. Because blood is usually not available in the prehospital setting, *lactated Ringer's* is the preferred solution for trauma resuscitation. In addition to sodium and chloride, lactated Ringer's solution contains small amounts of potassium, calcium, and lactate and is an effective volume expander. Crystalloid solutions, such as lactated Ringer's, do not replace the oxygen-carrying capacity of the lost RBCs or the lost platelets that are necessary for clotting and bleeding control. Therefore, rapid transportation of a severely injured patient to an appropriate facility is an absolute necessity.

En route to the receiving facility, the prehospital care provider places two large-bore (14- or 16-gauge) IV catheters in the patient's forearm or antecubital veins, if possible. In general, central IV lines (subclavian, internal jugular, or femoral) are not appropriate for the field management of

BOX 5-3   Critical Trauma Patient

Limit scene time to 10 minutes or less when any of the following life-threatening conditions are present:

- Inadequate or threatened airway
- Impaired ventilation, as demonstrated by the following:
  - Abnormally fast or slow ventilatory rate
  - Hypoxia (SpO_2 <95% even with supplemental oxygen)
  - Dyspnea
  - Open pneumothorax or flail chest
  - Suspected pneumothorax
- Significant external hemorrhage or suspected internal hemorrhage
- Abnormal neurologic status
  - GCS score ≤13
  - Seizure activity
  - Sensory or motor deficit
- Penetrating trauma to the head, neck, or torso, or proximal to elbow and knee in the extremities
- Amputation or near-amputation proximal to the fingers or toes
- Any trauma in the presence of the following:
  - History of serious medical conditions (e.g., coronary artery disease, chronic obstructive pulmonary disease, bleeding disorder)
  - Age >55 years
  - Hypothermia
  - Burns
  - Pregnancy

trauma patients. The rate of fluid administration depends on the clinical scenario, primarily whether or not the patient's hemorrhage has been controlled when the IV fluid is initiated, or if the patient has evidence of CNS injury. Chapter 7 provides guidelines for fluid resuscitation.

Starting an IV line at the scene only prolongs on-scene time and delays transport. As addressed previously, the definitive treatment for the trauma patient can only be accomplished in the hospital. For example, a patient with an injury to the spleen who is losing 50 mL of blood per minute will continue to bleed at that rate for each additional minute that delays arrival in the OR. Initiating IV lines on the scene instead of early transportation not only will increase blood loss, but also may decrease the patient's chance of survival. Exceptions exist, such as entrapment, when a patient simply cannot be moved immediately. Also, aggressive and continual volume replacement is not a substitute for manual hemorrhage control.

Basic Provider Level

At the basic provider level, the key steps in resuscitating a critically injured trauma patient include (1) immediate control of major external hemorrhage, (2) rapid packaging of the patient for transportation, and (3) quickly initiated, rapid but safe transport of the patient to the closest appropriate facility. If transport time is prolonged, it may be appropriate to call for aid from a nearby ALS service that can intercept the basic unit en route. Helicopter evacuation to a trauma center is another option. Both the ALS service and the flight service will allow advanced airway management, ventilatory management, and earlier fluid replacement.

Secondary Survey (Detailed History and Physical Examination)

The secondary survey is a head-to-toe evaluation of a patient. The prehospital care provider will complete the primary survey, identify and treat all life-threatening injuries, and initiate resuscitation before beginning the secondary survey. The objective of the secondary survey is to identify injuries or problems that were not identified during the primary survey. Because a well-performed primary survey will identify all life-threatening conditions, the secondary survey, by definition, deals with less serious problems. Therefore the prehospital care provider transports a critical trauma patient as soon as possible after conclusion of the primary survey and does not hold the patient in the field for either IV initiation or a secondary survey.

The secondary survey uses a "look, listen, and feel" approach to evaluate the skin and everything it contains. Rather than looking at the entire body at one time, returning to listen to all areas, and finally returning to palpate all areas, the prehospital care provider "searches" the body. The provider identifies injuries and correlates physical findings region by region, beginning at the head and proceeding through the neck, chest, and abdomen to the extremities, concluding with a detailed neurologic examination. The following phrases capture the essence of the entire assessment process:

See, don't just look.
Hear, don't just listen.
Feel, don't just touch.

The definition of the word *see* is "to perceive with the eye" or "to discover," whereas *look* is defined as "to exercise the power of vision." *Listen* is defined as "to monitor without participation," and *hear* is defined as "to listen with attention." While examining the patient, the prehospital care provider uses all information available to formulate a patient care plan. The provider not only provides the patient with transport, but also does everything possible to ensure survival of the patient.

See

- Examine all the skin of each region.
- Be attentive for external hemorrhage or signs of internal hemorrhage, such as marked tenseness of an extremity or an expanding hematoma.

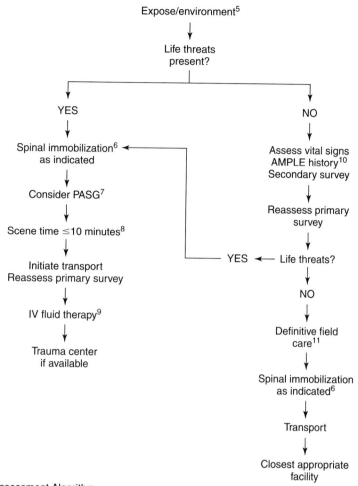

Notes for Assessment Algorithm

[1]Follow Airway Management algorithm (p. 125).

[2]Consider pleural decompression only if ALL are present:
- Diminished or absent breath sounds
- Increased work of breathing or difficulty ventilating with bag-valve-mask
- Decompensated shock/hypotension (SBP <90 mm Hg)
**Perform bilateral pleural decompression only if patient is receiving positive pressure ventilation.

[3]External hemorrhage control:
- Direct pressure/pressure dressing
- Tourniquet
*Consider topical hemostatic agent for prolonged transport.

[4]Shock: tachycardia; cool, diaphoretic, pallorous skin; anxiety; diminished or absent peripheral pulses.

[5]Quick check for other life-threatening conditions; cover patient to preserve body heat.

[6]See Indications for Spinal Immobilization algorithm (p. 235).

[7]PASG should be considered for: SBP <60 mm Hg; suspected pelvic fracture; suspected intraperitoneal hemorrhage; suspected retroperitoneal hemorrhage with decompensated shock (SBP <90 mm Hg).

[8]Scene time should be limited to 10 minutes or less for patients with life-threatening injuries unless extenuating circumstances exist.

[9]Transport should not be delayed to initiate IV fluid therapy. Initiate two large-bore IV lines; see Managing Volume Resuscitation algorithm (p. 188).

[10]AMPLE: allergies, medications, past medical/surgical history, last meal, events leading up to injury.

[11]Splint fractures and dress wounds as needed.

- Make note of soft tissue injuries, including abrasions, burns, contusions, hematomas, lacerations, and puncture wounds.
- Make note of any masses or swelling or deformation of bones that should not be present.
- Make note of abnormal indentations on the skin and the skin's color.
- Make note of anything that does not "look right."

Hear

- Make note of any unusual sounds when the patient inhales or exhales.
- Make note of any abnormal sounds when auscultating the chest.
- Verify whether the breath sounds are equal in both lung fields.
- Auscultate over the carotid arteries and other vessels.
- Make note of any unusual sounds (bruits) over the vessels that would indicate vascular damage.

Feel

- Carefully move each bone in the region. Note whether this produces crepitus, pain, or unusual movement.
- Firmly palpate all parts of the region. Note whether anything moves that should not, whether anything feels "squishy," where pulses are felt, whether pulsations are felt that should not be present, and whether all pulses are present.

Vital Signs

The prehospital care provider continually reevaluates the quality of the pulse and ventilatory rates and the other components of the primary survey because significant changes can occur rapidly. The provider measures quantitative vital signs and evaluates motor and sensory status in all four extremities as soon as possible, although this is normally not accomplished until the conclusion of the primary survey. Depending on the situation, a second provider may obtain vital signs while the first provider completes the primary survey, to avoid further delay. However, exact "numbers" for pulse rate, ventilatory rate, and blood pressure are not critical in the initial management of the patient with severe multisystem trauma. Therefore the measurement of the exact numbers can be delayed until completion of the essential steps of resuscitation and stabilization.

A set of complete vital signs includes blood pressure, pulse rate and quality, ventilatory rate (including breath sounds), and skin color and temperature. The prehospital care provider evaluates and records a complete set of vital signs every 3 to 5 minutes, as often as possible, or at the time of any change in condition or a medical problem. Even

if an automated, noninvasive blood pressure device is available, the initial blood pressure should be taken manually. Automatic blood pressure devices may be inaccurate when the patient is significantly hypotensive.

AMPLE History

The prehospital care provider will perform a quick history on the patient. This information should be documented on the patient care report and passed on to the medical personnel at the receiving facility. The mnemonic AMPLE serves as a reminder for the key components, as follows:

- *Allergies:* Primarily to medications.
- *Medications:* Prescription and nonprescription drugs that the patient takes regularly.
- *Past medical and surgical history:* Significant medical problems for which the patient receives ongoing medical care; includes prior surgeries.
- *Last meal:* Many trauma patients will require surgery, and recent food intake increases the risk of aspiration during induction of anesthesia.
- *Events:* Leading up to the injury.

Head

Visual examination of the head and face will reveal contusions, abrasions, lacerations, bone asymmetry, hemorrhage, bony defects of the face and supportive skull, and abnormalities of the eye, eyelid, external ear, mouth, and mandible. The prehospital care provider does the following during a head examination:

- Searches thoroughly through the patient's hair for any soft tissue injuries
- Checks pupil size for reactivity to light, equality, accommodation, roundness, and irregular shape
- Carefully palpates the bones of the face and skull to identify crepitus, deviation, depression, or abnormal mobility (this is extremely important in the nonradiographic evaluation for head injury)

Figure 5-4 reviews the normal anatomic structure of the face and skull.

Neck

Visual examination of the neck for contusions, abrasions, lacerations, and deformities will alert the prehospital care provider to the possibility of underlying injuries. Palpation may reveal subcutaneous emphysema of a laryngeal, tracheal, or pulmonary origin. Crepitus of the larynx, hoarseness, and subcutaneous emphysema constitute a triad classically indicative of laryngeal fracture. Lack of tenderness of the cervical spine may help rule out cervical spine fractures

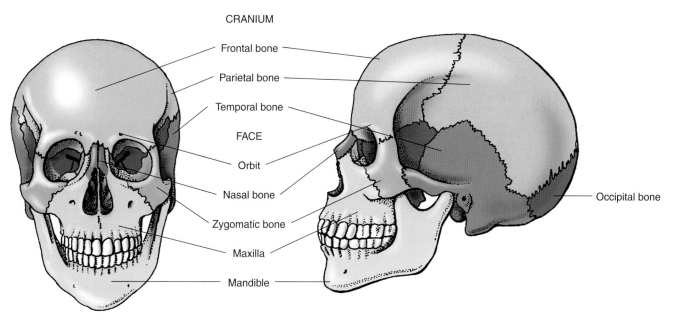

CRANIUM

Frontal bone

Parietal bone

Temporal bone

FACE

Orbit

Nasal bone

Zygomatic bone

Maxilla

Mandible

Occipital bone

FIGURE 5-4   Normal anatomic structure of the face and skull.

(when combined with strict criteria), whereas tenderness may frequently indicate the presence of a fracture, dislocation, or ligamentous injury. The prehospital care provider performs such palpation carefully, ensuring that the cervical spine remains in a neutral, inline position.

Figure 5-5 reviews the normal anatomy of the neck.

Chest

Because the thorax is strong, resilient, and elastic, it can absorb a significant amount of trauma. Close visual examination of the chest for deformities, areas of paradoxical movement, contusions, and abrasions is necessary to identify underlying injuries. Other signs for which the prehospital care provider should watch closely include splinting and guarding, unequal bilateral chest excursion, and intercostal, suprasternal, or supraclavicular bulging or retraction.

For example, a contusion over the sternum may be the only indication of a cardiac injury. A stab wound near the sternum may indicate cardiac tamponade. A line traced from the fourth intercostal space anteriorly, to the sixth intercostal space laterally, and to the eighth intercostal space posteriorly defines the upward excursion of the diaphragm at full expiration (Figure 5-6). A penetrating injury that occurs below this line or with a path that may have taken it below this line should be considered to have traversed the thoracic and abdominal cavities.

Except for the eyes and hands, the stethoscope is the most important instrument a prehospital care provider can use for chest examination. A patient will most often be in a supine position so that only the anterior and lateral chest is available for auscultation. It is important that a prehospital care provider learn to recognize normal and decreased

Paranasal sinuses

Turbinates

Pharyngeal tonsil (adenoids)

Nose

Pharynx

Larynx

Tongue

Esophagus

Trachea

Thyroid gland

FIGURE 5-5   Normal anatomy of the neck.

breath sounds with a patient in this position. A small area of rib fractures may indicate a severe underlying pulmonary contusion. Any type of compression injury to the chest can result in a pneumothorax (Figure 5-7). Diminished or absent breath sounds indicate a possible pneumothorax, tension pneumothorax, or hemothorax. Crackles heard posteriorly (when the patient is logrolled) or laterally

Lateral view of diaphragm position

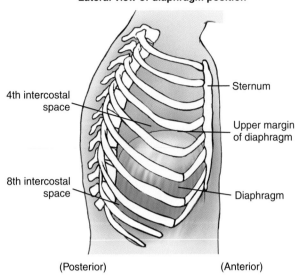

4th intercostal space

Sternum

Upper margin of diaphragm

8th intercostal space

Diaphragm

(Posterior)   (Anterior)

FIGURE 5-6   Lateral view of diaphragm position at full expiration.

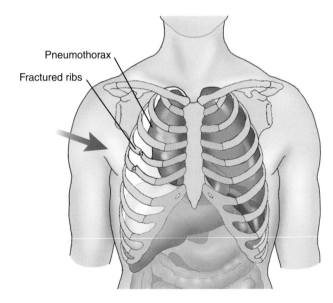

Pneumothorax

Fractured ribs

FIGURE 5-7   Compression injury to the chest can result in rib fracture and subsequent pneumothorax.

may indicate pulmonary contusion. Cardiac tamponade is characterized by distant heart sounds; however, these may be difficult for the prehospital care provider to ascertain given the commotion at the scene or road noise during transport. The provider also feels the thorax for subcutaneous emphysema.

Abdomen

The prehospital care provider initiates abdominal examination, as with the other parts of the body, by visual evaluation. Abrasions and ecchymosis indicate the possibility of

underlying injury. The prehospital care provider should examine the abdomen carefully, near the umbilicus, for a telltale transverse contusion, which suggests that an incorrectly worn seat belt has caused underlying injury. Almost 50% of patients with this sign will have an intestinal injury. Lumbar spine fractures may also be associated with the "seat belt sign."

Examination of the abdomen also includes palpation of each quadrant to evaluate tenderness, abdominal muscle guarding, and masses. When palpating, the prehospital care provider notes whether the abdomen is soft and whether rigidity or guarding is present. There is no need to continue palpating after discovering abdominal tenderness or pain. Additional information will not alter prehospital management, and the only outcomes of a continued abdominal examination are further discomfort to the patient and delayed transportation to the receiving facility. Similarly, auscultation of the abdomen adds virtually nothing to the assessment of a trauma patient.

Pelvis

The prehospital care provider evaluates the pelvis by observation and palpation. The provider visually examines for abrasions, contusions, lacerations, open fractures, and signs of distention. Pelvic fractures can produce massive internal hemorrhage, resulting in rapid deterioration of a patient's condition.

The pelvis is palpated only once for instability as part of the secondary survey. Because palpation can aggravate hemorrhage, the prehospital care provider will not repeat this examination step. Palpation is accomplished by gently first applying anterior-to-posterior pressure with the heels of the hands on the symphysis pubis and then medial pressure to the iliac crests bilaterally, evaluating for pain and abnormal movement. The provider should suspect hemorrhage with any evidence of instability.

Back

The back of the torso should be examined for evidence of injury. This is best accomplished when logrolling the patient for placement onto the long backboard. Breath sounds can be auscultated over the posterior thorax, and the spine should be palpated for tenderness and deformity.

Extremities

The prehospital care provider begins examination of the extremities with the clavicle in the upper extremity and the pelvis in the lower extremity, then proceeds toward the most distal portion of each extremity. Each individual bone and joint is evaluated by visual examination for deformity, hematoma, or ecchymosis and by palpation to determine the presence of crepitus, pain, tenderness, or unusual movements. Any suspected fracture should be immobilized until radiographic confirmation of its presence or absence is possible. The provider also checks circulation and motor and sensory nerve function at the distal end of each extremity. If an extremity is immobilized, pulses, movement, and sensation should be rechecked after splinting.

Neurologic Examination

As with the other regional examinations described, the prehospital care provider conducts the neurologic examination in the secondary survey in much greater detail than in the primary survey. Calculation of the GCS score, evaluation of motor and sensory function, and observation of pupillary response are all included. When examining a patient's pupils, the provider checks for equality of response as much as for equality of size. A small but significant portion of the population has pupils of differing sizes as a normal condition *(anisocoria).* Even in these patients, however, the pupils should react to light in a similar manner. Pupils that react at differing speeds to the introduction of light are considered to be unequal. Unequal pupils in an unconscious trauma patient may indicate increased intracranial pressure or pressure on the third cranial nerve, caused by either cerebral edema or a rapidly expanding intracranial hematoma (Figure 5-8). Direct eye injury can also cause unequal pupils.

A gross examination of sensory capability and response will determine the presence or absence of weakness or loss of sensation in the extremities and will identify areas that require further examination. The prehospital care provider needs to immobilize the entire length of the spine and thus the entire patient. Use of a long backboard, cervical collar, head pads, and straps is required. The provider does not immobilize the head only. If the body is not immobilized, a shift in the patient's body resulting from lifting or ambulance movement will cause the body to move and not the head, potentially causing further injury to the spinal cord. Protection of the entire spinal cord is required at all times.

Definitive Care in the Field

Included in assessment and management are the skills of packaging, transportation, and communication. Definitive care is the end phase of patient care. The following are examples of definitive care:

- For a patient with cardiac arrest, definitive care is defibrillation with resultant normal rhythm; cardiopulmonary resuscitation (CPR) is just a holding pattern until defibrillation can be accomplished.

FIGURE 5-8   A, Pupil dilation. **B,** Pupil constriction. **C,** Unequal pupils. **D,** Normal pupils.

- For a patient in a diabetic hypoglycemic coma, definitive care is IV glucose and a return to normal blood glucose levels.
- For a patient with an obstructed airway, part of the definitive care is the jaw thrust and assisted ventilation.
- For the patient with severe bleeding, definitive care is hemorrhage control and resuscitation from shock.

In general, definitive care for the trauma patient can only be provided in the OR. Anything that delays the administration of that definitive care will lessen the patient's chance for survival. The care given to the trauma patient in the field is similar to CPR for the cardiac arrest patient. It keeps the patient alive until something definitive can be done. For the trauma patient, the care given in the field is frequently only temporizing—buying additional minutes to reach the OR.

Packaging

As discussed previously, the prehospital care provider suspects spinal injury in all trauma patients. Therefore, when indicated, stabilization of the spine should be an integral component of packaging the trauma patient. If time is available, the prehospital care provider does the following:

- Carefully stabilizes extremity fractures using specific splints

- If the patient is in critical condition, immobilizes all fractures as the patient is stabilized on a long backboard ("trauma" board)
- Bandages wounds as necessary and appropriate

Transport

Transportation should begin as soon as the patient is loaded and stabilized. As discussed previously, delay at the scene to start an IV line or to complete the secondary survey only extends the period before the receiving facility can administer blood and control hemorrhage. Continued evaluation and further resuscitation occur en route to the receiving facility. *For some critically injured trauma patients, initiation of transport is the most important aspect of definitive care in the field.*

A patient whose condition is not critical can receive attention for individual injuries before transportation, but even this patient should be transported rapidly before a hidden condition becomes critical.

Revised Trauma Score

The Trauma Score (TS), originally developed by surgeon Howard Champion and colleagues, is a good predictor of survival of blunt trauma patients. The Revised Trauma Score (RTS), published in 1989, eliminated two components of the older TS and is equally useful in predicting survival after serious injury.[5] The RTS is composed of scores for the GCS, systolic blood pressure, and ventilatory rate (Figure 5-9). Each of these three components is assigned a value from 4 (best) to 0 (worst). The combined score indicates the patient's condition. The lowest possible com-

bined score, 0, is obviously the most critical; the highest, 12, is the least critical. The combined score is valuable to analyze the care given to a patient, but it is not necessarily a prehospital triage tool. In many prehospital systems, the score is calculated and recorded at the receiving facility based on information provided in the radio report, but prehospital care providers are neither required nor expected to compute it before arrival.

Field Triage Scheme

The Triage Decision Scheme, originally published by the American College of Surgeons (ACS) Committee on Trauma, is more useful than the RTS in making prehospital patient triage decisions (Figure 5-10).[6] In some systems the Triage Decision Scheme is used in the process of determining the most appropriate receiving facility for a trauma patient. As with any schematic tool, however, it should be used as a guideline and not as a replacement for good judgment. The Triage Decision Scheme divides triage into three prioritized steps that will assist in the decision as to when it is best to transport a patient to a trauma center, if available: (1) physiologic criteria, (2) anatomic criteria, and (3) mechanism of injury (kinematics). Following this scheme results in *overtriage* (not all patients taken to the trauma center will actually need a trauma center level of care), but this outcome is better than *undertriage* (patients needing a trauma center level of care are taken to nontrauma centers). Medical directors or local medical control boards should establish local protocols to familiarize prehospital field personnel with trauma centers. The field triage decision scheme on page 109 was revised by an expert panel representing emergency medical services, emergency medicine, trauma surgery,

			Score	Start of Transport	End of Transport
A. Ventilatory rate	10-29/min		4		
	>29/min		3		
	6-9/min		2		
	1-5/min		1		
	0		0		
B. Systolic blood pressure	>89 mm Hg		4		
	76-89 mm Hg		3		
	50-75 mm Hg		2		
	1-49 mm Hg		1		
	No pulse		0		
C. Glasgow Coma Scale score	13-15	=	4		
	9-12	=	3		
	6-8	=	2		
	4-5	=	1		
	<4	=	0		
Trauma score total = A + B + C					

FIGURE 5-9 Revised Trauma Score (RTS). A trauma score can be numerically calculated en route to the hospital. Such information is extremely helpful in preparing to manage a patient.
(Modified from Champion HR, Sacco WJ, Copes WS, et al: A revision of the trauma score, *J Trauma* 29(5):624, 1989.)

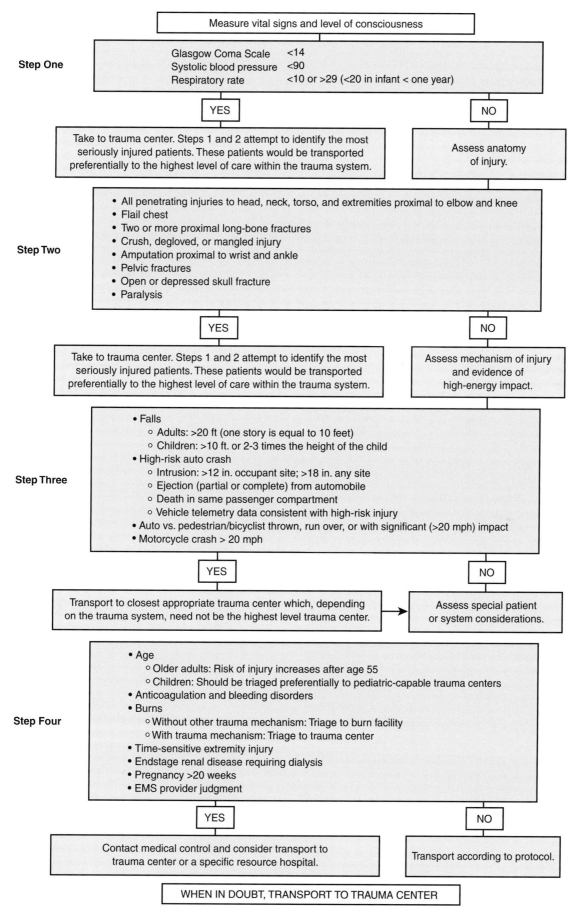

FIGURE 5-10 Deciding where to transport a patient is critical, with consideration of the type and location of available facilities. Situations that will most likely require an in-house trauma team are detailed in the Triage Decision Scheme.

and public health. The panel was convened by the Centers for Disease Control and Prevention (CDC) with support from the National Highway Traffic Safety Administration (NHTSA). Its contents are those of the expert panel and do not necessarily represent the official views of CDC and NHTSA.

Duration of Transport

The prehospital care provider should choose a receiving facility according to the severity of the patient's injury. In simple terms, the patient should be transported to the closest appropriate facility (i.e., the closest facility most capable of managing the patient's problems). If the patient's injuries are severe or indicate the possibility of continuing hemorrhage, the provider can take the patient to a facility that will provide definitive care as quickly as possible (i.e., a trauma center, if available).

For example, if an ambulance responds to a call in 8 minutes and the prehospital team spends 6 minutes on the scene to package and load the patient into the transporting unit, 14 minutes of the Golden Period have passed. The closest hospital is 5 minutes away, and the trauma center is 14 minutes away. On arrival at the trauma center, the surgeon is in the emergency department (ED) with the emergency physician and the entire trauma team. The OR is staffed and ready. After 10 minutes in the ED for resuscitation and necessary radiographs and blood work, the patient is taken to the OR. The total time since the incident is now 38 minutes. In comparison, the closest hospital has an available emergency physician, but the surgeon and OR team are out of the hospital. The patient's 10 minutes in the ED for resuscitation could stretch to 45 minutes by the time the surgeon arrives and examines the patient. Another 30 minutes could elapse while waiting for the OR team to arrive once the surgeon has examined the patient and decided to operate. The total time is 94 minutes, or $2^1/_2$ times longer than the first scenario. The 9 minutes saved by the shorter ambulance ride actually cost 57 minutes, during which operative management could have been started and hemorrhage control achieved.

In a rural community, the transport time to an awaiting trauma team may be 45 to 60 minutes or even longer. In this situation, the closest hospital with an on-call trauma team is the appropriate receiving facility.

Method of Transport

Another aspect in the transportation decision is the transportation method. Some systems offer an alternative option of air transportation. Air medical services may offer a higher level of care than ground units. Air transportation may also be quicker and smoother than ground transportation in some circumstances. As previously mentioned, if air transportation is available in a community, the prehospital care provider can anticipate its use early in the assessment process to benefit the patient.

Monitoring and Reassessment (Ongoing Assessment)

After the primary survey and initial care are complete, the prehospital care provider will continue to monitor the patient, reassess vital signs, and repeat the primary survey several times while en route to the receiving facility, or at the scene if transport is delayed. Continual reassessment of the points in the primary survey will help ensure that unrecognized compromise of vital functions does not occur. The provider pays particular attention to any significant change in a patient's condition and reevaluates management if the patient's condition changes. Furthermore, the continued monitoring of a patient helps reveal conditions or problems that may have been overlooked during the primary survey. Often the patient's condition will be obvious, and looking at and listening to the patient provide much information. How the information is gathered is not as important as ensuring that *all* the information is gathered. Reassessment should be conducted as quickly and thoroughly as possible. Monitoring during a prolonged transport situation is described later.

Communication

The prehospital care provider begins communication with medical direction and the receiving facility as soon as possible. The information transmitted about a patient's condition, management, and the expected time of arrival will give the receiving facility time to prepare. The prehospital team also transmits information about the mechanism of injury, the characteristics of the scene, the number of patients, and other pertinent facts to allow the receiving facility staff to best coordinate its resources and meet each patient's needs.

Equally important is the written *prehospital care report* (PCR). A good PCR is valuable for the following two reasons:

1. It gives the receiving facility staff a thorough understanding of the events that occurred and of the patient's condition should any questions arise after the prehospital care providers have left.
2. It helps ensure quality control throughout the prehospital system by making case review possible.

For these reasons, it is important that the prehospital care provider fill out the PCR accurately and completely and provide it to the receiving facility. The report should stay with the patient; the report is of little use if it does not arrive until hours or days after the patient arrives.

The PCR often becomes a part of the patient's medical record. It is a legal record of what was found and what was done and can be used as part of a legal action. The report is considered to be a complete record of the injuries found and the actions taken. A good adage to remember is, "If it is not on the report, it was not done." The prehospital care provider records in the report all that he or she knows, has seen, and has done to the patient. Another important reason for providing a copy of the PCR to the receiving facility is that most trauma centers maintain a "trauma registry," a database of all trauma patients admitted to their facility. The prehospital information is an important aspect of this database and may aid in valuable research.

The prehospital care provider also verbally transfers responsibility for a patient ("sign off," "report off," or "transfer over") to the physician or nurse who takes over the patient's care at the receiving facility. This verbal report is typically more detailed than the radio report and less detailed than the written record, providing an overview of the significant history of the incident, the action taken by the prehospital care providers, and the patient's response to this action. The report must highlight any significant changes in the patient's condition that have taken place since transmitting the radio report. Transfer of important prehospital information further emphasizes the team concept of patient care.

Special Considerations

Traumatic Cardiopulmonary Arrest

Cardiopulmonary arrest resulting from trauma differs from that caused by medical problems in three significant ways, as follows:

1. Most medical cardiac arrests are the result of either a respiratory problem, such as a foreign body airway obstruction, or a cardiac dysrhythmia that prehospital care providers may be able to treat fairly easily. Cardiac arrest resulting from injury most often results from exsanguination or, less often, a problem incompatible with life, such as a devastating brain or spinal cord injury, and the patient cannot be appropriately resuscitated in the field.
2. Medical arrests are best managed with attempts at stabilization at the scene (e.g., removal of airway foreign body, defibrillation). In contrast, traumatic cardiopulmonary arrest is best managed with immediate transport to a facility that offers immediate blood and emergent surgery.
3. Because of the differences in etiology and management, patients with traumatic cardiopulmonary arrest in the

prehospital setting have an extremely low likelihood of survival. Less than 4% of trauma patients who require CPR in the prehospital setting survive to be discharged from the hospital, with most studies documenting that victims of penetrating trauma have a slightly increased chance of survival over those of blunt trauma. Of the small percentage of patients who are discharged from the hospital alive, many sustain significant neurologic impairment.

In addition to the extremely low survival rate, resuscitation attempts in patients who are extremely unlikely to survive put prehospital care providers at risk from exposure to blood and body fluids and injuries sustained in motor vehicle crashes during transport. Such unsuccessful attempts at resuscitation may divert resources away from patients who are viable and have a greater likelihood of survival. For these reasons, the prehospital care provider needs to exercise good judgment regarding the decision to initiate resuscitation attempts for victims of traumatic cardiopulmonary arrest.

The National Association of EMS Physicians collaborated with the ACS Committee on Trauma to develop guidelines for withholding or terminating CPR in the prehospital setting. Victims of drowning, lightning strike, or hypothermia and patients in whom the mechanism of injury does not correlate with the clinical situation (suggesting a nontraumatic cause) deserve special consideration before a decision is made to withhold or terminate resuscitation. A patient found in cardiopulmonary arrest at the scene of a traumatic event may have experienced the arrest because of a medical problem (e.g., myocardial infarction), especially if the patient is elderly and evidence of injury is minimal.

Withholding Cardiopulmonary Resuscitation

If, during the primary survey, patients are found to meet the following criteria, CPR may be withheld and the patient declared dead[7]:

- For victims of blunt trauma, resuscitation efforts may be withheld if the patient is pulseless and apneic on arrival of prehospital care providers.
- For victims of penetrating trauma, resuscitation efforts may be withheld if there are no signs of life (no pupillary reflexes, no spontaneous movement, no organized cardiac rhythm on ECG >40/min).
- Resuscitation efforts are not indicated when the patient has sustained an obviously fatal injury (e.g., decapitation) or when evidence exists of dependent lividity, rigor mortis, and decomposition.

Basic Life Support

Guidelines for managing cardiopulmonary arrest have recently been revised and published by the American Heart Association.[8] After opening the airway with a jaw thrust, ventilatory effort is assessed. If the patient is apneic, the prehospital care provider delivers two rescue breaths. These breaths are delivered slowly to prevent gastric inflation. Any obvious, exsanguinating hemorrhage should be controlled. The carotid pulse is then assessed for up to 10 seconds. If no pulse is present, chest compressions are initiated. Cycles of compressions and ventilations are given, with a brief pause in compressions to deliver the two breaths. Once an advanced airway is in place, compressions are delivered at 100 per minute without pausing for ventilations; ventilations are administered at a rate of 8 to 10 per minute. The individual delivering chest compressions is changed every 2 minutes to prevent fatigue. If an automatic external defibrillator (AED) is available, the patient's cardiac rhythm is assessed and defibrillation performed if ventricular fibrillation is present.

Advanced Life Support

The airway is secured, ideally with endotracheal intubation while simultaneously ensuring inline stabilization of the cervical spine. Breath sounds should be auscultated and the possible presence of a tension pneumothorax ruled out. A tension pneumothorax may be present when a decrease in breath sounds is noted, with inadequate chest excursion during ventilation. If any doubt exists that the patient may have a tension pneumothorax, chest decompression is performed. Bilateral chest decompression should be performed only if the patient is receiving positive pressure ventilation.

Large-bore venous access is obtained, and isotonic crystalloid solution is delivered through a wide-open line if hypovolemic shock is a possible cause of the cardiac arrest. Electrocardiogram (ECG) monitoring is performed and cardiac rhythm assessed. The following dysrhythmias may be noted:

- *Pulseless electrical activity* (PEA). A patient found in PEA should be assessed for the presence of hypovolemia, hypothermia, tension pneumothorax, and cardiac tamponade. Fluids, warming, and chest decompression should be performed if indicated. Epinephrine and atropine may be administered.
- *Bradyasystole.* A patient found in this rhythm should be assessed for severe hypoxia and hypovolemia. The location of the airway should be confirmed and volume resuscitation initiated. Epinephrine and atropine may be administered.
- *Ventricular fibrillation/pulseless ventricular tachycardia.*
  The primary therapy for these dysrhythmias is defibrillation. If the available defibrillator is biphasic, a shock of 120 to 200 joules is delivered. If a monophasic defibrillator is present, a shock of 360 joules is used. Epinephrine, antidysrhythmics (amiodarone or lidocaine), and magnesium may be used in the management of this rhythm.

Terminating Cardiopulmonary Resuscitation

Termination of CPR and ALS measures may be considered in the prehospital setting in the following circumstances[7]:

- Trauma patients with an EMS-witnessed cardiopulmonary arrest and 15 minutes of unsuccessful resuscitation and CPR.
- Patients with traumatic cardiopulmonary arrest who would require transport longer than 15 minutes to reach an ED or trauma center.

Pain Management

Pain management *(analgesia)* is often used in the prehospital setting for pain caused by angina or myocardial infarction. Traditionally, pain management has had a limited role in the management of trauma patients, primarily because of the concern that side effects (decreased ventilatory drive and vasodilation) of narcotics may aggravate preexisting hypoxia and hypotension. This concern has resulted in pain relief being denied to some patients with appropriate indications, such as an isolated limb injury or spinal fracture. The prehospital care provider may consider pain management in such patients, particularly if prolonged transport occurs, provided that signs of ventilatory impairment or shock are not present.

Chapter 12 devotes a section to pain management as it relates to isolated extremity injuries and fractures. Morphine sulfate is typically the agent of choice and should be titrated intravenously in 1-mg to 2-mg increments until some degree of pain relief is obtained or a change in the patient's vital signs occurs. The prehospital care provider will monitor pulse oximetry and serial vital signs if any narcotics are administered to a trauma patient. Sedation with an agent such as a benzodiazepine should be reserved for exceptional circumstances, such as a combative intubated patient, because the combination of a narcotic and benzodiazepine may result in respiratory arrest. Prehospital personnel can collaborate with their medical control to develop appropriate protocols.

Abuse

A prehospital care provider is often the first person on the scene, allowing the provider to observe a potentially abusive situation. The provider inside a house can relay the details at the scene to the receiving facility so that the appropriate services in the area can be alerted. The prehospital care provider is usually the first, and sometimes the only, person to suspect and relay information about this silent danger.

Anyone at any age can be a potential abuser or victim of abuse. A pregnant woman, infant, toddler, child, adolescent, young adult, middle-age adult, and older adult are all at risk for abuse. Several different types of abuse exist, including physical, psychological (emotional), and financial.

Abuse may occur by *commission,* in which a purposeful act results in an injury (physical abuse or sexual abuse), or by *omission* (e.g., neglectful care of a dependent). This section does not discuss types of abuse and only introduces the reader to general characteristics and heightens a prehospital care provider's awareness and suspicion of abuse.

General characteristics of a potential abuser include dishonesty, the "story" not correlating with the injuries, a negative attitude, and abrasiveness with prehospital personnel. General characteristics of the abused patient include quietness, not wanting to elaborate on details of the incident, constant eye contact or lack of eye contact with someone at the scene, and minimization of personal injuries. Abuse, abusers, and the abused can take many different forms, and prehospital care providers need to keep suspicion high if the scene and the story do not correlate. The provider is required to relay suspicions and any information to the proper authorities.

Prolonged Transport

Although most urban or suburban EMS transports take 30 minutes or less, many prehospital care providers in rural and frontier settings routinely manage patients for much longer periods during transport. Additionally, providers are called on to manage patients during transfer from one medical facility to another, either by ground or air. These transfers may take up to several hours.

Special preparations need to be taken when prehospital care providers are involved in the prolonged transport of a trauma patient. The issues that must be considered before undertaking such a transport can be divided into those dealing with the patient, the prehospital crew, and equipment.

Patient Issues

Of preeminent importance is providing a safe, warm, and secure environment in which the patient is transported. The gurney should be appropriately secured to the ambulance, and the patient should be secured to the gurney. As emphasized throughout this text, hypothermia is a potentially deadly complication in a trauma patient, and the patient compartment must be sufficiently warm. The patient should be secured in a position that allows maximum access to the patient, especially the injured areas. Before transport, the security of all IV lines and catheters should be double-checked, and adjuncts (e.g., monitors, oxygen tanks) should be secured so that they do not become projectiles in the event that the ambulance has to swerve in an evasive action or is involved in a motor vehicle crash. Adjuncts should not rest on the patient, because pressure ulcers might be created during a prolonged transport.

The patient should receive serial assessments of the primary survey and vital signs at routine intervals. Pulse oximetry and ECG are monitored continuously for virtually all patients, as well as end-tidal CO_2, if available, in an intubated patient. The prehospital care providers should be trained at a level appropriate to the anticipated needs of the patient. Critically injured patients should generally be managed by providers with advanced training. If the patient is anticipated to require blood transfusion during transport, an individual should be in attendance whose scope of practice allows this procedure; in the United States, this generally requires a registered nurse.

Two management plans should be devised. The first, a medical plan, is developed to manage either anticipated or unexpected problems with the patient during transport. Necessary equipment, medications, and supplies should be readily available. The second plan involves identifying the most expeditious route to the receiving hospital. Weather conditions, road conditions (e.g., construction), and traffic concerns should be identified. Additionally, the providers should be knowledgeable of medical facilities along the transport route in case a problem arises that cannot be managed en route.

Crew

The safety of the EMS crew is as important as that of the patient. The prehospital crew needs to have appropriate safety devices, such as seat belts, and they should be secured during transport unless an issue involving patient care prevents this. The crew members use Standard Precautions and ensure that sufficient gloves and other personal protective equipment (PPE) are available for the trip.

Equipment

Equipment issues during prolonged transport involve the ambulance, supplies and medications, monitors, and communications. The ambulance must be in good working order, including an adequate amount of fuel and a spare tire. The crew must make sure that sufficient supplies and medications are available and accessible for the transport, including gauze and pads for reinforcing dressings, IV fluids, oxygen, and pain medications. Drug supplies are based on anticipated patient needs and include sedatives, paralytic agents, and antibiotics. A good rule of thumb is to provision the ambulance with about 50% more supplies and medications than the anticipated need, in case a significant delay is encountered. Patient care equipment must be in good working order, including monitors (with functioning alarms), oxygen regulators, and suction devices. Also, success of a prolonged transport may depend on functional communications, including the ability to communicate with other crew members, medical control, and the destination facility.

The management of specific injuries during prolonged transport is discussed in the subsequent corresponding chapters of this text.

SUMMARY

In the care of the trauma patient, a missed problem is a missed opportunity to aid potentially in an individual's survival. Chances of survival for a patient with traumatic injuries depend on the immediate identification and mitigation of conditions that interfere with tissue perfusion. The identification of these conditions requires a systematic, prioritized, logical process of collecting information and acting on it. This process is referred to as *patient assessment*. Patient assessment begins with scene assessment and includes the formation of a general impression of the patient, a primary survey, and when the patient's condition and availability of additional EMS personnel permit, a secondary survey. The prehospital care provider analyzes the information obtained through this process and uses it as the basis for patient care and transport decisions.

Life depends on adequate perfusion: the circulation of oxygenated blood to the tissues of the body and the release of oxygen to the cells of the tissues. Impairment of perfusion may occur during the patient's Golden Period, the length of which depends on the degree of impairment. After the simultaneous determination of scene safety and general impression of the situation, the prehospital care provider focuses the priorities of patient assessment on the patency of the patient's airway, the ventilatory status, and the circulatory status. Once the provider has responded to these immediate threats to the patient's life, further assessment is necessary to identify the patient's neurologic status and the presence of other injuries. This primary survey follows the ABCDE format for evaluation of the patient's airway, breathing, circulation, disability (initial neurologic examination), and exposure (removing the patient's clothing to discover additional significant injuries).

Although the sequential nature of language limits the ability to describe the simultaneity of these actions, the prehospital care provider understands that the primary survey of the patient is a process of actions that occur at the same time. For a patient with any impairment or potential for impairment of perfusion, the prehospital care provider will quickly intervene in a "find and fix" manner for immediate threats to the patient's life. Once the provider manages the patient's airway and breathing and controls exsanguinating hemorrhage, he or she packages the patient and begins transportation without additional treatment at the scene. The prehospital care provider needs to understand the limitations of the field management of trauma and make his or her goal the safe, expedient delivery of the patient to definitive care.

SCENARIO SOLUTION

You have been on the scene for 1 minute, yet you have obtained much important information to guide further assessment and treatment of the patient. In the first 15 seconds of patient contact, you have developed a general impression of the patient, determining that resuscitation is not necessary. With a few simple actions you have evaluated the A, B, C, and D of the initial assessment. The patient spoke to you without difficulty, indicating that her airway is open and she is breathing, with no signs of distress. At the same time, with an awareness of the mechanism of injury, you have stabilized the cervical spine. You have noted no obvious bleeding, your partner has assessed the radial pulse, and you have observed the patient's skin color, temperature, and moisture. These findings indicate no immediate threats to the patient's circulatory status. Additionally, you have simultaneously found no initial evidence of disability because the patient is awake, is alert, and answers questions appropriately. This information, along with information about the speed of the vehicle at the time of impact and the damage to the vehicle at the point of impact, will help you determine the need for additional resources, the type of transportation indicated, and to what type of facility you should deliver the patient.

Now that you have completed these steps and no immediate lifesaving intervention is necessary, you will proceed with step E of the primary survey early in the evaluation process and then obtain vital signs. You will expose the patient to look for additional injuries and bleeding that may have been concealed by clothing, then cover the patient to protect her from the environment. During this process, you will perform a more detailed examination, noting less serious injuries. The next steps you will take are packaging the patient, including splinting extremity injuries and bandaging wounds if time allows; initiating transportation; and communicating with medical direction and the receiving facility. During the trip to the hospital, you will continue to reevaluate and monitor the patient. Your knowledge of kinematics and the patient's witnessed loss of consciousness will generate a high index of suspicion for traumatic brain injury, lower-extremity injuries, and injuries to the chest and abdomen. In an advanced life support (ALS) system, intravenous (IV) access will be established en route to the receiving facility. ∎

References

1. Advanced Trauma Life Support (ATLS) Subcommittee, Committee on Trauma: Initial assessment and management. In *Advanced trauma life support course for doctors, student course manual,* ed 7, Chicago, 2004, ACS.
2. First Aid Science Advisory Board: First aid, *Circulation* 112(III):115, 2005.
3. Teasdale G, Jennett B: Assessment of coma and impaired consciousness: a practical scale, *Lancet* 2:81, 1974.
4. Healey C, Osler TM, Rogers FB, et al: Improving the Glasgow Coma Scale score: motor score alone is a better predictor, *J Trauma* 54:671, 2003.
5. Champion HR, Sacco WJ, Copes WS, et al: A revision of the Trauma Score, *J Trauma* 29(5):623, 1989.
6. Committee on Trauma: *Resources for optimal care of the injured patient: 1999,* Chicago, 1998, American College of Surgeons.
7. Hopson LR, Hirsh E, Delgado J, et al: Guidelines for withholding or termination of resuscitation in prehospital traumatic cardiopulmonary arrest, *Prehosp Emerg Care* 7:141, 2003.
8. American Heart Association: 2005 guidelines for cardiopulmonary resuscitation and emergency cardiovascular care, *Circulation* 112(IV):1, 2005.

Suggested Reading

American Heart Association: Cardiac arrest associated with trauma, *Circulation* 112(IV):146, 2005.

Chapter Objectives

*At the completion of this chapter, the reader
will be able to do the following:*

✓ Integrate the principles of ventilation and gas exchange with the
pathophysiology of trauma to identify patients with inadequate
perfusion.

✓ Relate the concepts of minute volume and oxygenation to the
pathophysiology of trauma.

✓ Explain the mechanisms by which supplemental oxygen and
ventilatory support are beneficial to the trauma patient.

✓ Given a scenario that involves a trauma patient, select the most
effective means of providing a patent airway to suit the needs of the
patient.

✓ Given a scenario that involves a patient who requires ventilatory
support, select the most effective means available to suit the needs
of the trauma patient.

✓ Given situations that involve various trauma patients, formulate a
plan for airway management and ventilation.

✓ Given current research, understand the risks versus benefits when
discussing new invasive procedures.

CHAPTER 6

Airway and Ventilation

SCENARIO

You are dispatched to a motor vehicle crash. On arrival, you observe that an SUV has struck a tree on the driver's side, which has sustained substantial damage. The driver of the SUV, a 30-year-old male, is lying in the grass approximately 30 feet (9 meters) from the incident site. Fire department first responders have logrolled the patient onto a long backboard and applied a cervical collar. They report that the patient has been unresponsive since their arrival. Periorbital ecchymosis ("raccoon eyes") is already present. You observe bleeding from both nares and the right ear. Frequent suctioning is required to maintain a patent airway. Ventilations are irregular, and snoring sounds are audible. The patient's skin is pale, and cyanosis is present around the lips.

What indicators of airway compromise are evident in this patient? What other information, if any, would you seek from witnesses or the first responders? Describe the sequence of actions you would take to manage this patient before and during transport. ■

Airway management plays a prominent role in the management of trauma patients. Its importance is recognized now even more than in years past. The failure to maintain oxygenation and ventilation causes secondary brain injury, compounding the primary brain injury produced by the initial trauma. Ensuring patency of the airway and maintaining the patient's oxygenation and supporting ventilation, when necessary, are critical steps in minimizing the overall brain injury and improving the likelihood of good outcome.

Cerebral oxygenation and oxygen delivery to other parts of the body provided by adequate airway management and ventilation remain the most important components of prehospital patient care. Because techniques and adjunct devices are changing and will continue to change, keeping abreast of these changes is important.

The respiratory system serves three primary functions, as follows:

1. The system provides oxygen to the red blood cells, which carry the oxygen to all the cells in the body.
2. In *aerobic metabolism* the cells use this oxygen as fuel to produce energy.
3. The system removes carbon dioxide (CO_2) from the body.

Inability of the respiratory system to provide oxygen to the cells or inability of the cells to use the oxygen supplied results in *anaerobic metabolism* and can quickly lead to death. Failure to eliminate CO_2 can lead to coma.

Anatomy

The respiratory system is composed of the upper airway and the lower airway, including the lungs (Figure 6-1). Each part of the system plays an important role in ensuring gas exchange—the process by which oxygen enters the bloodstream and CO_2 is removed.

Upper Airway

The airway system is an open path that leads atmospheric air through the nose, mouth, pharynx, trachea, and bronchi to the alveoli. With each breath the average adult takes in approximately 500 mL of air. The airway system holds up to 150 mL of air that never actually reaches the alveoli to participate in the critical gas exchange process. The space in which this air is held is known as *dead space*. The air inside this dead space is not available to the body to be used for oxygenation because it never reaches the alveoli.

The upper airway consists of the nasal cavity and the oral cavity (Figure 6-2). Air entering the nasal cavity is warmed, humidified, and filtered to remove impurities. Beyond these cavities is the area known as the *pharynx*, which runs from the back of the soft palate to the upper end of the esophagus. The pharynx is composed of muscle lined with mucous membranes. The pharynx is divided into three discrete sections: the *nasopharynx* (upper portion), the *oropharynx* (middle portion), and the *hypopharynx* (lower or distal end of the pharynx).

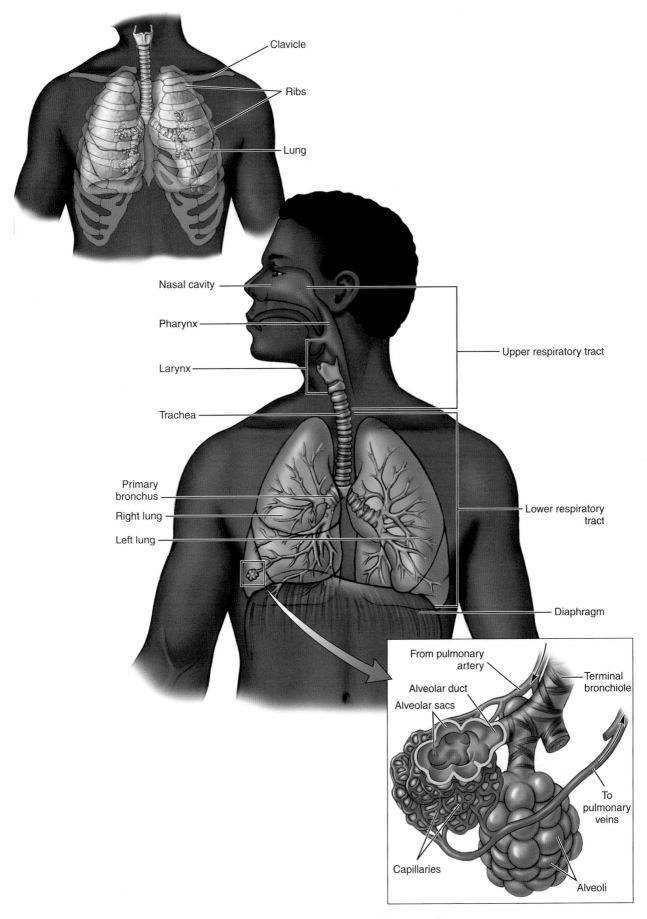

FIGURE 6-1   Organs of the respiratory system: upper respiratory tract and lower respiratory tract.
(From Herlihy B, Maebius WK: *The human body in health and disease,* Philadelphia, 2000, Saunders.)

FIGURE 6-2   Sagittal section through the nasal cavity and pharynx viewed from the medial side.

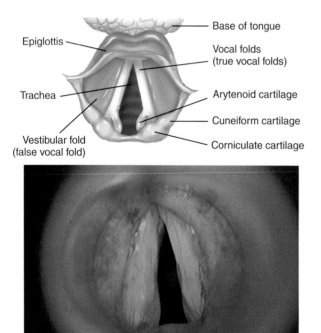

FIGURE 6-3   Vocal cords viewed from above, showing their relationship to the paired cartilages of the larynx and the epiglottis.
(*Bottom,* Custom Medical Stock photo, from Thibodeau GA: *Structure and function,* ed 9, St Louis, 1992, Mosby.)

Below the pharynx are the *esophagus,* which leads to the stomach, and the *trachea,* at which point the lower airway begins. Above the trachea is the *larynx* (Figure 6-3), which contains the vocal cords, and the muscles that make them work, housed in a strong cartilaginous box. The vocal cords are folds of tissue that meet in the midline. The false cords, or *vestibular folds,* direct the airflow through the vocal cords. Supporting the cords posteriorly is the arytenoid cartilage. Directly above the larynx is a leaf-shaped structure called the *epiglottis.* Acting as a gate or flapper valve, the epiglottis directs air into the trachea and solids and liquids into the esophagus.

Lower Airway

The lower airway consists of the trachea, its branches, and the lungs. On inspiration, air travels through the upper airway and into the lower airway before reaching the alveoli, where the actual gas exchange occurs (Figure 6-4). The trachea divides into the right and left *mainstem bronchi.* Each of the mainstem bronchi subdivides into several primary bronchi and then into bronchioles. *Bronchioles* (very small bronchial tubes) terminate at the *alveoli,* which are tiny air sacs surrounded by capillaries. The alveoli are the site of gas exchange where the respiratory and circulatory systems meet.

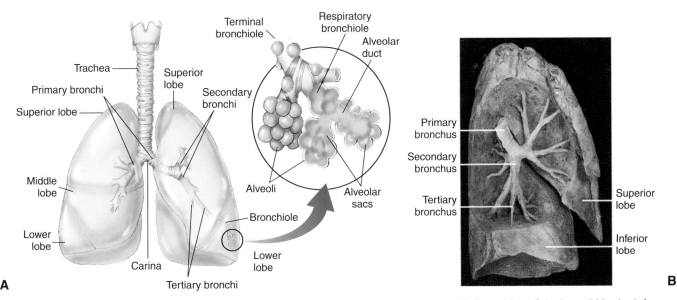

FIGURE 6-4   A, Trachea and lungs. *Inset,* Terminal bronchiole and its associated alveoli. **B,** Branching of the bronchi in the left lung.

Physiology

With each breath, air is drawn into the lungs. When atmospheric air reaches the alveoli, oxygen moves from the alveoli, across the alveolar-capillary membrane, and into the red blood cells (RBCs). The circulatory system then delivers the oxygen-carrying RBCs to the body tissues, where oxygen is used as fuel for metabolism.

As oxygen is transferred from inside the alveoli to the RBCs, CO_2 is exchanged in the opposite direction, from the plasma to the alveoli. Carbon dioxide, which is carried in the plasma, not in the RBCs, moves from the bloodstream, across the alveolar-capillary membrane, and into the alveoli, where it is eliminated during exhalation (Figure 6-5). On completion of this exchange, the oxygenated RBCs and plasma with a low CO_2 level return to the left side of the heart to be pumped to all the cells in the body.

Once at the cell, the oxygenated RBCs deliver their oxygen, which the cells then use as fuel for aerobic metabolism. Carbon dioxide, a byproduct of aerobic metabolism, is released into the blood plasma. Deoxygenated blood returns to the right side of the heart. The blood is pumped to the lungs, where it is again supplied with oxygen, and the CO_2 is eliminated by diffusion.

The alveoli must be constantly replenished with a fresh supply of air that contains an adequate amount of oxygen. This replenishment of air, known as *ventilation,* is essential for the elimination of CO_2. Ventilation is measurable. The size of each breath, called the *tidal volume,* multiplied by the ventilatory rate for 1 minute equals the *minute volume:*

Minute volume =

Tidal volume $\times$ Ventilatory rate per minute

During normal resting ventilation, about 500 mL of air is taken into the lungs. As mentioned previously, part of this volume, 150 mL, remains in the airway system as dead space and does not participate in gas exchange. If the tidal volume is 500 mL and the ventilatory rate is 14 breaths/min, the minute volume can be calculated as follows:

Minute volume = 500 mL $\times$ 14 breaths/min
Minute volume = 7000 mL/min, or 7 L/min

Therefore, at rest, about 7 liters of air must move in and out of the lungs each minute to maintain adequate CO_2 elimination and oxygenation. If the minute volume falls below normal, the patient has inadequate ventilation, a condition called *hypoventilation.* Hypoventilation leads to a buildup of CO_2 in the body. Hypoventilation is common when head or chest trauma causes an altered breathing pattern or an inability to move the chest wall adequately. For example, a patient with rib fractures who is breathing quickly and shallowly because of the pain of the injury may have a tidal volume of 100 mL and a ventilatory rate of 40 breaths/min. This patient's minute volume can be calculated as follows:

Minute volume = 100 mL $\times$ 40 breaths/min
Minute volume = 4000 mL/min, or 4 L/min

If 7 L/min is necessary for adequate gas exchange in a nontraumatized person at rest, 4 L/min is much less than what the body requires to eliminate CO_2 effectively, indicating hypoventilation. Furthermore, 150 mL of air is necessary to overcome dead space. If tidal volume is 100 mL, oxygenated air will never reach the alveoli. If left untreated,

FIGURE 6-5   Oxygen *(O₂)* moves into the red blood cells from the alveoli. The O₂ is transferred to the tissue cell on the hemoglobin molecule. After leaving the hemoglobin molecule, the O₂ travels into the tissue cell. Carbon dioxide *(CO₂)* travels in the reverse direction, but not on the hemoglobin molecule. It travels in the plasma as CO_2.

this hypoventilation will quickly lead to severe distress and ultimately death.

In the previous example the patient is hypoventilating even though the ventilatory rate is 40 breaths/min. Evaluating a patient's ability to exchange air involves assessing both ventilatory rate and depth. A common mistake is assuming that any patient with a fast ventilatory rate is hyperventilating. A much better measure of ventilatory status is the amount of CO_2 eliminated, which can be determined using CO_2 monitors. The effect of CO_2 elimination on metabolism is discussed with the Fick principle and aerobic and anaerobic metabolism in Chapter 7.

Assessment of ventilatory function always includes an evaluation of how well a patient is taking in, diffusing, and delivering oxygen. Without proper intake and processing of oxygen, anaerobic metabolism will begin. In addition, effective ventilation must also be assured. A patient may accomplish ventilation completely, partially, or not at all. Aggressive assessment and management of these inadequacies in both oxygenation and ventilation are paramount to a successful outcome.

Oxygenation and Ventilation of the Trauma Patient

The oxygenation process within the human body involves the following three phases:

1. *External respiration* is the transfer of oxygen (O₂) molecules from the atmosphere to the blood. All alveolar oxygen exists as free gas; therefore each O₂ molecule exerts pressure. Increasing the percentage of oxygen in the inspired atmosphere will increase alveolar O₂ tension.
2. *Oxygen delivery* is the result of an O₂ transfer from the atmosphere to the RBC during ventilation and the transportation of these RBCs to the tissues via the cardiovascular system. This process primarily involves cardiac output, hemoglobin concentration, and oxyhemoglobin saturation. The volume of oxygen consumed by the body in 1 minute is known as *oxygen consumption.* One could describe the RBCs as the body's "oxygen tankers." These tankers move along the vascular system "highways" to "off-load" their O₂ supply at the body's distribution points, the capillary beds.
3. *Internal (cellular) respiration* is the movement, or diffusion, of oxygen from the RBCs into the tissue cells. Metabolism normally occurs through glycolysis and the Krebs cycle to produce energy. Because the actual exchange of oxygen between the RBCs and the tissues occurs in the thin-walled capillaries, oxygen available for consumption will be decreased if fraction of inspired oxygen (Fio_2) is low (interruption in supply) or if circulation to the capillary beds is compromised ("roadblocked"). The tissues cannot consume adequate oxygen if adequate amounts are not available.

Adequate oxygenation depends on all three of these phases. Although the ability to assess tissue oxygenation in prehospital situations is improving rapidly, appropriate ventilatory support for all trauma patients begins by providing supplemental oxygen to help ensure that hypoxia is corrected or averted entirely.

Pathophysiology

Trauma can affect the respiratory system's ability to adequately provide oxygen and eliminate carbon dioxide in the following ways:

1. Hypoventilation can result from loss of ventilatory drive, usually because of decreased neurologic function, most often after a traumatic brain injury.
2. Hypoventilation can result from obstruction of airflow through the upper and lower airways.
3. Hypoventilation can be caused by decreased expansion of the lungs.
4. *Hypoxemia* (decreased oxygen level in the blood) can result from decreased diffusion of oxygen across the alveolar-capillary membrane.
5. *Hypoxia* (deficient tissue oxygenation) can be caused by decreased blood flow to the alveoli.
6. Hypoxia can result from the inability of the air to reach the capillaries, usually because the alveoli are filled with fluid or debris.
7. Hypoxia can be caused at the end cellular level by decreased blood flow to the tissue cells.

The first three ways involve hypoventilation as a result of the reduction of minute volume. If left untreated, hypoventilation results in CO_2 buildup, acidosis, and eventually death. Management involves improving the patient's ventilatory rate and depth by correcting existing airway problems and assisting ventilation as appropriate.

The following sections discuss the first two causes of inadequate ventilation: decreased neurologic function and mechanical obstruction. The third cause, a reduction in minute volume as a result of decreased pulmonary expansion, is discussed in Chapter 10. The last four causes are discussed in Chapter 7.

Decreased Neurologic Function

Decreased minute volume can be caused by two clinical conditions related to decreased neurologic function: flaccidity of the tongue and a decreased level of consciousness (LOC).

Flaccidity of the tongue associated with a reduced LOC allows the tongue to fall into a dependent position (toward the lowest area of the body). If a patient is supine, the base of the tongue will fall backward and occlude the hypopharynx (Figure 6-6). This complication commonly presents as snoring with respirations. To prevent the tongue from occluding the hypopharynx or correct the problem when it occurs, the airway patency must be assured in any supine patient with a diminished LOC, regardless of whether signs of ventilatory compromise exist. Such patients may also require periodic suctioning because secretions, saliva,

FIGURE 6-6   In an unconscious patient the tongue has lost its muscle tone and falls back into the hypopharnyx, occluding the airway and preventing passage of oxygen into the trachea and lungs.

blood, or vomitus may accumulate in the oropharynx. A decreased LOC will also affect ventilatory drive and may reduce the rate of ventilation, the volume of ventilation, or both. This reduction in minute volume may be temporary or permanent.

Mechanical Obstruction

Another cause of decreased minute volume is mechanical airway obstruction. The source of these obstructions may be neurologically influenced or purely mechanical in nature. Neurologic insults that alter the LOC may disrupt the "controls" that normally hold the tongue in an anatomically neutral (nonobstructing) position. If these "controls" are compromised, the tongue falls rearward, occluding the hypopharynx (see Figure 6-6).

Foreign bodies in the airway may be objects that were in the patient's mouth at the time of the injury, such as false teeth, chewing gum, tobacco, real teeth, and bone. Outside materials, such as glass from a broken windshield or any object that is near the patient's mouth on injury, may also threaten airway patency. Upper and lower airway obstructions may also be caused by bone or cartilage collapse as a result of a fractured larynx or trachea, by a mucous membrane avulsed from the hypopharynx or tongue, or by facial damage in which blood and fragments of bone and tissue create an obstruction.

Management of mechanical airway obstructions can be extremely challenging. Foreign bodies in the oral cavity may become lodged and create occlusions in the hypopharynx or the larynx. Crush injuries to the larynx and edema of the vocal cords may be present. Patients with facial injuries present with two of the most common foreign body obstructions, blood and vomit. Treatment of these problems is aimed at immediate recognition of the obstruction and the steps taken to ensure airway patency.

Management

Airway Control

Ensuring a patent airway is the first priority of trauma management and resuscitation, and no action is more crucial in airway management than appropriate assessment of the airway (Figure 6-7). Regardless of how the airway is managed, a cervical spine injury is possible. The use of any of these methods of airway control requires simultaneous manual stabilization of the cervical spine in a neutral position until the patient has been completely immobilized (see Chapter 9).

Essential Skills

Management of the airway in trauma patients takes precedence over all other procedures because without an adequate airway, a positive outcome cannot be achieved. Management of the airways can be challenging, but in most patients, basic-level procedures may be sufficient initially.[1] Even prehospital care providers who have been trained in more advanced airway techniques need to maintain their ability to perform these essential skills, because these methods provide an acceptable alternative when more advanced techniques fail. Providers with advanced skills always weigh the risk versus the benefit of performing these highly invasive procedures. Furthermore, maintenance of advanced skill proficiency, quality assurance, and close oversight by the medical director are necessary.

Manual Clearing of the Airway. The first step in airway management is a quick visual inspection of the oropharyngeal cavity. Foreign material (e.g., pieces of food) or broken teeth and blood may be found in the mouth of a trauma patient. These are swept out of the mouth using a gloved finger or, in the case of blood or vomitus, may be suctioned away.

Manual Maneuvers. In unresponsive patients the tongue becomes flaccid, falling back and blocking the hypopharynx (see Figure 6-6). The tongue is the most common cause of airway obstruction. Manual methods to clear this type of obstruction can easily be accomplished because the tongue is attached to the mandible (jaw) and moves forward with it. Any maneuver that moves the mandible forward will pull the tongue out of the hypopharynx:

- *Trauma jaw thrust.* In patients with suspected head, neck, or facial trauma, the cervical spine is maintained in a neutral inline position. The trauma jaw thrust maneuver allows the prehospital care provider to open the airway with little or no movement of the head and cervical spine (Figure 6-8). The mandible is thrust forward by placing the thumbs on each zygoma (cheekbone), placing the index and long fingers on the

mandible, and at the same angle, pushing the mandible forward.
- *Trauma chin lift.* The trauma chin lift maneuver is used to relieve a variety of anatomic airway obstructions in patients who are breathing spontaneously (Figure 6-9). The chin and lower incisors are grasped and then lifted to pull the mandible forward. The prehospital care provider wears gloves to avoid body fluid contamination.

Both these techniques result in movement of the lower mandible anteriorly (upward) and slightly caudal (toward the feet), pulling the tongue forward, away from the posterior airway, and opening the mouth. The trauma jaw thrust pushes the mandible forward, whereas the trauma chin lift pulls the mandible. The trauma jaw thrust and the trauma chin lift are modifications of the conventional jaw thrust and chin lift. The modifications provide protection to the patient's cervical spine while opening the airway by displacing the tongue from the posterior pharynx.

Suctioning. A trauma patient may not be capable of effectively clearing the buildup of secretions, vomitus, blood, or foreign objects from the trachea. Providing suction is an important part of maintaining a patent airway.

The most significant complication of suctioning is that suctioning for prolonged periods will produce hypoxemia, which may manifest as a cardiac abnormality (e.g., tachycardia). Preoxygenation of the trauma patient by providing supplemental oxygen will help prevent hypoxemia. In addition, during an extended period of suctioning, cardiac dysrhythmias may occur from arterial hypoxemia, and lead to myocardial hypoxemia or vagal stimulation secondary to tracheal irritation. True vagal stimulation may lead to profound bradycardia and hypotension.

The trauma patient not yet intubated may require aggressive suctioning of the upper airway. Much larger amounts of blood and vomit may be in the airway on the arrival of emergency medical services (EMS) than a suction unit can quickly clear. If so, the patient may be rolled onto his or her side while maintaining cervical spine stabilization; gravity will then assist in clearing the airway. A rigid suction device is preferred to clear the oropharynx. Although hypoxia can result from prolonged suctioning, a totally obstructed airway will provide no air exchange. Aggressive suctioning and patient positioning are done until the airway is at least partially clear. At that point, hyperoxygenation followed by repeated suctioning can be performed.

When suctioning intubated patients using the *endotracheal tube* (ET), the suction catheter should be made of soft material to limit trauma to the tracheal mucosa and to minimize frictional resistance. It needs to be long enough to pass the tip of the artificial airway (20-22 inches [50-55 cm]) and should have smooth ends to prevent mucosal trauma. The soft catheter will probably not be effective

AIRWAY MANAGEMENT

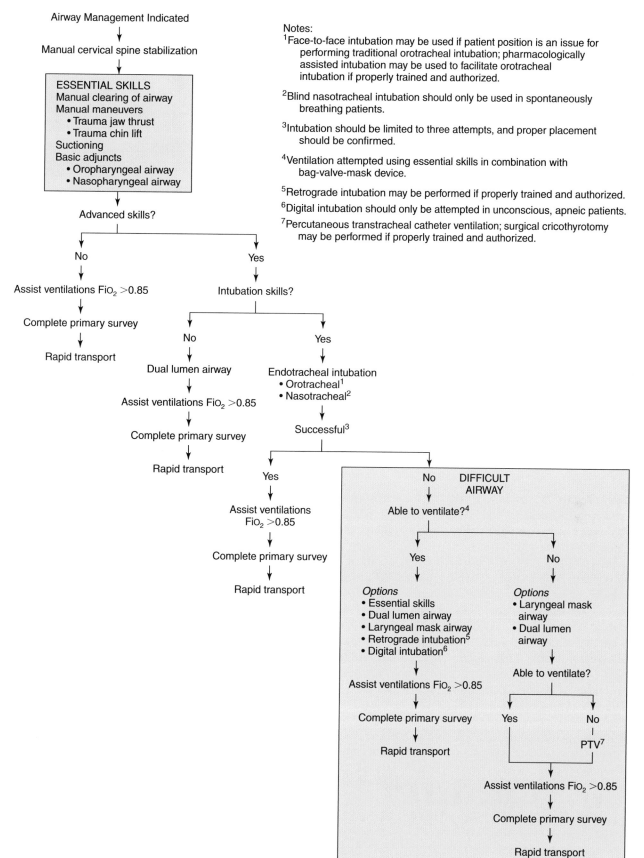

Notes:
[1] Face-to-face intubation may be used if patient position is an issue for performing traditional orotracheal intubation; pharmacologically assisted intubation may be used to facilitate orotracheal intubation if properly trained and authorized.

[2] Blind nasotracheal intubation should only be used in spontaneously breathing patients.

[3] Intubation should be limited to three attempts, and proper placement should be confirmed.

[4] Ventilation attempted using essential skills in combination with bag-valve-mask device.

[5] Retrograde intubation may be performed if properly trained and authorized.

[6] Digital intubation should only be attempted in unconscious, apneic patients.

[7] Percutaneous transtracheal catheter ventilation; surgical cricothyrotomy may be performed if properly trained and authorized.

FIGURE 6-7 Airway management algorithm.

FIGURE 6-8 Trauma jaw thrust. The thumb is placed on each zygoma with the index and long fingers at the angle of the mandible. The mandible is lifted superiorly.

FIGURE 6-9 Trauma chin lift. The chin lift performs a function similar to that of the trauma jaw thrust. It moves the mandible forward by moving the tongue.

in suctioning copious amounts of foreign material or fluid from the pharynx of a trauma patient, in which case the device of choice will be one with a tonsil-tip design.

While suctioning an intubated patient, aseptic procedures are vital. This technique includes the following steps:

1. Preoxygenate the trauma patient with 100% oxygen (Fio_2 of 1.0).
2. Prepare equipment while maintaining sterility.
3. Insert the catheter without suction. Suctioning is then initiated and continued for up to 15 to 30 seconds while withdrawing the catheter.
4. Reoxygenate the patient, and ventilate for at least five assisted ventilations.
5. Repeat as necessary, allowing time for reoxygenation to take place between procedures.

Basic Adjuncts. When manual airway maneuvers are unsuccessful or when continued maintenance of an open airway is necessary, the use of an artificial airway is the next step.

Oropharyngeal Airway. The most frequently used artificial airway is the oropharyngeal airway (OPA) (Figure 6-10). The OPA is inserted in either a direct or an inverted manner.

Indications
- Patient who is unable to maintain his or her airway
- To prevent an intubated patient from biting an ET tube

Contraindications
- Patient who is conscious or semiconscious

Complications
- Because it stimulates the gag reflex, use of the OPA may lead to gagging, vomiting, and laryngospasm in patients who are conscious.

FIGURE 6-10 Oropharyngeal airways.
(From McSwain NE Jr, Paturas JL: *The basic EMT: comprehensive prehospital patient care*, ed 2, St Louis, 2001, Mosby.)

Nasopharyngeal Airway. The nasopharyngeal airway (NPA) is a soft, rubberlike device that is inserted through one of the nares and then along the curvature of the posterior wall of the nasopharynx and oropharynx (Figure 6-11).

Indications
- Patient who is unable to maintain his or her airway

Contraindications
- No need for an airway adjunct

Complications
- Bleeding caused by insertion may be a complication

Dual-Lumen Airways

Dual-lumen airways offer a functional alternative airway to endotracheal intubation. Many jurisdictions allow the

FIGURE 6-11   Nasopharyngeal airways.
(From McSwain NE Jr, Paturas JL: *The basic EMT: comprehensive prehospital patient care,* ed 2, St Louis, 2001, Mosby.)

FIGURE 6-12   Endotracheal tube.

use of these devices because minimal training is required to achieve and retain competency. These devices are also a useful backup airway when endotracheal intubation attempts are unsuccessful, even when rapid-sequence intubation has been attempted. The primary advantage of dual-lumen airways is that they may be inserted independent of the patient's position, which may be especially important in trauma patients with a high suspicion of cervical injury. The use of these airways is typically limited to patients 16 years of age or older who are at least 5 feet tall.

Indications
- *Basic providers.* If the provider is trained and authorized, a dual-lumen airway is the primary airway device for an unconscious trauma patient who lacks a gag reflex and is apneic or ventilating at a rate of less than 10 breaths/min.
- *Advanced providers.* A dual-lumen airway is the alternative airway device when the provider is unable to perform endotracheal intubation and cannot easily ventilate the patient with a bag-valve-mask (BVM) device and an OPA or NPA.

Contraindications
- Intact gag reflex
- Known esophageal disease
- Recent ingestion of caustic substances

Complications
- Gagging and vomiting, if gag reflex is intact
- Damage to the esophagus
- Hypoxia if ventilated using the incorrect lumen

Endotracheal Intubation
Endotracheal intubation has been the preferred method for achieving maximum control of the airway in trauma patients who are either apneic or require assisted ventilation (Figures 6-12 and 6-13). Recent studies, however, have

FIGURE 6-13 Equipment for endotracheal intubation.
(From McSwain NE Jr, Paturas JL: *The basic EMT: comprehensive prehospital patient care,* ed 2, St Louis, 2001, Mosby.)

As with any advanced life support skill, prehospital care providers need to have the proper equipment. The standard components of an intubation kit should include the following:

- Laryngoscope with adult- and pediatric-sized straight and curved blades
- Extra batteries and spare light bulbs
- Suction machine
- Adult- and pediatric-sized endotracheal tubes
- Stylet
- 10-mL syringe
- Water-soluble lubricant
- Magill forceps
- End-tidal detection device (ETDD) for end-tidal carbon dioxide detection
- Tube-securing device

shown that in an urban environment, critically injured trauma patients with endotracheal intubation had no better outcome than those transported with a BVM and OPA.[1] Despite this, endotracheal intubation still remains the preferred method of airway control because it does the following:

- Isolates the airway
- Allows for ventilation with 100% oxygen (Fio_2 of 1.0)
- Eliminates the need to maintain an adequate mask-to-face seal
- Significantly decreases the risk of aspiration (vomitus, foreign material, blood)
- Facilitates deep tracheal suctioning
- Prevents gastric insufflation
- Provides an additional route for medication administration

Indications
- Patient who is unable to protect his or her airway
- Patient with significant oxygenation problem, requiring administration of high concentrations of oxygen
- Patient with significant ventilatory impairment requiring assisted ventilation

Contraindications
- Lack of training in technique
- Lack of proper indications
- Proximity to receiving facility (relative contraindication)

Complications
- Hypoxemia from prolonged intubation attempts
- Trauma to the airway with resultant hemorrhage
- Right mainstem bronchus intubation
- Esophageal intubation
- Vomiting leading to aspiration
- Loose or broken teeth
- Injury to the vocal cords
- Conversion of a cervical spine injury without neurologic deficit to one with neurologic deficit

Research studies have shown that practice increases the likelihood of success when intubating. Although no correlation was found between success rate and length of time as a paramedic, there was a correlation between the number of patients intubated by the paramedic and the success rate. Experience with the procedure increases the likelihood of successful performance.[2]

As with all procedures, the prehospital care provider, along with the system medical director, makes a risk/benefit judgment when using any advanced procedures. Performing procedures simply because "the protocols allow it" is inappropriate. Think of the possible benefits and the possible risks, and form a plan based on the best interest of the patient in a given situation. Situations differ drastically based on transport time, location (urban vs. rural), and provider level of comfort in performing a given procedure.

Alternative Methods. Several alternative methods are available for performing endotracheal intubation. The method of choice depends on such factors as the patient's needs, the level of urgency (orotracheal vs. nasotracheal), patient positioning (face to face), or training and scope of practice (pharmacologically assisted intubation). Regardless of the method selected, the patient's head and neck should be stabilized in a neutral position during the procedure and until spinal immobilization is completed. In general, if intubation is not successful after three attempts, consider a backup technique.

Orotracheal Intubation. Orotracheal intubation involves placing an ET tube into the trachea through the mouth. The nontrauma patient is often placed in a "sniffing" position to facilitate intubation. Because this position hyperextends the cervical spine at C1-C2 (the second most common site for cervical spine fractures in the trauma patient) and hyperflexes it at C5-C6 (the most common site for cervical spine fractures in the trauma patient), it should not be used for trauma patients (Figure 6-14).

Nasotracheal Intubation. In conscious trauma patients or in those with an intact gag reflex, endotracheal intubation may be difficult to accomplish. If spontaneous ventilations are present, blind nasotracheal intubation (BNTI) may be attempted if the benefit outweighs the risk. Although nasotracheal intubation is often more difficult to perform than direct visualization and oral intubation, a 90% success rate has been reported in traumatized patients. During BNTI the patient should be breathing to ensure that the ET tube is passed through the vocal cords. Many texts suggest that BNTI is contraindicated in the presence of midface trauma

FIGURE 6-14 Placing the patient's head in the "sniffing" position provides ideal visualization of the larynx through the mouth. However, such positioning hyperextends the patient's neck at C1 and C2 and hyperflexes it at C5 and C6. These are the two most common points of fracture of the cervical spine.

or fractures, but an exhaustive literature search reveals no documentation of an ET tube entering the cranial vault. Apnea is a contraindication specific to BNTI. In addition, no stylet is used when BNTI is performed.

Face-to-Face Intubation. Face-to-face intubation is indicated when standard trauma intubation techniques cannot be used because of the inability of the rescuer to assume the standard position at the head of the trauma patient. These situations include but are not limited to the following:

- Vehicle entrapment
- Pinning of the patient in rubble

Pharmacologically Assisted Intubation. Intubation using pharmacologic agents may occasionally be required to facilitate ET tube placement in injured patients. In skilled hands, this technique can facilitate effective airway control when other methods fail or are otherwise not acceptable. To maximize the effectiveness of this procedure and ensure patient safety, personnel using drugs to assist with intubation need to be familiar with applicable local protocols, medications, and indications for use of the technique. The use of drugs to assist with intubation, particularly rapid-sequence intubation, does have risks. Pharmacologically assisted intubation is a procedure of necessity, not convenience. Intubation using drugs falls into the following two categories:

1. *Intubation using sedatives or narcotics.* Medications such as diazepam, midazolam, fentanyl, or morphine are used alone or in combination, with the goal being to relax the patient enough to permit intubation but not to abolish protective reflexes or breathing. The effectiveness of a single pharmacologic agent, such as midazolam, has been well documented.[3]
2. *Rapid-sequence intubation (RSI) using paralytic agents* (Box 6-1). The patient is chemically paralyzed after first being sedated. This provides complete muscle paralysis but removes all protective reflexes and causes apnea. Studies of this method of airway management have demonstrated successful performance of the technique in the field, with intubation success rates reported in the mid-90% range. However, few studies have critically evaluated whether or not patient outcome is affected.[4] One center reported its experience with RSI in the field and documented that patients with traumatic brain injury who underwent RSI had a poorer outcome than those who did not require RSI.[5] Subsequent analysis has shown that unrecognized hyperventilation leading to hypocarbia and unrecognized hypoxia were major contributors to the poor outcome.[6]

Also, pharmacologically assisted intubation of any type requires time to accomplish. In every trauma patient for whom this intubation is contemplated, the benefits of securing an airway are weighed against the additional time spent on the scene to perform the procedure.

Indications
- A patient who requires a secure airway and is difficult to intubate because of uncooperative behavior (as induced by hypoxia, traumatic brain injury, hypotension, or intoxication)

Relative Contraindications
- Availability of an alternative airway (e.g., dual lumen)
- Severe facial trauma that would impair or preclude successful intubation
- Neck deformity or swelling that complicates or precludes placement of a surgical airway
- Known allergies to indicated medications
- Medical problems that would preclude use of indicated medications
- Inability to intubate

Complications
- Inability to insert the ET tube in a sedated or paralyzed patient no longer able to protect his or her airway or breathe spontaneously; patients who are medicated and then cannot be intubated require prolonged BVM ventilation until the medication wears off
- Development of hypoxia or hypercarbia during prolonged intubation attempts
- Aspiration
- Hypotension; virtually all the drugs have the side effect of decreasing blood pressure

Patients who are mildly or moderately hypovolemic but compensating may have a profound drop in blood pressure associated with the intravenous administration of many of these drugs. Exercise caution whenever the use of medications for intubation is considered (Table 6-1).

Verification of Endotracheal Tube Placement. Once intubation has been performed, take specific measures to ensure that the tube has been properly placed in the trachea. An improperly positioned ET tube, if unrecognized for only a brief period, may result in profound hypoxia, with resultant brain injury (hypoxic encephalopathy) and even death. Therefore it is important that proper placement be confirmed. Techniques to verify intubation include the use of both clinical assessments and adjunct devices.[7] Clinical assessments include the following:

- Direct visualization of the ET tube passing through the vocal cords
- Presence of bilateral breath sounds (auscultate laterally below the axilla) *and* absence of air sounds over the epigastrium

---

BOX 6-1   Sample Protocol for Rapid-Sequence Intubation (RSI)

1. Ensure availability of required equipment.
   a. Oxygen supply
   b. Bag-valve-mask (BVM) of appropriate size and type
   c. Nonrebreathing mask
   d. Laryngoscope with blades
   e. Endotracheal (ET) tubes
   f. Surgical and alternative airway equipment
   g. RSI medications
   h. Materials or devices to secure ET tube after placement
   i. Suction equipment
2. Ensure that at least one (but preferably two) patent intravenous (IV) line is present.
3. Preoxygenate the patient using a nonrebreathing mask or BVM with 100% oxygen. Preoxygenation for 3 to 4 minutes is preferred.
4. Apply cardiac and pulse oximetry monitors.
5. If the patient is conscious, strongly consider the use of sedative agents.
6. Consider the administration of sedative agents and lidocaine in the presence of potential or confirmed traumatic brain injury (TBI).
7. After administration of paralytic agents, use the Sellick (cricoid pressure) maneuver to decrease the potential for aspiration.
8. Confirm tube placement immediately after intubation. Continuous cardiac and pulse oximeter monitoring is required during and after RSI. Reconfirm tube placement periodically throughout transport and each time the patient is moved.
9. Use repeat doses of paralytic agents as needed to maintain paralysis.

PROCEDURE

1. Assemble the required equipment.
2. Ensure the patency of the IV lines.
3. Preoxygenate the patient with 100% oxygen for approximately 3 to 4 minutes if possible.
4. Place the patient on cardiac and pulse oximeter monitors.
5. Administer a sedative, such as midazolam, if appropriate.
6. In the presence of confirmed or potential TBI, administer lidocaine (1.5 mg/kg) 2 to 3 minutes before administration of a paralytic agent.
7. For pediatric patients, administer atropine (0.01-0.02 mg/kg) 1 to 3 minutes before paralytic administration to minimize the vagal response to intubation.
8. Administer a short-acting paralytic agent intravenously, such as succinylcholine. Paralysis and relaxation should occur within 30 seconds.
   a. Adult: 1 to 2 mg/kg
   b. Pediatric: 1 to 2 mg/kg
9. Insert an ET tube. If initial attempts are unsuccessful, precede repeat attempts with preoxygenation.
10. Confirm ET tube placement.
11. If repeated attempts to achieve endotracheal intubation fail, consider placement of an alternative or surgical airway.
12. Use doses of a long-acting paralytic agent, such as vecuronium, to continue paralysis.
    a. Initial dose: 0.1 mg/kg IV push
    b. Subsequent doses: 0.01 mg/kg every 30 to 45 minutes

Note: Requirements vary with individual patients.

- Visualization of the chest rising and falling during ventilation
- Fogging (water vapor condensation) in the ET tube on expiration

Unfortunately, none of these techniques is 100% reliable *by itself* for verifying proper tube placement. Therefore, prudent practice involves assessing and documenting *all* these clinical signs, if possible. On rare occasions, because of difficult anatomy, visualization of the ET tube passing through the vocal cords may not possible. In a moving vehicle (ground or aeromedical), engine noise may make auscultation of breath sounds almost impossible. Obesity and chronic obstructive pulmonary disease (COPD) may interfere with the ability to see chest movement during ventilation.

Adjunct devices include the following:

- Esophageal detector device
- Colorimetric CO_2 detector
- End-tidal CO_2 monitoring (capnography)
- Pulse oximetry

As with the clinical assessments, none of these adjuncts is 100% accurate in all patients. In a patient with a perfusing rhythm, end-tidal CO_2 monitoring (capnography) serves as the "gold standard" for determining ET tube placement. This technique should be used in the prehospital setting whenever available. Patients in cardiopulmonary arrest do not exhale CO_2, and therefore neither colorimetric detectors nor capnography may be useful in patients who lack a perfusing cardiac rhythm.

TABLE 6-1   Common Drugs Used for Pharmacologically Assisted Intubation

Drug	Dose (Adult)	Dose (Pediatric)	Indications	Complications/ side effects
PRETREATMENT				
Oxygen	High flow Assist ventilation as needed to achieve oxygen saturation of 100% if possible	High flow Assist ventilation as needed to achieve oxygen saturation of 100% if possible	All patients undergoing pharmacologically assisted intubation	—
Lidocaine	1.5 mg/kg	1.5 mg/kg IV	Brain injury	Seizure
Atropine	—	0.01-0.02 mg/kg IV	Pediatric intubation, prevention of bradycardia and excess secretions	Tachycardia
INDUCTION OF SEDATION				
Midazolam (Versed)	0.1-0.15 mg/kg up to 0.3 mg/kg IV	0.1-0.15 mg/kg up to 0.3 mg/kg IV	Sedation	Respiratory depression/ apnea, hypotension
Fentanyl (Sublimaze)	2-3 μg/kg IV	1-3 μg/kg IV	Sedation	Respiratory depression/ apnea, hypotension, bradycardia
Etomidate	0.2-0.3 mg/kg IV	Not approved for patients <10 years of age	Sedation, induced anesthesia	Apnea, hypotension, vomiting
CHEMICAL PARALYSIS				
Succinylcholine	1-2 mg/kg	1-2 mg/kg	Muscle relaxation and paralysis (short duration)	Hyperkalemia, muscle fasciculations
Vecuronium (Norcuron)	0.1 mg/kg	0.1 mg/kg	Muscle relaxation and paralysis (intermediate duration)	Hypotension
Pancuronium (Pavulon)	0.04-0.1 mg/kg	0.04-0.1 mg/kg	Muscle relaxation and paralysis (long duration)	Tachycardia, hypertension, salivation

Because none of these techniques is universally reliable, all the clinical assessments noted previously should be performed, unless impractical, followed by use of at least one of the adjunct devices. If any of the techniques used to verify proper placement suggests that the ET tube may not be properly positioned, the tube should be immediately removed and reinserted, with placement verified again. All the techniques used to verify tube placement should be noted on the patient care report.

Securing an Endotracheal Tube. Once endotracheal intubation has been performed and proper tube placement verified, the depth of tube insertion at the central incisors (front teeth) should be noted. Next, the ET tube is secured in place. The most common method used is to tape the tube to the patient's face. Unfortunately, blood and secretions often prevent the tape from adhering satisfactorily, allowing

movement and potential dislodging of the ET tube. Several commercially available products may serve to secure the ET tube adequately. Ideally, if sufficient personnel are present, someone should be assigned the task of manually holding the tube in proper position to ensure that it does not move.

Continuous pulse oximetry should be considered *necessary* for all patients who require endotracheal intubation. Any decline in the pulse oximetry reading (Sp_{O_2}), or development of cyanosis, requires reverification of ET tube placement. Additionally, an ET tube may also become dislodged during any movement of the patient. Reverify tube position after every move of a patient, such as logrolling to a long backboard or carrying the patient down a staircase.

Backup Techniques

If endotracheal intubation has been unsuccessful after three attempts, consideration of airway management using the essential skills described previously and ventilating with a BVM device are appropriate. *If the receiving facility is reasonably close, these techniques may be the most prudent option for airway management when faced with a brief transport time.* If the nearest appropriate facility is more distant, one of the following backup techniques may be considered.

Retrograde Intubation. In the prehospital setting, retrograde tracheal intubation (RI) is potentially useful because the presence of blood or secretions does not hinder insertion as it may in more traditional intubation methods. RI, although comparatively time-consuming, is a less invasive (and less risky) procedure than surgical cricothyrotomy when the cervical spine is properly stabilized and when orotracheal or nasotracheal intubation attempts have failed.

RI is a fairly straightforward procedure. A needle (large enough to accommodate the guide wire) is inserted into the caudal aspect of the cricothyroid membrane. A guide wire is advanced through the needle into the oropharynx, and the end of the wire is brought out of the mouth. An ET tube is then advanced over the guide wire and into the oropharynx. When resistance at attempts to advance the tube is encountered, the guide wire is then pulled completely out of the neck, and the ET tube is advanced as the guide wire exits the neck. Because these procedures are often difficult to perform expeditiously, RI is not recommended for use in apneic patients.

Indications
■ Patients in whom endotracheal intubation failed but for whom ventilations can be assisted with a BVM device.

Relative Contraindications
■ Apneic patient
■ Proximity to receiving facility
■ Insufficient training

Complications
■ Damage to the vocal cords and larynx
■ Bleeding at the puncture site
■ Esophageal intubation
■ Hypoxia or hypercarbia during the procedure

Digital Intubation. Digital, or *tactile,* intubation was a precursor to the current use of laryngoscopes for endotracheal intubation. Essentially, the intubator's fingers act similar to a laryngoscope blade by manipulating the epiglottis and acting as a guide for placement of the ET tube.

Indications
■ Patients in whom endotracheal intubation failed but for whom ventilations can be assisted with a BVM device
■ When laryngoscope is unavailable or fails

■ When the airway is obscured or blocked because of large volumes of blood or vomitus
■ Entrapment with inability to perform face-to-face intubation

Contraindications
■ Any patient who is not comatose and may bite the intubator's fingers (dental clamp or bite stick may be used to hold the patient's mouth open)

Complications
■ Esophageal intubation
■ Lacerations or crush injuries to the prehospital care provider's fingers
■ Hypoxia or hypercarbia during the procedure
■ Damage to the vocal cords

Laryngeal Mask Airway. The laryngeal mask airway (LMA) is another alternative for unconscious or seriously obtunded adult and pediatric patients. The device consists of an inflatable silicone ring attached diagonally to a silicone tube (Figure 6-15). When inserted, the ring creates a low-pressure seal between the LMA and the glottic opening, without direct insertion of the device into the larynx.

Advantages of the LMA include the following:

1. The device is designed for blind insertion. Direct visualization of the trachea and vocal cords is unnecessary.
2. With proper cleaning and storage, the LMA can be reused multiple times.
3. Disposable LMAs are now available.
4. The LMA is available in a range of sizes to accommodate both pediatric and adult patient groups.

Prehospital use of the LMA thus far has been more prevalent in Europe than in North America. A recent development is the introduction of an "intubating LMA." This device is inserted similar to the original LMA, but a flexible ET tube is then passed though the LMA, intubating the trachea. This secures the airway without the need to visualize the vocal cords.

FIGURE 6-15   Laryngeal mask airway.

Indications

- When unable to perform endotracheal intubation and the patient cannot be ventilated using a BVM device

Contraindications

- When endotracheal intubation can be performed
- Insufficient training

Complications

- Aspiration, because LMA does not completely prevent regurgitation and protect the trachea
- Laryngospasm

Percutaneous Transtracheal Ventilation. In rare cases a trauma patient's airway obstruction cannot be relieved by the methods previously discussed. In these patients a needle tracheostomy may be performed using a percutaneously placed catheter. It has been shown that adequate oxygenation can be achieved using percutaneous transtracheal ventilation (PTV), with acceptable levels of CO_2 maintained for 30 minutes.[8]

Advantages of PTV include the following:

1. Ease of access (landmarks usually easily recognized)
2. Ease of insertion
3. Minimal equipment required
4. No incision necessary
5. Minimal training required

Indications

- When all other alternative methods of airway management fail or are impractical and the patient cannot be ventilated with a BVM device

Contraindications

- Insufficient training
- Lack of proper equipment
- Ability to secure airway by another technique (as described previously), or ability to ventilate with a BVM device

Complications

- Hypercarbia from prolonged use (CO_2 elimination not as effective as with other methods of ventilation)[8]
- Damage to surrounding structures, including the larynx, thyroid gland, carotid arteries, jugular veins, and esophagus

Surgical Cricothyrotomy. Surgical cricothyrotomy involves the creation of a surgical opening in the *cricothyroid membrane,* which lies between the larynx (thyroid cartilage) and the cricoid cartilage. In most patients the skin is very thin in this location, making it amenable to immediate access to the airway.[9] Consider this a technique of "last resort" in prehospital airway management.

The use of this surgical airway in the prehospital arena is controversial. Proficient endotracheal intubation skills should minimize the need even to consider its use. *Surgical cricothyrotomy should never be the initial airway control method.* Insufficient data exist at this time to support a recommendation that surgical cricothyrotomy be established as a national standard for routine use in prehospital airway management. Local protocols should govern the implementation of surgical cricothyrotomy.

Indications

- Massive midface trauma precluding the use of a BVM device
- Inability to control the airway using less invasive maneuvers
- Ongoing tracheobronchial hemorrhage

Contraindications

- Any patient who can be safely intubated, either orally or nasally
- Patients with laryngotracheal injuries
- Children under 10 years of age
- Patients with acute laryngeal disease of traumatic or infectious origin
- Insufficient training

Complications

- Prolonged procedure time
- Hemorrhage
- Aspiration
- Misplacement or false passage of the ET tube
- Injury to neck structures or vessels
- Perforation of the esophagus

Continuous Quality Improvement

The ambulance service medical director or his or her designee should individually review all out-of-hospital uses of medications for intubation or invasive airway techniques. Specific points include the following:

- Adherence to protocol and procedures
- Proper indications for the use of medications
- Proper documentation of drug dosage routes and monitoring of the patient during and after intubation
- Confirmation of tube placement procedures
- Outcome and complications

Ventilatory Devices

All trauma patients receive appropriate ventilatory support with supplemental oxygen to ensure that hypoxia is corrected or averted entirely. In deciding which method or equipment to use, prehospital care providers should consider the following devices and their respective oxygen concentrations (Table 6-2).

TABLE 6-2 **Ventilatory Devices and Oxygen Concentration**

Device	Liter flow (L/min)	Oxygen concentration*
WITHOUT SUPPLEMENTAL OXYGEN		
Mouth-to-mouth	N/A	16%
Mouth-to-mask	N/A	16%
Bag-valve-mask (BVM)	N/A	21%
WITH SUPPLEMENTAL OXYGEN		
Nasal cannula	1-6	24%-45%
Mouth-to-mask	10	50%
Simple face mask	8-10	40%-60%
BVM without reservoir	8-10	40%-60%
BVM with reservoir	10-15	90%-100%
Nonrebreather mask with reservoir	10-15	90%-100%
Demand valve	N/A	90%-100%
Ventilator	N/A	21%-100%

*Percentages indicated are approximate.
N/A, Not applicable.

Pocket Masks

Regardless of which mask is chosen to support ventilation of the trauma patient, the ideal mask has the following characteristics:

1. Is a good fit.
2. Is equipped with a one-way valve.
3. Is made of a transparent material.
4. Has a supplemental oxygen port.
5. Is available in infant, pediatric, and adult sizes.

Mouth-to-mask ventilation satisfactorily delivers adequate tidal volumes by ensuring a tight face seal even when performed by those who do not use this skill often.

Bag-Valve-Mask

The BVM consists of a self-inflating bag and a nonrebreathing device; it can be used with basic (OPA, NPA) or advanced (endotracheal, nasotracheal) airway devices. Most BVM devices currently on the market have a volume of 1600 mL and can deliver an O_2 concentration of 90% to 100%. Some models also have a built-in colorimetric CO_2 detector. However, a *single* provider attempting to ventilate with a BVM may create poor tidal volumes secondary to the inability to create a tight face seal and to squeeze the bag adequately.

Ongoing practice of this skill is necessary to ensure that the technique is effective and that the trauma patient receives adequate ventilatory support.

Manually Triggered (Oxygen-Powered) Devices

Manually triggered devices can deliver O_2 concentrations of 100%. Because these devices do not permit the provider to feel the compliance of the chest during the ventilation process, care is taken not to overinflate the lungs. Maintaining a tight face seal with the device is easy because the trigger mechanism requires only one hand to operate. Complications may include gastric distention, overinflation of the lung, barotrauma, and lung rupture. These devices should not be used in the field except in unusual circumstances.

Positive-Pressure Ventilators

Positive-pressure volume ventilators during prolonged transport have long been used in the aeromedical environment. However, more ground units are now adopting the use of mechanical ventilation as a means of controlling rate, depth, and minute volume in trauma patients. Importantly, only volume ventilators with appropriate alarms and pressure control/relief should be used. These ventilators do not need to be as sophisticated as those used in the hospital and only have a few simple modes of ventilation:

Assist Control (A/C). A/C ventilation is probably the most widely used mode of ventilation in prehospital transport from the scene to the emergency department. The A/C setting delivers ventilations at a preset rate and tidal volume. If patients initiate a breath on their own, an additional ventilation of the full tidal volume is delivered.

Intermittent Mandatory Ventilation (IMV). IMV delivers a set rate and tidal volume to patients. If patients initiate their own breath, only the amount that they actually pull on their own will be delivered.

Positive End-Expiratory Pressure (PEEP). PEEP provides an elevated level of pressure at the end of expiration, thus keeping the alveolar sacs and small airways open and filled with air for a longer time. This intervention provides greater oxygenation. However, by increasing the end-expiratory pressure and therefore the overall intrathoracic pressure, PEEP may decrease blood return to the heart. In hemodynamically unstable patients, PEEP may further decrease blood pressure. PEEP should also be avoided in patients with traumatic brain injuries. The increase in thoracic pressure can cause an elevation in intracranial pressure.

Evaluation

Pulse Oximetry

Over the past few years, use of pulse oximetry has increased in the prehospital environment. Appropriate use of pulse oximetry devices allows early detection of pulmonary

FIGURE 6-16 Pulse oximeter.
(From Sanders MJ: *Mosby's paramedic textbook,* ed 3, St Louis, 2005, Mosby.)

FIGURE 6-17 Handheld end-tidal carbon dioxide detector.
(From Saunders MJ: *Mosby's paramedic textbook,* ed 3, St Louis, 2005, Mosby.)

compromise or cardiovascular deterioration before physical signs are evident. Pulse oximeters are particularly useful in prehospital applications because of their high reliability, portability, ease of application, and applicability across all age ranges and races (Figure 6-16).

Pulse oximeters provide measurements of arterial oxyhemoglobin saturation (Spo_2) and pulse rate. Spo_2 is determined by measuring the absorption ratio of red and infrared light passed through tissue. A small microprocessor correlates changes in light absorption caused by the pulsation of blood through vascular beds to determine arterial saturation and pulse rate. Normal Spo_2 is between 93% and 95% at sea level. When Spo_2 falls below 90%, severe compromise of oxygen delivery to the tissues is most likely present.

To ensure accurate pulse oximetry readings, the following general guidelines should be followed:

1. Use the appropriate size and type of sensor.
2. Ensure proper alignment of sensor light.
3. Ensure that sources and photodetectors are clean, dry, and in good repair.
4. Avoid sensor placement on grossly edematous sites.

Common problems that can produce inaccurate Spo_2 measurement include the following:

- Excessive motion
- Moisture in Spo_2 sensors
- Improper sensor application and placement
- Poor patient perfusion or vasoconstriction from hypothermia
- Anemia

In a critical trauma patient, pulse oximetry may be less than accurate because of poor capillary perfusion status. Therefore, pulse oximetry is only a valuable addition to the prehospital care provider's "toolbox" when combined with a thorough knowledge of trauma pathophysiology and strong assessment and intervention skills.

Capnography

Capnography, or end-tidal carbon dioxide ($ETco_2$) monitoring, has been used in critical care units for many years. Recent advances in technology have allowed smaller, more durable units to be produced for prehospital use (Figure 6-17). Capnography measures the partial pressure of carbon dioxide (Pco_2, or $ETco_2$) in a sample of gas. If this sample is taken at the end of exhalation, it correlates closely to arterial Pco_2 ($Paco_2$).

Most critical care units within the hospital setting use the *mainstream technique.* This technique places a sensor directly into the "main stream" of the exhaled gas. In the patient being ventilated with a BVM, the sensor is placed between the BVM and the ET tube. In the critical patient the $Paco_2$ is generally 2 to 5 mm Hg higher than the $ETco_2$. (A normal $ETco_2$ reading in a critical trauma patient is 30 to 40 mm Hg.) Although these readings may not totally reflect the patient's $Paco_2$, maintaining readings between normal levels will usually be beneficial to the patient.

Although capnography correlates closely with $Paco_2$, certain conditions will cause variations in accuracy. These conditions are often seen in the prehospital environment and include severe hypotension, high intrathoracic pressure, and any increase in dead space ventilation, as with pulmonary embolism. Therefore, following trends in $ETco_2$ levels may be more important than focusing on specific readings.

Continuous capnography provides another tool in the prehospital management of a trauma patient and is correlated with all other information about a patient. Initial transport decisions are based on physical and environmental conditions. For example, it would be inappropriate to take time to place the patient on monitors if the patient is losing blood. Instead, capnography should be used to monitor ET tube placement and continuously monitor patient status during transport. A sudden drop in expired CO_2 may result either from dislodgement of the ET tube or decreased perfusion and should prompt a reevaluation of patient status and ET tube position.[10]

Prolonged Transport

Airway management of a patient prior to and during a prolonged transport requires complex decision making on the part of the prehospital care provider. Intervention to control and secure the airway, especially with advanced techniques, depends on numerous factors, including the patient's injuries, the clinical skills of the prehospital care provider, the equipment available, and the distance and transport time to definitive care. Risks and benefits of all the airway options available should be considered prior to making a final airway decision. Both a longer distance of transport and a longer transport time lower the threshold for securing the airway with endotracheal intubation. For transports of 15 to 20 minutes, essential skills, including an oral airway and bag-valve-mask ventilation, may be sufficient. Use of air medical transport also lowers the threshold to perform endotracheal intubation, as a cramped, noisy environment makes ongoing airway assessment and management difficult.

Any patient requiring airway management or ventilatory support requires ongoing patient monitoring. Continuous pulse oximetry should be performed on all trauma patients during transport, and capnography should be strongly considered for all intubated patients. Loss of end-tidal CO_2 ($ETCO_2$) indicates that the ventilator circuit has become disconnected or, more importantly, the endotracheal tube has been dislodged, or the patient's perfusion has decreased

significantly. All of these possible causes require immediate action. Serial vital signs should also be recorded on patients requiring airway or ventilation interventions. Confirmation of endotracheal intubation, as described above, should be performed each time the patient is moved or repositioned. It is also a good idea to frequently confirm the security of any airway device.

Any patient who requires increasing Fio_2 or PEEP in order to maintain oxygenation needs to be carefully re-evaluated. Possible etiologies include the development of a pneumothorax or worsening of pulmonary contusions. Any known or suspected pneumothorax must be monitored closely for the development of a tension pneumothorax, and pleural decompression should be performed if hemodynamic compromise occurs. Burn patients should receive supplemental oxygen to maintain $Spo_2 \geq 95\%$, while those with known or suspected carbon monoxide poisoning should receive 100% oxygen. Remember that positive pressure ventilation can convert a simple pneumothorax to a tension pneumothorax. If the patient has had an open pneumothorax sealed, the dressing should be opened to release any pressure that may have accumulated. Prior to embarking on a prolonged transport of a patient, potential oxygen needs should be calculated, and sufficient amounts of oxygen should be available for the transport. A good rule of thumb is to bring 50% more oxygen than anticipated.

Intermittent sedation may be required for an agitated intubated patient. Sedation may also decrease the work of breathing, and any "fighting the ventilator" when mechanical ventilation is being used. Small doses of benzodiazepines should be titrated intravenously. The use of neuromuscular blocking agents may also be considered if the patient is significantly combative, the airway is secured with an endotracheal tube, *and* prehospital care personnel are properly trained and credentialed.

SUMMARY

The trauma patient is susceptible to various injuries that may impair ventilation and gas exchange. Trauma to the chest, airway obstruction, central nervous system injury, and hemorrhage can all result in inadequate tissue perfusion. Understanding the pathophysiology of inadequate tissue perfusion and the mechanisms by which it occurs will aid in recognizing the patient in need of airway management and ventilatory support.

The quality and timeliness of airway assessment and treatment in the field directly affect a patient's long-term

outcome and length of hospital stay. Therefore the first action in caring for any patient, once the scene assessment is complete, is to assess the status of airway and breathing. Aggressive airway management is the highest priority of care of the trauma patient and provides for the best possible outcome. To achieve this, prehospital care providers continually practice airway management skills and stay abreast of new research, techniques, and technology related to airway management. Sound critical thinking skills need to be in place to make the best judgments for the trauma patient.

SCENARIO SOLUTION

Physical evidence at the scene suggests that the driver has likely been subjected to kinetic forces capable of creating life-threatening injuries. The position of the patient suggests that multiple impacts have occurred.

The driver exhibits several signs of airway compromise and ventilatory insufficiency. His ventilations are sonorous and irregular, he has an altered level of consciousness, and he requires frequent suctioning. Bleeding from the nares and ears and the early presence of "raccoon eyes" strongly suggest the presence of a basilar skull fracture. The primary survey indicates a rapidly deteriorating patient who requires aggressive airway care and rapid transport.

First-responder personnel are already administering oxygen with ventilatory assistance using a BVM. Continue ventilatory support and cervical spine stabilization while preparing for endotracheal intubation. Be careful to ensure that the airway remains clear and that manual ventilations are effective.

You orally intubate the patient with an appropriately sized endotracheal (ET) tube. Cervical spine stabilization is continued before, during, and after the intubation attempt. Once the ET tube is placed, ensure proper positioning of the tube through auscultation of breath sounds, use of an esophageal intubation detector, end-tidal capnometry (if available), or another adjunctive device. Thoroughly suction the patient before transport and as often as needed thereafter.

After the patient is completely immobilized and the ET tube is secured, transport is initiated without delay. Establish intravenous access while the patient is en route to a trauma receiving facility. Take care to maintain the effectiveness of immobilization efforts and frequently reassess the patient's condition. To ensure proper activation of the receiving facility's trauma response, notify the trauma center during transport. On arrival at the trauma center, concisely convey all pertinent information regarding the incident, the patient, and medical interventions to the receiving physician or other appropriate trauma team member. ■

References

1. Stockinger ZT, McSwain NE Jr: Prehospital endotracheal intubation for trauma does not improve survival over bag-valve-mask ventilation, *J Trauma* 56(3):531, 2004.
2. Garza AG, Gratton MC, Coontz D, et al: Effect of paramedic experience on orotracheal intubation success rates, *J Emerg Med* 25(3):251, 2003.
3. Dickinson ET, Cohen JE, Mechem CC: The effectiveness of midazolam as a single pharmacologic agent to facilitate endotracheal intubation by paramedics, *Prehosp Emerg Care* 3(3):191, 1999.
4. Wang HE, Davis DP, O'Connor RE, Domeier RM: Drug-assisted intubation in the prehospital setting, *Prehosp Emerg Care* 10(2):261, 2006.
5. Davis DP, Hoyt DB, Ochs M, et al: The effect of paramedic rapid sequence intubation on an outcome in patients with severe trauma brain injury, *J Trauma* 54:444, 2003.
6. Davis DP, Dunford JV, Poste JC, et al: The impact of hypoxia and hyperventilation on outcome after paramedic rapid sequence intubation of severely head-injured patient, *J Trauma* 57:1, 2004.
7. O'Connor RE, Swor RA: Verification of endotracheal tube placement following intubation, *Prehosp Emerg Care* 3:248, 1999.
8. Frame SB, Simon JM, Kerstein MD, McSwain NE, Jr: Percutaneous transtracheal catheter ventilation (PTCV) in complete airway obstruction: a canine model, *J Trauma* 29:774, 1989.
9. American College of Surgeons Committee on Trauma: Airway management and ventilation. In *Advanced trauma life support for doctors, student course manual*, ed 7, Chicago, 2004, ACS.
10. Silvestri S, Ralis GA, Krauss B, et al: The effectiveness of out-of-hospital use of continuous end-tidal carbon dioxide monitoring on the rate of unrecognized misplaced intubations within a regional emergency medical services system, *Ann Emerg Med* 45:497, 2005.

Suggested Reading

American College of Surgeons Committee on Trauma: *Advanced trauma life support for doctors, student course manual*, ed 7, Chicago, 2004, ACS.

Brainard C: Whose tube is it? *JEMS* 31:62, 2006.

Dunford JV, David DP, Ochs M, et al: The incidence of transient hypoxia and heart rate reactivity during paramedic rapid sequence intubation, *Ann Emerg Med* 42:721, 2003.

Soubani AO: Noninvasive monitoring of oxygen and carbon dioxide, *Am J Emerg Med* 19:141, 2001.

Weitzel N, Kendal J, Pons P: Blind nasotracheal intubation for patients with penetrating neck trauma, *J Trauma* 56(5):1097, 2004.

Airway Management and Ventilation Skills

Manual Inline Stabilization

Principle: To maintain the cervical spine in a neutral inline position until the patient is completely immobilized.

Behind

From behind the patient, the prehospital care provider places his or her hands over the patient's ears without moving the patient's head. The thumbs are placed against the posterior aspect of the patient's skull. The little fingers are placed just under the angle of the mandible. The remaining fingers are spread on the flat lateral planes of the patient's head. Pressure is applied in such a manner as to maintain the head in a stable position. If the head is not in a neutral inline position, the provider slowly moves the head until it is, unless contraindicated (see Chapter 9). The provider brings his or her arms in and rests them against the seat, headrest, or torso for additional support.

Side

Standing at the side of the patient, the prehospital care provider passes his or her arm over the patient's shoulder closest to the provider and cups the back of the patient's head with his or her hand, being careful not to move the patient's head. The thumb and first finger of one hand are placed on either side of the patient's face. The thumb and finger should rest in the notch formed where the patient's teeth and maxilla join. Enough pressure is applied to support and stabilize the patient's head. If the patient's head is not in a neutral inline position, the provider slowly moves the head until it is, unless contraindicated (see Chapter 9). The provider braces his or her elbows on the patient's torso for additional support.

Front

Standing directly in front of the patient, the prehospital care provider places his or her hands on both sides of the patient's head as shown. The little fingers are placed at the posterior aspect of the patient's skull. One thumb is placed in the notch between the patient's upper teeth and the maxilla on each cheek. The remaining fingers are spread on the flat lateral planes of the patient's head. Pressure is applied in such a manner as to maintain the head in a stable position. If the patient's head is not in a neutral inline position, the provider slowly moves the head, unless contraindicated (see Chapter 9). The provider brings his or her arms in and braces the elbows against the patient's torso for additional support.

Note: The provider can also use this method when kneeling alongside the thorax of a supine patient and facing toward his or her head. The forearms are braced on the clavicle for additional stability.

Supine Patient

The prehospital care provider positions himself or herself above the supine patient's head, either kneeling or lying. The hands are placed on either side of the patient's head, covering the patient's ears with the palms. The fingers are spread so as to stabilize the patient's head with the fingers pointing toward the patient's feet (caudal). The fourth and fifth digits of each hand should wrap around the posterior portion of the patient's skull. The elbows and forearms can be rested on either the ground or the provider's knees for additional support.

Trauma Jaw Thrust

Principle: To open the airway without moving the cervical spine.

In both the trauma jaw thrust and the trauma chin lift, manual neutral inline stabilization of the head and neck is maintained while the mandible is moved anteriorly (forward). This maneuver moves the tongue forward, away from the hypopharynx, and holds the mouth slightly open.

From a position above the patient's head, the prehospital care provider positions his or her hands on either side of the patient's head, fingers pointing caudad (toward the patient's feet). Depending on the size of the provider's hands, the fingers are spread across the face and around the angle of the patient's mandible. Gentle, equal pressure is applied with these digits to move the patient's mandible anteriorly (forward) and slightly downward (toward the patient's feet).

The trauma jaw thrust can also be performed while positioned beside the patient, facing toward the patient's head. The provider's fingers point cephalad (toward the top of the patient's head). Depending on the size of the provider's hands, the fingers are spread across the face and around the angle of the patient's mandible. Gentle, equal pressure is applied with these digits to move the patient's mandible anteriorly (forward) and slightly downward (toward the patient's feet).

Trauma Chin Lift

Principle: To open the airway without moving the cervical spine.

From a position above the patient's head, the patient's head and neck are moved into a neutral inline position, and manual stabilization is maintained. The prehospital care provider positions himself or herself at the patient's side between the patient's shoulders and hips, facing the patient's head. With the hand closest to the patient's feet, the provider grasps the patient's teeth or the lower mandible between his or her thumb and first two fingers beneath the patient's chin. The provider now pulls the patient's chin anteriorly and slightly caudad, elevating the mandible and opening the mouth.

Bag-Valve-Mask Ventilation

Principle: The preferred method of providing assisted ventilation.

Ventilation using a bag-valve-mask (BVM) system has an advantage over other ventilatory support systems because it gives a prehospital care provider feedback by the feel of the bag (compliance). Positive feedback ensures the operator of successful ventilations; changes in the feedback indicate a loss of mask seal, the presence of a pathologic airway, or a thoracic problem interfering with the delivery of successful ventilations. This "feel" and the control it provides also make the BVM suitable for assisting ventilations. The BVM's portability and ability for immediate use make it useful for immediate delivery of ventilations on identification of the need.

Without supplemental oxygen, however, a BVM provides an oxygen concentration of only 21%, or fraction of inspired oxygen (Fio_2) of 0.21; as soon as time allows, an oxygen reservoir and high-concentration supplemental oxygen should be connected to the BVM. When oxygen is connected without a reservoir, the Fio_2 is limited to 0.50 or less; with a reservoir, the Fio_2 is 0.85 or greater.

If the patient being ventilated is unconscious without a gag reflex, a properly sized oropharyngeal airway should be inserted before attempting to ventilate with the BVM. If the patient has an intact gag reflex, a properly sized nasopharyngeal airway should be inserted before attempting to assist ventilations.

Various BVM devices are available, including disposable single-patient-use models that are relatively inexpensive. Different brands have varying bag, valve, and reservoir designs. All the parts used should be of the same model and brand because these parts are usually not safely interchangeable.

BVM units are available in adult, pediatric, and neonatal sizes. Although an adult bag can be used with the properly sized pediatric mask in an emergency, use of the correct bag size is recommended as a safe practice. Adequate ventilations of an adult patient are achieved when a minimum of 800 mL/breath is delivered (1000-1200 mL/breath preferred).

When ventilating with any positive-pressure device, inflation should stop once the chest has risen maximally. When using the BVM, the chest should be visualized for maximum inflation and the bag felt to recognize any marked increased resistance in the bag when lung expansion is at its maximum. Adequate time for exhalation is needed (1:3 ratio between time for inhalation and time for exhalation). If enough time is not allowed, "stepped breaths" occur, providing a greater volume of inspiration than expiration. Stepped breaths produce poor air exchange and result in hyperinflation, increased pressure, opening of the esophagus, and gastric distention.

Single-Provider Method

On many occasions it is difficult for a single provider to maintain a proper mask seal and provide adequate ventilations when using a BVM device. In ideal situations at least two prehospital care providers should be used to provide ventilations with a BVM. In most prehospital conditions, however, multiple experienced and trained providers may not be readily available. In these situations a single provider is relied on to give adequate ventilatory support to a patient until additional help arrives or until the patient is delivered to the appropriate facility.

The prehospital care provider kneels above the patient's head, providing manual stabilization of the patient's head and neck in a neutral inline position with his or her knees. After insertion of an airway adjunct, the mask is fitted over the patient's nose and mouth and held in place with firm downward pressure while keeping the airway open. This can be accomplished by placing the third, fourth, and fifth fingers around the mandible and applying slight upward pressure, wrapping the thumb and first finger around the mask at the mask and bag attachment point forming a C. Either adequate hand pressure is used or the bag is pressed against one's own body (e.g., the thigh) to squeeze the air or oxygen from the bag and into the patient's lungs.

Two-Provider Method

Two or more prehospital care providers performing ventilations with a BVM device is easier than with only one provider. The first provider can focus attention on maintaining an adequate mask seal while the second provides good delivery volume by using both hands to squeeze (deflate) the bag.

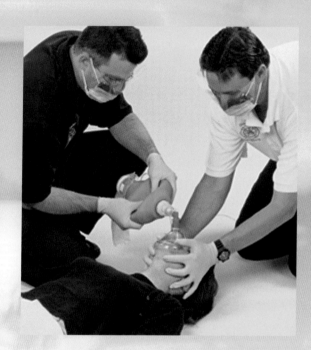

The first provider kneels above the patient's head and maintains manual stabilization of the patient's head and neck in a neutral inline position. The facemask is placed over the patient's nose and mouth, and the mask is held in place with the thumbs on the lateral portion of the mask while pulling the mandible up into the mask. The other fingers provide the manual stabilization and maintain a patent airway. The second provider kneels at the side of the patient and squeezes the bag with both hands to inflate the lungs. If an adequate volume cannot be provided (initiation of chest rise, about 500 mL/breath), the second provider should attempt to deflate the bag against his or her body.

Oropharyngeal Airway

Principle: An adjunct used to maintain an open airway mechanically in a patient without a gag reflex.

The oropharyngeal airway (OPA) is designed to hold the patient's tongue anteriorly out of the pharynx. The OPA is available in various sizes. Proper sizing to the patient is required to ensure a patent airway. *Placement of an OPA in the hypopharynx is contraindicated in patients who have an intact gag reflex.*

Two methods for insertion of the OPA are effective: the tongue jaw lift insertion method and the tongue blade insertion method. Regardless of which method is used, the first provider stabilizes the patient's head and neck in a neutral inline position while the second provider measures and inserts the OPA.

Tongue Jaw Lift Insertion Method

The first provider brings the patient's head and neck into a neutral inline position and maintains stabilization while opening the patient's airway with a trauma jaw thrust maneuver. The second provider selects and measures for a properly sized OPA. The accompanying illustration shows a workable method for measuring the OPA (the first provider's hands have been removed for clarification). The distance from the corner of the patient's mouth to the earlobe is a good estimate for proper size.

The patient's airway is opened with the chin lift maneuver. The OPA is turned so that the distal tip is pointing toward the top of the patient's head (flanged end pointing toward patient's head) and tilted toward the mouth opening (the first provider's hands have been removed for clarification).

The OPA is inserted into the patient's mouth and rotated to fit the contours of the patient's anatomy (the first provider's hands have been removed for clarification).

The OPA is rotated until its inside curve is resting against the tongue and holding it out of the posterior pharynx. The flanges of the OPA should be resting against the outside surface of the patient's teeth (the first provider's hands have been removed for clarification).

Tongue Blade Insertion Method

The tongue blade insertion method is probably a safer method than the tongue jaw lift because it eliminates the accidental tearing or puncturing of gloves or the skin by sharp, pointed, or broken teeth. This method also eliminates the possibility of being bitten if the patient's level of consciousness (LOC) is not as deep as previously assessed or if any seizure activity occurs.

The first provider brings the patient's head and neck into a neutral inline position and maintains stabilization while opening the patient's airway with the trauma jaw thrust maneuver. The second provider selects and measures for a properly sized OPA. The second provider pulls the patient's mouth open by the chin and places a tongue blade into the patient's mouth to move the tongue forward in place and keep the airway open. With the flanged end pointing toward the patient's head and the distal tip pointing into the patient's mouth, the second provider continues to insert the OPA following the curvature of the airway until the flanged end of the OPA rests against the outside surface of the patient's teeth.

Nasopharyngeal Airway

Principle: An adjunct used to maintain an open airway mechanically in a patient with or without a gag reflex.
The nasopharyngeal airway (NPA) is a simple airway adjunct that provides an effective way to maintain a patent airway in patients who may still have an intact gag reflex. Most patients will tolerate the NPA if properly sized. NPAs are available in a range of diameters (internal diameters of 5-9 mm), and the length varies appropriately with the size of the diameter. NPAs are usually made of a flexible, rubberlike material. Ridged NPAs are not recommended for field use.

The first provider brings the patient's head and neck into a neutral inline position and maintains stabilization while opening the patient's airway with the trauma jaw thrust maneuver. A second provider examines the patient's nostrils with a light and selects the one that is the largest and least deviated or obstructed (usually the right nostril). The second provider selects the appropriately sized NPA for the patient's nostril, a size slightly smaller in diameter than the size of the nostril opening (frequently the diameter of the patient's little finger). The length of the NPA is also important. The NPA needs to be long enough to supply an air passage between the patient's tongue and the posterior pharynx. An acceptable method for measuring the NPA for proper length is shown in the accompanying illustration (the first provider's hands have been removed for clarification). The distance from the patient's nose to the earlobe is a good estimate for proper size.

The distal tip (nonflanged end) of the NPA is lubricated liberally with a water-soluble jelly and slowly inserted into the nostril of choice. Insertion should be in an anterior-to-posterior direction along the floor of the nasal cavity, not in a superior-to-inferior direction. If resistance is met at the posterior end of the nostril, a gentle back-and-forth rotation of the NPA between the fingers will usually aid in passing beyond the turbinate bones of the nasal cavity without damage. Should the NPA continue to meet with resistance, the NPA should not be forced past the obstruction but rather should be withdrawn, and the distal tip should be relubricated and inserted into the other nostril. (The first provider's hands have been removed for clarification.)

The second provider continues insertion until the flange end of the NPA is next to the anterior nares or until the patient gags. If the patient gags, the NPA is withdrawn slightly. (The first provider's hands have been removed for clarification.)

Dual-Lumen Airway

Principle: A mechanical device used for opening and maintaining an airway when unable to intubate.

The dual-lumen airway provides prehospital care providers with a functional alternative airway. These combination airways are an acceptable prehospital field device and typically do not require extensive training to achieve competency. The airway's greatest advantage is that it can be inserted independent of the patient's position ("blindly" inserted), which may be especially important in trauma patients with high suspicion of cervical injury. The indications for placement of a dual-lumen airway are the same as for the placement of any airway: the necessity of obtaining a patent airway in a patient. Each manufacturer of the dual-lumen airway will identify age and size requirements pertinent to their airway. The provider should always follow the manufacturer's recommendations for size selection, contraindications, and specific insertion procedures.

As with any other invasive airway, the patient is preoxygenated with a high concentration of oxygen using a simple airway adjunct or manual airway procedure before insertion of a dual-lumen airway.

As with any other piece of medical equipment, the dual lumen should be inspected and each part tested before insertion. The distal end of the airway should be lubricated with a water-soluble lubricant.

Note: The Combitube is used in the following illustrations for demonstration purposes only. Other brands of dual-lumen airways are also effective.

The provider stops ventilations and removes all other airway adjuncts. If the patient is supine, the tongue and lower jaw are lifted upward with one hand (chin lift). The distal end of the tube is inserted (tearing the cuff when inserting the airway past broken teeth or dental appliances should be avoided). The Combitube is inserted until the marker rings line up with the patient's teeth.

Using the large syringe, the pharyngeal cuff is inflated with 100 mL of air and the syringe removed. The device should seat itself in the posterior pharynx just behind the hard palate.

Using the small syringe, the distal cuff is inflated with 15 mL of air and the syringe removed. Typically the balloon will be placed (inflated) in the patient's esophagus. The provider begins ventilation through the esophageal tube (generally marked with a #1). If auscultation of breath sounds is positive and gastric insufflation is negative, the provider continues ventilation through the esophageal tube.

If auscultation of breath sounds is negative and gastric insufflation is positive, the provider immediately ventilates with the shortened tracheal tube (generally marked with a #2), after which reauscultation of breath sounds and gastric sounds is done to affirm proper tube placement. The provider continues to ventilate the patient and initiate immediate transport to an appropriate facility.

All esophageal airways require the patient to have no gag reflex. If the patient regains consciousness and begins to gag or vomit, these devices are removed immediately. Extubation of esophageal airways almost always causes vomiting or regurgitation. Consequently, suction equipment must be readily available when the device is removed. Observe Standard Precautions.

SPECIFIC SKILLS

Visualized Orotracheal Intubation of the Trauma Patient

Principle: To secure a definitive airway without manipulating the cervical spine.

Visualized orotracheal intubation of the trauma patient is done with the patient's head and neck stabilized in a neutral inline position. Orotracheal intubation while maintaining manual inline stabilization requires additional training and practice beyond that for intubation of nontrauma patients. As with all skills, training requires observation, critique, and certification initially and at least twice a year by the medical director or designee.

In hypoxic trauma patients who are not in cardiac arrest, intubation should not be the initial airway maneuver. The provider should perform intubation only after he or she has preoxygenated the patient with a high concentration of oxygen using a simple airway adjunct or manual maneuver. Contact with the deep pharynx when intubating a severely hypoxic patient without preoxygenation can easily produce vagal stimulation, resulting in a dangerous bradycardia.

The provider should not interrupt ventilation for more than 20 seconds when intubating the patient. Ventilation should never be interrupted for more than 30 seconds for any reason.

Visualized orotracheal intubation is extremely difficult in conscious patients or patients with an intact gag reflex. The provider should consider use of topical anesthesia or paralytic agents after additional training, protocol development, and approval by the EMS medical director.

For the novice provider, the use of a straight laryngoscope blade tends to produce less rotary force (pulling the patient's head toward a "sniffing" position) than that produced by the use of a curved blade. However, because the success rate of intubation is often related to the provider's comfort with a given design, the style of blade selection for the laryngoscope remains a matter of individual preference.

Note: The cervical collar will limit forward motion of the mandible and complete opening of the mouth. Therefore, after adequate spinal immobilization is ensured, the cervical collar is removed, manual stabilization of the cervical spine is held, and intubation is attempted.

Before attempting intubation, the providers should assemble and test all required equipment and follow Standard Precautions. The first provider kneels at the patient's head and ventilates the patient with a BVM and high-concentration oxygen. The second provider, kneeling at the patient's side, provides manual stabilization of the patient's head and neck.

After preoxygenation, the first provider stops ventilations and grasps the laryngoscope in the left hand and the endotracheal (ET) tube (with syringe attached to pilot valve) in the right hand. If a stylet is used, this should have been inserted when the equipment was inspected and tested. The distal end of the stylet should be inserted just short of the ET tube's distal opening.

The laryngoscope blade is inserted into the right side of the patient's airway to the correct depth, sweeping toward the center of the airway while observing the desired landmarks.

After identification of desired landmarks, the ET tube is inserted between the patient's vocal cords to the desired depth. The laryngoscope is then removed while holding the ET tube in place; the depth marking on the side of the ET tube is noted. If a malleable stylet has been used, it should be removed at this time.

The pilot valve is inflated with enough air to complete the seal between the patient's trachea and the cuff of the ET tube (usually 8-10 mL of air), and the syringe is removed from the pilot valve. The first provider attaches the bag-valve system with a reservoir attached to the proximal end of the ET tube, and ventilation is resumed while observing the rise of the patient's chest with each delivered breath. Manual stabilization of the patient's head and neck is maintained throughout the process. Bilateral breath sounds and absence of air sounds over the epigastrium and other indications of proper ET tube placement are checked. Once tube placement is confirmed, the ET tube is secured in place. Although the use of tape or other commercially available devices is adequate in controlled situations in which the patient is not moved, *the best way to guard against displacement of the ET tube in the prehospital situation is to physically hold onto the tube at all times.*

Alternative Methods for Orotracheal Intubation of the Trauma Patient

Alternative Positioning

An alternative method to perform orotracheal intubation is for the prehospital care provider to provide stabilization of the patient's head and neck while performing the intubation. The provider sits on the ground above the patient's head and places his or her legs over the top of the patient's shoulders, holding the patient's head and neck in a neutral inline position with the inner thighs. While placing the laryngoscope into the patient's airway, the provider leans back, lifts the mandible without lifting the patient's head with the laryngoscope, and observes for desired landmarks. After identification of desired landmarks, the provider introduces the ET tube into the airway and confirms placement.

Another alternative method is for the prehospital care provider to kneel above the patient's head, scooting forward until the patient's head is between the provider's knees. Lateral pressure is applied to the patient's head to maintain stabilization of the head and neck in a neutral inline position. The provider leans back after inserting the laryngoscope into the patient's airway to the desired depth, without lifting forward or upward with the laryngoscope, and observes for the desired landmarks.

Face-to-Face Orotracheal Intubation

Principle: An alternative method of securing a definitive airway when patient positioning limits use of traditional methods.

Situations may arise in the prehospital setting in which the provider cannot take a position above the patient's head to initiate endotracheal intubation in a traditional manner. The face-to-face method for intubation is a viable option in these situations. The basic concepts of intubation still apply with face-to-face intubation: preoxygenate the patient with a BVM and high-concentration oxygen before attempting intubation, maintain manual stabilization of the patient's head and neck throughout the intubation, and do not interrupt ventilation for longer then 20 to 30 seconds at a time.

While manual stabilization of the patient's head and neck in a neutral inline position is held, the prehospital care provider positions himself or herself in front of the patient, "face to face." The laryngoscope is held in the right hand with the blade on the patient's tongue. The blade moves the tongue down and out rather than up and out. The patient's airway is opened with the left hand, and the laryngoscope is placed into the patient's airway.

After the laryngoscope blade is placed in the patient's airway, the desired landmarks are found. Looking into the airway from a position above the open airway provides the best view.

After identification of desired landmarks, the ET tube is passed between the patient's vocal cords to the desired depth with the left hand. The cuff is inflated with air to form the seal, and the syringe is removed. A bag-valve device is attached, and placement of the ET tube is confirmed.

After confirmation of ET tube placement, the patient is ventilated while the provider holds onto the ET tube and maintains manual stabilization of the patient's head and neck. The ET tube should then be secured into place.

An alternative method for face-to-face intubation is to hold the laryngoscope in the left hand and place the ET tube with the right hand. This method may block the visualization of the lower airway as the ET tube is placed.

Blind Nasotracheal Intubation

Principle: To secure a definitive airway without manipulating the cervical spine.

Blind nasotracheal intubation (BNTI) depends on the patient's spontaneous ventilation to ensure proper alignment when passing the ET tube between the vocal cords and into the trachea. Therefore, BNTI is limited to use with spontaneously breathing patients and in an environment that allows for the hearing and feeling of air exchange at the external (proximal) end of the ET tube.

This technique should only be attempted by personnel who are qualified in endotracheal intubation and who, after practice, have demonstrated their ability to their medical director or his or her designee.

Before attempting BNTI, the prehospital care provider should gather all required equipment and check for proper operating condition. Using a light source, the patient's nostrils are inspected, and the larger one with the lesser deviation or obstruction is selected. The appropriately sized ET tube is one slightly smaller than the diameter of the nostril. The distal end of the ET tube should be lubricated with a generous amount of a water-soluble lubricant before insertion. Use of a stylet during nasotracheal intubation requires more than casual experience.

Manual stabilization of the patient's head and neck in a neutral inline position is held while a second prehospital care provider is positioned above the patient and preoxygenates the patient with high-concentration oxygen and BVM-assisted ventilation.

The ET tube is taken in one hand. The other hand applies slight superior traction to the tip of the patient's nose. This traction will help ensure that the tube follows the anatomy of the nasal airway. The tube is placed into the patient's nostril (usually the right one) in an anterior-to-posterior direction (from the nose to the back of the head).

The prehospital care provider should place his or her ear over the proximal (external) opening of the ET tube and listen for breathing sounds. The ET tube is passed down the hypopharynx until the breath sounds are the loudest. At this point, progress is paused until the next inhalation begins. With a quick motion, the tube is passed through the vocal cords. If breath sounds stop, the tube has gone into the esophagus. The tube is then withdrawn until breath sounds are heard loudly again, and another attempt is made.

After passing the ET tube to the desired depth, the cuff is inflated with enough air to create a seal, and the syringe is removed. Tube placement is confirmed, the ET tube is secured with tape and manual holding, and ventilation with a BVM and high-concentration oxygen is begun.

Verification of Endotracheal Tube Placement

Once intubation has been performed, take specific measures to ensure that the tube has been properly placed in the trachea. An improperly positioned ET tube, if unrecognized for only a brief period, may result in profound hypoxia with resultant brain injury (hypoxic encephalopathy) and even death. Therefore, reasonable efforts must be made to ensure proper placement. Techniques to verify intubation include the use of both clinical assessments and adjunctive devices. Clinical assessments include the following:

- Direct visualization of the ET tube passing through the vocal cords.
- Presence of bilateral breath sounds (auscultate laterally below the axilla) *and* absence of air sounds over the epigastrium.
- Visualization of the chest rising and falling during ventilation.
- Fogging (water vapor condensation) in the ET tube on expiration.

Unfortunately, none of these techniques is 100% reliable *by itself* for verifying proper tube placement. Therefore, prudent practice involves assessing and documenting *all* these clinical signs, if possible. On rare occasions, because of difficult anatomy, visualization of the ET tube passing through the vocal cords may not be possible. In a moving vehicle (ground or aeromedical), engine noise may make auscultation of breath sounds almost impossible. Obesity and chronic obstructive pulmonary disease (COPD) may interfere with the ability to see chest movement during ventilation.

Adjunctive devices include the following:

- Esophageal detector device
- Carbon dioxide (CO_2) monitoring
- Colorimetric CO_2 detector
- End-tidal CO_2 monitoring (capnography)
- Pulse oximetry

As with the clinical assessments, none of these adjuncts is 100% accurate in all patients. In a patient with a perfusing rhythm, end-tidal CO_2 monitoring (capnography) serves as the "gold standard" for determining ET tube placement of an airway in the operating room. This technique should be used in the prehospital setting if it is available. Patients in cardiopulmonary arrest do not generate CO_2, and therefore neither colorimetric detectors nor capnography may be useful in patients who lack a perfusing cardiac rhythm.

Because none of these techniques is universally reliable, all the clinical assessments noted previously should be performed, unless impractical, followed by use of at least one of the adjunctive devices. Because of the cost of performing capnography, most EMS systems require a combination of clinical assessments and a colorimetric CO_2 detector or esophageal detector device. In any instance, if any of the techniques used to verify proper placement suggests that the ET tube may not be properly positioned, the tube should be immediately removed and reinserted, with placement verified again. All the techniques used to verify tube placement should be noted on the patient care report.

Percutaneous Transtracheal Ventilation

Principle: A method of providing oxygenation to a patient who cannot be intubated or ventilated with a BVM. All parts except the needle, tank, and regulator should be modified as needed, preassembled, and packaged for ready availability in the field. This will ensure successful assembly. When percutaneous transtracheal ventilation (PTV) is needed, time will be of the essence. The equipment should be ready to use, requiring only connection to the regulator and needle. The prehospital care provider can use a commercially available product that contains all the necessary equipment. If this is not available, the following equipment is required:

- Syringe: 10 to 30 mL
- To allow for inflation and deflation of the lung while there is constant flow from the oxygen source, some type of bypass is necessary. The following are two examples:
  1. A hole approximately 40% of the circumference of the oxygen delivery tube, cut in the side, which can be occluded by the thumb.
  2. A plastic T or Y connector of a size compatible with the oxygen tubing used and connected to the oxygen source with a length of standard universal oxygen tubing.
- A short piece of tubing that will fasten over the lower end of the T or Y and snugly fit into the hub of the needle (this leaves one opening of the T or Y connector free with nothing attached to it).
- An oxygen tank with a regulator that has a 50-psi delivery pressure at its supplemental oxygen nipple.
- Strips of $1/2$-inch adhesive tape

The patient should be in the supine position while manual inline stabilization is maintained.

The larynx and trachea are stabilized with the fingers of one hand. The needle, attached to the syringe, is placed midline over the cricothyroid membrane or directly into the trachea at a slightly downward angle. As the needle is inserted into the trachea, the plunger of the syringe is withdrawn to create a negative pressure. Once the needle enters into the trachea, air will be sucked into the syringe, confirming that the tip of the needle is properly located. The needle is advanced an additional centimeter, and then the syringe is removed from the needle. The inner needle is removed, leaving the catheter in place. The provider quickly forms a loop with adhesive tape around the needle or the hub of the catheter and places the ends of tape on the patient's neck to secure the airway. The provider should use caution when securing the catheter to prevent kinking the catheter.

The oxygen delivery tube with a vent is connected to the hub of the needle while the hand that initially stabilized the trachea is moved to hold the needle in place. Ventilation is begun by occluding the opening of the tubing assembly with the thumb for 1 second. The patient's chest may or may not rise to indicate that inhalation is occurring. To stop the flow of oxygen into the lungs, the thumb is removed from the opening.

Note: The passive process of exhalation takes three to four times as long as inhalation with a normal airway. In this process, exhalation will require a longer time because of the smaller opening.

The patient is oxygenated by alternately closing the hole to provide the positive flow of oxygen for inhalation and opening the same hole to stop the oxygen flow and allow deflation. The proper time sequence for these maneuvers is 1 second of occlusion of the opening for inhalation and 4 seconds of leaving the hole open for passive deflation. This process is continued until a more definitive airway is established.

After PTV of 45 to 60 minutes, this technique can provide a high $Paco_2$ level because of carbon dioxide retention as a result of the restricted expirations. Therefore the patient should have a more definitive airway established as soon as possible.

Warning: Patients receiving PTV may remain hypoxic and unstable. Prehospital care providers should initiate transportation to a suitable facility without delay because the patient is in urgent need of a more definitive surgical transtracheal procedure (cricothyrotomy) for adequate ventilation and oxygenation.

Chapter Objectives

*At the completion of this chapter, the reader
will be able to do the following:*

✓ Define shock.

✓ Classify shock on an etiologic basis.

✓ Explain the pathophysiology of shock and its progression through
phases.

✓ Describe the physical findings in shock.

✓ Clinically differentiate the different types of shock.

✓ Discuss the limitations of the field management of shock.

✓ Recognize the need for rapid transport and early definitive
management in various forms of shock.

✓ Apply principles of management of shock in the trauma patient.

CHAPTER 7

Shock

You have arrived at the scene of a motor vehicle crash (MVC) involving a car and an SUV. You recognize a side impact on the driver's side of the car with about 12 inches (30 cm) of intrusion into the passenger compartment and very little damage to the SUV. All other passengers have left the vehicles without injury except the driver of the car, a 20-year old white male slumped over the steering wheel with obvious contact of the steering wheel to his anterior chest.

The patient is awake, anxious, diaphoretic, and breathing rapidly (30 breaths/min). He has a weak, thready, rapid radial pulse. There is tenderness and bruising over the left upper quadrant of his abdomen.

What injuries do you expect in this patient? How would you manage this patient in the field? You are 30 minutes away from the nearest trauma center. How does this alter your management plans? ■

Although shock following trauma has been recognized for more than three centuries, its description by Samuel Gross in 1872 as a "rude unhinging of the machinery of life"[1] and John Collins Warren as "a momentary pause in the act of death"[2] emphasizes its continuing central role in the causes of major morbidity and mortality in the trauma patient. Prompt diagnosis, resuscitation, and definitive management are all essential in determining patient outcome after shock resulting from trauma. The prehospital care provider faces significant challenges in all these essential actions for shock. To improve survival from shock, a clear understanding of the definition, pathophysiology, and clinical features is essential.

In the prehospital setting the therapeutic challenge posed by the patient in shock is compounded by the need to assess and manage such patients in a relatively primitive environment where sophisticated diagnostic and management tools are either unavailable or impractical to apply. To assist prehospital health care providers in their approach to the shock patient, this chapter defines and classifies shock and describes the pathophysiologic changes to help direct management strategies.

Definition of Shock

Although it has many definitions, shock is most often regarded as a state of generalized cellular hypoperfusion in which delivery of oxygen at the cellular level is inadequate to meet metabolic needs. Based on this definition, shock can be classified in terms of the determinants of cellular perfusion and oxygenation. An understanding of the cellular changes arising from this state of hypoperfusion, as well as the endocrine, microvascular, cardiovascular, tissue, and end organ effects, will also assist in directing treatment strategies.

Classification of Shock

The prime determinants of cellular perfusion are: the heart (acting as the pump or the motor of the system), fluid volume (acting as the hydraulic fluid), the blood vessels (serving as the conduits or plumbing) and finally the cells of the body. Based on these components of the perfusion system, shock may be classified into the following categories:

1. *Hypovolemic,* primarily hemorrhagic in the trauma patient, related to loss of circulating blood volume. This is the most common cause of shock in the trauma patient.
2. *Distributive* (or vasogenic), related to abnormality in vascular tone arising from several different causes.
3. *Cardiogenic,* related to interference with the pump action of the heart.

By far the most common cause of shock in the trauma patient is hemorrhage, and the safest approach in managing the trauma patient in shock is to consider the cause of the shock as being hemorrhagic until proven otherwise.

More detailed descriptions of these different types of shock follow after a discussion of the relevant anatomy and pathophysiology of shock.

Anatomy and Pathophysiology

Cardiovascular, Hemodynamic, and Endocrine Responses
Heart

The heart consists of two receiving chambers *(atria)* and two major pumping chambers *(ventricles)*. The function of the

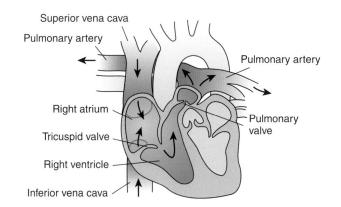

FIGURE 7-1 With each contraction of the right ventricle, blood is pumped through the lungs. Blood from the lungs enters the left side of the heart, and the left ventricle pumps it into the systemic vascular system.

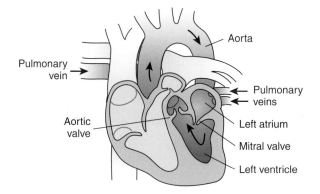

FIGURE 7-2 Blood returning from the lungs is pumped out of the heart and through the aorta to the rest of the body by left ventricular contraction.

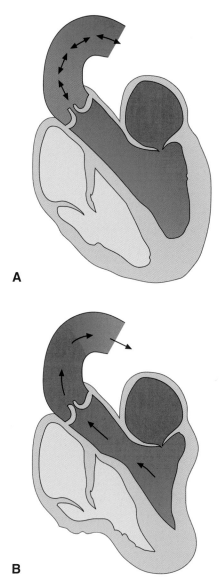

FIGURE 7-3 In a relaxed position (diastole), the ventricle fills with blood from the contractions of the atrium. During this time, blood is gradually flowing out of the major vessels as the pressure gradually decreases. During the contraction of the ventricle (systole), a large amount of blood flows into the vascular system, which raises the pressure. Cardiac action and blood flow is demonstrated in **A** and the pulse wave is seen in **B**.

atria is to accumulate and store blood so that the ventricles can fill rapidly, minimizing delay in the pumping cycle. The right atrium receives blood from the veins of the body and pumps it to the right ventricle. With each contraction of the right ventricle, blood is pumped through the lungs for oxygenation (Figure 7-1). The blood from the lungs is returned to the left atrium. From there, blood is pumped into the left ventricle, which then pumps it throughout the arteries of the body (Figure 7-2). Blood is forced through the system by the contraction of the left ventricle; a pressure rise occurs in the blood vessels greater than the normal resting pressure. This sudden pressure increase produces a pulse wave to push blood through the system. The peak of pressure increase is the systolic blood pressure and represents the force of the blood produced by ventricular contraction *(systole)*. The resting pressure in the vessels between ventricular contractions is the diastolic blood pressure and represents the residual force remaining in the system while the heart is refilling *(diastole)*. This is an indirect estimate of vascular resistance (Figure 7-3). Thus

more information can be obtained if both systolic and diastolic pressures are determined during the secondary survey by auscultating with a stethoscope. In some patients, however, the provider determines only the systolic pressure using palpation (feeling for a pulse with the fingers). The difference between the systolic and diastolic pressures is called *pulse pressure.*

Another term used in the discussion of shock management but often not emphasized in the prehospital setting is *mean arterial pressure* (MAP). The MAP is the average pressure in the vascular system and is calculated as follows:

MAP = Diastolic pressure + 1/3 Pulse pressure

For example, the MAP of a patient with a blood pressure of 120/80 mm Hg is calculated as follows:

$$\text{MAP} = 80 + ([120 - 80]/3)$$
$$= 80 + (40/3)$$
$$= 80 + 13.3$$
$$= 93.3, \text{ rounded to } 93$$

Many automatic, noninvasive blood pressure devices report the MAP in addition to the systolic and diastolic pressures.

The volume of fluid pumped into the system with each contraction of the ventricle is called the *stroke volume,* and the volume of blood pumped into the system over 1 minute is called the *cardiac output.* The formula for cardiac output (CO) is as follows:

Cardiac output (CO) =
Heart rate (HR) × Stroke volume (SV)

Cardiac output is reported in liters per minute (LPM, or L/min). Cardiac output is not measured in the prehospital environment. However, understanding cardiac output and its relationship to stroke volume is important in understanding shock management.

For the heart to work effectively, an adequate volume of blood must be present in the vena cava and pulmonary veins to fill the ventricles. *Starling's law* of the heart is an important concept explaining how this relationship works: the more the ventricles fill, the greater the strength of contraction of the heart. This pressure *(preload)* that fills the heart stretches the myocardial muscle fibers so that ventricular filling is adequate. Significant hemorrhage or relative hypovolemia decreases cardiac preload so that a reduced volume of blood is present and the fibers are not stretched effectively, resulting in a lower stroke volume. If the filling pressure of the heart is too great, the cardiac muscle fibers become overstretched and can fail to deliver a satisfactory stroke volume. This is often the case with congestive heart failure (CHF).

The resistance to blood flow that the left ventricle must overcome to pump blood out into the arterial system is called *afterload,* which can be thought of as a function of the systemic vascular resistance (SVR). As peripheral arterial vasoconstriction increases, the heart has to generate a greater force to pump blood into the arterial system. Conversely, widespread peripheral vasodilation decreases afterload.

Although one organ, the heart actually has two subsystems, which is an important concept in understanding the cardiovascular system. The right atrium, which receives

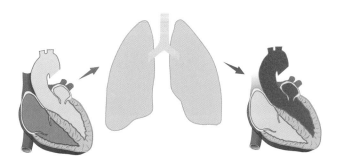

FIGURE 7-4 Although the heart seems to be one organ, it functions as if it were two organs. Unoxygenated blood is received into the "right heart" from the superior and inferior venae cavae and pumped through the pulmonary artery into the lungs. The blood is oxygenated in the lungs, flows back into the heart through the pulmonary vein, and is pumped out of the left ventricle.

blood from the body, and the right ventricle, which pumps blood to the lungs, are referred to as the "right heart." The left atrium, which receives blood from the lungs, and the left ventricle, which pumps blood to the body, are referred to as the "left heart." Preload and afterload of the right heart *(pulmonary)* and left heart *(systemic)* pumping systems are important concepts in the discussion and management of shock (Figure 7-4).

The systemic circulation contains more capillaries and a greater length of blood vessels than the pulmonary circulation. Therefore the left (or *left-sided*) heart system works at a higher pressure and bears a greater load than the right (or *right-sided*) heart system. Anatomically, the muscle of the left ventricle is thicker and stronger than that of the right ventricle.

Blood Vessels

The blood vessels contain the blood and route it to the various areas and cells of the body. They are the "highways" of the physiologic process of circulation. The single, large exit tube from the heart, the *aorta,* cannot serve every individual cell in the body and therefore splits into multiple arteries of decreasing size, the smallest of which are the capillaries (Figure 7-5). A capillary may be only one cell wide; therefore, oxygen and nutrients carried by red blood cells (RBCs) and plasma are able to diffuse easily through the walls of the capillary into the tissue cell (Figure 7-6). Each tissue cell has a membranous covering called the *cell membrane.* Interstitial fluid is located between the cell membrane and the capillary wall. The amount of interstitial fluid varies tremendously. If little interstitial fluid is present, the cell membrane and the capillary wall are close together, and oxygen can easily diffuse between them (Figure 7-7).

The size of the vascular "container" is controlled by muscles in the walls of the arteries and arterioles and, to a lesser extent, by muscles in the walls of the venules and veins. These muscles respond to signals from the brain via

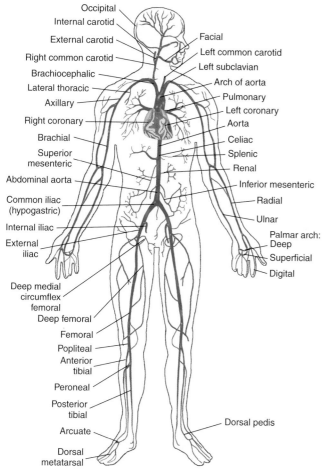

FIGURE 7-5 Principal arteries of the body.

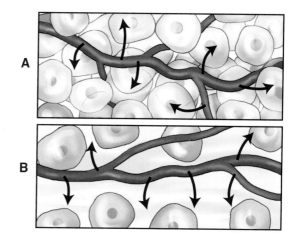

FIGURE 7-6 **A,** If the tissue cells are close to the capillary, oxygen can easily diffuse into them, and carbon dioxide can diffuse out. **B,** If tissue cells are separated from capillary walls by increased edema (interstitial fluid), it is much more difficult for the oxygen and carbon dioxide to diffuse.

FIGURE 7-7 Oxygen and nutrients diffuse from the red blood cells through the capillary wall, the interstitial fluid, and the cell membrane into the cell. Acid production is a byproduct of cellular energy production during the Krebs cycle. By way of the buffer system of the body, this acid is converted into carbon dioxide and travels with the red blood cells and in the plasma to be eliminated from the circulatory system by the lungs.

the sympathetic nervous system, to the circulating hormones epinephrine and norepinephrine, and to other chemicals, such as nitric oxide (NO). These muscle fibers in the walls of the vessels, depending on whether they are being stimulated or allowed to relax, result in either the constriction or dilation of the blood vessels, thus changing the size of the container component of the cardiovascular system.

Blood

The fluid component of the circulatory system, the blood, contains not only RBCs but also infection-fighting factors (white blood cells [WBCs] and antibodies), platelets essential for clotting, protein for cellular rebuilding, nutrition in the form of glucose, and other substances necessary for metabolism and survival. The volume of fluid within the vascular system must equal the capacity of the blood vessels if it is to adequately fill the container. Any variance in the size of the vascular system compared with the amount of blood in the system will affect the flow of blood either positively or negatively.

Human body weight is 60% water, which is the base of all body fluids. A person who weighs 154 pounds (70 kg)

contains approximately 40 L of water. Body water is present in two components: intracellular and extracellular fluid. Each type of fluid has specific, important properties (Figure 7-8). *Intracellular fluid*, the fluid within the cells, accounts for approximately 45% of body weight. *Extracellular fluid*, the fluid outside the cells, can be further classified into two subtypes: interstitial fluid and intravascular fluid. *Interstitial fluid*, which surrounds the tissue cells and also includes cerebrospinal fluid (found in the brain) and synovial fluid (found in the joints), accounts for approximately 10.5% of body weight. *Intravascular fluid*, which is found in the

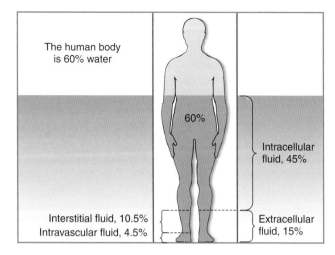

FIGURE 7-8 Body water represents 60% of body weight. This water is divided into intracellular and extracellular fluid. The extracellular fluid is further divided into interstitial and intravascular fluid.

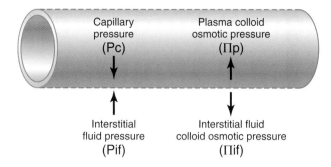

FIGURE 7-9 Forces governing fluid flux across capillaries. (From Guyton AC, Hall JE: *Textbook of medical physiology,* ed 10, Philadelphia, 2000, Saunders.)

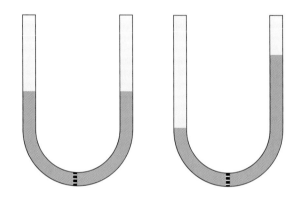

FIGURE 7-10 A U-tube, in which the two halves are separated by a semipermeable membrane, contains equal amounts of water and solid particles. If a solute that cannot diffuse through the semipermeable membrane is added to one side but not to the other, fluid will flow across to dilute the added particles. The pressure difference of the height of fluid in the U-tube is known as *osmotic pressure.*

vessels and carries the formed components of blood as well as oxygen and other vital nutrients within the blood vessels, accounts for approximately 4.5% of body weight.

A review of some key concepts is helpful in this discussion of how fluids operate in the body. Besides movement of fluid through the vascular system, there are two major types of fluid movement: (1) movement between the plasma and interstitial fluid (across capillaries) and (2) movement between the intracellular and interstitial fluid compartments (across cell membranes).

The rate of fluid movement *(flux)* across the capillaries is determined by (1) the difference between the hydrostatic pressure within the capillary (Pc, tending to push fluid out) and the hydrostatic pressure outside the capillary (Pif, tending to push fluid in), (2) the difference in the oncotic pressure from protein concentration within the capillary (πp, tending to keep fluid in) and the oncotic pressure outside the capillary (πif, tending to pull fluid out), and (3) the "leakiness" or permeability (δ) of the capillary (Figure 7-9). Hydrostatic pressure, oncotic pressure, and capillary permeability are all affected by the shock state itself, as well as by the type and volume of fluid resuscitation, leading to alterations in circulating blood volume, hemodynamics, and tissue or pulmonary edema.

Movement of fluid between the intracellular and interstitial space occurs across cellular membranes, which is determined primarily by osmotic effects. *Osmosis* is the process by which solutes separated by a membrane to which the solutes are impermeable govern the movement of water across that semipermeable membrane based on the concentration of the solute. Water moves from the compartment of low solute concentration to that of higher solute concentration to maintain osmotic equilibrium across the semipermeable membrane (Figure 7-10).

Nervous System

The *autonomic nervous system* directs and controls the involuntary functions of the body, such as respiration, digestion, and cardiovascular function. It is divided into two subsystems, the sympathetic and parasympathetic nervous systems. These systems oppose each other to keep vital body systems in balance.

The *sympathetic nervous system* produces the fight-or-flight response. This response simultaneously causes the heart to beat faster and stronger, increases the ventilatory rate, and constricts the blood vessels to nonessential organs (skin and gastrointestinal tract) while dilating vessels and improving blood flow to muscles. The goal of this response is to maintain sufficient amounts of oxygenated blood to critical tissues so that an individual can respond to an emergency situation, while shunting blood away from nonessential areas. The sensitivity of the body's cells to the lack of oxygen varies from organ system to organ system; this *ischemic sensitivity* is greatest in the brain, heart, and lungs. Only 4 to 6 minutes of hypoxia may be necessary

TABLE 7-1 Organ Tolerance to Ischemia

Organ	Warm ischemia time
Heart, brain, lungs	4-6 minutes
Kidneys, liver, gastrointestinal tract	45-90 minutes
Muscle, bone, skin	4-6 hours

before one or more of these vital organs is damaged. Skin and muscle tissues have significantly longer ischemic sensitivity, 6 to 8 hours. The abdominal organs (kidneys and liver) generally fall between these two groups and are able to survive 45 to 90 minutes of hypoxia (Table 7-1).

The cardiovascular system is regulated by the vasomotor center in the medulla. Stimuli travel via cranial nerves IX and X from stretch receptors in the carotid sinus and the aortic arch in response to a transient fall in blood pressure. This leads to increased sympathetic nervous system activity, with increased peripheral vascular resistance resulting from arteriolar constriction and increased cardiac output from an increased rate and force of cardiac contraction. Increased venous tone enhances circulatory blood volume. Blood is thus diverted from the extremities, bowel, and kidney to more vital areas, that is, the heart and brain, where vessels constrict very little under intense sympathetic stimulation. These responses result in cold, cyanotic extremities with decreased urine output and decreased bowel perfusion.

A decrease in the left atrial filling pressure, a fall in blood pressure, and changes in plasma osmolality cause release of antidiuretic hormone (ADH) from the pituitary gland and aldosterone from the adrenal glands, which enhances retention of sodium and water by the kidneys.

Cellular Changes

The *Fick principle* expresses the relationship between cardiac output (Q), oxygen consumption (Vo_2), and the difference in oxygen content of arterial (Cao_2) and mixed venous (Cvo_2) blood: $Q = Vo_2/(Cao_2 - Cvo_2)$. As cardiac output decreases, oxygen consumption is maintained by increasing oxygen extraction at the cellular level; this is reflected in a decrease in the oxygen content of mixed venous blood. However, this relationship is maintained only to a critical point when oxygen delivery (the product of cardiac output and arterial oxygen content) cannot be maintained beyond this critical level to support the oxygen needs of the cells. Oxygen extraction and oxygen consumption therefore decrease, leading to cellular hypoxia. The oxygen content of arterial blood is related to the loading of oxygen on the RBCs at the alveolar level. This is related to the hemoglobin concentration, the inspired oxygen concentration, and to a lesser extent the oxygen diffusion gradient.

Many factors, such as temperature, hydrogen ion concentration (pH), and level of 2,3-diphosphoglyceric acid

(DPG) in the RBCs, affect this affinity of hemoglobin for oxygen.[3] All these factors can be affected in the shock state. Normally, oxygen consumption is maintained within a very narrow range, but it can be increased in stress. In shock and with the decreased oxygen delivery occurring in the shock state, oxygen debt also occurs, resulting in tissue hypoxia.[4] Oxygen is required to metabolize glucose with the production of adenosine triphosphate (ATP), which is the source of energy for cellular function. Cellular hypoxia leads to *anaerobic metabolism* (metabolism in the presence of decreased oxygen), with a reduction in ATP generation and accumulation of acids (primarily lactic acid) resulting in metabolic acidosis.

Metabolic acidosis in the shock state has several deleterious effects at the cellular level. The maintenance of a high sodium concentration in the extracellular space and a high potassium concentration in the intracellular space is a process that requires energy. With the lack of ATP, this function at the cellular membrane cannot be maintained, resulting in sodium and water entering the cells and potassium and lactic acid entering the serum, leading to lactic acidosis and hyperkalemia as well as cellular edema, which then compounds the loss of circulating blood volume in hypovolemic shock. At low pH levels, enzyme systems and lysosomal membranes are disrupted, releasing lysozymes, which result in autodigestion of the cells, and leading to death of the cells, multiorgan failure, and eventually death of the organism if the process is not halted.

Microcirculatory Changes

Initially, as intravascular hydrostatic pressure falls, fluid tends to enter the vascular space (plasma refill phase) in an attempt to maintain circulating blood volume. This is enhanced by precapillary and postcapillary vasoconstriction: the *ischemic phase* of shock (Figure 7-11). As plasma pH decreases further with acidosis, the precapillary sphincters relax while the postcapillary sphincters remain contracted, with resultant pooling of fluid in the capillaries (the *stagnant, or irreversible, phase* of shock). The third phase consists of worsening of the pH with dilation of both precapillary and postcapillary sphincters, resulting in the *washout phase,* during which there is increased liberation of acid in the circulation.

Types of Shock

Hypovolemic Shock

When acute blood volume loss occurs through dehydration (loss of plasma) or hemorrhage (loss of plasma and RBCs), the relationship of fluid volume to the size of the container becomes unbalanced. The container retains its normal size, but the fluid volume is decreased. *Hypovolemic shock* is

FIGURE 7-11 The cellular pathophysiologic process of shock is divided into three phases: **A,** ischemic; **B,** stagnant (irreversible); and **C,** washout.

the most common cause of shock encountered in the prehospital environment, and blood loss is by far the most common cause of shock in trauma patients.

When blood is lost from the circulation, the heart is stimulated to increase cardiac output by increasing the strength and rate of contractions through the release of *epinephrine* from the adrenal glands. The sympathetic nervous system releases *norepinephrine* to trigger constriction of the blood vessels to reduce the size of the container and bring it more into proportion with the volume of remaining fluid. Vasoconstriction results in closing of the peripheral capillaries, as discussed previously, and prompts the switch from aerobic to anaerobic metabolism at the cellular level.

These compensatory defense mechanisms work well up to a point. When defense mechanisms can no longer overcome the volume reduction, a patient's blood pressure drops. A decrease in blood pressure marks the switch from compensated to decompensated shock—a sign of impending death. A patient who has signs of compensation is already in shock, not "going into shock." Unless aggressive resuscitation occurs, the patient who enters decompensated shock has only one more stage of decline left—death.

Hemorrhagic Shock

Hemorrhagic shock (hypovolemic shock resulting from blood loss) can be categorized into four classes, depending on the severity of hemorrhage, as follows (Table 7-2):

1. *Class I hemorrhage* represents a loss of up to 15% of blood volume in the adult (up to 750 mL). This stage has few clinical manifestations. Tachycardia is often minimal, and no measurable changes in blood pressure, pulse pressure, or ventilatory rate occur. Most healthy patients sustaining this amount of hemorrhage only require maintenance fluid as long as no further blood loss occurs. The body's compensatory mechanisms restore intravascular fluid.

2. *Class II hemorrhage* represents a loss of 15% to 30% of blood volume (750-1500 mL). Most adults are capable of compensating for this amount of blood loss by activation of the sympathetic nervous system and maintaining their blood pressure. Clinical findings include increased ventilatory rate, tachycardia, and a narrowed pulse pressure. The patient often demonstrates anxiety or fright. Urine output drops slightly, to between 20 and 30 mL/hr in the adult. On occasion, these patients may require blood transfusion; however, most will respond well to crystalloid infusion.

3. *Class III hemorrhage* represents a loss of 30% to 40% of blood volume (1500-2000 mL). When blood loss reaches this point, most patients are no longer able to compensate for the volume loss, and hypotension occurs. The classic findings of shock are obvious and include tachycardia (heart rate >120 beats/min), tachypnea (ventilatory rate 30-40 breaths/min), and severe anxiety or confusion. Urine output falls to 5 to 15 mL/hr. Many of these patients will require blood transfusion and surgical intervention for adequate resuscitation.

4. *Class IV hemorrhage* represents a loss of more than 40% of blood volume (>2000 mL). This stage of severe shock is characterized by marked tachycardia (heart rate >140 beats/min), tachypnea (ventilatory rate >35 breaths/min), profound confusion or lethargy, and greatly decreased systolic blood pressure, typically in the range of 60 mm Hg. These patients truly have only minutes to live. Survival depends on immediate control of hemorrhage (surgery for internal hemorrhage) and aggressive resuscitation, including blood transfusions.

The definitive management for volume deficit is to stop the fluid loss and replace the lost fluid. A dehydrated patient needs fluid replacement with water and salt, whereas a trauma patient who has lost blood needs to have the source of blood loss stopped and consideration for blood replacement. Mild to moderate dehydration can be treated with an electrolyte solution that a conscious patient

TABLE 7-2   Classifications of Hemorrhagic Shock

	Class I	Class II	Class III	Class IV
Amount of blood loss (% total blood volume)	<750 mL (<15%)	750-1500 mL (15%-30%)	1500-2000 mL (30%-40%)	>2000 mL (>40%)
Heart rate (beats/min)	Normal or minimally increased	>100	>120	>140
Ventilatory rate (breaths/min)	Normal	20-30	30-40	>35
Systolic blood pressure (mm Hg)	Normal	Normal	Decreased	Greatly decreased
Urine output (mL/hr)	Normal	20-30	5-15	Minimal

Modified from American College of Surgeons Committee on Trauma: *Advanced trauma life support for doctors, student course manual,* ed 7, Chicago, 2004, ACS.

can drink. An unconscious or severely dehydrated patient should receive the replacement intravenously. Because blood replacement is usually not available in the prehospital environment, trauma patients who have lost blood should undergo measures to control external blood loss and receive an intravenous electrolyte solution and rapid transportation to the hospital, where blood and emergent surgery are available.

Shock research has demonstrated that for lost blood, the replacement ratio with electrolyte solution should be 3 L of replacement for each liter of blood lost. This is because only about one third of the volume of an isotonic crystalloid solution remains in the intravascular space 1 hour after infusing it. For moderate and severe shock, this research has shown that replacement with both a crystalloid solution and blood was better than with blood alone.[5] The use of a limited volume of electrolyte solution before blood replacement is the correct approach. The best crystalloid solution for treating hemorrhagic shock is lactated Ringer's solution. Normal saline is another isotonic crystalloid solution that can be used for volume replacement, but its use may produce hyperchloremia (marked increase in the blood chloride level), leading to acidosis.

A *pneumatic antishock garment* (PASG) may provide short-term assistance with managing severe hemorrhagic shock by increasing vascular resistance, reducing container size, and tamponading abdominal and pelvic hemorrhage. The most important use of the PASG is in intraabdominal and pelvic hemorrhage control in patients with blood pressure below 60 mm Hg. However, as the PASG increases the patient's blood pressure, hemorrhage from injury sites outside the confines of the garment may increase.[6] (See Management section for further discussion of PASG.)

Distributive (Vasogenic) Shock

Distributive shock, or vasogenic shock, occurs when the vascular container enlarges without a proportional increase in fluid volume. Relatively less fluid will be available for

the size of the container. As a result, the volume of fluid available to the heart as preload decreases, and cardiac output falls. In most situations, fluid has not been lost from the vascular system. This form of shock is not a case of hypovolemia, where fluid has been lost through hemorrhage, vomiting, or diarrhea; the problem is with the size of the container. For this reason, this condition is sometimes referred to as *relative hypovolemia.* Although some of the presenting signs and symptoms may closely mimic those of hypovolemic shock, the cause of the two conditions is different.

In distributive shock, resistance to flow is decreased because of the relatively larger size of the blood vessels. This reduced resistance decreases the diastolic blood pressure. When this reduced resistance is combined with the reduced preload and therefore a reduced cardiac output, the net result is a decrease in both systolic and diastolic blood pressures, but tissue oxygenation may remain adequate.

Distributive shock can result from loss of autonomic nervous system control of the smooth muscles that control the size of the blood vessels or release of chemicals that result in peripheral vasodilation. This loss of control can stem from spinal cord trauma, simple fainting, severe infections, or allergic reactions. Management of distributive shock is directed toward improving oxygenation of the blood and improving or maintaining blood flow to the brain and vital organs.

Septic Shock

Septic shock, seen in patients with life-threatening infections, is another condition that exhibits vascular dilation. Cytokines, released in response to the infection, cause damage to the walls of the blood vessels, causing peripheral vasodilation and a leakage of fluid from the capillaries into the interstitial space. Thus, septic shock has characteristics of both distributive shock and hypovolemic shock. Preload is diminished because of the vasodilation and loss of fluid, and hypotension occurs when the heart can no longer compensate. Septic shock is virtually never encountered within

TABLE 7-3   Signs Associated with Types of Shock

Vital Sign	Hypovolemic	Neurogenic	Septic	Cardiogenic
Skin temperature	Cool, clammy	Warm, dry	Cool, clammy	Cool, clammy
Skin color	Pale, cyanotic	Pink	Pale, mottled	Pale, cyanotic
Blood pressure	Drops	Drops	Drops	Drops
Level of consciousness	Altered	Lucid	Altered	Altered
Capillary refilling time	Slowed	Normal	Slowed	Slowed

minutes of an injury; however, the prehospital care provider may be called on to care for a trauma patient in septic shock during an interfacility transfer, or if a patient sustains an injury to the gastrointestinal tract and did not promptly seek medical attention.

Neurogenic "Shock"

Neurogenic shock occurs when the injury interrupts the spinal cord sympathetic nervous system pathway. In the spinal cord, this usually involves injury to the thoracolumbar area. Because of the loss of sympathetic control of the vascular system, which controls the smooth muscles in the walls of the blood vessels, the peripheral vessels dilate below the level of injury. The marked decrease in systemic vascular resistance and peripheral vasodilation that occurs as the container for the blood volume increases results in relative hypovolemia. The patient is not hypovolemic, but the normal blood volume insufficiently fills an expanded container. This decrease in blood pressure does not alter perfusion or compromise energy production and therefore is *not* shock.

Decompensated hypovolemic shock and neurogenic shock both produce a decreased systolic blood pressure. However, the other vital signs vary significantly, and the treatment for each is also different (Table 7-3). Decreased systolic and diastolic pressures and a narrow pulse pressure characterize hypovolemic shock. Neurogenic shock also displays decreased systolic and diastolic pressures, but the pulse pressure remains normal or is widened. Hypovolemia produces cold, clammy, pale, or cyanotic skin and delayed capillary refilling time. In neurogenic shock the patient has warm, dry skin, especially below the area of injury. The pulse in hypovolemic shock patients is weak, thready, and rapid. Because of unopposed parasympathetic activity on the heart in neurogenic shock, bradycardia is typically seen rather than tachycardia, but the pulse quality may be weak. Hypovolemia produces a decreased level of consciousness (LOC), or at least anxiety and often combativeness. In the absence of a traumatic brain injury, the patient with neurogenic shock is alert, oriented, and lucid when in the supine position (Box 7-1).

BOX 7-1   Neurogenic Shock versus Spinal Shock

As discussed in this chapter, the term *neurogenic shock* refers to a disruption of the sympathetic nervous system, typically from injury to the spinal cord, that results in significant dilation of the peripheral arteries. If untreated, this may result in impaired perfusion to the body's tissues. This condition should not be confused with *spinal shock,* a term that refers to an injury to the spinal cord that results in *temporary* loss of sensory and motor function. Thus, spinal shock indicates that the spinal cord has been damaged ("shocked") and is not working properly. Strictly speaking, spinal shock does not represent a defect in organ or tissue perfusion. The prehospital care provider should be aware that both neurogenic shock and spinal shock can simultaneously occur in the same patient.

Patients with neurogenic shock may have associated injuries that produce severe hemorrhage. Therefore a patient who has neurogenic shock and signs of hypovolemia, such as tachycardia, should be treated appropriately.

Psychogenic (Vasovagal) "Shock"

Psychogenic shock is typically mediated through the parasympathetic nervous system. Stimulation of the tenth cranial nerve (vagus nerve) produces bradycardia. The increased parasympathetic activity may also result in transient peripheral vasodilation and hypotension. If the bradycardia and vasodilation are severe enough, cardiac output falls dramatically, resulting in insufficient blood flow to the brain. Vasovagal syncope (fainting) occurs when the patient loses consciousness. Compared with neurogenic shock, the periods of bradycardia and vasodilation are generally limited to minutes, whereas neurogenic shock may last up to several days. In psychogenic shock patients, normal blood pressure is quickly restored when the patient is placed in a horizontal position. Because it is self-limited, a vasovagal episode is unlikely to result in true "shock" and the body quickly recovers before significant systemic impairment of perfusion occurs.

Cardiogenic Shock

Cardiogenic shock, or failure of the heart's pumping activity, results from causes that can be categorized as either intrinsic (a result of direct damage to the heart itself) or extrinsic (related to a problem outside the heart).

Intrinsic Causes

Heart Muscle Damage. Any process that weakens the cardiac muscle will affect its output. The damage may result from an acute interruption of the heart's own blood supply (as in a myocardial infarction from coronary artery disease) or from a direct bruise to the heart muscle (as in a blunt cardiac injury). A recurring cycle will ensue: decreased oxygenation causes decreased contractibility, which results in decreased cardiac output and therefore decreased systemic perfusion. Decreased perfusion results in a continuing decrease in oxygenation and thus a continuation of the cycle. As with any muscle, the cardiac muscle does not work as efficiently when it becomes bruised or damaged.

Dysrhythmia. The development of a cardiac dysrhythmia can affect the efficiency of contractions, resulting in impaired systemic perfusion. Hypoxia may lead to myocardial ischemia and cause dysrhythmias, such as premature contractions and tachycardia. Because cardiac output is determined by the stroke volume multiplied by the number of contractions per minute, any dysrhythmia that results in a slow rate of contractions (bradycardia) or shortens the left ventricle's fill time (tachycardia), resulting in decreased stroke volume, could decrease cardiac output. Blunt cardiac injury may also result in dysrhythmias, the most common of which is a mild, persistent tachycardia.

Valvular Disruption. A sudden, forceful compressing blow to the chest or abdomen (see Chapter 3) may damage the valves of the heart. Severe valvular injury results in acute regurgitation, where a significant amount of blood leaks back into the chamber from which it was just pumped. These patients often rapidly develop CHF, manifested by pulmonary edema and cardiogenic shock. The presence of a new heart murmur is an important clue in making this diagnosis.

Extrinsic Causes

Cardiac Tamponade. Fluid in the pericardial sac will prevent the heart from refilling completely during the diastolic (relaxation) phase. According to Starling's law, inadequate filling results in a diminished strength of cardiac contraction. In the case of penetrating cardiac trauma, more blood may enter the pericardial sac with each contraction, further compromising the cardiac output. Severe shock and death may rapidly follow.

Tension Pneumothorax. A tension pneumothorax shifts the mediastinum away from the injury. Compression and kinking of the superior and inferior venae cavae and increased pulmonary vascular resistance because of increased intrathoracic pressure drastically impede venous return to the heart, producing a significant drop in preload. Because of its impaired filling, the heart loses its efficiency as a pump, and shock rapidly ensues.

Complications of Shock

Several complications may result in patients with persistent or inadequately resuscitated shock, which is why early recognition and aggressive management of shock are essential. Many prehospital care providers fail to realize that the quality of care delivered in the prehospital setting can alter a patient's hospital course and outcome. *Failure to recognize shock and initiate proper treatment in the prehospital setting may extend the patient's hospital length of stay.* Although the following complications of shock are not often seen in the prehospital setting, a prehospital care provider may encounter them while transferring patients between facilities.

Acute Renal Failure

Impaired circulation to the kidneys, resulting from inappropriate care of shock leading to prolonged shock, can lead to temporary or permanent renal failure. The cells that make up the renal tubules are most sensitive to ischemia and may die if their oxygen delivery is impaired for more than 45 to 60 minutes. This *acute tubular necrosis* (ATN) may cause the kidneys to fail. Because the kidneys are no longer functioning, excess fluid is not excreted, and volume overload may result. Also, the kidneys lose their ability to excrete metabolic acids and electrolytes, leading to a metabolic acidosis and hyperkalemia (increased blood potassium). These patients often require dialysis for several weeks to months. Most patients who develop ATN resulting from shock will eventually recover normal renal function, provided they survive.

Acute Respiratory Distress Syndrome

Acute respiratory distress syndrome (ARDS) is the result of damage to the lining of the capillaries in the lung, leading to the leakage of fluid into the interstitial spaces and alveoli of the lungs. This makes it much more difficult for oxygen to diffuse across the alveolar walls and into the capillaries and bind with the RBCs. Although these patients do have pulmonary edema, it is not the result of impaired cardiac function, as in CHF (*cardiogenic* pulmonary edema). ARDS represents *noncardiogenic* pulmonary edema, and patients generally do not improve with diuretic therapy. Many factors have been associated with the development of ARDS, including shock, massive blood transfusions, aspiration, and severe infection. ARDS is associated with a mortality rate of about 40%, and the patients who survive may require mechanical ventilation for up to several months.

Hematologic Failure

The term *coagulopathy* refers to impairment in the normal blood-clotting capabilities. This may result from hypothermia (decreased body temperature), dilution of clotting factors from transfusion of fluids, or depletion of the clotting substances as they are used in an effort to control bleeding (*consumptive* coagulopathy). The normal blood-clotting cascade involves several enzymes and eventually results in the creation of fibrin molecules that serve as a matrix to trap platelets and form a plug in a vessel wall. These enzymes function best in a narrow temperature range (i.e., near-normal body temperature). As the core temperature of the body falls, this dramatically slows down blood clotting, leading to continued hemorrhage. The blood-clotting factors may also be used up as they form blood clots in an effort to slow and control hemorrhage. Another manifestation of hematologic failure is a marked decrease in the number of WBCs, predisposing the shock patient to infection. The decreased body temperature worsens the clotting problems, which exacerbates hemorrhage, which further reduces the body temperature. Thus, with inadequate resuscitation, this becomes an ever-worsening cycle.

Hepatic Failure

Severe damage to the liver is a less common result of prolonged shock, but it may occur. Liver failure is manifested by persistent hypoglycemia (low blood sugar), a persistent lactic acidosis, and jaundice. Because the liver produces many of the clotting factors necessary for hemostasis, a coagulopathy may accompany liver failure.

Multiple Organ Failure

Shock, if not successfully treated, can lead to dysfunction in one organ followed by several organs simultaneously with sepsis being a common accompaniment leading to the multiple organ dysfunction syndrome.

Failure of one major body system (e.g., lungs, kidneys, blood-clotting cascade, liver) is associated with a mortality rate of about 40%. As an organ system fails, the shock state worsens. By the time four organ systems fail, the mortality rate is essentially 100%.[7] Cardiovascular failure, in the form of cardiogenic and septic shock, can only occasionally be reversed.

Assessment

Shock was defined earlier as a state of generalized hypoperfusion. In assessing for the presence of shock, a provider therefore seeks evidence of this state of hypoperfusion. In the prehospital setting, this requires the assessment of organs and systems that are immediately accessible for such assessment. Signs of hypoperfusion will manifest as a malfunction of these accessible organs or systems. Such systems are the brain and central nervous system (CNS), heart and cardiovascular system, respiratory system, skin and extremities, and the kidneys. Thus the signs of hypoperfusion would include the following:

- Decreased LOC, anxiety, disorientation, belligerence, bizarre behavior (brain and CNS)
- Tachycardia, decreased systolic and pulse pressure (heart and cardiovascular system)
- Rapid, shallow breathing (respiratory system)
- Cold, pale, clammy, diaphoretic or even cyanotic skin with decreased capillary refill time (skin and extremities)
- Decreased urine output (kidneys), identified only rarely in the prehospital setting in situations of prolonged or delayed transport when a urinary catheter may be present

Because hemorrhage is the most common cause of shock in the trauma patient, the prehospital care provider's approach should be to consider all shock as hemorrhagic until proven otherwise. The provider should first examine for external sources of hemorrhage and control this as directly as possible. This may involve such techniques as application of pressure dressing, tourniquets, or splinting of extremity fractures. If there is no evidence of external hemorrhage, internal hemorrhage should be suspected. Although definitive management of internal hemorrhage is not practical in the prehospital setting, identification of an internal source would further facilitate the process of rapid transport to the definitive care institution. Internal hemorrhage can occur in the chest, abdomen, pelvis, or retroperitoneum. Evidence of blunt or penetrating chest injury, with decreased breath sounds and dullness to percussion, would suggest a thoracic source. The provider would suspect the abdomen, pelvis, and retroperitoneum as a source of bleeding with evidence of blunt trauma (e.g., ecchymosis) or penetrating trauma, abdominal distention or tenderness, pelvic instability, leg inequality, pain in the pelvic area aggravated by movement, perineal ecchymosis, and blood at the urethral meatus.

If the assessment does not suggest hemorrhage as the cause of the shock, nonhemorrhagic causes should be suspected. These include cardiac tamponade and tension pneumothorax (both evident by distended neck veins vs. collapsed neck veins in hemorrhagic shock) and neurogenic shock. Decreased breath sounds and hyperresonance on the side of the chest injury with possible tracheal deviation would suggest tension pneumothorax, which requires immediate needle decompression. The provider would suspect different sources of cardiogenic shock with blunt or penetrating chest trauma, muffled heart sounds (probably not discernible in the prehospital setting), and dysrhythmias and sources of neurogenic shock with signs of spinal trauma, bradycardia, and warm extremities. Most, if not all, of these features can be detected by the astute prehospital care provider who can determine the cause of the shock and the need for appropriate intervention when feasible in the field.

Simultaneous evaluation is an important part of patient assessment as the prehospital care provider continues to gather and process information from different sources simultaneously. If the provider finds that all systems are functioning normally, no alarm is set off.

Areas of patient evaluation include status of the airway, ventilation, perfusion, skin color and temperature, capillary refilling time, and blood pressure. Each is presented separately here in the context of both the primary survey (initial assessment) and the secondary survey (focused history and physical examination).

Primary Survey

The following signs identify the need for continued suspicion of life-threatening conditions:

- Mild anxiety, progressing to confusion or altered LOC
- Mild tachypnea, leading to rapid, labored ventilations
- Mild tachycardia, progressing to marked tachycardia
- Weakened radial pulse, progressing to an absent radial pulse
- Pale or cyanotic skin color
- Capillary refilling time longer than 2 seconds

Any compromise or failure of the airway, breathing, or circulatory system must be managed before proceeding. The following steps are described in an ordered series. When performing these in the field, however, the provider does them all more or less simultaneously.

Airway

Assessment should include evaluation of the airway to ensure its patency (see Chapter 6).

Breathing

As noted earlier, the anaerobic metabolism associated with decreased cellular oxygenation will produce an increase in lactic acid. The hydrogen ions (H^+) from the acidosis and hypoxia lead to stimulation of the respiratory center to increase the rate and depth of ventilation. Thus, tachypnea is frequently one of the earliest signs of shock. In the primary survey, time is not taken to measure a ventilatory rate. Instead, ventilations should be estimated to be slow, normal, fast, or very fast. A slow ventilatory rate, in conjunction with shock, generally indicates that a patient is in profound shock and may be moments away from cardiac arrest. Any fast ventilatory rate is a concern and should serve as an impetus to search for the cause of shock. A patient who tries to remove an oxygen mask, particularly when such action is associated with anxiety and belligerence, is displaying another sign of cerebral ischemia. This patient has "air hunger" and feels the need for more ventilation. The presence of a mask over the nose and mouth creates a psychological feeling of ventilatory restriction. This action should be a clue that the patient is not receiving enough oxygen and is hypoxic. Decreased oxygen saturation, as measured by the pulse oximeter, will confirm this suspicion. Any pulse oximeter reading below 95% is worrisome and should serve as a stimulus to identify the cause of hypoxia.

Circulation

The prehospital care provider can check the following vital signs and conditions rapidly and assimilate the data to make a quick initial determination of the patient's volume and perfusion status.

Hemorrhage. Assessment of circulation should begin with a rapid scan for significant external hemorrhage. No efforts at restoring perfusion will be effective in the face of ongoing hemorrhage. The patient can lose a significant volume of blood from scalp lacerations because of the high concentration of blood vessels and from wounds that damage major blood vessels (subclavian, axillary, brachial, radial, ulnar, carotid, femoral, or popliteal).

Pulse. The next important assessment point for perfusion is the pulse. Initial evaluation of the pulse determines whether it is palpable at the artery being examined. In general, loss of a radial pulse indicates severe hypovolemia or vascular damage to the arm, especially when a central pulse, such as in the carotid or femoral artery, is weak, thready, and extremely fast. If the pulse is palpable, its character and strength should be noted, as follows:

- Is the rate strong or weak and thready?
- Is the rate normal, too fast, or too slow?
- Is the rate regular or irregular?

Although many individuals involved in the management of trauma patients focus on blood pressure, precious time should not be spent during the primary survey to obtain a blood pressure. Significant information can be determined from the pulse rate and character. In one series of trauma patients, a radial pulse characterized by prehospital care providers as "weak" was associated with blood pressure that averaged 26 mm Hg lower than a pulse thought to be "normal." More importantly, trauma patients with a weak radial pulse were 15 times more likely to die than those with a normal pulse.[8] Although generally obtained at the beginning of the secondary survey, blood pressure can be palpated or auscultated earlier in the assessment if sufficient assistance is present, or once the primary survey has been completed and life-threatening issues are being addressed during transport.

Level of Consciousness. Next, the patient's LOC is assessed. Mental status is generally considered part of the disability evaluation, but altered mental status can represent impaired cerebral perfusion. An anxious, belligerent patient should be assumed to have cerebral ischemia and anaerobic metabolism until another cause is identified. Drug and alcohol overdose and cerebral contusion are conditions that cannot be treated rapidly, but cerebral ischemia can be treated. Therefore, all patients in whom cerebral ischemia might be present should be managed as if it is present.

Skin Color. Pink skin color generally indicates a well-oxygenated patient without anaerobic metabolism. Blue (cyanotic) or mottled skin indicates unoxygenated hemoglobin and a lack of adequate oxygenation to the periphery. Pale, mottled, or cyanotic skin has inadequate blood flow resulting from one of the following three causes:

1. Peripheral vasoconstriction (most often associated with hypovolemia)
2. Decreased supply of RBCs (acute anemia)
3. Interruption of blood supply to that portion of the body, such as might be found with a fracture

Pale skin may be a localized or generalized finding with different implications. Other findings, such as tachycardia, should be used to resolve these differences and to determine if the pale skin is a localized, regional, or systemic condition. Also, cyanosis may not develop in hypoxic patients who have lost a significant number of their RBCs from hemorrhage. In patients who have dark-pigmented skin, cyanosis may be noted in the lips and gums and in the palms.

Skin Temperature. As the body shunts blood away from the skin to more important parts of the body, skin temperature decreases. Skin that is cool to the touch indicates decreased cutaneous perfusion and decreased energy production and therefore shock. Because a significant amount of heat can be lost during the assessment phase, steps should be taken to preserve the patient's body temperature.

A good sign of adequate resuscitation is a warm, dry, pink toe. The environmental conditions in which the provider finds the patient when performing this test can affect the results.

Capillary Refilling Time. The ability of the cardiovascular system to refill the capillaries after the blood has been "removed" represents an important support system. Analyzing this support system's level of function by compressing the capillaries to remove all the blood and then measuring the refilling time may provide insight into the perfusion of the capillary bed being assessed. Generally, the body shuts down circulation in the most distal parts of the body first and restores this circulation last. Evaluation of the nail bed of the big toe or thumb provides the earliest possible indication that hypoperfusion is developing. Additionally, it provides a strong indication when resuscitation is complete. However, as with many other signs that a patient may exhibit, several conditions, both environmental and physiologic, can alter the results. A test of the capillary refilling time is a measurement of the time required to reperfuse the skin and therefore an indirect measurement of the actual perfusion of that part of the body. It is not a diagnostic test of any specific disease process or injury.

Capillary refilling time has recently been described as a poor test of shock. However, it is not a test of shock, but rather a test of perfusion of the capillary bed being analyzed. Arterial interruption from a fracture, a gunshot wound of the vessel, hypothermia, and even arteriosclerosis are conditions that produce poor perfusion and decreased capillary refilling time. Another cause of poor capillary refilling is decreased cardiac output resulting from hypovolemia. It is a helpful diagnostic sign that can also be used to monitor the progress of resuscitation.

Disability

One body system that can be readily evaluated in the field is brain function. At least five conditions can produce an altered LOC or change in behavior (combativeness or belligerence) in trauma patients, as follows:

1. Hypoxia
2. Shock with impaired cerebral perfusion
3. Traumatic brain injury
4. Intoxication with alcohol or drugs
5. Metabolic processes such as diabetes, seizures, and eclampsia

Of these five conditions, the easiest to treat—and the one that will kill the patient most quickly if not treated—is hypoxia. Any patient with an altered LOC should be treated as if decreased cerebral oxygenation is the cause. An altered LOC is usually one of the first visible signs of shock.

Brain injury may be considered *primary* (caused by direct trauma to brain tissue) or *secondary* (caused by the effects of hypoxia, hypoperfusion, etc.). There is no effective treatment in the prehospital setting for the primary brain injury, but secondary brain injury can essentially be prevented by maintaining oxygenation and perfusion.

The brain's function decreases as perfusion and oxygenation drop and ischemia develops. This decreased function evolves through various stages as different areas of the brain become affected. Anxiety and belligerent behavior are usually the first signs, followed by a slowing of the thought processes and a decrease of the body's motor and sensory functions. The level of cerebral function is an important and measurable prehospital sign of shock. A belligerent, combative, anxious patient or one with a decreased LOC should be assumed to have a hypoxic, hypoperfused brain until another cause can be identified. Hypoperfusion and cerebral hypoxia frequently accompany brain injury and make the long-term result even worse. Even brief episodes of hypoxia and shock may worsen the original brain injury and result in poorer outcomes.

Body Exposure/Environment

The prehospital care provider exposes the patient's body to look for less obvious sites of external blood loss and clues that may indicate internal hemorrhage. The possibility of hypothermia is also considered.

Secondary Survey
Vital Signs

Measurement of an accurate set of vital signs is one of the first steps taken by the prehospital care provider in the secondary survey or, after reassessing the primary survey, when a few minutes are available during transport.

Ventilatory Rate. A rate of 20 to 30 breaths/min indicates a borderline abnormal rate and the need for supplemental oxygen. A rate greater than 30 breaths/min indicates a late stage of shock and the need for assisted ventilation because it is generally associated with a decreased tidal volume.

Both these rates indicate the need to look for the potential sources of impaired perfusion.

Pulse. In the secondary survey the pulse rate is determined more precisely. The normal pulse range for an adult is 60 to 100 pulsations/min. With rates below this, except in extremely athletic individuals, an ischemic heart or a pathologic condition such as complete heart block should be considered. A pulse in the range of 100 to 120/min identifies a patient who has early shock, with an initial cardiac response toward tachycardia. A pulse above 120/min is a definite sign of shock unless it is caused by pain or fear, and a pulse over 140/min is considered extremely critical and near-death.

Blood Pressure. Blood pressure is one of the least sensitive signs of shock. Blood pressure does not begin to drop until a patient is profoundly hypovolemic (from either true fluid loss or container-enlarged relative hypovolemia). In otherwise healthy patients, blood loss must exceed 30% of blood volume before the patient's compensatory mechanisms fail and systolic blood pressure drops below 90 mm Hg. For this reason, ventilatory rate, pulse rate and character, capillary refilling time, and LOC are more sensitive indicators of hypovolemia than blood pressure.

When the patient's pressure has begun to drop, an extremely critical situation exists, and rapid intervention is required. In the prehospital environment, a patient who is found to be hypotensive has already lost a significant volume of blood. The presence of a hypotensive patient means that earlier signs of shock may have been overlooked.

The severity of the situation and the appropriate type of intervention vary based on the cause of the condition. For example, low blood pressure associated with neurogenic shock is not nearly as critical as low blood pressure with hypovolemic shock. Table 7-4 presents the signs used to assess compensated and decompensated hypovolemic shock.

One important pitfall to avoid involves equating systolic blood pressure with cardiac output and tissue perfusion. As emphasized in this chapter, significant blood loss is typically required before the patient becomes hypotensive (Class III hemorrhage). Thus, patients will have decreased

TABLE 7-4   Shock Assessment in Compensated and Decompensated Hypovolemic Shock

Vital sign	Compensated	Decompensated
Pulse	Increased; tachycardia	Greatly increased; marked tachycardia that can progress to bradycardia
Skin	White, cool, moist	White, cold, waxy
Blood pressure range	Normal	Decreased
Level of consciousness	Unaltered	Altered, ranging from disoriented to coma

cardiac output and impaired tissue oxygenation when they have lost 15% to 30% of their blood volume despite having a normal systolic blood pressure.

When assessing patients with multiple trauma, the prehospital care provider should remember that brain injuries do not cause hypotension until the cerebellum begins to herniate through the incisura and foramen magnum. Therefore, if a patient with a brain injury is hypotensive, the prehospital care provider should assume that this condition is caused by hypovolemia (usually blood loss) from other injuries and not from the brain injury. Young infants (<6 months) are the exception to this rule because they may bleed into hypovolemic shock inside their head as a result of open sutures and fontanelles.

Musculoskeletal Injuries

Significant internal hemorrhage can occur with fractures (Table 7-5). Of greatest concern are fractures to the femur and pelvis. A single femoral fracture may be associated with up to 2 to 4 units (1000-2000 mL) of blood loss into a thigh. This injury alone could potentially result in the loss of 30% to 40% of an adult's blood volume, resulting in decompensated hypovolemic shock. Pelvic fractures, especially those resulting from significant falls or crushing mechanisms, can be associated with massive internal hemorrhage into the retroperitoneal space. Occasionally a victim of blunt trauma has multiple fractures and Class III or IV shock but no evidence of external blood loss, hemothoraces, intraabdominal bleeding, or pelvic fracture. For example, an adult pedestrian struck by a vehicle and sustaining four rib fractures, a humerus fracture, a femur fracture, and bilateral tibia/fibula fractures may experience internal bleeding of 3000 to 5500 mL of blood. This potential blood loss is enough for the patient to die from shock if it is unrecognized and inappropriately treated.

Confounding Factors

Numerous factors can confound assessment because they obscure the usual signs of shock in the trauma patient.

TABLE 7-5 Approximate Internal Blood Loss Associated with Fractures

Type of fracture	Internal blood loss (mL)
Rib	125
Radius or ulna	250-500
Humerus	500-750
Tibia or fibula	500-1000
Femur	1000-2000
Pelvis	1000-massive

Age

Patients at the extremes of life—the very young (neonates) and the elderly—have diminished capability to compensate for acute blood loss and other shock states. Thus a relatively minor injury may produce decompensated shock in these individuals. On the other hand, children and young adults have a tremendous ability to compensate for blood loss and may appear relatively normal on a quick scan. A closer look may reveal subtle signs of shock, such as mild tachycardia and tachypnea, pale skin with delayed capillary refilling time, and anxiety. Because of their powerful compensatory mechanisms, children found in decompensated shock represent dire emergencies. Elderly individuals may be more prone to certain complications of prolonged shock, such as acute renal failure.

Athletic Status

Well-conditioned athletes often have enhanced compensatory capabilities. Many have resting heart rates in the range of 40 to 50 beats/min. Thus a heart rate of 100 to 110 beats/min or hypotension in a well-conditioned athlete may be warning signs that indicate significant hemorrhage.

Pregnancy

During pregnancy, a woman's blood volume may increase by up to 48%. Heart rate and cardiac output during pregnancy are also increased. Because of this, a pregnant female may not demonstrate signs of shock until her blood loss exceeds 30% to 35% of her blood volume. Also, well before the mother demonstrates signs of hypoperfusion, the fetus may be affected because the placental circulation is more sensitive to the vasoconstrictive effects of catecholamines released in response to the shock state. During the third trimester, the gravid uterus may compress the inferior vena cava, greatly diminishing venous return to the heart and resulting in hypotension. Elevation of the patient's right side once she has been immobilized to a long backboard may alleviate this. Hypotension in a pregnant female that persists after performing this maneuver typically represents life-threatening blood loss.

Preexisting Medical Conditions

Patients with serious preexisting medical conditions, such as coronary artery disease and chronic obstructive pulmonary disease (COPD), are typically less able to compensate for hemorrhage and shock. These patients may experience angina as their heart rate increases in an effort to maintain their blood pressure. Patients with implanted fixed-rate pacemakers are typically unable to develop the compensatory tachycardia necessary to maintain blood pressure.

Medications

Numerous medications may interfere with the body's compensatory mechanisms. Beta-adrenergic blocking agents and calcium channel blockers used to treat hypertension may prevent an individual from developing a compensatory tachycardia that may maintain blood pressure. Additionally, nonsteroidal antiinflammatory drugs (NSAIDs), used in the treatment of arthritis and musculoskeletal pain, may impair platelet activity and blood clotting, resulting in increased hemorrhage.

Time Between Injury and Treatment

In situations where the emergency medical services (EMS) response time has been brief, patients may be encountered with life-threatening internal hemorrhage but have not yet lost enough blood to manifest severe shock (Class III or IV hemorrhage). Even patients with penetrating wounds to their aorta, venae cavae, or iliac vessels may arrive at the receiving facility with a normal systolic blood pressure if the EMS response, scene, and transport times are brief. The prehospital care provider should never assume that patients are not bleeding internally just because they "look good." Patients should be thoroughly assessed for even the subtlest signs of shock, and internal hemorrhage should be assumed to be present until it is definitively ruled out. This is one reason why continued reassessment of trauma patients is essential.

Management

In addition to securing the airway and providing ventilation to maintain oxygenation, the prime goals of treatment of shock include identifying the source or cause, treating the cause as specifically as possible, and supporting the circulation. In the prehospital setting the external source of bleeding can frequently be identified and immediately and directly controlled. Internal causes of shock usually cannot be definitively treated in the prehospital setting; therefore the approach should be to transfer the patient rapidly to the definitive care setting while supporting the circulation in the best way possible. Resuscitation in the prehospital setting includes the following:

- Improve oxygenation of the RBCs in the lungs through appropriate airway management.
- Provide ventilatory support with a bag-valve-mask (BVM), and deliver a high concentration of oxygen.
- Control both external hemorrhage and internal hemorrhage, to the extent possible in the prehospital setting. *Every red blood cell counts.*
- Improve circulation to deliver the oxygenated RBCs more efficiently to the systemic tissues, and improve oxygenation at the cellular level.
- Reach definitive care as soon as possible for hemorrhage control and replacement of lost RBCs.

If the prehospital care provider does not take appropriate measures, a patient will continue to deteriorate rapidly until he or she reaches the ultimate stable condition—death.

The following four questions should be asked when deciding what treatment to provide for a patient in shock:

1. What is the cause of the patient's shock?
2. What is the definitive care for the patient's shock?
3. Where can the patient best receive this definitive care?
4. What interim steps can be taken to manage the patient's condition while the patient is being transported to definitive care?

Although the first question may be difficult to answer accurately, identification of the source of the shock would assist in defining which facility is best suited to meet the patient's need and what measures may be necessary during transport to improve the patient's chances of survival.

Airway

The airway should be evaluated initially in all patients. Patients in need of immediate management of their airway include those with the following conditions, in order of importance:

1. Patients who are not breathing.
2. Patients who have obvious airway compromise.
3. Patients who have ventilatory rates in excess of 20 breaths/min.
4. Patients who have noisy sounds of ventilation.

Advanced techniques for securing the airway and maintaining ventilation may be required in the prehospital setting, as outlined in Chapter 6, but the prehospital care provider should not underestimate the importance of essential airway skills, especially when transport times are brief.

Breathing

Once a patent airway is ensured, patients in shock or those at risk for developing shock (almost all trauma patients) should initially receive an oxygen concentration as close to 100% (Fio_2 of 1.0) as possible. This type of oxygenation can be achieved only with a device that has a reservoir attached to the oxygen source, not a nasal cannula or a simple facemask. *Oxygen saturation (Spo_2) should be monitored by pulse oximetry in virtually all trauma patients.* Once the prehospital care provider has addressed the patient's acute problems and stabilized the patient's condition, the provider may titrate the oxygen downward while maintaining an Spo_2 reading of at least 95%.

If the patient is not breathing or is not breathing with an adequate depth and rate, the prehospital care provider should begin ventilatory assistance using a BVM unit immediately. Care must be taken to ensure that the patient is not hyperventilated when ventilations are assisted, especially in the patient with hypovolemic shock. Ventilating too deeply and too quickly can make the patient alkalotic, which shifts the oxyhemoglobin curve to the right, which increases the affinity of hemoglobin for oxygen, thereby decreasing oxygen delivery to the tissue. Recent data from animal experiments utilizing a hypovolemic shock model suggest that normal or higher ventilatory rates in animals with even moderate hemorrhage impaired hemodynamic functioning, as exhibited by lower systolic blood pressure and cardiac output. The presumed mechanism was increased intrathoracic pressure, which impaired venous return to the heart, resulting in hypotension.[9,10] The increased intrathoracic pressure could result from either large tidal volumes (10-12 mL/kg body weight) or from the creation of "auto-PEEP" (positive end-expiratory pressure) when ventilated too quickly (inadequate exhalation leads to air trapping in the lungs). One retrospective study of prehospital intubation found an association between prehospital intubation and lower blood pressure on arrival at the trauma center, although a cause-and-effect relationship was far from conclusive.[11]

For an adult patient, giving a reasonable tidal volume (350-500 mL) at a rate of 10 ventilations/min is probably sufficient. If available, end-tidal carbon dioxide ($ETCO_2$) monitoring may be used in conjunction with pulse oximetry to maintain the patient in a eucapneic state (normal blood CO_2 level) with satisfactory oxygenation.

Circulation: Hemorrhage Control

Control of obvious external hemorrhage immediately follows securing the airway and initiating oxygen therapy and ventilatory support, or it is performed simultaneously with these steps if sufficient assistance is present. Early recognition and control of external bleeding in the trauma patient help preserve the patient's blood volume and RBCs and ensure continued perfusion of tissues. Even a small trickle of blood can add up to substantial blood loss if it is ignored for a long period. Thus, in the multisystem trauma patient, *no bleeding is minor, and every red blood cell counts* toward ensuring continued perfusion of the body's tissues.

External Hemorrhage

Control of external hemorrhage should proceed in a stepwise fashion, escalating if initial measures fail to control bleeding.

Pressure. Direct pressure, applied over a bleeding site, is the initial technique employed to control external hemorrhage. The ability of the body to respond to and control bleeding from a lacerated vessel is a function of (1) the size of the vessel, (2) the pressure within the vessel, (3) the

presence of clotting factors, and (4) the ability of the injured vessel to go into spasm. Vessels, especially arteries, that are completely divided (transected) often retract and go into spasm. Because of this, there is often less hemorrhage from the stump of an extremity with a complete amputation than from an extremity with severe trauma but with blood vessels that are damaged but not completely transected. For damaged blood vessels, the rate of blood loss is directly related to the size of the hole in the blood vessel and the *transmural pressure* (difference between the pressure inside the vessel and the pressure outside the vessel). This relationship was first described in an equation developed by Bernoulli, a Swiss mathematician. The specifics of the equation are not as important as understanding the underlying principle—how the size of the hole and the transmural pressure relate to hemorrhage—and how direct pressure controls blood loss.

Imagine the blood vessels as plumbing inside a home and the blood inside the vessels as water in the pipes. If the plumbing has a leak, the amount of water lost is directly related to the size of the hole and the transmural pressure inside and outside the pipe. For example, if the hole in the pipe is 1 inch (2.5 cm) in diameter and the pressure inside the plumbing is 100 psi, more water will leak out than if the hole is 1 inch in diameter and the pressure inside the plumbing is 50 psi. Similarly, the blood flow from a wound in a vessel is proportional to the difference between the size of the hole in the vessel wall and the difference between intraluminal (inside the vessel) and extraluminal (outside the vessel) pressures.

Direct pressure over the site of hemorrhage increases the extraluminal pressure and therefore reduces the transmural pressure, helping to slow or stop bleeding. Direct pressure also serves a second and equally important function. Unlike the pipes inside a home, blood vessels are compressible. Compressing the sides of the torn vessel reduces the size (area) of the opening and further reduces blood flow out of the vessel. Even if blood loss is not completely stemmed, it may be diminished to the point that the blood-clotting system can stop the hemorrhage. This is why direct pressure is almost always successful at controlling bleeding. Multiple studies involving hemorrhage from femoral artery puncture sites after cardiac catheterization have documented that direct pressure is an effective technique.[12-15]

Three additional points about direct pressure should be emphasized. First, when managing a wound with an impaled object, pressure should be applied on either side of the object rather than over the object. Impaled objects should not be removed in the field because the object may have damaged a vessel, and the object itself could be tamponading the bleeding. Removal of the object could result in uncontrolled internal hemorrhage. Second, if hands are required to perform other lifesaving tasks, a pressure (compression) dressing can be created using gauze pads and an elastic roller bandage or a blood pressure cuff inflated until hemorrhage stops. This dressing is placed directly over the bleeding site. Third, applying direct pressure to exsanguinating hemorrhage takes precedence over insertion of intravenous (IV) lines and fluid resuscitation. For example, the prehospital care provider would make a serious error to deliver a well-packaged shooting victim to the receiving facility who has two IV lines inserted and neatly taped in place, but who is hemorrhaging to death from a gunshot wound to the femoral artery and has only trauma dressings taped in place and no direct pressure applied.

Tourniquets. In the past, emphasis has been placed on elevation of an extremity and compression on a pressure point (proximal to the bleeding site) as intermediate steps in hemorrhage control. No research has been published on whether or not elevation of a bleeding extremity slows hemorrhage. If the extremity is fractured, this maneuver could potentially result in converting a closed fracture to an open one or in causing increased internal hemorrhage. Similarly, the use of pressure points for hemorrhage control has not been studied. Thus, in the absence of compelling data, these interventions can no longer be recommended for situations where direct pressure or a pressure dressing has failed to control hemorrhage.

If external bleeding from an extremity cannot be controlled by pressure, application of a tourniquet is the reasonable next step in hemorrhage control (Figure 7-12). Tourniquets had fallen out of favor because of concern about potential complications, including damage to nerves and blood vessels and potential loss of the limb if the tourniquet is left on too long. Although there is a small risk that all or part of a limb may be sacrificed, given the choice of losing a limb or saving the patient's life, the obvious decision

FIGURE 7-12 A fisherman who was run over by a motorboat suffered severe damage to his lower extremities. His life was saved by first responders who applied tourniquets to both thighs.

is to preserve life. Data from the military experience suggest that appropriately applied tourniquets could potentially prevent 7 of 100 combat deaths.[16,17] Tourniquets occluding arterial inflow have been widely used in the operating room (OR) by surgeons for many years, with satisfactory results. *Used properly, tourniquets are not only safe, but also lifesaving.*[18]

Device Options. Traditionally, a tourniquet has been devised from a cravat folded into a width of about 4 inches (10 cm) and wrapped twice around the extremity—the "Spanish windlass." A knot is tied in the bandage, and a metal or wooden rod is placed on top of the knot, and a second knot is tied. The rod is twisted until hemorrhage ceases, and the rod is secured in place. Tourniquets that are narrow and bandlike should be avoided. Wider tourniquets are more effective at controlling bleeding, and they control hemorrhage at a lower pressure. An inverse relationship exists between tourniquet width and the pressure required to occlude arterial inflow. A very narrow band is also more likely to result in damage to arteries and superficial nerves. A blood pressure cuff represents another alternative that can be used as a tourniquet.

Because of the U.S. military's interest in an effective, easy-to-use tourniquet (especially one that a soldier could apply with one hand if the other arm was injured), many commercial tourniquets have been developed and marketed. One military study concluded that only three products were 100% effective in occluding distal arterial blood flow in a laboratory study: the Combat Application Tourniquet (C-A-T, Phil Durango, Golden Colo), the Emergency Military Tourniquet (EMT, Delfi Medical Innovations, Vancouver, Can), and the Special Operations Force Tactical Tourniquet (SOFTT, Tactical Medical Solutions, Anderson, S. C.).[19] Of these, the Committee on Tactical Combat Casualty Care (COTCCC) recommends use of the C-A-T.

Application Site. A tourniquet should be applied just proximal to the hemorrhaging wound. Traditionally, tourniquets have not been placed distal to the knee or elbow because of the risk of damaging more superficial nerves and vessels. The flaw in this approach, however, is that more tissue of the limb is made ischemic, especially if the wound is at the level of the wrist or ankle. Once applied, the tourniquet site should not be covered so that it can be monitored for recurrent hemorrhage.

Application Tightness. A tourniquet should be applied tight enough to block arterial flow. A device that only occludes venous outflow from a limb will actually increase hemorrhage from a wound. A direct relationship exists between the amount of pressure required to control hemorrhage and the size of the limb. Thus, on average, a tourniquet will need to be placed more tightly on a leg to achieve hemorrhage control than on an arm.

Time Limit. To minimize damage to tissue, many authorities recommended periodic loosening of a tourniquet to perfuse the tissue distal to the device. Because hemorrhage control had not been obtained, the net result of this practice was increased hemorrhage and risk of exsanguination. Arterial tourniquets have been used safely for up to 120 to 150 minutes in the OR without significant nerve or muscle damage. Even in suburban and rural settings, many EMS transport times are significantly less than this period. In general, a tourniquet placed in the prehospital setting should remain in place until the patient reaches definitive care at the closest appropriate hospital. One potential exception to this principle is in the prolonged-transport situation (see later discussion).

If application of a tourniquet is required, the patient will most likely need emergent surgery to control hemorrhage. Thus the ideal receiving facility for such a patient is one with surgical capabilities. A tourniquet can be painful for a conscious patient to tolerate, and pain management should be considered, provided that the patient does not have signs of Class III or IV shock (see Chapter 12). Box 7-2 provides a sample protocol for tourniquet application.

Topical Hemostatic Agents. The U.S. Food and Drug Administration (FDA) has approved the following topical hemostatic agents for use:

- HemCon dressing (Hemorrhage Control Technologies, Portland, Ore), made of chitosan, a protein derived from shrimp shells. There have been no reported cases of cross-reactivity in individuals with shellfish allergy. This product performed efficaciously in laboratory studies of severe hemorrhage conducted by the U.S.

Army Institute for Surgical Research (USAISR).[20] Anecdotal reports have documented its effectiveness in humans.[21] HemCon is the first-line topical hemostatic agent recommended by COTCCC.

- QuikClot (Z-Medica, Wallingford, Conn), composed of Zeolite, a proprietary formulation of a mineral derived from volcanic rock. QuikClot rapidly absorbs water, thereby concentrating clotting factors at the bleeding site. Although it is probably the most effective topical hemostatic agent at controlling hemorrhage, it is associated with an exothermic (heat-producing) reaction, with temperatures up to about 150° F (65° C), sufficient to cause thermal injury to surrounding structures, such as skin and nerves.[22]
- TraumaDex (Medafor, Inc., Minneapolis, Minn), made of microporous "beads" from a plant-derived biomaterial. It is believed to dehydrate the blood, resulting in accelerated blood clotting. Scientific data available on the company's website are limited. One published study of a model of lethal groin injury in laboratory animals demonstrated that TraumaDex was no better than a standard dressing (absorbent pad).[23]

The data demonstrating the effectiveness of the HemCon dressing and QuikClot often include injuries (e.g., liver and aortic trauma) that correlate poorly with the types of injuries that prehospital care providers encounter. To date, no published data exist about the use of topical hemostatic agents in the civilian setting, and only anecdotal reports exist for the military experience. A prehospital care provider might be tempted to delay transport to use one of these novel but unproven technologies. In the civilian setting, no data show that these products are superior to direct pressure and rapid transport to an appropriate receiving facility. Application of HemCon and QuikClot may be appropriate in a prolonged-transport situation (see following discussion).

Internal Hemorrhage

Internal hemorrhage from fracture sites should also be considered. Rough handling of an injured extremity not only may convert a closed fracture to an open one, but also may significantly increase internal bleeding from bone ends, adjacent muscle tissue, or damaged vessels. All suspected extremity fractures should be immobilized in an effort to minimize this hemorrhage. Time may be taken to splint several fractures individually if the patient has no evidence of life-threatening conditions. If the primary survey identifies threats to the patient's life, however, the patient should be immobilized rapidly on a long backboard, thereby immobilizing all the extremities in an anatomic manner, and transported to a medical facility. For patients with decompensated shock (hypotension) and suspected intraabdominal hemorrhage or a suspected pelvic fracture, the PASG may tamponade internal hemorrhage, as detailed later.

BOX 7-2   Protocol for Tourniquet Application

1. Attempt at direct pressure or pressure dressing must fail to control hemorrhage.
2. A commercially manufactured tourniquet, blood pressure cuff, or "Spanish windlass" is applied to the extremity just proximal to the bleeding wound.
3. The tourniquet is tightened until hemorrhage ceases, and then it is secured in place.
4. The time of tourniquet application is written on a piece of tape and secured to the tourniquet ("TK 21:45" indicates that the tourniquet was applied at 9:45 PM).
5. The tourniquet should be left uncovered so that the site can be monitored for recurrent hemorrhage.
6. Pain management should be considered unless the patient is in Class III or IV shock.
7. The patient should ideally be transported to a facility that has surgical capability.

Disability

There are no unique, specific interventions for altered mental status in the shock patient. If the patient's abnormal neurologic status is the result of cerebral hypoxia and poor perfusion, efforts to restore perfusion throughout the body should result in improved mental status. In assessing a patient's prognosis after traumatic brain injury, an "initial" Glasgow Coma Scale (GCS) score is typically considered the score following adequate resuscitation and restoration of cerebral perfusion. Assessing a patient's GCS score while still in shock may result in an overly grim prognosis.

Body Exposure and Environment

Maintaining the patient's body temperature within a normal range is important. Hypothermia results in myocardial dysfunction, coagulopathy, hyperkalemia, vasoconstriction, and a host of other problems that negatively affect a patient's chance of survival.[24] Although cold temperatures preserve tissue for a short time, the temperature drop must be very rapid and very low for preservation to occur. Such a rapid change is unacceptable for the patient in shock.

In the prehospital setting, increasing the core temperature once hypothermia has developed can be difficult; therefore all steps that can be taken in the field to preserve normal body temperature should be initiated. A patient's temperature decreases as a result of reduced energy production and loss of heat to the surrounding environment. Once exposed and examined, the patient must be protected from the environment and body temperature maintained. Any wet clothing, including that saturated with blood, is removed from the patient because wet clothing increases heat loss. The patient is covered with warm blankets. An alternative involves covering the patient with plastic sheets, such as heavy, thick garbage bags. They are inexpensive, easily stored, disposable, and effective devices for heat retention. Heated, humidified oxygen, if available, may help preserve body heat, especially in intubated patients.

Once assessed and packaged, the shock patient is moved into the warmed patient compartment of the ambulance. Ideally, the patient compartment of an ambulance is kept at 85° F (29° C) or more when transporting a severely injured trauma patient. The patient's rate of heat loss into a cold compartment is very high. The conditions must be ideal for the patient, not for the providers, because the patient is the most important person in any emergency.

Patient Transport

Effective treatment of a patient in severe hemorrhagic shock requires a surgeon with access to an OR and blood. Because neither is routinely available in the prehospital trauma setting, rapid transportation to a facility that is capable of managing the patient's injuries is extremely important.

Rapid transport does not mean disregarding or neglecting the treatment modalities that are important in patient care (doing the old-fashioned "scoop and run"). However, it does mean that the prehospital care provider quickly institutes key, potentially lifesaving measures, such as airway management, ventilatory support, and hemorrhage control. Time must not be wasted on an inappropriate assessment or with unnecessary immobilization maneuvers. When caring for a critically injured patient, many steps, such as warming the patient, starting IV therapy, and even performing the secondary survey, are accomplished in the ambulance while en route.

Patient Positioning

In general, trauma patients who are in shock should be transported in the supine position, immobilized on a long backboard. Special positioning, such as the Trendelenburg position (placed on an incline with the feet elevated above the head) or the "shock" position (head and torso supine with legs elevated), is no longer recommended. The Trendelenburg position may aggravate already-impaired ventilatory function by placing the weight of the abdominal organs on the diaphragm and may increase intracranial pressure in patients with traumatic brain injury. More importantly, patients who are in severe hypovolemic shock are generally maximally vasoconstricted. Thus the use of the Trendelenburg position is no longer believed to result in a significant autotransfusion of blood to the vital organs from the lower extremities and should not be used.[25,26] Both the Trendelenburg and the shock position are contraindicated in patients with a suspected spine injury.

Pneumatic Antishock Garment

The PASG remains one of the most controversial devices ever introduced to prehospital care. One large study from the Houston EMS system failed to demonstrate a benefit of using the PASG in hypotensive trauma patients in an urban setting with brief transport times to trauma centers with in-house trauma surgeons.[27] A similar study at the same institution also demonstrated the same outcome when IV fluids were used for resuscitation.[28] Both studies should be considered when developing protocols for the use of either IV fluids or the PASG. The PASG is mainly a device for controlling blood loss and not for resuscitation, except in a few situations of extreme hypotension. Although the PASG has not been adequately studied in suburban and rural settings, many EMS services have removed it from their units. This approach overlooks some patients in shock who may benefit from the use of the PASG.

Physiology

Pressure applied by the PASG to the legs and abdomen is transmitted directly through the skin, fat, muscle, and other soft tissues to the blood vessels themselves. As the vessels are compressed, their diameters are reduced in size. The primary physiologic result is that the vascular container in body areas beneath the device is decreased in size, increasing the SVR and thereby raising the systolic and diastolic blood pressures. Virtually every study of PASG application in both experimental animals and humans has documented a rise in the systolic blood pressure with the application of this device for hemorrhagic shock.[29,30] The MAP is also increased, which is probably beneficial to improving tissue perfusion. In addition to the increase in SVR, a small amount of blood is shifted from the veins in the lower extremities to the central organs. Venous return is increased with inflation of the PASG, resulting in improved cardiac output. The clinical significance of this "autotransfusion" has been questioned because research has shown that the amount of blood shifted is in the range of only several hundred milliliters.

Use in Hemorrhagic Shock

In the following four situations, the PASG may have significant benefit in patients with shock from blood loss:

1. *Suspected pelvic fractures with hypotension* (systolic blood pressure of 90 mm Hg). Pelvic fractures caused by anterior-posterior compression and by falls may result in severe hemorrhage into the pelvic soft tissues and retroperitoneal space. Inflation of the entire PASG may decrease the volume of the pelvis and result in tamponade of the associated hemorrhage.[31] If a PASG is not available, consideration should be given to wrapping a sheet tightly around the pelvis and tying it as a sling. This should be accomplished so that the lower extremities are maintained in an adducted and internally rotated position.

2. *Profound hypotension.* Some data suggest that patients with severe hypotension (systolic blood pressure <50 to 60 mm Hg) may have an improved outcome when the PASG is used.[30] The increased perfusion of the brain and heart that results from PASG inflation may contribute to the improved survival.

3. *Suspected intraperitoneal hemorrhage with hypotension.* Inflation of the entire PASG compresses intraperitoneal organs. This may result in a slowing or cessation of hemorrhage (tamponade) from the solid organs, such as the liver and spleen, and the mesenteric vessels. Several studies have demonstrated improved survival in animals receiving the PASG in models of uncontrolled intraabdominal hemorrhage.[30]

4. *Suspected retroperitoneal hemorrhage with hypotension.* Inflation of the entire device compresses the retroperitoneal organs. Because of the increased pressure, the device may tamponade bleeding from the kidneys, aorta, and venae cavae.[32]

The PASG is probably significantly *less effective* than direct pressure or a pressure dressing with gauze and an elastic bandage for control of external hemorrhage from the lower extremities. The prehospital care provider uses a PASG in this manner only when direct pressure cannot be applied because of assistance limitations.

Contraindications

- *Penetrating thoracic trauma.* Application and inflation of the PASG increase the rate of hemorrhage from damaged blood vessels in the upper half of the body (outside the confines of the device) as the patient's blood pressure significantly increases. In the Houston PASG study, hypotensive patients with penetrating thoracic trauma clearly had a higher mortality rate when the PASG was used.[27]

- *Splinting of lower extremity fractures.* The PASG could be thought of as a large air splint, and its use has been suggested to immobilize fractures of the femur, tibia, and fibula. A traction splint is a much better immobilization device for fractures of the midshaft femur because it reduces the bone ends back into anatomic alignment and treats pain by combating the severe muscle spasm that develops in the thigh. The PASG has been associated with the development of compartment syndromes of the calf, especially when fractures are present. Use of the PASG solely as a splint for isolated lower extremity fractures where shock is not present is not recommended.

- *Evisceration of abdominal organs*
- *Impaled objects in the abdomen*
- *Pregnancy*
- *Traumatic cardiopulmonary arrest*

Application

The PASG should be applied to a patient as quickly as possible once indication for its use is identified. The PASG is positioned under the patient in one of several ways. In many cases, it may be easiest to logroll the patient onto the device after spreading it out on a long backboard. Another alternative involves one prehospital care provider placing each arm into the foot ends of each of the patient's trouser legs. As one provider grabs the patient's ankles and lifts up on the legs, a second provider slides the PASG onto the patient's legs. The patient's pelvis is then gently lifted to complete proper placement of the garment beneath the patient. The top of the garment should come up to the lower rib margin laterally.

The straps of the PASG are securely fastened and the device is inflated, typically beginning with the legs, followed by the abdomen. All three compartments may be inflated simultaneously; however, the abdominal compartment should never be inflated before the leg compartments. When the Velcro straps begin to crackle, the pressure inside the PASG is generally between 60 and 80 mm Hg. A well-trained crew can apply the device rapidly, and several studies demonstrated no increase in scene time when a PASG was used.

Deflation

Prehospital deflation of the PASG should *not* be done except in extreme circumstances, such as evidence of a ruptured diaphragm. In this patient the blunt trauma ruptured the diaphragm, and application and inflation of the device result in herniation of abdominal organs into the thoracic cavity, leading to marked respiratory distress. This may mimic the development of a tension pneumothorax; however, patient deterioration will occur almost immediately after inflation of the device.

The decision to deflate the PASG should be made in consultation with online medical direction. Except in the unusual circumstances in which inflation of the device resulted in rapid deterioration of the patient's condition, the PASG should not be deflated unless the patient's vital signs are within normal limits. Even when vital signs are within normal ranges, the patient's blood volume might still be significantly depleted. The inflated PASG may have reduced the size of the patient's container (vessels) to match the available blood volume. As the PASG is deflated, the patient's container size will increase. Unless a sufficient amount of fluid is infused, cardiac preload and SVR may drop dramatically, resulting in severe hypotension and profound shock.

Volume Resuscitation

Vascular Access

Intravenous Route. The prehospital care provider routinely obtains IV access in a trauma patient who has known or suspected serious injuries so that the provider can initiate volume resuscitation. Except in unusual circumstances where a patient is undergoing extrication from a vehicle or prehospital care providers are awaiting the arrival of a helicopter, IV access should be obtained after the patient has been placed in the ambulance and transportation has been initiated to the closest appropriate facility.

Although volume resuscitation of a trauma patient in shock makes empiric sense, no research has demonstrated improved survival of critically injured trauma patients when IV fluid therapy has been administered in the prehospital setting. In fact, one physiologic computer model of prehospital IV fluid administration found that IV fluid is only beneficial when three conditions exist: (1) the patient is bleeding at a rate of 25 to 100 mL/min; (2) the IV fluid administration rate is equal to the bleeding rate; and (3) the scene time and transport time exceed 30 minutes.[33] Therefore, *transport of the trauma patient should never be delayed to initiate IV lines.*

For patients in shock or with potentially serious injuries, two large-bore (14- or 16-gauge), short (1-inch) IV catheters should be inserted by percutaneous puncture. The rate of fluid administration is directly proportional to the fourth power of the radius of the catheter and inversely proportional to its length (i.e., more fluid will rapidly flow through a short, large-diameter catheter than through a longer, smaller-diameter catheter). The preferred site for percutaneous access is a vein of the forearm. Alternative sites for IV access are the veins of the antecubital fossa, the hand, and the upper arm (cephalic vein). If two attempts at percutaneous access are unsuccessful in a child, inserting an intraosseous line should be considered. Central venous lines or venous cutdowns are not generally considered appropriate venous access in the prehospital setting and are rarely needed.

Intraosseous Route. Another alternative for vascular access in adults is the intraosseous route.[34,35] This can be accomplished by the sternal technique using appropriately designed devices[36,37] (e.g., F.A.S.T.1, Pyng Medical Corporation, Richmond, BC). Specially designed devices such as the Bone Injection Gun ("BIG," WaisMed, Houston, Tex) and the EZ-IO (Vidacare Corp., San Antonio, Tex) may also be used to establish access through sites in the distal tibia above the ankle.[38] Such techniques have justifiably not been used routinely in the prehospital setting, where the focus should be on rapid transport rather than IV fluid administration. For delayed or prolonged transport to definitive care, intraosseous vascular access may have a role in adult trauma patients.

Intravenous Solutions

Because of its ability to transport oxygen, blood remains the fluid of choice for the resuscitation of a patient in severe hemorrhagic shock. Unfortunately, blood is impractical for use in the prehospital setting because of issues related to blood typing and because blood is perishable when not refrigerated. Alternative solutions for volume resuscitation fall into one of four categories: (1) isotonic crystalloids, (2) hypertonic crystalloids, (3) synthetic (artificial) colloids, and (4) blood substitutes.

Isotonic Crystalloid Solutions. Isotonic crystalloids are balanced salt solutions comprised of electrolytes (substances that separate into charged ions when dissolved in solutions). They act as effective volume expanders for a short time, but they possess no oxygen-carrying capacity. Immediately after infusion, crystalloids fill the vascular space that was depleted by blood loss, improving preload and cardiac output. *Lactated Ringer's* (LR) solution remains the isotonic crystalloid solution of choice for the management of shock because its composition is most similar to the electrolyte composition of blood plasma. It contains specific amounts of sodium, potassium, calcium, chloride, and lactate ions. *Normal saline* (NS, 0.9% sodium chloride [NaCl] solution) remains an acceptable alternative, although hyperchloremia (a marked increase in the blood chloride level) may occur with massive volume resuscitation with NS administration. Solutions of dextrose in water (e.g., D_5W) are not effective volume expanders and have no place in the resuscitation of trauma patients.

One hour after administration of a crystalloid solution, only about one-third remains in the cardiovascular system. The rest has shifted into the interstitial space because both the water and the electrolytes in the solution can freely cross the capillary membranes. A rule of thumb (the 3:1 rule) is that most patients with hemorrhagic shock generally only achieve adequate resuscitation when about 300 mL of crystalloid solution has been infused for every 100 mL of blood volume that has been lost. If possible, IV fluids should be warmed to about 102° F (39° C) before infusion. Infusion of large amounts of room temperature or cold IV fluid contributes to hypothermia and increased hemorrhage.

Hypertonic Crystalloid Solutions. Hypertonic crystalloid solutions have extremely high concentrations of electrolytes compared with blood plasma. The most common of these is *hypertonic saline,* a 7.5% NaCl solution, which is more than eight times the concentration of NaCl in NS. This is an effective plasma expander, especially in that a small, 250-mL infusion often produces the same effect as infusing 2 to 3 L of isotonic crystalloid solution.[39,40] Although hypertonic solutions are somewhat more costly than isotonic crystalloids, they are considered advantageous in military situations where medics are limited in the amount of IV fluid they can carry. An analysis of several studies of hypertonic saline failed to demonstrate improved survival rates over the use of isotonic crystalloids.[41]

Synthetic Colloid Solutions. Proteins are large molecules produced by the body and are composed of amino acids. They have countless functions; however, one type of protein found in the blood, *albumin,* helps maintain fluid in the intravascular space. Administration of human albumin is costly and has been associated with the transmission of infectious diseases, such as hepatitis. When administered to a patient in hemorrhagic shock, synthetic colloid solutions draw fluid from the interstitial and intracellular spaces into the intravascular space, thereby producing expansion of the blood volume. As with crystalloids, colloid plasma expanders do not transport oxygen.

Gelofusine is a 4% gelatin solution produced from bovine protein and is occasionally used in Europe and Australia for fluid resuscitation. It is moderately expensive and carries a risk of severe allergic reactions. A small infusion of gelofusine produces expansion of the intravascular volume for several hours.

Hetastarch (Hespan) and dextran (Gentran) are synthetic colloids that have been created by linking numerous starch (amylopectin) or dextrose molecules together until they are similar in size to an albumin molecule. These solutions are also moderately expensive compared with crystalloids and have been associated with allergic reactions and impairment of blood typing.

The use of crystalloids versus colloids has been a long-standing debate in the management of trauma patients.[42] A recent study of almost 7000 patients admitted to intensive care units demonstrated no difference in outcome when patients were resuscitated with colloid (albumin) versus normal saline.[43] Virtually no research exists involving the use of these synthetic colloid solutions in the prehospital setting, and no data exist from their use in the hospital that shows them to be superior to crystalloid solutions. These products are not recommended for the prehospital management of shock.

Blood Substitutes. Blood has several undesirable qualities, including the need to type and crossmatch, a short shelf life, perishability when not refrigerated, a potential of transmission of infectious disease, and an increasing shortage of donated units. This has led to intense research in blood substitutes in the last two decades. The military has played a central role in this research because a blood substitute that would not need refrigeration and did not require blood typing could be carried to a wounded soldier on the battlefield and infused rapidly to combat shock.

Perfluorocarbons (PFCs) are synthetic compounds that have high oxygen solubility. These inert materials can dissolve approximately 50 times more oxygen than can blood plasma. PFCs contain no hemoglobin or protein; they are completely free of biologic materials, thereby greatly reducing the threat of infectious agents being found in them; and oxygen is transported by being dissolved in the plasma portion. First-generation PFCs experienced limited usefulness because of numerous problems, including a short half-life and the need for a concurrent high-Fio_2 administration. Newer PFCs have fewer of these disadvantages, but their role as oxygen carriers remains undetermined.

Most *hemoglobin-based oxygen carriers* (HBOCs) use the same oxygen-carrying molecule (hemoglobin) found in human blood cells; however, one under investigation uses bovine hemoglobin. The major difference between HBOCs and human blood is that the hemoglobin in HBOCs is not contained within a cell membrane. This removes the need for conducting type and crossmatch studies because the antigen-antibody risk is removed. Additionally, many of these HBOCs can be stored for long periods, making them the ideal solution for mass-casualty incidents. Early problems with hemoglobin-based oxygen-carrying solutions included toxicity from hemoglobin. Of the several HBOCs currently involved in clinical trials, most cause vasoconstriction and gastrointestinal symptoms. Although some look promising for use in the hospital, only the product made from bovine hemoglobin does not require refrigeration, and thus their applicability in the prehospital setting is limited.[44,45] A large, multicenter trial is ongoing in the United States comparing blood substitutes to placebo in trauma patients in the prehospital setting.

Warming Intravenous Fluids. Any IV fluid given to a shock patient should be warm, not room temperature or cold. The ideal temperature for such fluids is 102° F (39° C). Most ambulances do not have conventional rapid fluid warmers, but other steps can keep fluids at an adequate temperature. A convenient storage area for fluids is in a box in the engine compartment. Wrapping heat packs around the bag can also warm fluid. Commercially available fluid warmer units for the patient care compartment provide an easy and reliable means to keep fluids at the correct temperature. These units are costly but justifiable for prolonged transports.

Managing Volume Resuscitation

As noted earlier, significant controversy surrounds prehospital fluid administration for a trauma patient who is in shock. When basic and advanced prehospital trauma life support (PHTLS) was first introduced in the United States, prehospital care providers adopted the approach used by emergency physicians and surgeons in most hospitals and trauma centers: administer an IV crystalloid solution until the vital signs had returned to normal (typically, pulse <100 beats/min and systolic blood pressure >100 mm Hg).

A major contribution of PHTLS over the past two decades has been to establish the conceptual change that, in the critically injured trauma patient, *transportation should never be delayed while IV lines are placed and fluid is infused.* These actions can be performed in the back of the ambulance en route to the closest appropriate facility. The critically injured trauma patient who is in shock generally requires blood and surgical intervention to control internal hemorrhage, neither of which can be accomplished in the field.

When sufficient crystalloid solution is infused to restore vital signs to normal, the patient's perfusion should be improved. Experts believed that such rapid intervention would clear lactic acid and restore energy production in the cells of the body and also decrease the risk of developing irreversible shock and kidney failure. However, no study of trauma patients in the prehospital setting has shown that the administration of IV fluid decreases complications and death.

Recent research, primarily in experimental models of shock, has shown that IV volume resuscitation may have detrimental side effects when administered before surgical control of the source of hemorrhage. In experimental animals, internal hemorrhage often continues until the animal is hypotensive, at which point bleeding slows and a blood clot (thrombus) typically forms at the site of injury. In one sense, this hypotension is protective in that it is associated with a dramatic slowing or cessation of internal hemorrhage. When aggressive IV fluids were administered to the animals in an attempt to restore perfusion, internal hemorrhage again started, and the thrombus was disrupted. In addition, crystalloid infusions may also dilute coagulation factors. These animals often had a worse outcome compared with animals that received resuscitation *after* surgical control of the injury site.[46-48] In a similar animal model, improved survival was noted with "hypotensive resuscitation," where the blood pressure was purposefully kept low until hemorrhage was controlled, then resuscitation took place.[49-51]

Clearly, these studies have potential implications on fluid resuscitation in the prehospital setting. Theoretically, aggressive volume resuscitation could return the blood pressure to normal. This in turn may dislodge blood clots that had formed at bleeding sites in the peritoneal cavity or elsewhere and may result in renewed hemorrhage that cannot be controlled until the patient reaches the OR. On the other hand, withholding IV fluid from a patient in profound shock only leads to further tissue hypoxia and failure of energy production. If the prehospital care provider does not provide fluid therapy, the patient may slip from decompensated shock into irreversible shock.

A single clinical study conducted in an urban prehospital setting demonstrated a worse outcome in trauma patients who received crystalloid solutions before control of internal hemorrhage (mortality rate of 62% vs. 70% in the delayed-treatment group).[28] The findings of this single study have not been replicated in other prehospital systems, and the findings cannot be generalized to rural EMS systems. In a survey of trauma surgeons, fewer than 4% opted for an approach that involved withholding IV fluid from a patient in Class III shock. Almost two thirds of the surgeons recommended that such a patient be maintained in a relatively hypotensive state during transport.[52]

Prehospital volume resuscitation should be tailored to the clinical situation.

Uncontrolled Hemorrhage. For patients with suspected internal hemorrhage in their chest, abdomen, or retroperitoneum (pelvis), sufficient IV crystalloid solution should be titrated to maintain a systolic blood pressure in the range of 80 to 90 mm Hg or MAP of 60 to 65 mm Hg. This should maintain adequate perfusion to the kidneys with less risk of worsening internal hemorrhage. A fluid bolus should not be administered because this may "overshoot" the target blood pressure range, resulting in recurrent intrathoracic, intraabdominal, or retroperitoneal bleeding.

Central Nervous System Injuries. Hypotension has been associated with increased mortality in the setting of traumatic brain injury (TBI). Patients with certain conditions (e.g., TBIs) appear to benefit from a more aggressive fluid resuscitation.[53] Guidelines published by the Brain Trauma

Foundation recommend maintaining the systolic blood pressure (SBP) above 90 mm Hg in patients with suspected TBI.[54] Consensus guidelines focusing on the management of acute spinal cord injury also recommend avoiding hypotension (SBP <90 mm Hg), but also recommend maintaining a MAP of at least 85 to 90 mm Hg in hopes of improving spinal cord perfusion. To accomplish, fairly aggressive volume resuscitation may be required, increasing the risk of recurrent bleeding from associated internal injuries.[55]

Controlled Hemorrhage. Patients with significant external hemorrhage that has been controlled can be managed with a more aggressive volume resuscitation strategy, provided the prehospital care provider has no reason to suspect associated intrathoracic, intraabdominal, or retroperitoneal injuries. Examples include a large scalp laceration or a wound in an extremity involving major blood vessels, but when the bleeding has been controlled with a pressure dressing. Adult patients who fall in this category and present in Class II, III, or IV shock should receive an initial rapid bolus of 1 to 2L of warmed crystalloid solution, preferably LR. Pediatric patients should receive a bolus of 20 mL/kg of warmed crystalloid solution. As noted previously, this should always occur during transport to the closest appropriate facility. Vital signs, including pulse and ventilatory rates and blood pressure, should be monitored to assess the patient's response to the initial fluid therapy. In most urban settings the patient will be delivered to the receiving facility before the initial fluid bolus is completed.

The initial fluid bolus elicits three possible responses, as follows:

1. *Rapid response.* The vital signs return to and remain normal. This typically indicates that the patient has lost less than 20% of blood volume and that the hemorrhage has stopped.
2. *Transient response.* The vital signs initially improve (pulse slows and blood pressure increases); however, during continued assessment, these patients show deterioration with recurrent signs of shock. These patients have typically lost between 20% and 40% of their blood volume.
3. *Minimal or no response.* These patients show virtually no change in the profound signs of shock after a 1- to 2-L bolus.

Patients who have a rapid response are candidates for continued volume resuscitation, until vital signs have returned to normal and all clinical indicators of shock have resolved. Patients who fall into either the transient response or minimal/no response groups have ongoing hemorrhage that is probably internal. These patients are then best managed in a state of relative hypotension, and IV fluid should be titrated to SBP in the range of 80 to 90 mm Hg (MAP of 60-65 mm Hg).

¹ Suspected intrathoracic, intraabdominal or retroperitoneal hemorrhage
² KVO = keep vein open (about 30 mL/hr)
³ Consider MAP 85-90 mm Hg for spinal cord injury
⁴ External hemorrhage controlled with pressure dressing, topical hemostatic agent, or tourniquet
⁵ Warmed crystalloid solution (102° F if possible)
⁶ Rapid response = vital signs return to normal
⁷ HR < 120/min; SBP > 90 mm Hg for adult
⁸ Transient response = vital signs initially improve, then deteriorate
⁹ Minimal or no response = little or no change in vital signs

Prolonged Transport

During prolonged transport, it is important that perfusion is maintained to the vital organs. Airway management should be optimized before a long transport, and endotracheal intubation is performed if there any question regarding airway patency. Ventilatory support is provided, with care taken to ensure that ventilations are of a reasonable tidal volume and rate so as not to compromise a patient with already tenuous perfusion. Pulse oximetry should be monitored continuously. Capnography provides information regarding

SHOCK MANAGEMENT ALGORITHM

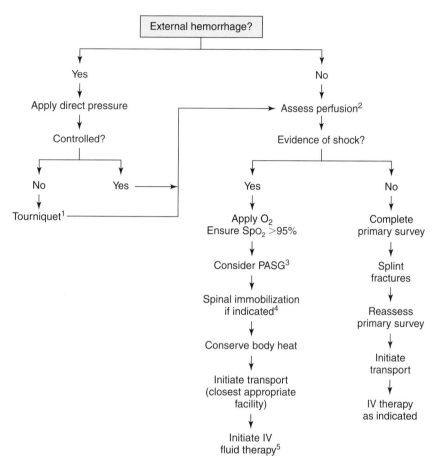

Notes:

[1]A manufactured tourniquet, blood pressure cuff, or cravat should be placed just proximal to the bleeding site and tightened until bleeding stops. The application time is marked on the tourniquet.

[2]Assessment of perfusion includes, presence, quality, and location of pulses; skin color, temperature, and moisture; and capillary refilling time.

[3]PASG should be considered for decompensated shock (SBP <90 mm Hg), and suspected pelvic, intraperitoneal, or retroperitoneal hemorrhage, and in patients with profound hypotension (SBP <60 mm Hg). PASG is contraindicated in penetrating thoracic trauma, abdominal evisceration, pregnancy, impaled object in the abdomen, and traumatic cardiopulmonary arrest, or for splinting the lower extremity fractures.

[4]See Indications for Spinal Immobilization algorithm (p. 235)

[5]Initiate two large-bore (14- or 16-guage) IV catheters en route. See Managing Volume Resuscitation algorithm (p. 188).

the position of the endotracheal tube, as well as information on the patient's perfusion status. A marked drop in ET_{CO_2} indicates that the airway has become dislodged or that the patient has experienced a significant drop in perfusion. A suspected tension pneumothorax is decompressed, or the equipment is kept at the bedside should the patient develop hypotension.

Direct pressure is impractical during a long transport, so significant external hemorrhage should be controlled with pressure dressings. If these efforts fail, a tourniquet should be applied. In situations where a tourniquet has been applied and transport time is expected to exceed 2 hours, attempts should be made to remove the tourniquet after more aggressive attempts at local hemorrhage control. This can be accomplished by removing the pressure dressing from over the wound once the tourniquet has controlled hemorrhage. Next, any blood clot is manually wiped from the wound. A topical hemostatic agent (first a HemCon dressing, followed by QuikClot if HemCon fails) should be applied and a pressure dressing reapplied. The tourniquet should then be slowly loosened while observing the dressing for signs of hemorrhage. If no rebleeding occurs, the tourniquet is completely loosened but left in place in case hemorrhage recurs. Conversion of a tourniquet back to a dressing should not be attempted in the following situations: (1) presence of Class III or IV shock; (2) complete amputation; (3) inability to observe the patient for rebleeding; and (4) tourniquet in place longer than 6 hours.[18] Internal hemorrhage control should be optimized by splinting all fractures and applying the PASG or pelvic binder, as indicated for intraabdominal or retroperitoneal hemorrhage.

Techniques for maintaining normal body temperature, as previously described, are even more important in the setting of prolonged transport time. In addition to a warmed patient compartment, the patient should be covered with blankets or materials that preserve body heat; even large, plastic garbage bags help prevent loss of heat. IV fluids should be warmed before administration. The U.S. Army Ranger Regiment often uses the Thermal Angel (Estill Medical Technologies, Dallas), a battery-powered, disposable fluid warmer. Experience with the flameless heater pack from a Meal Ready to Eat (MRE) appears very encouraging as a means of warming crystalloid fluids during patient transport.[56]

In prolonged-transport circumstances, vascular access for fluid administration may be critical, and two large-bore IV lines should be established. For both children and adults, inability to obtain vascular percutaneous venous access may necessitate use of the IV route even for adults, as described previously. For patients with suspected ongoing hemorrhage, maintaining SBP in the range of 80 to 90 mm Hg or MAP of 60 to 65 mm Hg can usually accomplish the goal of maintaining perfusion to vital organs with less risk of renewing internal hemorrhage. Patients with suspected TBIs or spinal cord injuries should have SBP maintained above 90 to 100 mm Hg.

Vital signs should be reassessed frequently to monitor response to resuscitation. The following should be documented at serial intervals: ventilation rate, pulse rate, blood pressure, skin color and temperature, capillary refill, GCS score, SpO_2, and $ETCO_2$, if available.

Although insertion of a urinary catheter is not usually required in rapid transport circumstances, monitoring urine output is an important tool that can help guide decisions regarding the need for additional fluid therapy during prolonged transport. Insertion of a urinary catheter should be considered so that urine output can be monitored. Adequate urine outputs include 0.5 mL/kg/hr for adults, 1 mL/kg/hr for pediatric patients, and 2 mL/kg/hr for infants younger than 1 year. A urine output less than these amounts may be a key indicator that the patient requires further volume infusion.

If time permits during prolonged transport, placement of a nasogastric (NG) catheter should be considered for all intubated patients unless fractures of the patient's midface are suspected. In the latter case, placement of an orogastric (OG) catheter should be considered. Gastric distention may cause unexplained hypotension and dysrhythmias, especially in children. Placement of an NG or OG tube may also decrease the risk of vomiting and aspiration.

During prolonged transport, assessing the patient's clinical status and the response to resuscitation is key in determining outcome. There are encouraging reports supporting the use of the Life Support for Trauma and Transport (LSTAT, Integrated Medical Systems) for monitoring critically injured patients during transport. This "mobile ICU" has shown promising results in the military for transport of critically injured patients, as well as in the transfer of critically injured patients in civilian practice.[57] Disadvantages of using such devices are the cost and weight. If these obstacles could be overcome, there may be a wider application for these devices when prolonged transport of the critically injured trauma patient is necessary.

SUMMARY

Shock causes a state of generalized hypoperfusion, resulting in cellular hypoxia, anaerobic metabolism, lactic acidosis, and death if not appropriately treated. In the trauma patient, hemorrhage is the most common cause of this shock state, and the primary goal of therapy is to identify the source of hemorrhage and treat it specifically. In the prehospital setting, this approach is most effective when the bleeding source is external. Internal hemorrhage can be treated definitively only in the hospital environment. In some cases, nonhemorrhagic sources of shock in the trauma patient (e.g., tension pneumothorax) can be temporarily corrected. However, all trauma patients in shock, in addition to maintenance of adequate oxygenation, require rapid extrication and expeditious transport to a definitive care institution where the cause of the shock can be specifically identified and treated. Institution of such measures as IV access and volume infusion should not delay transport of these patients and should be done in the ambulance during transport. Overaggressive fluid infusion should be avoided to minimize further bleeding in the patient with hemorrhagic shock after trauma.

SCENARIO SOLUTION

Based on the mechanism, you should have a high suspicion for thoracic and abdominal injuries leading to hemorrhagic shock, as well as the possibility of nonhemorrhagic shock. Because this patient is in shock, rapid extrication is required with spinal control. High oxygen concentration should be delivered to the most appropriate airway device based on the level of consciousness and ability to maintain a secure airway after suctioning the airway. External sources of hemorrhage should be sought and controlled by direct pressure. The status of the neck veins would help differentiate hemorrhagic from nonhemorrhagic causes of the shock.

Transport should be rapid, and establishing two large-bore IV lines for fluid administration should be done en route. Transport should not be delayed to establish IV access. If you suspect intraabdominal bleeding, and the patient's status is deteriorating in the absence of penetrating thoracic injury, consider PASG use en route if available. The major focus of management is rapid extrication and transport to the trauma center, where definitive control of hemorrhage would prevent progression through the various stages of shock, leading to death or complications of hypoperfusion, such as renal failure, respiratory failure, and multiorgan dysfunction syndrome. ■

References

1. Gross SD: *A system of surgery: pathological, diagnostic, therapeutic, and operative,* Philadelphia, 1859, Blanchard and Lea.
2. Thal AP: *Shock: a physiologic basis for treatment,* Chicago, 1971, Yearbook Medical Publishers.
3. Bunn HF, Jandl JH: Control of hemoglobin function within the red cell, *N Engl J Med* 282:1414, 1970.
4. Marini JJ: Monitoring during mechanical ventilation, *Clin Chest Med* 9:73, 1988.
5. McClelland RN, Shires GT, Baxter CR, et al: Balanced salt solutions in the treatment of hemorrhagic shock, *JAMA* 199:830, 1967.
6. Ali J, Vanderby B, Purcell C: The effect of the pneumatic antishock garment (PASG) on hemodynamics, hemorrhage and survival in penetrating thoracic aortic injury, *J Trauma* 31(6):846, 1991.
7. Marshall JC, Cook DJ, Christou NV, et al: The multiple organ dysfunction score: a reliable descriptor of a complex clinical syndrome, *Crit Care Med* 23:1638, 1995.
8. McManus J, Yershov AL, Ludwig D, et al: Radial pulse character relationship to systolic blood pressure and trauma outcomes, *Prehosp Emerg Care* 9:423, 2005.
9. Pepe PE, Raedler C, Lurie KG, et al: Emergency ventilatory management in hemorrhagic states: elemental or detrimental? *J Trauma* 54:1048, 2003.
10. Pepe PE, Roppolo LP, Fowler RL: The detrimental effects of ventilation during low-blood-flow states, *Curr Opin Crit Care* 11:212, 2005.
11. Shafi S, Gentilello L: Prehospital endotracheal intubation and positive pressure ventilation is associated with hypotension and decreased survival in hypovolemic trauma patients: an analysis of the National Trauma Data Bank, *J Trauma* 59:1140, 2005.
12. Koreny M, Riedmuller E, Nikfardjam M, et al: Arterial puncture closing devices compares with standard manual compression after cardiac catheterization: systematic review and meta analysis, *JAMA* 291:350, 2004.
13. Walker SB, Cleary S, Higgins M: Comparison of the FemoStop device and manual pressure in reducing groin puncture site complications following coronary angioplasty and coronary stent placement, *Int J Nurs Pract* 7:366, 2001.
14. Simon A, Baumgarner B, Clark K, et al: Manual versus mechanical compression for femoral artery hemostasis after cardiac catheterization, *Am J Crit Care* 7:308, 1998.
15. Lehmann KG, Heath-Lange SJ, Ferris ST: Randomized comparison of hemostasis techniques after invasive cardiovascular procedures, *Am Heart J* 138:1118, 1999.
16. Bellamy RF: The causes of death in conventional land warfare: implications for combat casualty care research, *Mil Med* 149:55, 1984.
17. Mabry RL, Holcomb JB, Baker AM, et al: United States Army Rangers in Somalia: an analysis of combat casualties on an urban battlefield, *J Trauma* 49:515, 2000.
18. Walters TJ, Mabry RL: Use of tourniquets on the battlefield: a consensus panel report, *Mil Med* 170:770, 2005.
19. Walters TL, Wenke JC, Kauvar DS, et al: Laboratory evaluation of battlefield tourniquets in human volunteers, US Army Institute of Surgical Research (unpublished).
20. Pusateri AE, McCarthy S, Gregory KW, et al: Effect of a chitosan-based hemostatic dressing on blood loss and survival in a model of severe venous hemorrhage and hepatic injury in swine, *J Trauma* 54:177, 2003.
21. Uniformed Services University of the Health Sciences: News Release No 03-03-05, March 11, 2003.
22. Alam HB, Chen Z, Jaskille A, et al: Application of a Zeolite hemostatic agent achieves 100% survival in a lethal model of complex groin injury in swine, *J Trauma* 56:974, 2004.
23. Alam HB, Uy GB, Miller D, et al: Comparative analysis of hemostatic agents in a swine model of lethal groin injury, *J Trauma* 54:1077, 2003.
24. Gentilello LM: Advances in the management of hypothermia, *Surg Clin North Am* 75:2, 1995.

25. Marino PL: *The ICU book,* ed 2, Baltimore, 1998, Williams & Wilkins.

26. Johnson S, Henderson SO, Myth L: The Trendelenburg position improves circulation in cases of shock, *Can J Emerg Med* 6:48, 2004.

27. Mattox KL, Bickell WH, Pepe PE, et al: Prospective MAST study in 911 patients, *J Trauma* 29:1104, 1986.

28. Bickell WH, Wall MJ Jr, Pepe PE, et al: Immediate versus delayed fluid resuscitation for hypotensive patients with penetrating torso injuries, *N Engl J Med* 331:1105, 1994.

29. Ali J, Duke K: Pneumatic antishock garment decreases hemorrhage and mortality from splenic injury, *Can J Surg* 34(5):496, 1991.

30. McSwain NE Jr: Pneumatic antishock garment: state of the art, *Ann Emerg Med* 17:506, 1988.

31. Flint LM, Brown A, Richardson JD, et al: Definitive control of bleeding from severe pelvic fractures, *Ann Surg* 189:709, 1979.

32. Ali J, Purcell C, Vanderby B: The effect of intraabdominal pressure and saline infusion on abdominal aortic hemorrhage, *J Cardiovasc Surg* 32:653, 1991.

33. Lewis FR: Prehospital intravenous fluid therapy: physiologic computer modeling, *J Trauma* 26:804, 1986.

34. Deboer S, Seaver M, Morissette C: Intraosseous infusion: not just for kids anymore, *J Emerg Med Serv* 34:54, 2005.

35. Glaeser PW, Hellmich TR, Szewczuga D, et al: Five-year experience in prehospital intraosseous infusions in children and adults, *Ann Emerg Med* 22:1119, 1993.

36. Sawyer RW, Bodai BI, Blaisdell FW, McCourt M: The current status of intraosseous infusion, *J Am Coll Surg* 179:353, 1994.

37. Macnab A, Christenson J, Findlay J, et al: A new system for sternal intraosseous infusion in adults, *Prehosp Emerg Care* 4:173, 2000.

38. Hubble MW, Trigg DC: Training prehospital personnel in saphenous vein cut down and adult intraosseous techniques, *Prehosp Emerg Care* 5(2):181, 2001.

39. Vassar MJ, Fischer RP, Obrien PE, et al: A multicenter trial of resuscitation of injured patients with 7.5% sodium chloride: the effect of added dextran 70, *Arch Surg* 128:1003, 1993.

40. Vassar MJ, Perry CA, Holcroft JW: Prehospital resuscitation of hypotensive trauma patients with 7.5% NaCl versus 7.5% NaCl with added dextran: a controlled trial, *J Trauma* 34:622, 1993.

41. Wade CE, Kramer GC, Grady JJ: Efficacy of hypertonic 7.5% saline and 6% dextran in treating trauma: a meta analysis of controlled clinical trials, *Surgery* 122:609, 1997.

42. Rizoli SB: Crystalloids and colloids in trauma resuscitation: a brief overview of the current debate, *J Trauma* 54:S82, 2003.

43. SAFE Study Investigators: A comparison of albumin and saline for fluid resuscitation in the intensive care unit, *N Engl J Med* 350:2247, 2004.

44. Gould SA, Moore EE, Hoyt DB, et al: The first randomized trial of human polymerized hemoglobin as a blood substitute in acute trauma and emergent surgery, *J Am Coll Surg* 187:113, 1998.

45. Ketchan EM, Cairns CB: Hemoglobin based oxygen carriers: development and clinical potential, *Ann Emerg Med* 33:326, 1999.

46. Solomonov E, Hirsh M, Yahiya A, Krausz MM: The effect of vigorous fluid resuscitation in uncontrolled hemorrhagic shock after massive splenic injury, *Crit Care Med* 28:749, 2000.

47. Krausz MM, Horn Y, Gross D: The combined effect of small volume hypertonic saline and normal saline solutions in uncontrolled hemorrhagic shock, *Surg Gynecol Obstet* 174:363, 1992.

48. Bickell WH, Bruttig SP, Millnamow, et al: The detrimental effects of intravenous crystalloid after aortotomy in swine, *Surgery* 110:529, 1991.

49. Kowalenko T, Stern S, Dronen SC, et al: Improved outcome with hypotensive resuscitation of uncontrolled hemorrhagic shock in a swine model, *J Trauma* 33:349, 1992.

50. Sindlinger JF, Soucy DM, Greene SP, et al: The effects of isotonic saline volume resuscitation in uncontrolled hemorrhage, *Surg Gynecol Obstet* 177:545, 1993.

51. Capone AC, Safar, Stezoski W, et al: Improved outcome with fluid restriction in treatment of uncontrolled hemorrhagic shock, *J Am Coll Surg* 180:49, 1995.

52. Salomone JP, Ustin JS, McSwain NE, Feliciano DV: Opinions of trauma practitioners regarding prehospital interventions for critically injured patients, *J Trauma* 58:509, 2005.

53. York J, Abenamar A, Graham R, Miller R: Fluid resuscitation of patients with multiple injuries and severe closed head injury: experience with an aggressive fluid resuscitation strategy, *J Trauma* 48(3):376, 2000.

54. Brain Trauma Foundation: *Guidelines for prehospital management of traumatic brain injury,* New York, 2000, The Foundation.

55. American Association of Neurological Surgeons and Congress of Neurological Surgeons Joint Section on Disorders of the Spine and Peripheral Nerves: Blood pressure management after acute spinal cord injury. In Guidelines for the management of acute cervical spine and spinal cord injuries, *Neurosurgery* 50:S58, 2002.

56. Garcia GD, Modesto VL, Lee KT: Avoiding hypothermia in trauma: use of the Flameless Heater Pack, Meal Ready to Eat, as a field expedient means of warming crystalloid fluids, *Mil Med* 165(12):903, 2000.

57. Velmahos GC, Demetriades D, Ghilardi M, et al: Life Support for Trauma and Transport: a mobile ICU for safe in-hospital transport of critically injured patients, *J Am Coll Surg* 199:62, 2004.

Suggested Reading

American College of Surgeons Committee on Trauma: Shock. In *Advanced trauma life support for doctors, student course manual,* ed 7, Chicago, 2004, ACS.

Allison KP, Gosling P, Jones S, et al: Randomized trial of hydroxyethyl starch versus gelatine for trauma resuscitation, *J Trauma* 47:1114, 1999.

Moore EE: Blood substitutes: the future is now, *J Am Coll Surg* 196:1, 2003.

Novak L, Shackford SR, Bourgenignon P, et al: Comparison of standard and alternative prehospital resuscitation in uncontrolled hemorrhagic shock and head injury, *J Trauma* 47(5):834, 1999.

Proctor KG: Blood substitutes and experimental models of trauma, *J Trauma* 54:S106, 2003.

Revell M, Greaves I, Porter K: Endpoints for fluid resuscitation in hemorrhagic shock, *J Trauma* 54:S637, 2003.

Trunkey DD: Prehospital fluid resuscitation of the trauma patient: an analysis and review, *Emerg Med* 30(5):93, 2001.

Chapter Objectives

*At the completion of this chapter, the reader
will be able to do the following:*

✓ Relate the kinematics of trauma to the potential for traumatic brain injury (TBI).

✓ Incorporate the recognition of pathophysiologic manifestations and historical data significant for TBI into assessment of the trauma patient to formulate a field impression.

✓ Formulate a plan of field intervention for both short and prolonged transport times for patients with TBI.

✓ Compare and contrast the pathophysiology, management, and potential consequences of specific types of primary TBI and secondary brain injury.

✓ Identify criteria for patient care decisions with regard to mode of transport, level of prehospital care, and hospital resources needed for the appropriate management of the TBI patient.

CHAPTER 8

Head Trauma

SCENARIO

You and your partner are dispatched to a construction site where a 30-year-old male ironworker lost his balance and fell about 25 feet (8 m) to a concrete floor. Bystanders state that he was unconscious for about 10 minutes but has now awakened. The scene is safe. The primary survey reveals that the patient is maintaining his airway and breathing normally. A 3¼-inch (8-cm) laceration on the right side of his scalp is bleeding copiously but is readily controlled with direct pressure and a pressure dressing. His pulse rate is 116 beats/min, and his skin is warm, pink, and well perfused. He opens his eyes spontaneously and follows commands; however, he does not recall the events leading up to his fall. He exhibits some confusion as he attempts to answer questions (GCS 14). You apply oxygen using a nonrebreather mask. During spinal immobilization, he speaks incomprehensible words and now only opens his eyes and withdraws his extremities to painful stimuli (GCS 9).

How should you alter your care based on the change in the patient's level of consciousness? What injury is most likely present given the patient's presenting signs? What are your management priorities at this point? What actions may you need to take to combat increased intracranial pressure and maintain cerebral perfusion during a prolonged transport? ■

Approximately 1.6 million emergency department (ED) visits for head injury occur each year. About 500,000 of these patients sustain *traumatic brain injury* (TBI). Although 80% of these patients are categorized as having only mild injuries, about 50,000 patients with TBI are pronounced dead on arrival in the ED. TBI contributes significantly to the death of about half of all trauma victims. Moderate to severe brain injuries are identified in about 100,000 trauma patients annually. Mortality rates for moderate and severe brain injuries are about 10% and 30%, respectively. Of those who survive moderate and severe brain injuries, between 50% and 99% have some degree of permanent neurologic disability.

Motor vehicle crashes (MVCs) remain the leading cause of TBI in those under 65 years of age, and falls are the leading cause of TBI in the elderly population. The head is the most frequently injured part of the body in patients with multisystem injuries. The incidence of gunshot wounds to the brain has increased in recent years in urban areas, and up to 60% of these victims die from their injury.

Patients with TBI represent some of the most challenging trauma patients to treat. They may be combative, and attempts to intubate can be extremely difficult because of clenched jaw muscles and vomiting. Intoxication with drugs or alcohol or the presence of shock from other injuries can hinder assessment. Occasionally, serious intracranial injuries can be present with only minimal evidence of external trauma. Skilled care in the prehospital setting focuses on ensuring the adequate delivery of oxygen and nutrients to the brain and rapidly identifying patients at risk for herniation and elevated intracranial pressure. This approach can decrease mortality from TBI and also the incidence of permanent neurologic disability.

Anatomy

Knowledge of head and brain anatomy is essential to understand the pathophysiology of TBI. The scalp is the outermost covering of the head and offers some protection to the skull and brain. The scalp is composed of several layers, including skin, connective tissue, galea aponeurotica, and the periosteum of the skull. The galea is important because it provides the structural support to the scalp and is the key to its integrity. The scalp and soft tissues overlying the face are highly vascular.

The skull, or cranium, is composed of a number of bones that fuse into a single structure during childhood. Several small openings *(foramina)* through the base of the skull provide pathways for blood vessels and cranial nerves. One large opening, the foramen magnum, is located on the caudal aspect of the skull base and serves as a passageway for the brainstem to the spinal cord (Figure 8-1). In infancy, "soft spots" *(fontanelles)* can often be identified between the bones. The infant has no bony protection over these portions of the brain until the bones fuse, typically by 2 years of age.

Although most of the bones forming the cranium are thick and strong, the skull is especially thin in the temporal and ethmoid regions, which are more prone to fracture. The cranium provides significant protection to the brain, but the interior surface of the skull base is rough and irregular. When exposed to a blunt force, the brain may slide across these irregularities, producing cerebral contusions or lacerations.

Three separate membranes, the *meninges,* cover the brain (Figure 8-2). The outermost layer, the *dura mater,* is composed of tough fibrous tissue and is applied to the inner table, or inside, of the skull. Under normal circumstances,

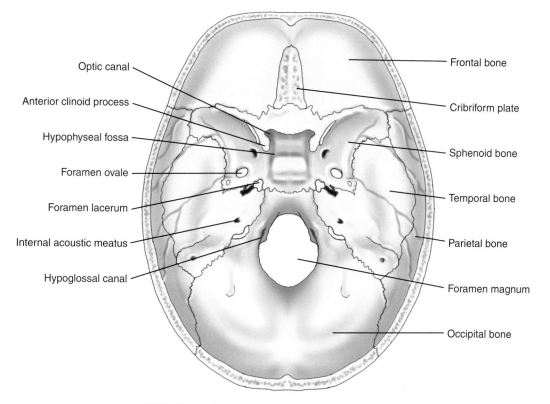

Optic canal

Anterior clinoid process

Hypophyseal fossa

Foramen ovale

Foramen lacerum

Internal acoustic meatus

Hypoglossal canal

Frontal bone

Cribriform plate

Sphenoid bone

Temporal bone

Parietal bone

Foramen magnum

Occipital bone

FIGURE 8-1   Internal view of the base of the skull.

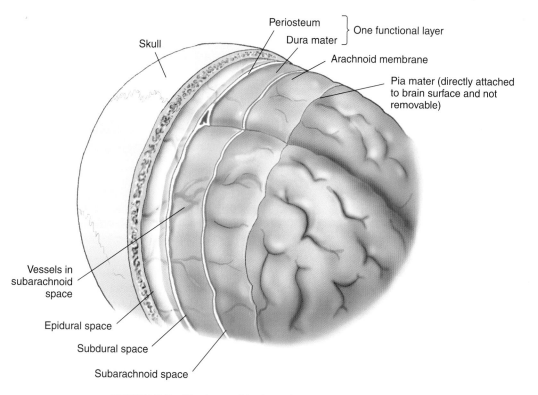

Skull

Periosteum

Dura mater

One functional layer

Arachnoid membrane

Pia mater (directly attached to brain surface and not removable)

Vessels in subarachnoid space

Epidural space

Subdural space

Subarachnoid space

FIGURE 8-2   Meninges. Meningeal coverings of the brain.

the space between the dura and the inside of the skull, the epidural space, does not exist; it is a potential space. The dura is applied to the skull similar to a laminate. The middle meningeal arteries are located in grooves in the temporal bones on either side of the head, outside the dura. A blow to the thin temporal bone can create a fracture and tear the middle meningeal artery, the common etiology for epidural hematomas.

Unlike the epidural space, which is a potential space, the subdural space is an actual space, between the dura and the brain. This space is spanned in places by veins, which create a vascular communication between skull and brain. The traumatic rupture of these veins often creates subdural hematomas, which, unlike epidural hematomas, are venous, of lower pressure, and often associated with brain injury. Along with the injury to these bridging veins, this TBI accounts for the morbidity of subdural hematomas.

On the other side of the subdural space lies the brain, which is closely covered with two additional meningeal layers, the arachnoid and the pia. The *pia mater* is closely adhered to the brain, again similar to a laminate, and is the final brain covering. On top of the pia run cerebral blood vessels, which emerge from the base of the brain and then cover its surface. Layered on top of these blood vessels is the *arachnoid membrane,* which more loosely covers the brain and its blood vessels, giving the appearance of a "cellophane wrap" around the brain when it is viewed from the subdural space. Before cellophane existed, this covering was thought to resemble a spiderweb, thus the name "arachnoid." Because the cerebral blood vessels run on the surface of the brain but beneath the arachnoid membrane, their rupture (usually from trauma or a ruptured cerebral aneurysm) will result in bleeding into the subarachnoid space, causing a subarachnoid bleed. This blood normally does not enter the subdural space but is contained beneath the arachnoid; it can be seen at surgery as a thin layer of blood on the surface of the brain, contained beneath this translucent membrane. Unlike epidural and subdural

---

BOX 8-1 The Brain

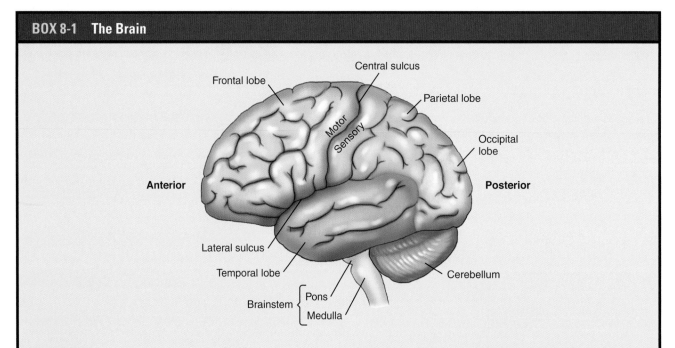

CEREBRUM

The cerebrum is composed of the right and left cerebral hemispheres. The dominant hemisphere is the one that contains the language center. This is the left hemisphere in virtually all right-handed individuals and about 85% of left-handed individuals. The cerebrum is composed of the following lobes:

- *Frontal.* Contains emotions, motor function, and expression of speech on the dominant side.
- *Parietal.* Contains sensory function and spatial orientation.

- *Temporal.* Regulates certain memory functions; contains the area for speech reception and integration in all right-handed and the majority of left-handed individuals.
- *Occipital.* Contains vision.

BRAINSTEM

- *Midbrain and upper pons.* Contain the reticular activating system (RAS), which is responsible for arousal and alertness.
- *Medulla.* Contains the cardiorespiratory centers.

CEREBELLUM

Controls coordination and balance.

hematomas, subarachnoid blood does not normally create mass effect but can be symptomatic of other serious injury to the brain.

The brain also is surrounded by *cerebrospinal fluid* (CSF), which is produced in the ventricular system of the brain and also surrounds the spinal cord. CSF helps cushion the brain and is contained in the subarachnoid space as well.

The brain occupies about 80% of the cranial vault and is divided into three main regions: the cerebrum, cerebellum, and brainstem (Box 8-1). The *cerebrum* consists of right and left hemispheres that can be subdivided into several lobes. The cerebrum houses sensory functions, motor functions, and higher intellectual functions such as intelligence and memory. The *cerebellum* is located in the posterior fossa of the cranium, behind the brainstem and beneath the cerebrum, and coordinates movement. The *brainstem* contains the medulla, an area that controls many vital functions, including breathing and heart rate. Much of the reticular activating system (RAS), the portion of the brain responsible for arousal and alertness, is also found in the brainstem. Blunt trauma can impair the RAS, leading to a transient loss of consciousness. The tentorium cerebelli, a portion of the dura mater, lies between the cerebrum and the cerebellum and contains an opening, the tentorial incisura, at the level of the midbrain.

The 12 cranial nerves originate from the brain and brainstem (Figure 8-3). The oculomotor nerve, cranial nerve III, controls pupillary constriction and provides an important tool in the assessment of a patient with a suspected brain injury.

Physiology

Cerebral Blood Flow

It is critical that the brain's neurons receive a constant flow of blood. This constant cerebral blood flow is maintained by ensuring (1) an adequate pressure (cerebral perfusion pressure) to force blood into the head and (2) a regulatory mechanism (autoregulation), which ensures a constant blood flow by varying the resistance to blood flow as the perfusion pressure changes.

Mean Arterial Pressure

The heart is a cyclic pump, and thus the pressure created by the heart is represented as two pressures. The *diastolic pressure* is the baseline pressure that the system maintains when the heart is not pumping, and the *systolic pressure* is the maximum pressure generated at the peak of cardiac contraction. Because such a dynamic characterization of the pressures generated by the heart can be difficult to work with, for the purposes of discussing cerebral perfusion pressure, we use an average pressure for the cardiac cycle, the *mean arterial pressure* (MAP), to characterize the pressure driving blood into the head.

Calculation of the MAP assumes that cardiac contraction (systole) takes up one third of the cardiac cycle and that the remaining two thirds of the cycle, the systemic pressure, remains at baseline (diastole). The MAP is therefore calculated by (1) averaging the additional pressure added to the

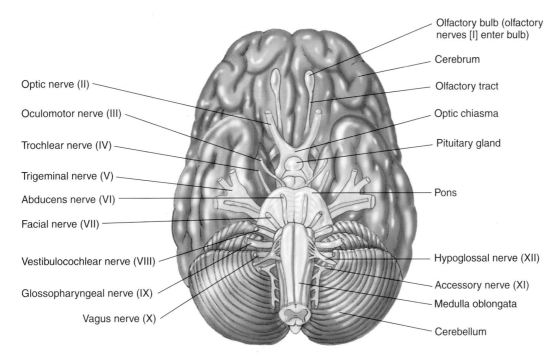

FIGURE 8-3 Inferior surface of the brain showing the origins of the cranial nerves.

system during cardiac contraction, or systole, over the entire cardiac cycle and (2) adding it to the diastolic pressure. This is done by calculating the additional pressure added to the system during systole, the *pulse pressure,* dividing it by 3, and adding this number to the diastolic pressure, as follows:

Pulse pressure = Systolic pressure – Diastolic pressure

and

MAP = Diastolic pressure + 1/3 Pulse pressure

Most blood pressure monitors calculate the MAP with a much more accurate method of calculation that uses the actual blood pressure waveform. Because the percentage of time the heart spends in systole increases as the heart rate increases, the assumption that systole is one third of diastole becomes less and less accurate as the patient becomes more tachycardic. Therefore the blood pressure monitor, in the vast majority of patients being transported for neurologic injury, will more accurately represent the MAP than the preceding calculation. The value in learning the calculation lies in the insights it provides into the nature of the MAP.

Cerebral Perfusion Pressure

Cerebral perfusion pressure (CPP) is the MAP minus the pressure in the head, the *intracranial pressure* (ICP):

CPP = MAP – ICP

Normal MAP ranges from about 85 to 95 mm Hg, and ICP is normally below 20 mm Hg. Therefore CPP is normally about 70 to 80 mm Hg.

Autoregulation of CBF

The most important factor for the brain, however, is not CPP, but cerebral blood flow (CBF). The best ways to measure CBF are not very convenient. The CPP is used to estimate the adequacy of CBF.

To understand autoregulation, we need to remember that for any flowing system:

Pressure = Flow × Resistance

In the case of the brain, this translates into:

**Cerebral perfusion pressure =
Cerebral blood flow × Cerebral vascular resistance**

CPP = CBF × CVR

Because the brain's principal concern is CBF, it is useful to rewrite this equation as:

CBF = CPP/CVR

Using this equation, it is evident how the brain keeps blood flow constant. If a person switches from lying down to standing, the CPP will fall. The only way to keep CBF constant is to also have the cerebral vascular resistance (CVR) fall. The brain accomplishes this decline in CVR by dilating the cerebral vasculature. The process of changing the caliber of the cerebral blood vessels to adjust CVR to compensate for changes in CPP is called *autoregulation.*

Autoregulation is crucial to the brain's normal function. In people who stand up too quickly and faint, their autoregulatory mechanisms simply did not react quickly enough to their change in position, resulting in a temporary but dramatic loss of cerebral function.

To function normally, the autoregulatory mechanism must have a certain minimum pressure. Clearly, at a pressure of 0 mm Hg, no amount of vasodilation will cause blood to flow, and there are limits to how much the blood vessels in the head can dilate. Therefore, below a CPP of about 50 mm Hg, the autoregulatory mechanisms can no longer compensate for the decreased CPP, and CBF starts to decrease. As CBF begins to fall, cerebral function declines, and the risk of permanent cerebral injury from ischemia increases.

To make matters worse, injured brains often require higher-than-normal CPPs to activate the autoregulatory mechanisms and keep CBF adequate. Although each individual patient probably has his or her own CPP threshold above which CBF is adequate, there is no way to determine this threshold in the field. Therefore, the best estimate of an adequate CPP is 60 to 70 mm Hg.

Measuring CPP requires both a blood pressure monitor and an ICP monitor. In the absence of an ICP monitor, the best practice is simply to try and maintain a high MAP. Because most literature on outcomes from TBI has used *systolic blood pressure* (SBP) instead of MAP to measure blood pressure, SBP is the value used to monitor the adequacy of cerebral perfusion in settings without ICP monitoring. Best evidence suggests that an SBP greater than 90 mm Hg is desirable for neurologically injured patients.[1-5]

Hyperventilation

Hyperventilation reduces ICP but also impacts CBF. In fact, data suggest that hyperventilation more reliably reduces CBF than ICP. Hyperventilation reduces ICP by reducing the arterial carbon dioxide partial pressure ($Paco_2$) by increasing the rate at which CO_2 is blown off by the lungs. This reduced $Paco_2$ changes the acid-base balance in the brain, resulting in vasoconstriction. This cerebral vasoconstriction reduces the intravascular volume of the brain, reducing cerebral blood volume and therefore, often ICP.[6,7]

Under normal circumstances, autoregulation ensures adequate CBF by making sure that CVR is correct for the available CPP to ensure continuing adequate CBF. It is important to note that hyperventilation of a patient is by-passing autoregulation. Therefore, hyperventilation causes cerebral vasoconstriction, which may reduce cerebral blood volume enough to reduce ICP, but it also increases CVR, whether or not CPP is adequate to maintain CBF. As a result, hyperventilation can reduce CBF, placing the injured brain at risk for ischemic injury. A $Paco_2$ less than 35 mm Hg increases the risk of cerebral ischemia, and a $Paco_2$ greater than the normal range of 35 to 45 mm Hg leads to dilation of cerebral arterioles, thus increasing CBF. (Management of hyperventilation is discussed later.)

Pathophysiology

TBI can be divided into two categories: primary and secondary.

Primary Brain Injury

Primary brain injury is the direct trauma to the brain and associated vascular injuries that occur at the time of the original insult. It includes lacerations and other direct mechanical injury to the brain, its vasculature, and coverings. Because neural tissue does not regenerate well, there is minimal expectation of recovery of the structure and function lost due to primary injury. Also, little possibility exists for repair.

Secondary Brain Injury

Secondary brain injury refers to the ongoing injury processes that are set in motion by the primary injury. At the time of injury, pathophysiologic processes are initiated that continue to injure the brain for hours, days, and weeks after the initial insult. The primary focus in the management of TBI is to identify and limit or stop these secondary injury mechanisms.

Before computed tomography (CT) was available, the principal secondary injury mechanism was "unidentified intracranial bleeds." The literature referred to "talk and die" patients, or those who were initially lucid after a trau-matic insult but then lapsed into a coma and died as an unidentified intracranial hematoma expanded, leading to fatal herniation. Clearly, in these patients, if the initiated pathologic process could be interrupted, the patient's life could be saved.[8-10] Pathologic mechanisms related to intracranial mass effect, elevated ICP, and herniation still are concerns as causes of secondary injury, but their management has been revolutionized by CT, ICP monitoring, and immediate surgery. In the prehospital environment, the identification of patients at high risk for herniation from mass effect and their rapid transport to a hospital with the facilities to address these issues are still the key priorities.

With the advent of CT, it became easier to identify and treat these hematomas. However, it also became clear that other mechanisms were present and continued to injure the brain after injury. Large studies in the late 1980s demonstrated that unrecognized and untreated hypoxia and hypotension were as damaging to the injured brain as elevated ICP. Subsequent observations have shown that impaired delivery of oxygen or energy substrate (e.g., glucose) to the injured brain has a much more devastating impact than in the normal brain. Therefore, in addition to hematoma, two other sources of secondary injury are hypoxia and hypotension.[4,5,11-13]

Ongoing research in the laboratory is revealing a fourth class of secondary injury mechanisms, those occurring at the cellular level. Studies have identified multiple destructive cellular mechanisms that are initiated by injury. The ability to understand, manipulate, and stop these mechanisms may lead to new therapies to limit brain injury, perhaps even a prehospital "cocktail." At present, the study of these mechanisms is limited to the laboratory.

Secondary injury mechanisms include the following:

1. Mass effect and the subsequent elevated ICP and mechanical shifting of the brain, which can lead to herniation and significant morbidity and mortality if not addressed.
2. Hypoxia, which results from inadequate delivery of oxygen to the injured brain caused by ventilatory or circulatory failure or mass effect.
3. Hypotension and inadequate CBF, which can cause inadequate oxygen delivery to the brain. Low CBF also reduces delivery of substrate (e.g., glucose) to the injured brain and results in inadequate substrate (e.g., glucose).
4. Cellular mechanisms, including energy failure, inflammation, and "suicide" cascades, which can be triggered at the cellular level and can lead to cell death, called *apoptosis*.

Intracranial Causes

Mass Effect and Herniation. The secondary injury mecha-nisms most often recognized are those related to mass effect. These mechanisms are the result of the complex inter-actions described by the Monro-Kellie doctrine.[14] The brain is encased in a space that is closed once the fontanelles are closed, and all the space within the cranium is taken up by brain, blood, or CSF. If any other mass, such as a hematoma, cerebral swelling, or a tumor, occupies any space within the cranial vault, some other structure needs to be forced out (Figure 8-4).

Normal state - ICP normal

Compensated state - ICP normal

Decompensated state - ICP elevated

FIGURE 8-4   Monro-Kellie doctrine: intracranial compensation for expanding mass. The volume of the intracranial contents remains constant. If the addition of a mass such as a hematoma results in the squeezing out of an equal volume of cerebrospinal fluid *(CSF)* and venous blood, the intracranial pressure *(ICP)* remains normal. However, when this compensatory mechanism is exhausted, an exponential increase occurs in ICP for even a small additional increase in the volume of the hematoma.

(From McSwain NE Jr, Paturas JL: *The basic EMT: comprehensive prehospital patient care,* ed 2, St Louis, 2001, Mosby.)

The dynamics of forcing blood, CSF, or brain out of the cranial vault in response to an expanding mass effect are the second part of the Monro-Kellie doctrine. At first, in response to the expanding mass, the volume of CSF surrounding the brain is reduced. The CSF naturally circulates within and around the neuroaxis, and as the mass expands, more CSF is forced out of the head, and the total CSF volume is reduced. Blood volume in the cranial vault is also reduced in a similar manner, with venous blood the principal volume reduced in the head.

As a result of the CSF and blood volumes being reduced, the pressure in the head does not rise during the early phases of the expansion of intracranial masses. During this phase, if the growing mass is the only intracranial pathology, patients can appear to be asymptomatic. Once the ability to force out CSF and blood has been exhausted, however, the pressure inside the cranium, the ICP, starts to rise rapidly, and the next structure to be forced out of the head is brain.

The brain has only one direction to move, down toward the foramen magnum. The consequences of this movement toward the foramen magnum are described as the various herniation syndromes.

If the expanding mass is along the convexity of the brain, as in the typical position for a temporal lobe epidural hematoma, the temporal lobe will be forced toward the center of the brain before attempting to move downward

FIGURE 8-5   Suspect injury to the brain whenever a patient's pupils are unequal in size.

toward the foramen magnum. This movement forces the medial portion of the temporal lobe, the *uncus,* into the third nerve, the motor tract, and the brainstem and RAS on that side. This is called *uncal herniation* and results in malfunction of the third cranial nerve, causing a dilated or blown pupil on the side of the herniation (Figure 8-5). It also results in loss of function of the motor tract on the same side, which causes weakness on the opposite of the body from the lesion. In the last stages of uncal herniation, the RAS is affected and the patient lapses into coma, an event associated with a much poorer prognosis.

Some convexity masses lead to *cingulate herniation,* either in conjunction with uncal herniation or in isolation. In cingulate herniation the cingulate gyrus along the medial surface of the cerebral hemispheres is forced under the falx, the dural division between the two hemispheres. This

Skull

Cerebrum

Swelling
causing
herniation

Cerebellum   Foramen magnum

FIGURE 8-6   The skull is a large, bony structure that contains the brain. The brain cannot escape the skull if it expands because of edema or if there is hemorrhage in the skull that presses on the brain.

can cause injury to the medial cerebral hemispheres and the midbrain.

Another type of herniation, called *tonsillar herniation*, occurs as the brain is pushed down toward the foramen magnum and pushes the cerebellum and medulla ahead of it. This can ultimately result in the most caudal part of the cerebellum, the cerebellar tonsils, and the medulla becoming wedged in the foramen magnum, with the medulla subsequently being crushed. Injury to the lower medulla results in cardiac and respiratory arrest, a common final event for patients with herniation. The process of forcing the posterior fossa contents into the foramen magnum is referred to as "coning"[15] (Figure 8-6).

Clinical Herniation Syndromes. Clinical features of the herniation syndromes can help identify a patient who is herniating. Traditionally, as just mentioned, uncal herniation will often result in dilation or sluggishness of the ipsilateral pupil, referred to as a "blown pupil." Abnormal motor findings can also accompany herniation. Contralateral weakness may be associated with uncal herniation. More extensive herniation can result in destruction of structures in the brain known as the red nucleus or the vestibular nuclei. This can result in *decorticate posturing,* which involves flexion of the upper extremities and rigidity and extension of the lower extremities. A more ominous finding is *decerebrate posturing,* in which all extremities are extended, and arching of the spine may occur. After herniation, the extremities become flaccid, and motor activity is absent.[16,17]

In the final stages, herniation often produces abnormal ventilatory patterns or apnea, with worsening hypoxia

and significantly altered blood CO_2 levels. *Cheyne-Stokes ventilations* are a repeating cycle of slow, shallow breaths that become deeper and more rapid and then return to slow, shallow breaths. Brief periods of apnea may occur between cycles. *Central neurogenic hyperventilation* refers to consistently rapid, deep breaths, and *ataxic breathing* refers to erratic ventilatory efforts that lack any discernible pattern. Spontaneous respiratory function ceases with compression of the brainstem, a common final pathway for herniation.[15]

As tissue hypoxia develops in the brain, reflexes are activated in an effort to maintain cerebral oxygen delivery. To overcome rising ICP, the autonomic nervous system is activated to increase systemic blood pressure, and therefore the MAP, to maintain a normal CPP. Systolic pressures can reach up to 250 mm Hg. However, as the baroreceptors in the carotid arteries and aortic arch sense a greatly increased blood pressure, messages are sent to the brainstem to activate the parasympathetic nervous system. A signal then travels via the tenth cranial nerve, the vagus nerve, to slow the heart rate. *Cushing's phenomenon* refers to this ominous combination of greatly increased arterial blood pressure and the resultant bradycardia that can occur with severely increased ICP.

Ischemia and Herniation. The herniation syndromes describe how the swelling brain, because it is contained in a fully enclosed space, can sustain mechanical damage. However, elevated ICP from cerebral swelling can also cause injury to the brain by creating cerebral ischemia as well as the resulting decreased oxygen delivery. As cerebral swelling increases, ICP also increases. Because CPP = MAP − ICP, as ICP increases, CPP decreases. Increases in ICP therefore threaten CBF. In addition to mechanical injury to the brain, cerebral swelling also can cause ischemic injury to the brain, compounding the ischemic insults the brain might sustain from other causes, such as systemic hypotension.

To complicate matters further, as these mechanical and ischemic insults create injury to the brain, they create more cerebral swelling. In this way, cerebral edema can cause injury that creates more cerebral edema, which in turn leads to further injury and edema in a downward spiral that can lead to herniation and death if not interrupted. Limiting this secondary injury and breaking this cycle of injury is the principal goal of TBI management.

Cerebral Edema.   Cerebral edema (brain swelling) often occurs at the site of a primary brain injury. Injury to the neuronal cell membranes allows intracellular fluid to collect within damaged neurons, leading to cerebral edema. In addition, injury can lead to inflammatory responses that injure the neurons and the cerebral capillaries, leading to fluid collection within the neurons as well as within the interstitial spaces, both leading to cerebral edema. As the edema develops, the mechanical and ischemic injury previously described occurs, which aggravates these processes and leads to further edema and injury.

Cerebral edema can occur in association with or as a result of intracranial hematomas, as a result of injury to the brain parenchyma in the form of cerebral contusion, or as a result of diffuse brain injury from hypoxia or hypotension.

Intracerebral Hematomas. In trauma, mass effect results from actual accumulation of blood in the intracranial space. Intracranial hematomas, such as epidural, subdural, or intracerebral hematomas, are major sources of mass effect. Because the mass effect from these hematomas is caused solely by their size, rapid removal of these hematomas can break the cycle of edema and injury described earlier. Unfortunately, these hematomas often have associated cerebral edema, and other means, in addition to removing the hematoma, are required to stop the cycle of injury and edema. (Specific cerebral hematomas are described later.)

Intracranial Hypertension. Intracranial hypertension results because cerebral edema occurs in an enclosed space. ICP is measured as a way to quantify and assess the degree of cerebral edema. ICP monitors are placed to allow providers to quantify the cerebral swelling, assess the risk of herniation, and monitor the effectiveness of therapies designed to combat cerebral edema. In this sense, elevated ICP is a sign of cerebral swelling.

Because elevated ICP, or intracranial hypertension, is part of the cycle previously described, it also causes cerebral injury in the form of mechanical compression of the brain and ischemic and hypoxic injury to the brain. For this reason, ICP is often discussed, correctly, both as a symptom and as a cause of cerebral edema.

ICP monitoring is not routinely available in the prehospital environment, but understanding it and the reasons for its control can help prehospital care providers with decision making for the brain-injured patient.

Extracranial Causes

Hypotension. As long known, brain ischemia is common in head injury. Evidence of ischemia is found in 90% of the patients who die of TBI, and even many of the survivors have evidence of ischemic injury.[18] Therefore the impact of low CBF on the outcome from TBI has been a primary focus for limiting secondary injury after TBI.

In the national TBI database, the two most significant predictors of poor outcome from TBI were the amount of time spent with an ICP greater than 20 mm Hg and with an SBP less than 90 mm Hg. In fact, a single episode of SBP less than 90 mm Hg can lead to a poorer outcome.[19] Several studies have confirmed the profound impact of low SBP on the outcome after TBI.

Many patients with TBI sustain other injuries, many of which involve hemorrhage and subsequent low blood pressure. Aggressive fluid resuscitation of these injuries in a focused effort to keep SBP greater than 90 mm Hg is essential to limiting the secondary injury to the brain that can result from failing to meet this goal.

In addition to hemorrhage, a second factor threatens CBF after TBI, especially in the most severe injuries. A typical cortical CBF is 50 mL/100 g of brain/min. After severe TBI, this value can drop to 30 mL or even as low as 20 mL/100 g/min in the most severe injuries. This decline may be caused by loss of autoregulation, or it may be a protective mechanism, downregulating the entire brain in response to injury. Whatever the cause, this effect, added to the impact of hemorrhagic shock, compounds the ischemic threat to the brain.[6,7,19,20]

In addition, as noted earlier, autoregulation in the injured brain is deranged. As a result, higher CPP is required to maintain adequate CBF. Severely injured areas of the brain can lose almost all ability to autoregulate. In these areas the blood vessels become dilated, causing hyperemia and shunting blood toward the most severely injured brain areas and possibly away from areas that could still be saved by adequate perfusion.[21,22] Lastly, aggressive hyperventilation can further threaten CBF and compound the ischemic threat.

This combination of physiologic downregulation, shunting, and hemorrhagic shock creates multiple ischemic threats to the brain and makes the aggressive management of hypotension an essential part of the management of TBI. For this reason, an aggressive approach in the prehospital environment, with fluid resuscitation aimed at keeping the SBP above 90 mm Hg, is essential to limit secondary injury in the brain-injured patient.

Hypoxia. One of the most critical substrates delivered to the injured brain by the circulation is oxygen. Irreversible brain damage can occur after only 4 to 6 minutes of cerebral anoxia. Studies have also demonstrated a significant impact of an oxygen partial pressure (Po_2) less than 60 mm Hg in TBI patients.[1,4,13] A significant number of TBI patients are not adequately resuscitated in the field.[13] In addition, several studies have demonstrated that significant numbers of TBI victims present with low or inadequate Po_2 or O_2 saturation.[12] The emphasis on prehospital airway management and oxygen delivery for brain-injured patients has partly been the result of these studies.

Elegant work with brain tissue oxygen monitors has demonstrated the impact of hemorrhagic shock on oxygen delivery to the brain. Limiting hypotension is a key component in ensuring that the brain receives an adequate supply of oxygen during the postinjury phase.[23]

Hemorrhage is common in patients with TBI, resulting not only in shock but also in loss of blood and therefore hemoglobin.

For oxygenated blood to be delivered to the brain, the lungs must be properly functioning, which they often are not after trauma. Patients with an inadequate airway, aspiration of blood or gastric contents, pulmonary contusions, or pneumothoraces have pathology that will interfere with good respiratory function and the ability to transfer oxygen from the atmosphere to the blood. In addition to ensuring oxygen transport to the brain through adequate hemoglobin and circulation, providers must ensure adequate oxygenation through an adequate airway and with adequate ventilation.

As with hypotension, aggressive limitation of cerebral hypoxia with appropriate management of airway, breathing, and circulation is essential for limiting secondary brain injury.

Anemia. Also critical to the delivery of oxygen to the brain is the oxygen-carrying capacity of the blood, which is determined by the amount of hemoglobin it contains. A 50% drop in hemoglobin has a much more profound effect on oxygen delivery to the brain than a 50% drop in P_{O_2}. For this reason, anemia can impact the outcome of TBI.

Hypoglycemia and Hyperglycemia. Hypotension makes it highly likely that CBF is also low. As CBF falls, oxygen delivery to the brain also falls, as does delivery of glucose and other necessary brain metabolites. The epidemiologic effects of low SBP and the physiology of low oxygen delivery to the brain have been well studied. However, the injured brain's use of glucose and the impact of glucose utilization and delivery on the injured brain are still the subjects of research.

The research available, however, offers a fascinating look into the brain's response to injury. It appears that after head injury, cerebral glucose metabolism can become deranged in complex ways. Some compelling evidence indicates that glucose metabolism and therefore cerebral glucose need actually increase after severe head injury, threatening a mismatch between glucose delivery and utilization.[24-26]

On the other hand, good clinical and laboratory data in stroke patients show that patients whose serum glucose is allowed to remain elevated for long periods in the intensive care unit (ICU) may have larger areas of infarction and less effective resuscitation of salvageable brain than patients whose glucose is better controlled. Limited studies seem to indicate that these same factors are present in the ischemia that occurs after head injury.

Elevated blood glucose levels in patients with TBI have also been associated with poorer neurologic outcome.

Both elevations (hyperglycemia) and decreases (hypoglycemia) in blood sugar can jeopardize ischemic brain tissue. The disastrous impact of significant hypoglycemia on the nervous system, during injury, and at other times is well known. Neurons are unable to store sugar and require a continual supply of glucose to carry out cellular metabolism. In the absence of glucose, ischemic neurons can be permanently damaged. However, it is also true that

a prolonged serum glucose level greater than 150 mg/dL and probably greater than 200 mg/dL may be harmful to the injured brain and should be avoided.[27,28]

In the prehospital environment the emphasis should be on avoiding hypoglycemia because the physiologic threat from low sugar is much more immediate than from elevated serum glucose. In addition, any induced hyperglycemia will be transient, and the tight glucose control required to manage these patients properly is unlikely to be established before resuscitation is completed in the ED.

Hypocapnia and Hypercapnia. Both hypocapnia (decreased Pa_{CO_2}) and hypercapnia (increased Pa_{CO_2}) can worsen brain injury. When cerebral blood vessels constrict, as results from significant hypocapnia, CBF is compromised, leading to a decrease in oxygen delivery to the brain. Hypercapnia can result from hypoventilation from many causes, including drug or alcohol intoxication and abnormal ventilation patterns seen in patients with increased ICP. Hypercapnia causes cerebral vasodilation, which can further increase ICP.

Seizures. A patient with acute TBI is at risk for seizures for several reasons. Hypoxia from either airway or breathing problems can induce generalized seizure activity, as can hypoglycemia and electrolyte abnormalities. Ischemic or damaged brain tissue can serve as an irritable focus to produce grand mal seizures or status epilepticus. Seizures, in turn, can aggravate preexisting hypoxia caused by impairment of respiratory function. Additionally, the massive neuronal activity associated with generalized seizures rapidly depletes oxygen and glucose levels, further worsening cerebral ischemia.

Assessment

A quick survey of the kinematics of the injury, combined with a rapid primary survey, will help identify potential life-threatening problems in a patient with a suspected TBI.

Kinematics

As with all trauma patients, assessment must include consideration of the mechanism of injury. Because many patients with severe TBI have an altered level of consciousness (LOC), key data about the kinematics will frequently come from observation of the scene or from bystanders. The windshield of the patient's vehicle may have a "spiderweb" pattern, suggesting an impact with the patient's head, or a bloody object may be present that was used as a weapon during an assault. This important information should be reported to personnel at the receiving facility because it may be essential for proper diagnosis and management of the patient.

Primary Survey
Airway

The patency of the patient's airway should be examined. In unconscious individuals the tongue may completely occlude the airway. Noisy ventilations indicate partial obstruction by either the tongue or foreign material. Emesis, hemorrhage, and swelling from facial trauma are common causes of airway compromise in patients with TBI.

Breathing

Evaluation of respiratory function must include an assessment of the rate, depth, and adequacy of breathing. As noted previously, several different breathing patterns can result from severe brain injury. In multisystem trauma patients, thoracic injuries can further impair both oxygenation and ventilation. Cervical spine fractures occur in about 2% to 5% of patients with TBI and may result in spinal cord injuries that significantly interfere with ventilation.

Adequate oxygen delivery to the injured brain is an essential part of the effort to limit secondary brain injury. Failure to keep the oxygen saturation of hemoglobin (Spo_2) above 90% appears to result in poorer outcomes for brain-injured patients; maintaining Spo_2 above 90% is critical. Assessing for adequate airway and ventilatory effort is crucial in the early stages of managing TBI.

Circulation

As noted previously, maintaining an SBP greater than 90 mm Hg is critical for limiting secondary brain injury in the victims of TBI. Therefore the control of hemorrhage and the prevention and treatment of shock are critical. The prehospital care provider will note and quantify evidence of external bleeding, if possible. In the absence of significant external blood loss, a weak, rapid pulse in a victim of blunt trauma suggests life-threatening internal hemorrhage in the pleural spaces, peritoneum, retroperitoneum, or soft tissues surrounding long-bone fractures. In an infant with open fontanelles, sufficient blood loss can occur inside the cranium to produce hypovolemic shock. A slow, forceful pulse may result from intracranial hypertension and indicate impending herniation (Cushing's phenomenon). In a patient with potentially life-threatening injuries, transport should not be delayed to measure blood pressure but should be performed en route as time permits.

Disability

During the primary survey and after the initiation of appropriate measures to treat problems identified in the airway, breathing, and circulation assessments, a baseline Glasgow Coma Scale (GCS) score should be calculated to assess the patient's LOC accurately (Table 8-1). As described in Chapter 5, the GCS score is calculated by using the best response noted while evaluating the patient's eyes, verbal response, and motor response. If a patient lacks spontaneous eye opening, a verbal command (e.g., "Open your eyes") should be used. If the patient does not respond to a verbal stimulus, a painful stimulus, such as nail bed pressure with a pen or squeezing of anterior axillary tissue, should be applied.

The patient's verbal response can be examined using a question such as, "What happened to you?" If fully oriented, the patient will supply a coherent answer. Otherwise, the patient's verbal response is scored as confused, inappropriate, unintelligible, or absent. If the patient is intubated, the score is calculated from only the eye and motor scales, and a "T" is added to note the inability to assess the verbal response, such as "8T."

The last component of the GCS is the motor score. A simple, unambiguous command should be given to the patient, such as, "Hold up two fingers" or "Show me a hitchhiker's sign." A patient who squeezes the finger of a prehospital care provider may simply be demonstrating

TABLE 8-1 Glasgow Coma Scale

Evaluation	Points
EYE OPENING	
Spontaneous eye opening	4
Eye opening on command	3
Eye opening to painful stimulus	2
No eye opening	1
BEST VERBAL RESPONSE	
Answers appropriately (oriented)	5
Gives confused answers	4
Inappropriate response	3
Makes unintelligible noises	2
Makes no verbal response	1
BEST MOTOR RESPONSE	
Follows command	6
Localizes painful stimuli	5
Withdrawal to pain (nonlocalizing movement to pain)	4
Responds with abnormal flexion to painful stimuli (decorticate)	3
Responds with abnormal extension to pain (decerebrate)	2
Gives no motor response	1

Note that the lowest possible score is 3 and the highest possible score is 15.

a grasping reflex as opposed to following a command purposefully. A painful stimulus is used if the patient fails to follow a command and the patient's *best* motor response scored. A patient who attempts to push away a painful stimulus is considered to be "localizing." Other possible responses to pain include withdrawal from the stimulus, abnormal flexion (decorticate) or extension (decerebrate) of the upper extremities, and absence of a motor function.

The pupils are examined quickly for symmetry and response to light. A difference of greater than 1 mm in pupil size is considered abnormal. A significant portion of the population has *anisocoria,* inequality of pupil size that is either congenital or acquired as the result of ophthalmic trauma. It is not always possible in the field to distinguish between pupillary inequality caused by trauma and congenital or preexisting posttraumatic anisocoria. Pupillary inequality should always be treated as secondary to the acute trauma until the appropriate workup has ruled out cerebral edema or motor or ophthalmic nerve injury.[29]

Expose/Environment

Patients who have sustained a TBI frequently have other injuries, which threaten life and limb as well as the brain. All such injuries must be identified. The entire body should be examined for other, potentially life-threatening problems.

Secondary Survey

Once life-threatening injuries have been identified and managed, a thorough secondary survey should be completed if time permits. The patient's head and face should be palpated carefully for wounds, depressions, and crepitus. Any drainage of clear fluid from the nose or ear canals may be CSF. When placed on a gauze pad or cloth, CSF may diffuse out from blood, producing a characteristic yellowish "halo." Although a positive halo is not always caused by CSF, this is an excellent test to use in the field if time permits, because it alerts crews that a CSF leak may be present.[30]

The pupillary size and response should be rechecked at this time. Because of the incidence of cervical spine fractures in patients with TBI, as noted previously, the neck should be examined for tenderness and bony deformities.

In a cooperative patient, a more thorough neurologic examination, assessing sensory and motor function in all extremities, should also be performed. Neurologic deficits, such as hemiparesis (weakness) or hemiplegia (paralysis), may be present on only one side of the body. These "lateralizing signs" tend to be indicative of TBI.

History

An AMPLE history can be obtained from the patient, family members, or bystanders (*a*llergies, *m*edications, *p*ast history, *l*ast meal, *e*vents). Diabetes mellitus, seizure disorders, and drug or alcohol intoxication can mimic TBI. Any evidence

of drug use or overdose should be noted. The patient may have a history of prior head injury and may complain of persistent or recurring headache, visual disturbances, nausea and vomiting, or difficulty speaking.[31]

Serial Examinations

About 3% of patients with apparently mild brain injury (GCS 14 or 15) may experience an unexpected deterioration in their mentation. During transport, the primary survey and assessment of the GCS should be repeated at frequent intervals. Patients whose GCS deteriorates by more than 2 points during transport are at particularly high risk for an ongoing pathologic process.[29,32,33] These patients need rapid transport to an appropriate facility. The receiving facility will use GCS trends during transport in the patient's early management. Trends in the GCS or vital signs should be reported to the receiving facility and documented on the patient care report. Responses to management should also be recorded.[34]

Specific Injuries

Head and Neck Injuries

Scalp

As noted in the anatomy section, the scalp is composed of multiple layers of tissue and is highly vascular; even a small laceration may result in copious hemorrhage. More complex injuries, such as a degloving injury, in which a large area of the scalp is torn back from the skull, can result in hypovolemic shock and even exsanguination (Figure 8-7). These types of injury often occur in an unrestrained front-seat occupant of a vehicle whose head impacts the windshield, as well as in workers whose long hair becomes caught in machinery. A serious blow to the head may result in the formation of a scalp hematoma, which may be confused with a depressed skull fracture while palpating the scalp.

Skull Fractures

Fractures of the skull can result from either blunt or penetrating trauma. *Linear fractures* account for about 80% of skull fractures; however, a powerful impact may produce a *depressed* skull fracture, where fragments of bone are driven toward or into the underlying brain tissue (Figure 8-8). Although simple linear fractures can be diagnosed only with a radiographic study, depressed skull fractures can often be palpated during a careful physical examination. A closed, nondepressed skull fracture by itself is of little clinical significance, but its presence increases the risk of an intracranial hematoma. Closed, depressed skull fractures may require neurosurgical intervention. Open skull fractures can result from a particularly severe impact or from a gunshot wound and serve as an entry

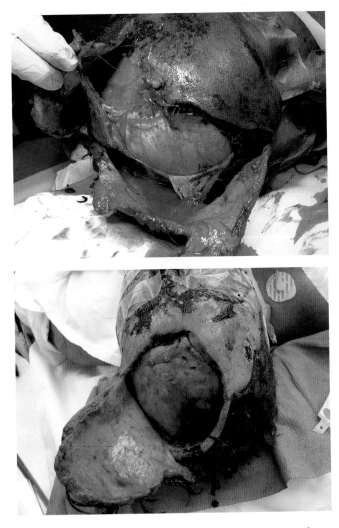

FIGURE 8-7 Extensive scalp injuries may result in massive external hemorrhage.

FIGURE 8-8 Depressed skull fracture may force particles of bone into the brain tissue.

site for bacteria, predisposing the patient to meningitis. If the dura mater is torn, brain tissue or CSF may leak from an open skull fracture. Because of the risk of meningitis, these wounds require immediate neurosurgical evaluation.

Basilar skull fractures (fractures of the floor of the cranium) should be suspected if CSF is draining from the nostrils or ear canals. Periorbital ecchymosis ("raccoon eyes") and Battle's sign, in which ecchymosis is noted over the mastoid area behind the ears, often occur with basilar skull fractures, although they may take several hours after injury to become apparent.

Facial Injuries

Injuries to the face range from minor soft tissue trauma to severe injuries associated with airway compromise or hypovolemic shock. The airway may be compromised by either structural changes resulting from the trauma or from fluid or other objects in the airway itself. Structural changes may result from deformities of the fractured facial bones or from hematomas that develop in the tissues. Because the head has a high concentration of blood vessels, many injuries to this region result in significant hemorrhage. Blood and blood clots may interfere with the patency of the airway. Facial trauma is often associated with alterations in consciousness and even severe trauma to the brain. Trauma to the face may result in fractures or displacement of teeth into the airway lumen, and TBIs and hypovolemic shock may lead to vomiting, which also leads to airway obstruction.

Mandibular Fractures. Following fractures of the nasal bones, mandibular fractures are the second most common type of facial fracture. In more than 50% of cases the mandible is broken in more than one location. The most common complaint of a patient with a mandibular fracture is malocclusion of the teeth; that is, the upper and lower teeth no longer meet in usual alignment. On palpation, a "step-off" type of deformity and crepitance may be noted.

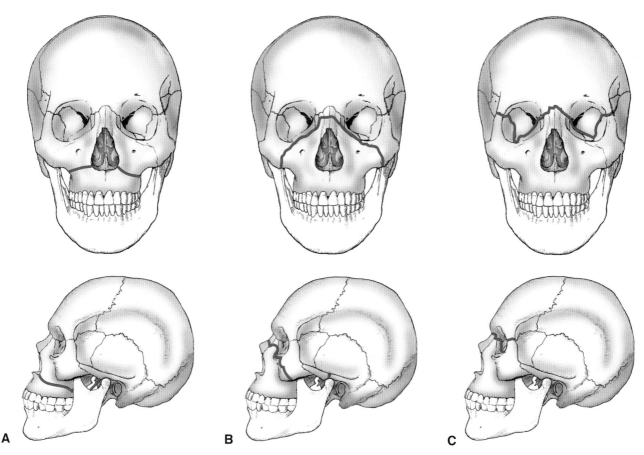

FIGURE 8-9   Types of Le Fort fractures of the midface. **A,** Le Fort I fracture. **B,** Le Fort II fracture. **C,** Le Fort III fracture. (From Sheehy S: *Emergency nursing,* ed 3, St Louis, 1992, Mosby.)

Nasal Fractures. Indications that a nasal fracture is present include ecchymosis, edema, and epistaxis. On palpation, bony abnormalities may be noted.

Midface Fractures. Midfacial fractures can be categorized as follows (Figure 8-9):

- *Le Fort I fracture* involves a horizontal detachment of the maxilla from the nasal floor. Although air passage through the nares may not be affected, the oropharynx may be compromised by a blood clot or edema in the soft palate.
- *Le Fort II fracture,* also known as a *pyramidal fracture,* includes the right and left maxillae, the medial portion of the orbital floor, and the nasal bones. The sinuses are well vascularized, and this fracture may be associated with airway compromise from significant hemorrhage.
- *Le Fort III fracture* involves the facial bones being fractured off the skull (craniofacial disjunction). Because of the forces involved, this injury may be associated with airway compromise, presence of TBI, and

injuries to the tear ducts, malocclusion of teeth, and CSF leakage from the nares.

Patients with a midface fracture generally have loss of normal facial symmetry. The face may appear flattened, and the patient may be unable to close the jaws or teeth. If conscious, the patient may complain of facial pain and numbness. On palpation, crepitus may be noted over fracture sites.

Laryngeal Injuries

Fractures of the larynx typically result from a blunt blow to the anterior neck, or a motorcycle or bicycle rider's anterior neck may be struck by an object. The patient may complain of a change in voice (usually lower in tone). On inspection, the provider may note a neck contusion or loss of the prominence of the thyroid cartilage (Adam's apple). A fracture of the larynx may result in the development of subcutaneous emphysema in the neck, which may be noted on palpation. Endotracheal intubation is generally contra-indicated in the presence of a laryngeal fracture because this procedure may dislodge fracture segments. If a patient with a suspected laryngeal fracture has a compromised airway, a surgical cricothyrotomy may be lifesaving.

Injuries to Cervical Vessels

A carotid artery and jugular vein traverse the anterior neck on either side of the trachea. The carotid arteries supply blood to the majority of the brain, and the jugular veins drain this region. Injury to one of these vessels can produce profound hemorrhage. An added danger from jugular vein injuries is air embolism. If a patient is sitting up or the head is elevated, venous pressure may fall below atmospheric pressure during inspiration, permitting air to enter the venous system. A large air embolus can be fatal because it can interfere with both cardiac function and cerebral perfusion.

Brain Injuries
Cerebral Concussion

The diagnosis of a "concussion" is made when an injured patient shows any transient alteration in neurologic function. Although most people associate a loss of consciousness with the diagnosis of concussion, loss of consciousness is not required to make a diagnosis of concussion; rather, posttraumatic amnesia is the hallmark of concussion. Other neurologic changes include the following[35]:

- Vacant stare (befuddled facial expression)
- Delayed verbal and motor responses (slow to answer questions or follow instructions)
- Confusion and inability to focus attention (easily distracted and unable to follow through with normal activities)
- Disorientation (walking in the wrong direction; unaware of time, date, and place)
- Slurred or incoherent speech (making disjointed or incomprehensible statements)
- Lack of coordination (stumbling, inability to walk tandem/straight line)
- Inappropriate emotions to the circumstances (distraught, crying for no apparent reason)
- Memory deficits (exhibited by patient repeatedly asking the same question that has already been answered)
- Inability to memorize and recall (e.g., 3 of 3 words or 3 of 3 objects in 5 minutes)

In all patients with concussion, head CT will be normal.

Severe headache, dizziness, and nausea and vomiting frequently accompany a concussion. Although most of these findings last several hours to a couple days, some patients experience a postconcussive syndrome with headaches, dizziness, and difficulty concentrating for weeks and even months after a severe concussion. Patients exhibiting signs of concussion and especially patients with nausea, vomiting, or neurologic findings on secondary survey should be immediately transported for further evaluation.

Intracranial Hematoma

Intracranial hematomas are divided into three general types: epidural, subdural, and intracerebral. Because the signs and symptoms of each of these have significant overlap, specific diagnosis in the prehospital setting (as well as the ED) is almost impossible, although the prehospital care provider may suspect an epidural hematoma based on the characteristic clinical presentation. Even so, a definitive diagnosis can only be made after a CT scan is performed at the receiving facility. Because these hematomas occupy space inside the rigid skull, they may produce rapid increases in ICP, especially if they are sizable.

Epidural Hematoma. Epidural hematomas account for about 2% of TBIs that require hospitalization. These hematomas often result from a low-velocity blow to the temporal bone, such as the impact from a punch or baseball. A fracture of this thin bone damages the middle meningeal artery, which results in arterial bleeding that collects between the skull and dura mater (Figure 8-10). This high-pressure arterial blood can start to dissect or peal the dura off of the inner table of the skull, creating an epidural space full of blood. Such an epidural hematoma has a characteristic lens shape, as seen on the CT scan, created by the dura holding the hematoma against the inner table of the skull. Because this hematoma is often created by skull fractures, there is often little direct damage to the brain beneath the hematoma. The principal threat to the brain is from the expanding mass of blood displacing the brain and threatening herniation. For this reason, patients whose epidural hematoma is rapidly evacuated often have excellent recoveries.

The classic history for an epidural hematoma is a patient experiencing a brief loss of consciousness, then regaining consciousness, and then experiencing a rapid decline in consciousness. During the period of consciousness, the *lucid interval,* the patient may be oriented, lethargic, or confused or may complain of a headache. Only about one third of patients with epidural hematomas actually experience this "lucid interval," however, and it may also occur with other intracranial bleeds, making it nonspecific for epidural hematoma. Nonetheless, a patient who experiences a "lucid interval," followed by a decline in GCS, is at risk for a progressive intracranial process and needs emergency evaluation.

As a patient's LOC worsens, examination may reveal a dilated and sluggish or nonreactive pupil on the side of the impact (ipsilateral side). Because motor nerves cross over to the other side above the spinal cord, hemiparesis or hemiplegia typically occurs on the side opposite the impact (contralateral side). The mortality rate for an epidural hematoma is about 20%; however, with rapid recognition

FIGURE 8-10   A, Epidural hematoma. **B,** CT scan of epidural hematoma.
(*B* from Cruz J: *Neurologic and neurosurgical emergencies,* Philadelphia, 1998, Saunders.)

and evacuation, the mortality rate can be as low as 2%. This is because an epidural hematoma is usually a "pure" space-occupying lesion, with little injury to the brain beneath. Once the hematoma is removed, the pathologic effect is also removed, and the patient can make an excellent recovery. Such rapid removal reduces not only mortality but also subsequent, significant neurologic morbidity. Epidural hematomas often occur in young people, who are just beginning their careers, emphasizing the societal value as well as the human value of their rapid identification and removal.

Subdural Hematoma. Subdural hematomas account for about 30% of severe brain injuries. In addition to being more common than epidural hematomas, they also differ in etiology, location, and prognosis. Unlike the epidural hematoma caused by arterial hemorrhage, a subdural hematoma generally results from a venous bleed from bridging veins that are torn during a violent blow to the head. In this injury the blood collects in the subdural space, between the dura mater and the arachnoid membrane (Figure 8-11).

Subdural hematomas present in two different ways. In some patients who have just experienced significant trauma, the disruption of the bridging veins results in relatively rapid accumulation of blood in the subdural space, with rapid onset of mass effect. Adding to this morbidity is injury to the brain parenchyma beneath the subdural hematoma, which occurs as part of the injury leading to the venous disruption. As a result, unlike epidural hematomas, the mass effect of subdural hematomas is often caused by both the accumulated blood and the swelling of the injured brain beneath. Patients presenting with such acute mass effect will have an acutely depressed mental status and will need emergency ICP monitoring and management and possibly surgery.

In some patient populations, however, clinically occult subdural hematomas can occur. In elderly or debilitated patients, such as those with chronic disease, the subdural space is enlarged secondary to brain atrophy. In such patients, blood may accumulate in the subdural space without inducing mass effect and thus may be clinically occult. Such subdural hematomas can occur during falls in elderly persons or during apparently minor trauma. At particular

FIGURE 8-11 **A,** Subdural hematoma. **B,** CT scan of subdural hematoma.
(**B** from Cruz J: *Neurologic and neurosurgical emergencies,* Philadelphia, 1998, Saunders.)

risk are patients receiving anticoagulants such as warfarin (Coumadin). Because these falls are minor, patients often do not present for evaluation, and the bleeds are not identified. Many patients in whom chronic subdural hematoma is eventually identified cannot recall the traumatic event.

In some patients in whom occult subdural hematoma *is* eventually identified, however, the subdural blood liquefies but is retained in the subdural space. Over time, through a mechanism that includes repeated small bleeds into the liquid hematoma, the now-chronic subdural hematoma can expand and slowly start to exert mass effect on the brain. Because the onset of the mass effect is slow, the patient will not have the dramatic presentation associated with an acute subdural hematoma and is more likely to present with headache, visual disturbances, personality changes, difficulty speaking (dysarthria), and hemiparesis or hemiplegia of a slowly progressive nature. Only when some of these symptoms become pronounced enough to prompt the patient or caregiver to seek help is the chronic subdural hematoma discovered. On CT scan a chronic subdural hematoma has a distinct appearance compared with the more emergent, acute subdural hematoma. Often the event precipitating transport for evaluation and care is the most recent of the small, repetitive subdural bleeds that create chronic subdural hematomas, and a small amount of acute blood may be found in a larger collection of chronic blood. The need for and the urgency of surgery are determined by the patient's symptoms, the amount of mass effect, and the patient's overall medical condition.

Prehospital personnel frequently encounter these patients when called to facilities that care for chronically ill populations. Because the symptoms are nonspecific, diagnosing a chronic subdural hematoma in the field is rarely possible, and the symptoms may be confused with those of a stroke, infection, or even a generalized decline in the patient.

Although many subdural hematomas in these patients will be chronic, patients taking Coumadin, after an apparently insignificant trauma, may have a subdural hematoma that expands over several hours and progresses to herniation resulting from the patient's inability to clot. These patients can have a benign presentation and then deteriorate several hours after arrival. Elderly patients, and especially patients receiving Coumadin, who have experienced apparently minor falls should be managed with a heightened sense of urgency and care.

Cerebral Contusions. Damage to the brain itself may produce cerebral contusions and, if this damage includes injury to the blood vessels within the brain, actual bleeding into the substance of the brain, or *intracerebral hematomas.* Cerebral contusions are relatively common, occurring in about 20% to 30% of severe brain injuries, but in a significant percentage of moderate head injuries as well. Although typically the result of blunt trauma, these injuries may also occur from penetrating trauma, such as a gunshot wound to the brain. In blunt trauma, cerebral contusions may be numerous. Cerebral contusions result from a complex pattern of transmission and reflection of forces within the skull. As a result, contusions often occur in locations remote from the site of impact, often on the opposite side of the brain, the familiar "contrecoup" injury.

Cerebral contusions often take 12 to 24 hours to appear on CT scans, and thus a patient with a cerebral contusion may have an initially normal head CT scan. The only clue to its presence may be a depressed GCS, with many patients showing moderate head injuries (GCS 9-13). As the contusion evolves after injury, it not only becomes more apparent on head CT, but also can cause increased mass effect and create increasing headache, or cause moderate head injuries to deteriorate to severe head injuries in about 10% of patients.[36]

Subarachnoid Hemorrhage. Subarachnoid hemorrhage is bleeding beneath the arachnoid membrane, which lies under the subdural space covering the brain. Blood in the subarachnoid space cannot enter the subdural space. Many of the brain's blood vessels are located in the subarachnoid space, so injury to these vessels will cause subarachnoid bleeding, a layering of blood beneath the arachnoid membrane on the surface of the brain. This layering of blood is thin and rarely causes mass effect.

Subarachnoid hemorrhage is usually thought to be associated with ruptured cerebral aneurysms. In fact, posttraumatic subarachnoid hemorrhage is the most common cause of subarachnoid bleeding. Because subarachnoid bleeding rarely causes mass effect, it does not require surgery for decompression. It is a marker for potentially severe brain injury, however, and its presence increases the risk for other space-occupying lesions. Patients with traumatic subarachnoid hemorrhage (tSAH) have a 63% to 73% increased risk of a cerebral contusion, and 44% will develop subdural hematomas. Patients with tSAH have an increased risk of elevated ICP and intraventricular hemorrhage. Patients with large amounts of tSAH (>1 cm of blood thickness, blood in suprasellar or ambient cisterns) have a positive predictive value of 72% to 78% for a poor outcome, and in the Trauma Coma Data Bank the presence of tSAH doubled the incidence of death in brain-injured patients.[37,38]

Management

Effective management of a patient with TBI begins with orderly interventions focused on treating any life-threatening problems identified in the primary survey. Once these problems are addressed, the patient should be rapidly packaged and transported to the nearest facility capable of caring for TBI.

Airway

Patients with a depressed LOC may be unable to protect their airway, and adequate oxygenation of the injured brain is critical to preventing secondary injury. As noted earlier, facial injuries can be associated with hemorrhage and edema that may compromise the airway. Hematomas in the floor of the mouth or in the soft palate may occlude the airway. The essential skills are appropriate initial airway interventions (see Chapter 6). Both oral and nasal airways may become occluded by edema or blood clots, and intermittent suctioning may be necessary. Patients with facial fractures and laryngeal or other neck injuries will typically assume a position that maintains their airway. Attempts to force a patient to lay supine or wear a cervical collar may be met with extreme combativeness if they become hypoxic as a result of positional airway impairment. In these situations, airway patency takes precedence over spinal immobilization, and patients may be transported in a sitting or semisitting position, as tolerated. Cervical collars may be deferred if thought to compromise the airway while manual stabilization is performed. Conscious patients can often assist in managing their airway by suctioning when they feel it is needed; the provider can allow them to hold and use the suction device. Facial trauma, including those injuries caused by GSWs, is not a contraindication to ET intubation.

An early study showed that victims of TBI who were intubated appeared to do better.[39] Recent studies, however, have yielded mixed results in TBI casualties intubated in the field.[40-44] The explanation for these conflicting data awaits further study. Under some circumstances, however, poorly performed intubation may be more harmful than no intubation at all. The deciding factors may be operator skill and length of transport. In urban settings, short transport times allow patients to be fairly urgently delivered to and intubated in an ED setting. Patients intubated in the field may do worse because of prolonged field times and a less experienced provider performing the intubation. Similarly, intubation in a system where providers perform only a few intubations a year may be more detrimental than other means of airway support during transport. Conversely, in systems with longer transport times, intubation may be more beneficial than no intubation at all, even when done by a less experienced operator. Future studies should help determine the best practice in the prehospital environment.

With these qualifiers in mind, all patients with a severe TBI (GCS ≤8) should be considered for intubation. Because this can be extremely challenging due to the patient's combativeness, clenched jaw muscles (trismus), vomiting, and the need to maintain inline cervical spine stabilization, intubation should be performed by the most skilled operator who can be available in a timely manner. The use of neuromuscular blocking agents as part of a rapid-sequence intubation (RSI) protocol may facilitate successful intubation.[45] Blind nasotracheal intubation (BNTI) can serve as an alternative technique, but the presence of midface trauma is a relative contraindication for this procedure. Suction equipment should be readily available. If initial attempts at intubation are unsuccessful, prolonged laryngoscopy should be avoided, especially with a short transport time. An oropharyngeal airway with bag-valve-mask (BVM) ventilation or percutaneous transtracheal ventilation (PTV) are reasonable alternatives. Patients with severe facial injuries and obvious airway compromise may require PTV or a surgical cricothyrotomy.

Breathing

All patients with suspected TBI should receive supplemental oxygen. The use of pulse oximetry is strongly recommended because hypoxia can worsen neurologic outcome. Oxygen concentration can be titrated when using pulse oximetry; Spo_2 should be at least 90%, with 95% or higher being optimal. If pulse oximetry is not available, oxygen should be provided via a nonrebreather facemask for a spontaneously breathing patient. For intubated patients, an oxygen concentration of 100% (Fio_2 of 1.0) should be maintained with a BVM device. If hypoxia persists despite oxygen therapy, the provider should attempt to identify and treat all likely etiologies, including aspiration and tension pneumothoraces. Use of positive end-expiratory pressure (PEEP) valves, if available, may be considered to improve oxygenation; however, levels of PEEP greater than 15 cm H_2O may increase ICP.[46,47]

Because both hypocapnia and hypercapnia can aggravate TBI, control of ventilatory rate is important. When arterial blood gases (ABGs) are available, $Paco_2$ should be maintained in the range of 35 to 40 mm Hg. In the hospital setting, end-tidal carbon dioxide ($ETco_2$) can be used to estimate serum $Paco_2$ in hemodynamically stable patients. Because the measured values for $ETco_2$ and $Paco_2$ vary widely from patient to patient, each in-hospital patient must have a unique "offset" between $Paco_2$ and $ETco_2$ determined by comparison with an ABG to obtain acceptable accuracy from the use of $ETco_2$. New ABGs are obtained each time the patient's condition changes.

In the prehospital environment, $Paco_2$ is not routinely available to determine its "offset" with $ETco_2$. In addition, other patient factors, such as changes in pulmonary perfusion, in cardiac output, and in patient temperature, all cause changes in $ETco_2$, which cannot be distinguished from $ETco_2$ changes that result from changes in $Paco_2$. Because physiologic changes occur rapidly in the prehospital phase as patients are resuscitated and warmed as well as ventilated, they are rarely stable enough to allow $ETco_2$ to be used with any accuracy. Although $ETco_2$ is an excellent tool for monitoring ventilation, it is not accurate enough to guide hyperventilation therapy meaningfully in the prehospital setting.[48-56]

It is simpler and as accurate simply to judge degree of ventilation by counting breaths per minute.

Normal ventilatory rates should be used when assisting ventilation in patients with TBI: 10 breaths/min for adults, 20 breaths/min for children, and 25 breaths/min for infants. Overaggressive hyperventilation produces cerebral vasoconstriction, which in turn leads to a decrease in cerebral oxygen delivery. Routine prophylactic hyperventilation has been shown to worsen neurologic outcome and should not be used. A subgroup analysis of patients enrolled in the San Diego Paramedic RSI trial showed that both hyperventilation and severe hypoxia in the prehospital setting were associated with an increase in mortality. For adult patients, ventilating with a tidal volume of 350 to 500 mL at a rate of 10 breaths/min should be sufficient to maintain adequate oxygenation without inducing hypocarbia.[57]

Circulation

Both anemia and hypotension are important causes of secondary brain injury, so efforts should be taken to prevent or treat these conditions. Hemorrhage control is essential. Direct pressure or pressure dressings should be applied to any external hemorrhage. Complex scalp wounds can produce significant external blood loss. Several gauze pads held in place by an elastic roller bandage creates an effective pressure dressing to control bleeding. If this fails to control bleeding, it can often be controlled by applying direct pressure along the wound edges, thereby compressing the scalp vasculature between the skin and soft tissues and the galea. Dramatic bleeding can often be controlled with this maneuver. A pressure dressing should not be applied to a depressed or open skull fracture unless significant hemorrhage is present, because it may aggravate brain injury and lead to an increase in ICP. Direct gentle pressure may also limit the size of extracranial (scalp) hematomas. Gentle handling and immobilization to a long backboard in anatomic alignment can minimize interstitial blood loss around fractures.

Hemorrhage from the carotid arteries and jugular veins may be massive. In most circumstances, direct pressure will control such external hemorrhage. Injuries to these vessels from penetrating trauma may be associated with internal bleeding presenting as an expanding hematoma. These hematomas may compromise the airway, and endotracheal intubation may be necessary. However, attempts to intubate a conscious patient with an expanding neck hematoma but no external bleeding may stimulate a cough, which may be sufficient to disrupt a clot that may have formed at a knife or bullet wound, resulting in massive external hemorrhage.

Because hypotension further worsens brain ischemia, standard measures should be employed to combat shock. In patients with TBI, the combination of hypoxia and hypotension is associated with a mortality rate of about 75%. If shock is present and major internal hemorrhage is suspected, prompt transport to a trauma center takes priority over brain injuries. Hypovolemic and neurogenic shock are aggressively treated by resuscitation with isotonic crystalloid solutions; however, transport should not be delayed to establish intravenous (IV) access. Although assessing blood volume is extremely difficult in the prehospital setting, the patient should be returned to a state of normal circulating blood volume (euvolemia) if possible. To preserve cerebral perfusion, attempts should be made to maintain an SBP of at least 90 to 100 mm Hg. For adult TBI patients with normal vital signs and no other suspected injuries, IV fluid at a rate of no more than 125 mL/hr should be administered and adjusted if signs of shock develop.[58] A randomized trial of patients with severe TBI showed that those who received prehospital resuscitation with hypertonic saline had almost identical neurologic functioning 6 months after injury compared to those treated with crystalloid.[59] Because of its increased cost and lack of benefit compared to normal saline or lactated Ringer's solution, hypertonic saline is not recommended for routine prehospital volume replacement.

Disability

Assessment of the GCS should be integrated into the routine evaluation of all trauma patients after circulation is addressed. Use of the GCS helps evaluate the patient's status and may impact transport and triage decisions, depending on the system in which the provider is working.

Prehospital management of TBI patients primarily consists of measures aimed at reversing and preventing factors that cause secondary brain injury. Prolonged or multiple grand mal seizures can be treated with IV administration of a benzodiazepine, such as diazepam, lorazepam, or midazolam. These drugs should be cautiously titrated because hypotension and ventilatory depression may occur.

Because of the significant incidence of cervical spine fractures, patients with suspected TBI should be placed in spinal immobilization. Some degree of caution must be exercised when applying a cervical collar to a patient with TBI. Some evidence suggests that a tightly fitted cervical collar can impede venous drainage of the head, thereby increasing ICP. *Application of a cervical collar is not mandatory as long as the head and neck are sufficiently immobilized.*

Transportation

To achieve the best possible outcome, patients with moderate and severe TBI should be transported directly to a trauma center that can perform a CT scan and ICP monitoring and provide prompt neurosurgical intervention. If such a facility is not available, aeromedical transport from the scene to an appropriate trauma center should be considered.[34]

The patient's pulse rate, blood pressure, SpO_2, and GCS should be reassessed and documented every 5 to 10 minutes during transport. PEEP valves may be used cautiously if persistent hypoxia exists because, as noted, levels of PEEP greater than 15 cm H_2O may increase ICP. The patient's body heat should be preserved during transport.

Controversy exists regarding the optimal position for a patient with TBI. In general, patients with TBI should be transported in a supine position because of the presence of other injuries.[60] Although elevating the head on the ambulance stretcher or long backboard (reverse Trendelenburg position) may decrease ICP, cerebral perfusion pressure may also be jeopardized, especially if the head is elevated higher than 30 degrees.

The receiving facility should be notified as early as possible so that appropriate preparations can be made before the patient's arrival. The radio report should include information regarding the mechanism of injury, initial GCS score and any changes en route, focal signs (e.g., motor exam asymmetry, unilaterally or bilaterally dilated pupils) and vital signs, other serious injuries, and response to management.[34]

Prolonged Transport

As with all patients with suspected TBI, efforts should focus on preventing secondary brain injury. A prolonged transport time may lower the threshold for performing endotracheal intubation. RSI may be used in this setting, especially if aeromedical transport is considered, because a combative patient in the confines of a helicopter threatens the crew, pilot, and himself. Efforts to control the airway should be performed while cervical spine stabilization is being applied. Oxygenation should be administered to maintain an appropriate SpO_2 level. Because of the risk of developing pressure ulcers from lying on a hard backboard, the patient may be placed on a padded long backboard, especially if the anticipated transport time is lengthy. Patients should be attached to continuous pulse oximetry, and serial vital signs, including ventilations, pulse, blood pressure, and GCS score, should be measured. Pupils should be periodically checked for response to light and symmetry.

When there is a delay in transport or a prolonged transport time to an appropriate facility, additional management options can be considered. For patients with an abnormal GCS score, the blood glucose level should be checked. If the patient is hypoglycemic, a 50% dextrose solution can be administered intravenously until the blood sugar is restored to a normal level. Benzodiazepines may be titrated intravenously if recurrent or prolonged seizures occur.

External hemorrhage should be controlled, and volume resuscitation is administered if signs of shock are apparent.

Fluids should be titrated to maintain the SBP greater than 90 mm Hg. Associated injuries should be managed while en route to the receiving facility. Fractures should be appropriately splinted to control both internal hemorrhage and pain.

Appropriate management of increased ICP in the prehospital setting is extremely challenging because the ICP is not monitored in the field unless the patient is undergoing interfacility transfer and an ICP monitor or ventriculostomy has been placed at the referring center. Although a declining GCS score may represent increasing ICP, it may also be the result of worsening cerebral perfusion from hypovolemic shock. Warning signs of possible increased ICP and herniation include the following:

- Decline in GCS score of two points or more
- Development of a sluggish or nonreactive pupil
- Development of hemiplegia or hemiparesis
- Cushing's phenomenon

The decision to intervene and manage increased ICP is based on written protocol or made in consultation with medical control at the receiving facility. Possible temporizing management options include sedation, chemical paralysis, osmotherapy (the use of osmotically active agents that may assist in the treatment of intracranial hypertension), and controlled hyperventilation. Small doses of benzodiazepine sedatives should be titrated cautiously because of the potential side effects of hypotension and ventilatory depression. Use of a long-acting neuromuscular blocking agent, such as vecuronium, may be considered if the patient is intubated. If the cervical collar is believed to be too tight, it may be loosened slightly or removed, provided that the head and neck are adequately immobilized with other measures.

Osmotherapy with mannitol (0.25-1.0 g/kg) can be given intravenously. However, aggressive diuresis may produce hypovolemia, which can worsen cerebral perfusion. Mannitol should be avoided for patients in whom systemic resuscitation has not been achieved, that is, patients with SBP less than 90 mm Hg. If an osmotic agent is used, the patient should be maintained in a euvolemic state. In addition, a Foley catheter should be placed if transport will be extremely prolonged.

Controlled, mild therapeutic hyperventilation may be considered for obvious signs of herniation. The following ventilatory rates should be used: 20 breaths/min for adults, 30 breaths/min for children, and 35 breaths/min for infants. *Prophylactic hyperventilation has no role in TBI, and therapeutic hyperventilation, if instituted, should be stopped if signs of intracranial hypertension resolve.* Steroids have not been shown to improve the outcome of patients with TBI and should not be administered.

The primary focus for the TBI patient during prolonged transport or in austere environments is the best possible maintenance of cerebral oxygenation and perfusion and the best efforts possible to control cerebral edema.

Brain Death and Organ Donation

The diagnosis of brain death is made when there is no clinical evidence of neurologic function in a patient who is warm, whose mental status is not impacted by sedating or paralyzing medications, and who is completely resuscitated with an SBP greater than 90 mm Hg and SpO_2 greater than 90%.

Assessment for clinical evidence of neurologic function consists of ensuring that there is no evidence of cortical function, followed by an assessment of midbrain and brainstem function down to the respiratory center in the lower medulla. This assessment consists of establishing the absence of response to deep pain, followed by the midbrain and brainstem assessment for nonreactive pupils, absence of a corneal reflex, and absence of response to cold caloric stimulation. A few patients can safely be tested for the absence of an oculocephalic reflex. In addition, absence of a gag reflex, absence of a cough reflex, and finally the absence of any effort to breathe, with $PaCO_2$ greater than 60 mm Hg and adequate PO_2, are all determined. This last observation is obtained with an apnea test. In the absence of any activity on these tests, the patient can be declared clinically "brain dead."

Many clinical protocols and some state statutes also require that brain death be confirmed by an ancillary test, such as radionucleotide CBF studies or electroencephalography (EEG).

The physiologic definition of brain death just described is the definition typically used in the United States. Philosophical, ethical, and legal issues remain about how much of the brain must be dead before "personhood" is lost, and thus the definition of brain death varies throughout the world. In addition, various hospitals and systems have differing methods for declaring brain death, and the states have varying legal statutes defining who may declare death and brain death and how it is to be declared. Those interested should ask within their local system.

It must be emphasized, however, that brain death is not the same as a "hopeless prognosis." Brain death is a *physiologic* event in which the brain dies while the heart and lungs are still functioning, usually through artificial support. As noted, how much brain must die before declaring brain death is debatable, but the fact that it is a physiologic event is not debatable.

In contrast, a hopeless prognosis is a medical judgment that a good outcome is not possible from the current injuries. This distinction is often blurred by health care providers, with the resulting confusion resulting in a loss of credibility on the part of the health care system.

This credibility is critical because the victims of TBI that progresses to brain death provide an important source of organs for transplantation. In 1999, TBI was the cause of brain death for more than 40% of individuals from whom organs were procured, with the majority of organs coming from those between 18 and 49 years of age. Despite the presence of a fatal brain injury, an individual's heart, lungs, liver, kidneys, pancreas, and corneas may benefit others with chronic illnesses. Enlisting the trust and support of the public in obtaining these organs is critical to ensuring their availability to those who so desperately need them. To gain this trust, the families of TBI victims first need to be sure that the resuscitation of the injured brain has been the first priority of the treating team, and second, when that resuscitation has failed, they need to understand the issues surrounding physiologic brain death versus a futile situation. A clear understanding of these issues empowers families to make good decisions for themselves and their loved one, decisions that they can live with as they gain more information in the aftermath of the event. Blurring or confusing these issues erodes the trust of the family and the credibility of the health care and organ procurement communities. It is essential that health care providers clearly understand the issues surrounding brain death and effectively communicate these issues to the family members of the victims of TBI.

MANAGEMENT OF SUSPECTED TRAUMATIC BRAIN INJURY

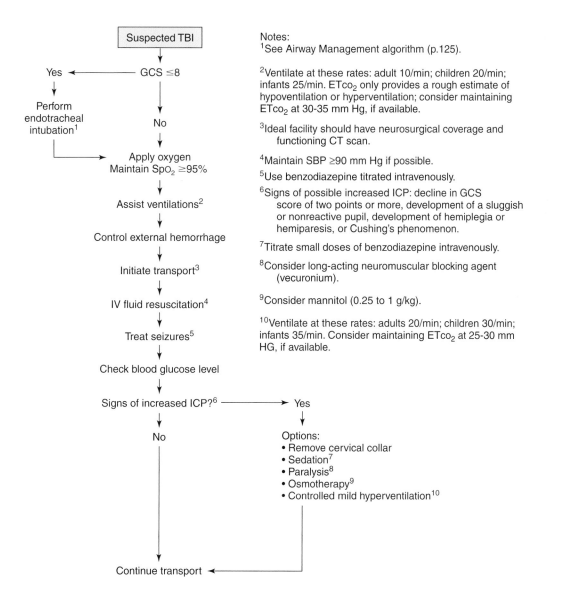

SUMMARY

Head injury is a common feature of trauma. Aggressive management to maintain cerebral perfusion and prevent secondary brain injury can make a difference in morbidity and mortality from traumatic brain injury (TBI). Unrecognized and untreated hypoxia and reduced cerebral blood flow in the field can make the difference between a good and an unacceptable outcome. Only the prehospital provider can intervene to prevent this injury in the early stages of trauma. Therefore the role of the prehospital care provider in determining the outcome for the patient with TBI cannot be overstated.

The severity of TBI may not be immediately apparent; therefore, the prehospital care provider needs to maintain a high index of suspicion based on mechanism of injury and to perform serial neurologic evaluations of the patient, including Glasgow Coma Scale scores and pupillary response.

TBI may be found concomitant with multisystem trauma, so all problems are addressed in the appropriate order of priority. Not only are airway, breathing, and circulation always the priorities of patient care, but they are specifically important in the management of TBI in preventing secondary brain injury.

The goals of immediate prehospital management of the TBI patient in the short term are accomplished by controlling hemorrhage from other injuries, maintaining a systolic blood pressure of at least 90 mm Hg, providing oxygenation to maintain oxygen saturation of at least 90%, and only hyperventilating patients with objective signs of herniation. When transport to an appropriate facility is prolonged, these goals are pursued more aggressively with sedation, chemical paralysis, osmotherapy, and controlled hyperventilation. The prehospital care provider not only has an important role in the prehospital care of the TBI patient, but also has a significant influence on in-hospital care by selecting the appropriate facility to which to transport the patient. Prehospital care providers also need to play a high-profile role in TBI prevention through patient and public education efforts.

SCENARIO SOLUTION

The rapid decrease in this patient's GCS score is extremely worrisome, so you need to transport the patient to a facility with neurosurgical coverage immediately on completion of spinal immobilization. Given the lucid interval demontrated by this patient, suspect the presence of an epidural hematoma. Examination of the eyes may reveal an enlarged, sluggishly reactive pupil on the right side, and weakness or paralysis may develop on the left side of the body. A CT scan at the receiving trauma center can confirm the diagnosis.

Once en route, reevaluate the patient's airway and breathing and apply a pulse oximeter. If his Spo$_2$ is less than 95%, you apply supplemental oxygen and assist ventilations with a BVM device. Additionally, given the mechanism of injury, consider a pneumothorax. If the GCS score further deteriorates, also consider intubating this patient, preferably using a rapid-sequence technique. Reassess the scalp wound to ensure that hemorrhage is adequately controlled and start two large-bore IV lines. Measure the patient's vital signs and take a blood pressure

reading. The mild tachycardia may suggest compensated shock from intraabdominal hemorrhage from the liver or spleen or retroperitoneal hemorrhage from a pelvic fracture. Perform a complete secondary survey to rule out additional injuries, and you determine blood glucose level. During transport, you frequently assess the patency of the patient's airway, measure his vital signs, and check his GCS score and papillary response. Notify the receiving facility of the patient's condition and update it if any significant changes occur.

If transport to an appropriate facility is prolonged and the patient's neurologic status continues to deteriorate, further measures can be taken. After endotracheal intubation, titrate a benzodiazepine sedative intravenously. Consider a dose of mannitol, as well as mild, controlled hyperventilation. When combined with appropriate neurosurgical intervention, aggressive prehospital care should improve the outcome of patients with moderate to severe TBI. ∎

References

1. Chestnut RM, Marshall LF, Klauber MR, et al: The role of secondary brain injury in determining outcome from severe head injury, *J Trauma* 34:216, 1993.
2. Fearnside MR, Cook RJ, McDougall P, et al: The Westmead Head Injury Project outcome in severe head injury: a comparative analysis of pre-hospital, clinical and CT variables, *Br J Neurosurg* 7:267, 1993.
3. Gentleman D: Causes and effects of systemic complications among severely head injured patients transferred to a neurosurgical unit, *Int Surg* 77:297, 1992.
4. Marmarou A, Anderson RL, Ward JL, et al: Impact of ICP instability and hypotension on outcome in patients with severe head trauma, *J Neurosurg* 75:S59, 1991.
5. Miller JD, Becker DP: Secondary insults to the injured brain, *J R Coll Surg Edinb* 27:292, 1982.
6. Obrist WD, Gennarelli TA, Segawa H, et al: Relation of cerebral blood flow to neurologic status and outcome in head injured patients, *J Neurosurg* 51:292, 1979.
7. Obrist WD, Langfitt TW, Jaggi JL, et al: Cerebral blood flow and metabolism in comatose patients with acute head injury, *J Neurosurg* 61:241, 1984.
8. Marshall LF, Toole BM, Bowers SA: Patients who talk and deteriorate. Part 2. Implications for treatment, *J Neurosurg* 59:285, 1983.
9. Reilly PL, Adams JH, Graham DI, Jennett B: Patients with head injury who talk and die, *Lancet* 2:375, 1975.
10. Rose J, Valtonen S, Jennett B: Avoidable factors contributing to death after head injury, *BMJ* 2:615, 1977.
11. Miller JD, Sweet RC, Narayan RK, et al: Early insults to the injured brain, *JAMA* 240:439, 1978.
12. Silverston P: Pulse oximetry at the roadside: a study of pulse oximetry in immediate care, *BMJ* 298:711, 1989.
13. Stochetti N, Furlan A, Volta F: Hypoxemia and arterial hypotension at the accident scene in head injury, *J Trauma* 40:764, 1996.
14. Kellie G: An account of the appearances observed in the dissection of two of three individuals presumed to have perished in the storm of the 3rd, and whose bodies were discovered in the vicinity of Leith on the morning of the 4th of November 1821 with some reflections on the pathology of the brain, *Trans Med Chir Sci Edinb* 1:84, 1824.
15. Plum F: *The diagnosis of stupor and coma,* ed 3, New York, 1982, Oxford University Press.
16. Langfitt TW, Weinstein JD, Kassell NF, Simeone FA: Transmission of increased intracranial pressure. I. Within the craniospinal axis, *J Neurosurg* 21:989, 1964.
17. Langfitt TW: Increased intracranial pressure, *Clin Neurosurg* 16:436, 1969.
18. Graham DI, Ford I, Adams JH, et al: Ischeaemic brain damage is still common in fatal non-missle head injury, *J Neurol Neurosurg Psychiatry* 52:346, 1989.
19. Marmarou A, Anderson RL, Ward JL, et al: Impact of ICP instability and hypotension on outcome in patients with severe head trauma, *J Neurosurg* 75:S59, 1991.
20. Obrist WD, Wilkinson WE: Regional cerebral blood flow measurement in humans by xenon-133 clearance, *Cerebrovasc Brain Metab Rev* 2:283, 1990.

21. Darby JM, Yonas H, Marion DW, et al: Local "inverse steal" induced by hyperventilation in head injury, *Neurosurgery* 23:84, 1988.

22. Marion DW, Darby J, Yonas H: Acute regional cerebral blood flow changes caused by severe head injuries, *J Neurosurg* 74:407, 1991.

23. Manley GT, Pitts LH, Morabito D, et al: Brain tissue oxygenation during hemorrhagic shock, resuscitation, and alterations in ventilation, *J Trauma Injury Infect Crit Care* 46:261, 1999.

24. Caron MJ, Hovda DA, Mazziotta JC, et al: The structural and metabolic anatomy of traumatic brain injury in humans: a computerized tomography and positron emission tomography analysis, *J Neurotrauma* 10(suppl 1):S58, 1993.

25. Caron MJ, Mazziotta JC, Hovda DA, Becker DP: Quantification of cerebral glucose metabolism in brain injured humans utilizing positron emission tomography, *J Cereb Blood Flow Metab* 13(suppl 1):S379, 1993.

26. Caron MJ: PET/SPECT imaging in head injury. In Narayan RK, Wilberger JE, Povlishock JT, editors: *Neurotrauma*, New York, 1996, McGraw-Hill.

27. Lam AM, Winn HR, Cullen BF, Sundling N: Hyperglycemia and neurological outcome in patients with head injury, *J Neurosurg* 75:545, 1991.

28. Young B, Ott L, Dempsey R, et al: Relationship between admission hyperglycemia and neurologic outcome of severely brain-injured patients, *Ann Surg* 210:466, 1989.

29. Brain Trauma Foundation: Glasgow Coma Score. In *Guidelines for prehospital management of traumatic brain injury*, New York, 2000, The Foundation.

30. Dula DJ, Fales W: The 'ring sign': is it a reliable indicator for cerebral spinal fluid? *Ann Emerg Med* 22:718, 1993.

31. American College of Surgeons: *Advanced trauma life support*, Chicago, 2004, The College.

32. Servadei F, Nasi MT, Cremonini AM: Importance of a reliable admission Glasgow Coma Scale score for determining the need for evacuation of post-traumatic subdural hematomas: a prospective study of 65 patients, *J Trauma* 44:868, 1998.

33. Winkler JV, Rosen P, Alfrey EJ: Prehospital use of the Glasgow Coma Scale in severe head injury, *J Emerg Med* 2:1, 1984.

34. Brain Trauma Foundation: Hospital transport decisions. In *Guidelines for prehospital management of traumatic brain injury*, New York, 2000, The Foundation.

35. American Academy of Neurology: The management of concussion in sports (summary statement), *Neurology* 48:581, 1997.

36. Rimel RW, Giordani B, Barth JT: Moderate head injury: completing the clinical spectrum of brain trauma, *Neurosurgery* 11:344, 1982.

37. Brain Trauma Foundation: CT scan features. In *Management and prognosis of severe traumatic brain injury,* ed 2, New York, 2000, The Foundation.

38. Kihtir T, Ivatury RR, Simon RJ, et al: Early management of civilian gunshot wounds to the face, *J Trauma* 35:569, 1993.

39. Winchell RJ, Hoyt DB: Endotracheal intubation in the field improves survival in patients with severe head injury, *Arch Surg* 132:592, 1997.

40. Davis DP, Hoyt DB, Ochs M, et al: The effect of paramedic rapid sequence intubation on outcome in patients with severe traumatic brain injury, *J Trauma Injury Infect Crit Care* 54:444, 2003.

41. Bochicchio GV, Ilahi O, Joshi M, et al: Endotracheal intubation in the field does not improve outcome in trauma patients who present without an acutely lethal traumatic brain injury, *J Trauma Injury Infect Crit Care* 54:307, 2003.

42. Davis DP, Peay J, Sise MJ, et al: The impact of prehospital endotracheal intubation in moderate to severe traumatic brain injury, *J Trauma* 58:933, 2005.

43. Bulger EM, Copass MK, Sabath DR, et al: The use of neuromuscular blocking agents to facilitate prehospital intubation does not impair outcome after traumatic brain injury, *J Trauma* 58:718, 2005.

44. Wang HE, Peitzman AB, Cassidy LD, et al: Out-of-hospital endotracheal intubation and outcome after traumatic brain injury, *Ann Emerg Med* 44:439, 2004.

45. Davis DP, Ochs M, Hoyt DB, et al: Paramedic-administered neuromuscular blockade improves prehospital intubation success in severely head-injured patients, *J Trauma Injury Infect Crit Care* 55:713, 2003.

46. Cooper KR, Boswell PA, Choi SC: Safe use of PEEP in patients with severe brain injury, *J Neurosurg* 63:552, 1985.

47. McGuire G, Crossley D, Richards J, Wong D: Effects of varying levels of positive end-expiratory pressure on intracranial pressure and cerebral perfusion pressure, *Crit Care Med* 25:1059, 1997.

48. Christensen MA, Bloom J, Sutton KR: Comparing arterial and end-tidal carbon dioxide values in hyperventilated neurosurgical patients, *Am J Crit Care* 4:116, 1995.

49. Grenier B, Dubreuil M: Noninvasive monitoring of carbon dioxide: end-tidal versus transcutaneous carbon dioxide, *Anesth Analg* 86:675, 1998.

50. Grenier B, Verchere E, Mesli A, et al: Capnography monitoring during neurosurgery: reliability in relation to various intraoperative positions, *Anesth Analg* 88:43, 1999.

51. Isert P: Control of carbon dioxide levels during neuroanaesthesia: current practice and an appraisal of our reliance upon capnography, *Anaesth Intensive Care* 22:435, 1994.

52. Kerr ME, Zempsky J, Sereika S, et al: Relationship between arterial carbon dioxide and end-tidal carbon dioxide in mechanically ventilated adults with severe head trauma, *Crit Care Med* 24:785, 1996.

53. Mackersie RC, Karagianes TG: Use of end-tidal carbon dioxide tension for monitoring induced hypocapnia in head-injured patients, *Crit Care Med* 18:764, 1990.

54. Russell GB, Graybeal JM: Reliability of the arterial to end-tidal carbon dioxide gradient in mechanically ventilated patients with multisystem trauma, *J Trauma Injury Infect Crit Care* 36:317, 1994.

55. Sanders AB: Capnometry in emergency medicine, *Ann Emerg Med* 18:1287-53, 1989.

56. Sharma SK, McGuire GP, Cruise CJE: Stability of the arterial to end-tidal carbon dioxide difference during anaesthesia for prolonged neuro-surgical procedures, *Can J Anaesthesiol* 42:498, 1995.

57. Davis DP, Dunford JV, Poste JC, et al: The impact of hypoxia and hyperventilation on outcome after paramedic rapid sequence intubation of severely head injured patients, *J Trauma* 57:1, 2004.

58. Brain Trauma Foundation: Treatment: fluid resuscitation. In *Guidelines for prehospital management of traumatic brain injury*, New York, 2000, The Foundation.

59. Cooper DJ, Myles PS, McDermott FT, et al: Prehospital hypertonic saline resuscitation of patients with hypotension and severe traumatic brain injury: a randomized controlled trial, *JAMA* 291:1350, 2004.

60. Feldman Z, Kanter MJ, Robertson CS: Effect of head elevation on intracranial pressure, cerebral perfusion pressure and cerebral blood flow in head-injured patients, *J Neurosurg* 76:207, 1992.

Suggested Reading

American College of Surgeons Committee on Trauma: Head trauma. In *Advanced trauma life support for doctors, student course manual,* ed 7, Chicago, 2004, ACS.

Atkinson JLD: The neglected prehospital phase of head injury: apnea and catecholamine surge, *Mayo Clin Proceed* 75:37, 2000.

Bertz JE: Maxillofacial injuries, *Clin Symp* 33:2, 1981.

Chi JH, Nemani V, Manley GT: Prehospital treatment of traumatic brain injury, *Sem Neurosurg* 14:71, 2003.

Guidelines for the determination of brain death, *JAMA* 246:2184, 1981.

Kolb JC, Summer RL, Galli L: Cervical collar–induced changes in intracranial pressure, *Am J Emerg Med* 17:135, 1999.

Muizelaar JP, Marmarou A, Ward JD, et al: Adverse effects of prolonged hyperventilation in patients with severe brain injury: a randomized clinical trial, *J Neurosurg* 75:731, 1991.

Rosner MJ, Coley IB: Cerebral perfusion pressure, intracranial pressure and head elevation, *J Neurosurg* 65:636, 1986.

Teasdale G, Jennett B: Assessment of coma and impaired consciousness: a practical scale, *Lancet* 2:81, 1974.

Valadka AB: Injury to the cranium. In Mattox KL, Feliciano DV, Moore EE: *Trauma,* ed 4, Norwalk, Conn, 2000, Appleton & Lange.

Chapter Objectives

*At the completion of this chapter, the reader
will be able to do the following:*

✓ Describe the epidemiology of spinal injuries.

✓ Compare and contrast the most common mechanisms that produce
spinal injury in adults with those in children.

✓ Recognize patients with the potential for spinal trauma.

✓ Relate the signs and symptoms of spinal injury and neurogenic
shock with their underlying pathophysiology.

✓ Integrate principles of anatomy and pathophysiology with
assessment data and principles of trauma management to formulate
a treatment plan for the patient with obvious or potential spinal
injury.

✓ Describe the indications for spinal immobilization.

✓ Discuss factors associated with prehospital findings and
interventions that may affect spinal injury morbidity and mortality.

CHAPTER 9

Spinal Trauma

SCENARIO

You have been dispatched to a pedestrian hit by a car. On arrival, you find a woman, approximately 25 years of age, lying supine in the road. The scene is safe. Police are already on the scene.

As you begin your primary survey, you find an unresponsive female patient who apparently was struck while trying to cross the street against the light. She has abrasions and an obvious deformity of the right femur. Her airway is open, and she is breathing, although her respirations do not appear to be regular. The patient has weak radial and carotid pulses. She shows no obvious signs of external blood loss. Her skin appears normal and warm in the lower extremities. Her upper extremities are pale, cool, and clammy.

What pathologic processes explain the patient's presentation? What intermediate interventions and further assessments are needed? What are the management goals for this patient? ■

Spinal trauma, if not recognized and properly managed, can result in irreparable damage and leave a patient paralyzed for life. Some patients sustain immediate spinal cord damage as a result of trauma. Others sustain an injury to the spinal column that does not initially damage the cord; cord damage may result later with movement of the spine. Because the central nervous system (CNS) is incapable of regeneration, a severed spinal cord cannot be repaired. The consequences of inappropriately moving a patient with a spinal column injury, or allowing the patient to move, can be devastating. Failure to detect and immobilize a fractured spine properly may produce a much worse outcome than, for example, failure to immobilize a fractured femur properly. Conversely, spinal immobilization of the patient who has no indications of injury also has consequences and should not be done without careful consideration of the risks versus the benefits.

Spinal cord injury can have profound effects on human physiology, lifestyle, and financial circumstances. Human physiology is affected because the use of extremities or other areas is severely limited or completely impaired as a result of cord damage. Lifestyle is affected because spinal cord injury usually results in profound changes to daily activity levels and independence. Spinal cord injury also impacts the financial circumstances of the patient as well as the population in general.[1] A patient with this injury requires both acute and long-term care. The lifetime cost of this care is estimated at approximately $1.25 million for a permanent spinal cord injury.

About 32 people per 1 million population will sustain some type of spinal cord injury annually. An estimated 250,000 to 400,000 people live with spinal cord injuries in the United States. Spinal cord injury can occur at any age; however, it usually occurs in those 16 to 35 years of age because this age group is involved in the most violent and high-risk activities. Most trauma patients are 16 to 20 years of age. The second largest group of patients is 21 to 25 years, and the third largest group is 26 to 35 years of age. Common causes are motor vehicle crashes (48%), falls (21%), penetrating injuries (15%), sports injuries (14%), and other injuries (2%). Overall, approximately 11,000 people sustain spinal cord injuries annually in the United States.[2]

Sudden violent forces acting on the body can move the spine beyond its normal limits of motion by either impacting on the head or neck or driving the torso out from under the head. The following four concepts help clarify the possible effect on the spine when evaluating the potential for injury:

1. The head is similar to a bowling ball perched on top of the neck, and its mass often moves in a different direction from the torso, resulting in strong forces being applied to the neck (cervical spine, spinal cord).
2. Objects in motion tend to stay in motion, and objects at rest tend to stay at rest.
3. Sudden or violent movement of the upper legs displaces the pelvis, resulting in forceful movement of the lower spine. Because of the weight and inertia of the head and torso, force in an opposite (contra) direction is applied to the upper spine.
4. Lack of neurologic deficit does not rule out bone or ligament injury to the spine or conditions that have stressed the spinal cord to the limit of its tolerance.

Some trauma patients with neurologic deficit will have a temporary or permanent spinal cord injury. Other patients have neurologic deficit caused by either a peripheral nerve injury or an extremity injury not associated with spinal cord injury. It should be assumed that any patient who has sustained any of the following injuries has a potential spinal injury[3,4]:

- Any mechanism that produced a violent impact on the head, neck, torso, or pelvis
- Incidents that produce sudden acceleration, deceleration, or lateral bending forces to the neck or torso

- Any fall from a height, especially in elderly persons
- Ejection or a fall from any motorized or otherwise powered transportation device
- Any victim of a shallow-water incident

Any such patient should be manually stabilized in a neutral inline position (unless contraindicated) until the need for spinal immobilization has been assessed.

Anatomy and Physiology

Vertebral Anatomy

The spinal column is composed of 33 bones called *vertebrae,* which are stacked on top of one another. Except for the first (C1) and second (C2) vertebrae (cervical) at the top of the spine and the fused sacral and coccygeal vertebrae at the lower spine, all the vertebrae are almost alike in form, structure, and motion (Figure 9-1). The largest part of each vertebra is the anterior part called the *body.* Each vertebral body bears most of the weight of the vertebral column and torso superior to it. Two curved sides called the *neural arches* are formed by the pedicle and posteriorly by the lamina. The posterior part of the vertebra is a tail-like structure called the *spinous process.* In the lower five cervical vertebrae, this posterior process points directly posterior, whereas in the thoracic and lumbar vertebrae, it points slightly downward in a caudad direction (toward the feet).

Most vertebrae also have similarly styled protuberances called *transverse processes* at each side near their anterior lateral margins. The transverse and spinous processes serve as points for muscle attachment and are therefore fulcrums for movement. The neural arches and the posterior part of each vertebral body form a near-circular shape with an opening in the center called the *vertebral foramen.* The spinal cord passes through this opening. The cord is protected somewhat from injury by the bony vertebrae surrounding it. Each vertebral foramen lines up with that of the vertebrae above and the vertebrae below to form the hollow spinal canal through which the spinal cord passes.

Vertebral Column

The individual vertebrae are stacked in an S-like shape (Figure 9-2). This organization allows extensive multidirectional movement while imparting maximum strength. The spinal column is divided into five individual regions for reference. Beginning at the top of the spinal column and descending downward, these regions are the cervical, thoracic, lumbar, sacral, and coccygeal regions. Vertebrae are identified by the first letter of the region in which they are found and their sequence from the top of that region. The first cervical vertebra is called *C1,* the third thoracic

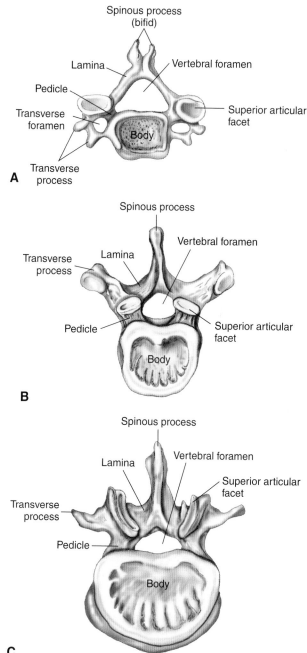

FIGURE 9-1 Except for the fused sacral and coccygeal vertebrae, each vertebra has the same parts as the other vertebrae. The body (anterior portion) of each vertebra becomes larger and stronger because it must support more weight nearing the pelvis. **A,** Fifth cervical vertebra. **B,** Thoracic vertebra. **C,** Lumbar vertebra.

vertebra *T3,* the fifth lumbar vertebra *L5,* and so on throughout the entire spinal column. Each vertebra supports increasing body weight as the vertebrae progress down the spinal column. Appropriately, the vertebrae from C3 to L5 become progressively larger to accommodate the increased weight and workload (Figure 9-3).

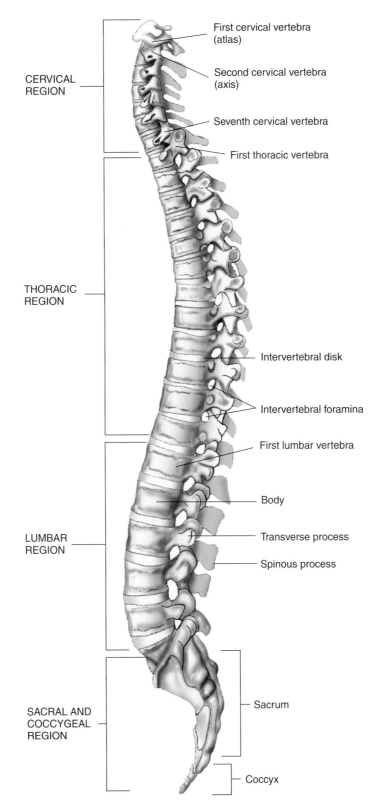

CERVICAL
REGION

First cervical vertebra
(atlas)

Second cervical vertebra
(axis)

Seventh cervical vertebra

First thoracic vertebra

THORACIC
REGION

Intervertebral disk

Intervertebral foramina

First lumbar vertebra

Body

LUMBAR
REGION

Transverse process

Spinous process

SACRAL AND
COCCYGEAL
REGION

Sacrum

Coccyx

FIGURE 9-2   The vertebral column is not a straight rod, but a series of blocks that are stacked to allow for several bends or curves. At each of the curves, the spine is more vulnerable to fractures, thus the origin of the phrase "breaking the S in a fall."

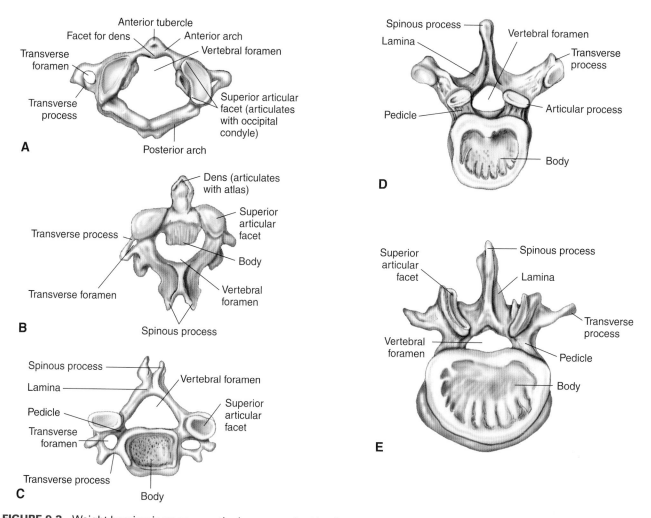

FIGURE 9-3 Weight bearing increases on the lower vertebral bodies, which are thick and stronger to carry this load. **A,** Atlas (C1). **B,** Axis (C2). **C,** Cervical. **D,** Thoracic. **E,** Lumbar.

Located at the top end of the spinal column are the seven *cervical* vertebrae that support the head. The cervical region is flexible to allow for total movement of the head. Next are 12 *thoracic* vertebrae. Each pair of ribs connects posteriorly to one of the thoracic vertebrae. Unlike the cervical spine, the thoracic spine is relatively rigid with less movement. Below the thoracic vertebrae are the five *lumbar* vertebrae. These are the most massive of all the vertebrae. The lumbar area is also flexible, allowing for movement in several directions. The five *sacral* vertebrae are fused, forming a single structure known as the *sacrum*. The four *coccygeal* vertebrae are also fused, forming the *coccyx* (tailbone). Approximately 55% of spinal injuries occur in the cervical region, 15% in the thoracic region, 15% at the thoracolumbar junction, and 15% in the lumbosacral area.

Ligaments and muscles tether the spine from the base of the skull to the pelvis. These ligaments and muscles form a web that sheathes the entire bony part of the spinal column, holding it in normal alignment and allowing for movement. If these ligaments and muscles are torn, excessive movement of one vertebra in relation to another occurs. In the presence of torn spinal ligaments, this excessive movement may result in dislocation of the vertebrae, which can compromise the space inside the spinal canal and thus damage the spinal cord.

The anterior and posterior longitudinal ligaments connect the vertebral bodies anteriorly and inside the canal. Ligaments between the spinous processes provide support for flexion-extension (forward and backward) movement, and those between the lamina provide support during lateral flexion (side bending).

The head balances on top of the spine, and the spine is supported by the pelvis (Figure 9-4). The skull perches on the ring-shaped first cervical vertebra (C1), referred to as the *atlas.* The *axis,* C2, is also basically ring shaped but has a spur (the odontoid process) that protrudes upward similar to a tooth, located just behind the anterior arch of the atlas. The axis allows the head approximately a 180-degree range of rotation (Figure 9-5).

The human head weighs between 16 and 22 lb (7-10 kg), approximately the same weight as an average bowling ball.

FIGURE 9-4 The spine is attached to the legs by attachments to the pelvis at the sacroiliac joints. The head resembles a bowling ball that balances on top of the spine.

The weight and position of the head atop the thin and flexible neck, the forces that act on the head, the small size of the supporting muscle, and the lack of ribs or other bones help make the cervical spine particularly susceptible to injury. At the level of C3, the spinal cord occupies approximately 95% of the spinal canal (the spinal cord occupies approximately 65% of the spinal canal area at its end in the lumbar region), and only 3 mm of clearance exists between the cord and the canal wall. Even a minor dislocation at this point can produce compression of the spinal cord. The posterior neck muscles are strong, permitting up to 60% of the range of flexion and 70% of the range of extension of the head without any stretching of the cord. However, when sudden violent acceleration, deceleration, or lateral force is applied to the body, the significant weight of the head on the narrow cervical spine can amplify the effects of sudden movement.

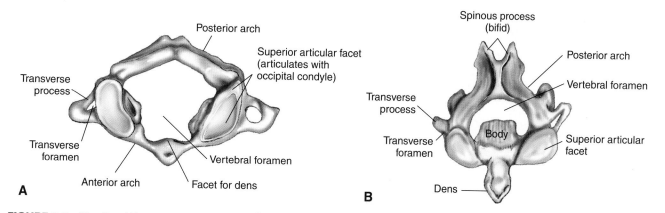

FIGURE 9-5 The first **(A)** and second **(B)** cervical vertebrae are shaped differently than the rest of the vertebrae of the spine. Their function is to support the skull and allow rotation and anterior-posterior motion of the head.

An example of this would be a rear-end collision without the headrest properly adjusted.

The *sacrum* is the base of the spinal column, the platform on which the spinal column rests. Between 70% and 80% of the body's total weight rests on the sacrum. The sacrum is a part of both the spinal column and the pelvic girdle, and it is joined to the rest of the pelvis by immovable joints.

Spinal Cord Anatomy

The spinal cord is continuous with the brain and starts from the base of the brainstem, passing through the foramen magnum (the hole at the base of the skull) and through each vertebra to the level of the second lumbar (L2) vertebra. Blood is supplied to the spinal cord by the vertebral and spinal arteries.

The spinal cord itself consists of gray matter and white matter. The white matter contains the anatomic spinal tracts. Spinal tracts are divided into two types: ascending and descending.

Ascending nerve tracts carry sensory impulses from body parts through the cord up to the brain. Ascending nerve tracts can be further divided into tracts that carry the different sensations of pain and temperature; touch and pressure; and sensory impulses of motion, vibration, position, and light touch. The nerve tracts that carry pain and temperature sensation "cross over" in the body, meaning that the nerve root with that information from the right side of the body crosses over to the left side of the spinal cord and then goes up to the brain. In contrast, the nerve tract that carries the sensory information for position, vibration, and light touch does *not* cross over in the spinal cord. Thus this sensory information is carried up to the brain on the same side of the spinal cord as the nerve roots.

Descending nerve tracts are responsible for carrying motor impulses from the brain through the cord down to the body, and they control all muscle movement and muscle tone. These descending tracts also do not cross over in the

spinal cord. Therefore the motor tract on the right side of the cord controls motor function on the right side of the body. These motor tracts *do* cross over in the brainstem, however, so the left side of the brain controls motor function on the right side of the body, and vice versa.

As the spinal cord continues to descend, pairs of nerves branch off from the cord at each vertebra and extend to the various parts of the body (Figure 9-6). The spinal cord has 31 pairs of spinal nerves, named according to the level from which they arise. Each nerve has two roots on each side. The *dorsal root* is for sensory impulses, and the *ventral root* is for motor impulses. Neurologic stimuli pass between the brain and each part of the body through the cord and particular pairs of these nerves. As they branch from the spinal cord, these nerves pass through a notch in the inferior lateral side of the vertebra, posterior to the vertebral body, called the *intervertebral foramen.* Cartilage-like inter- vertebral discs lie between the body of each vertebra and act as shock absorbers (Figure 9-7).

These nerve branches have multiple control functions, and their level in the spinal cord is represented by derma- tomes. A *dermatome* is the sensory area on the body for which a nerve root is responsible. Collectively, dermatomes allow the body areas to be mapped out for each spinal level (Figure 9-8). Dermatomes help determine the level of a spinal cord injury. Two landmarks to keep in mind are the *nipple level,* which is the T4 dermatome, and the *umbilicus level,* which is the T10 dermatome.

The process of inhalation and exhalation requires both chest excursion and proper changes in the shape of the diaphragm. The diaphragm is innervated by the phrenic nerves, which originate from the nerves arising from the cord between levels C2 and C5. If the cord above the level of C2 or the phrenic nerves are cut or the nerve impulses are otherwise disrupted, a patient will lose the ability to breathe spontaneously. A patient with this injury may asphyxiate before the arrival of providers unless bystanders initiate rescue breathing. Positive-pressure ventilation will need to be continued during transport.

FIGURE 9-6 The spinal nerves branch from each side of the spinal cord to provide motor and sensory innervation to the torso and extremities.

FIGURE 9-7 The cartilage between each vertebral body is called the *intervertebral disc.* These discs act as shock absorbers. If damaged, the cartilage may protrude into the spinal canal, compressing the cord or the nerves that come through the intervertebral foramina.

The spinal cord is surrounded by cerebrospinal fluid (CSF) and is encased in a dural sheath. This dural sheath covers the brain and continues down to the second sacral vertebra, where a saclike reservoir (the great cistern) exists. CSF produced by the brain passes around the cord and is absorbed in this cistern. CSF performs the same function for the cord as for the brain, acting as a cushion against injury during rapid and severe movement.

Pathophysiology

The bony spine can normally withstand forces of up to 1000 foot-pounds (1360 joules) of energy. High-speed travel and contact sports can routinely exert forces well in excess of this amount on the spine. Even in a low- to moderate-speed vehicle crash, the body of an unrestrained 150-lb (68-kg) person can easily place 3000 to 4000 foot-pounds (4080-5440 joules) of force against the spine as the head is suddenly stopped by the windshield or roof. Similar force can occur when a motorcyclist is thrown over the front of the motorcycle or when a high-speed skier collides with a tree.

Skeletal Injuries

Various types of injuries can occur to the spine, including the following[5]:

- Compression fractures of a vertebra that produce wedge compression or total body flattening of the vertebra.
- Fractures that produce small fragments of bone that may lie in the spinal canal near the cord.
- *Subluxation,* which is a partial dislocation of a vertebra from its normal alignment in the spinal column.
- Overstretching or tearing of the ligaments and muscles, producing instability between the vertebrae.

Any of these skeletal injuries may immediately result at the time of the traumatic injury in the irreversible transection of the cord, or the injury may compress or stretch the cord. In some patients, however, damage to the vertebrae or ligaments results in an *unstable* spinal column injury but does not produce an immediate spinal cord injury. In addition, patients who have cervical spine injuries also have a 10% chance of having another spinal fracture. Therefore the entire spine must be immobilized in patients who have indications for cervical spinal immobilization.

FIGURE 9-8 Dermatome map shows the relationship between areas of touch sensation on the skin and the spinal nerves that correspond to these areas. Loss of sensation in a specific area may indicate injury to the corresponding spinal nerve.

A lack of neurologic deficit does not rule out a bony fracture or an unstable spine. Although the presence of good motor and sensory responses in the extremities indicates that the cord is currently intact, it does not exclude a damaged vertebra or associated bony or soft tissue injury. A significant percentage of patients with spine fractures have no neurologic deficit. A full assessment is required to determine the need for immobilization.

Specific Mechanisms of Injury That Cause Spinal Trauma

Axial loading can occur in several ways. Most often, this compression of the spine occurs when the head strikes an object and the weight of the still-moving body bears against the stopped head, such as when the head of an unrestrained occupant strikes the windshield or when the head strikes an object in a shallow-water diving incident. Compression and axial loading also occur when a patient sustains a fall from a substantial height and lands in a standing position. This drives the weight of the head and thorax down against the lumbar spine while the sacral spine remains stationary. About 20% of falls from a height greater than 15 feet involve an associated lumbar spine fracture. During such an extreme energy exchange, the spinal column tends to exaggerate its

normal curves, and fractures and compressions occur at such areas. The spine is S shaped; therefore it can be said that the compressive forces tend to "break the patient's S." These forces compress the concave side and open the convex side of the spine.

Excessive flexion (hyperflexion), excessive extension (hyperextension), and *excessive rotation (hyperrotation)* can cause bone damage and tearing of muscles and ligaments, resulting in impingement on or stretching of the spinal cord.

Sudden or excessive lateral bending requires much less movement than flexion or extension before injury occurs. During lateral impact, the torso and the thoracic spine are moved laterally. The head tends to remain in place until it is pulled along by the cervical attachments. The center of gravity of the head is above and anterior to its seat and attachment to the cervical spine; therefore the head will tend to roll sideways. This movement often results in dislocations and bony fractures.

Distraction (overelongation of the spine) occurs when one part of the spine is stable and the rest is in longitudinal motion. This pulling apart of the spine can easily cause stretching and tearing of the cord. Distraction injury is a common mechanism in children's playground injuries and in hangings.

Although any one of these types of violent movements may be the dominant cause of spinal injury in a given patient, one or more of the others will usually also be involved.

Spinal Cord Injuries

Primary injury occurs at the time of impact or force application and may cause cord compression, direct cord injury (usually from sharp unstable bony fragments or projectiles), and interruption of the cord's blood supply. Secondary injury occurs after the initial insult and can include swelling, ischemia, or movement of bony fragments.[6]

Cord concussion results from the temporary disruption of the spinal cord functions distal to the injury. *Cord contusion* involves bruising or bleeding into the spinal cord's tissues, which may also result in a temporary loss of cord functions distal to the injury (spinal "shock"). Spinal shock is a neurologic phenomenon that occurs for an unpredictable, variable time after spinal cord injury, resulting in temporary loss of all sensory and motor function, flaccidity and paralysis, and loss of reflexes below the level of the spinal cord injury. Cord contusion is usually caused by a penetrating type of injury or movement of bony fragments. The severity of injury resulting from the contusion is related to the amount of bleeding into the tissue. Damage to or disruption of the spinal blood supply can result in local cord tissue ischemia. *Cord compression* is pressure on the spinal cord caused by swelling, which may result in tissue ischemia and in some cases may require decompression to prevent a permanent loss of function. *Cord laceration* occurs when cord tissue is torn or cut. Neurologic deficits may be reversed if the cord has sustained only slight damage; however, it usually results in permanent disability if all spinal tracts are disrupted.

Spinal cord transection can be categorized as complete or incomplete. In *complete cord transection*, all spinal tracts are interrupted, and all cord functions distal to the site are lost. Because of the effects of swelling, determination of the extent of loss of function may not be accurate until 24 hours after the injury. Most complete cord transections result in either paraplegia or quadriplegia, depending on the level of the injury. In *incomplete cord transection*, some tracts and motor/sensory functions remain intact. Prognosis for recovery is greater than with complete transections. Types of incomplete cord injuries include the following[7]:

- *Anterior cord syndrome* is a result of bony fragments or pressure on spinal arteries (Figure 9-9). Symptoms include loss of motor function and pain, temperature, and light touch sensations. However, some light touch, motion, position, and vibration sensations are spared.
- *Central cord syndrome* usually occurs with hyperextension of the cervical area (Figure 9-10). Symptoms include weakness or paresthesia in the upper extremities but normal strength in the lower extremities. This syndrome causes varying degrees of bladder dysfunction.

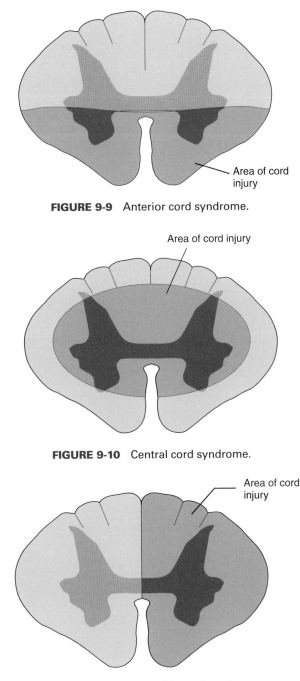

FIGURE 9-9 Anterior cord syndrome.

FIGURE 9-10 Central cord syndrome.

FIGURE 9-11 Brown-Séquard syndrome.

- *Brown-Séquard syndrome* is caused by penetrating injury and involves hemitransection of the cord, involving only one side of the cord (Figure 9-11). Symptoms include complete cord damage and loss of function on the affected side (motor, vibration, motion, and position) with loss of pain and temperature sensation on the side opposite the injury.

Neurogenic "shock" secondary to spinal cord injury represents a significant additional finding. Neurogenic shock from spinal cord injury is caused by different mechanisms that result from the neurologic deficits produced by injury to the spinal cord. Injury to the vasoregulatory fibers produces loss of sympathetic tone to the vessels or vasodilation. The skin will be warm and dry and the pulse rate will be slow, but the blood pressure will be low. When the cord is disrupted, the body's sympathetic compensatory mechanism cannot maintain control of the muscles in the walls of the blood vessels below the point of disruption. These arteries and arterioles dilate, enlarging the size of the vascular container and producing relative hypovolemia and partial loss of systemic vascular resistance (SVR). Instead of the tachycardia usually associated with hypovolemic shock, this type of injury is associated with a normal heart rate or a slight bradycardia. Although the patient may be hypotensive, neurogenic "shock" often does not cause impairment in oxygen delivery to peripheral tissues (see Chapter 7). High spinal cord injuries (C5 or above) are more likely to require cardiovascular interventions such as vasopressors and pacemakers.[8] A recent consensus statement recommends prompt correction of hypotension (SBP <90 mm Hg) in the setting of acute spinal cord injury. Ideally, the blood pressure of patients with suspected spinal cord injury should be maintained in a normal range (MAP 85-90 mm Hg).[9]

Assessment

Spinal injury, as with other conditions, should be assessed in the context of other injuries and conditions present. The primary survey is the first priority. However, often the patient first needs to be moved. Therefore a rapid scene assessment and history of the event should determine if the possibility of a spinal injury exists, in which case the patient's spine must be manually protected. The patient's head is brought into a neutral inline position, unless contraindicated (see later discussion). The head is maintained in that position until the assessment reveals no indication for immobilization, or the manual stabilization is replaced with a spine immobilization device, such as a half-spine board, long backboard, or vest-type device.

A rapid neurologic examination is performed to identify obvious deficits related to a spinal cord injury. The patient is asked to move the arms, hands, and legs, and any inability to do so is noted. Then the patient is checked for the presence or absence of sensation, beginning at the shoulders and moving down the body to the feet.

Using Mechanism of Injury to Assess Spinal Cord Injury

Traditionally, prehospital care providers have been taught that injury is based solely on the mechanism of injury and that spinal immobilization is required for any patient with a mechanism of injury. This generalization has caused a lack of clear clinical guidelines for assessment of spinal cord

injuries. However, assessment for spinal immobilization should also include assessment of the motor and sensory function, presence of pain or tenderness, and patient reliability as predictors of spinal cord injury. In addition, the patient may not complain of pain in the spinal column because of pain associated with a more distracting painful injury, such as a fractured femur.[8] Alcohol or drugs that the patient may have ingested may also blunt the patient's perception of pain and mask serious injury.

The primary focus of care should be to recognize the indications for spinal immobilization rather than to attempt to clear the spine.[10-17] Because many patients do not have spinal injury, a more selective approach to performing spinal immobilization is appropriate, especially in that spinal immobilization has been shown to produce adverse effects in healthy volunteers, including increases in respiratory effort, skin ischemia, and pain.[18] Providers should focus on appropriate indications for performing spinal immobilization.

If no indications are present after a careful and thorough examination, there may be no need for spinal immobilization. The cornerstone to proper spinal care is the same as with all trauma care: superior assessment, with appropriate and timely treatment.

Blunt Trauma

Major causes of spinal injury in adult patients include the following:

1. Motor vehicle crashes (MVCs)
2. Shallow-water incidents
3. Motorcycle crashes
4. All other injuries and fall
5. Sports injuries

Major causes of spinal injury in pediatric patients include the following:

1. Falls from heights (generally two to three times the patient's height)
2. Falls from a tricycle or bicycle
3. Being struck by a motor vehicle

As a guideline, the provider should assume the presence of spinal injury and an unstable spine with the following situations, and an assessment of the spine should be conducted to determine the need for immobilization:

■ Any mechanism that produced a violent impact on the head, neck, torso, or pelvis (e.g., assault, entrapment in a structural collapse).
■ Incidents that produce sudden acceleration, deceleration, or lateral bending forces to the neck or torso (e.g., moderate- to high-speed MVCs, pedestrians struck by vehicle, involvement in explosion).

- Any fall, especially in elderly persons.
- Ejection or a fall from any motorized or otherwise powered transportation device (e.g., scooters, skateboards, bicycles, motor vehicles, motorcycles, recreational vehicles).
- Any victim of a shallow-water incident (e.g., diving, body surfing).

Other situations often associated with spinal damage include the following:

- Head injuries with any alteration in level of consciousness
- Significant helmet damage
- Significant blunt injury to the torso
- Impacted or other deceleration fractures of the legs or hips
- Significant localized injuries to the area of the spinal column

These mechanisms of injury should mandate a thorough and complete examination to determine if indications are present to necessitate spinal immobilization.

The wearing of proper seat belt restraints has proved to save lives and reduce head, face, and thoracic injuries. However, the use of proper restraints does not rule out the possibility of spinal injury. In significant frontal-impact collisions when sudden severe deceleration occurs, the restrained torso stops suddenly, but the unrestrained head attempts to continue its forward movement. Held by the strong posterior neck muscles, the head can move forward only slightly. If the force of deceleration is strong enough, the head then rotates down until the chin strikes the chest wall, frequently rotating across the diagonal strap of the shoulder restraint. Such rapid, forceful hyperflexion and rotation of the neck can result in compression fractures of the cervical vertebrae, "jumped and locked" facets (dislocation of the articular processes), and stretching of the spinal cord. Different mechanisms can also cause spinal trauma in restrained victims of rear or lateral collisions. The amount of damage to the vehicle and the patient's other injuries are the key factors in determining if a patient needs to be immobilized.

The patient's ability to walk should not be a factor in determining whether a patient needs to be treated for spinal injury. A significant number of patients who required surgical repair of unstable spinal injuries were found "walking around" at the scene or walked into the emergency department at the hospital.

Penetrating Trauma

Penetrating injury represents a special consideration regarding the potential for spinal trauma.[19] In general, if a patient did not sustain definite neurologic injury at the moment that the trauma occurred, there is little concern for a spinal injury. This is because of the mechanism of injury and the kinematics associated with the force involved. Penetrating objects generally do not produce unstable spinal fractures, as does blunt force injury, because penetrating trauma produces minimal risk of unstable ligamentous or bony injury. A penetrating object causes injury along the path of penetration. If the object did not directly injure the spinal cord as it penetrated, the patient is unlikely to develop a spinal cord injury. Numerous studies have shown that unstable injuries rarely occur from penetrating trauma to the head, neck, or torso[21-26] and such injuries are not indications for spinal immobilization unless a neurologic deficit is identified. In general, the other injuries created by the penetrating trauma require a higher priority in management than those to the spine.

Indications for Spinal Immobilization

The mechanism of injury can be used as an aid to determine indications for spinal immobilization (Figure 9-12). The key point always is that a complete physical assessment coupled with good clinical judgment will guide decision making, and *if in doubt, immobilize.*

Patients with a penetrating injury (e.g., gunshot or stab wounds) to the head, neck, or torso should be considered to have a concerning mechanism of injury when they complain of neurologic symptoms or display such findings as numbness, tingling, and loss of motor or sensory function or actual loss of consciousness. However, if patients with penetrating injury have no neurologic complaints, secondary mechanism of injury, or findings, the spine does not need to be immobilized (although the backboard may still be used for lifting and transport purposes).

In the patient with blunt trauma, the following conditions should mandate spinal immobilization:

1. *Altered level of consciousness* (LOC), with Glasgow Coma Scale (GCS) score less than 15. Any factor that alters the patient's perception of pain will hinder the responder's assessment for injury; this includes the following:
   - Traumatic brain injury (TBI)
   - Altered mental status (AMS) other than TBI. For example, patients with psychiatric illness, with Alzheimer's disease, or under the influence of intoxicants may have impaired pain perception.
   - Acute stress reactions (ASRs) may cause "pain masking."
2. *Spinal pain or tenderness.* This includes pain or pain on movement, point tenderness, and deformity and guarding of the spinal area.
3. *Neurologic deficit or complaint.* This includes bilateral paralysis, partial paralysis, paresis (weakness), numbness, prickling or tingling, and neurogenic

INDICATIONS FOR SPINAL IMMOBILIZATION

Notes:
[1]Concerning Mechanisms of Injury
• Any mechanism that produced a violent impact to the head, neck, torso, or pelvis (e.g., assault, entrapment in structural collapse, etc.)
• Incidents producing sudden acceleration, deceleration, or lateral bending forces to the neck or torso (e.g., moderate- to high-speed MVC, pedestrian struck, involvement in an explosion, etc.)
• Any fall, especially in elderly persons
• Ejection or fall from any motorized or otherwise-powered transportation device (e.g., scooters, skateboards, bicycles, motor vehicles, motorcycles, or recreational vehicles)
• Victim of shallow-water diving incident

[2]Distracting Injury
   Any injury that may have the potential to impair the patient's ability to appreciate other injuries. Examples of distracting injuries include a) long bone fracture; b) a visceral injury requiring surgical consultation; c) a large laceration, degloving injury, or crush injury; d) large burns, or e) any other injury producing acute functional impairment.
   (Adapted from Hoffman JR, Wolfson AB, Todd K, Mower WR: Selective cervical spine radiography in blunt trauma: methodology of the National Emergency X-Radiography Utilization Study [NEXUS], *Ann Emerg Med* 461, 1998.)

[3]Inability to communicate. Any patient who, for reasons not specified above, cannot clearly communicate so as to actively participate in their assessment. Examples: speech or hearing impaired, those who only speak a foreign language, and small children.

FIGURE 9-12   Indications for spinal immobilization.

spinal shock below the level of the injury. In males, a continuing erection of the penis (priapism) may be an additional indication of spinal cord injury.

4. *Anatomic deformity of the spine.* This includes any deformity noted on physical examination of the patient.

However, the absence of these signs does not rule out bony spinal injury (Box 9-1).

When a patient has a concerning mechanism of injury in the absence of the conditions just listed, the reliability of the patient must be assessed. A reliable patient is calm, cooperative, and sober. An unreliable patient may exhibit any of the following:

- *Intoxication.* Patients who are under the influence of drugs or alcohol are immobilized and managed as if they had spinal injury until they are calm, cooperative, and sober.
- *Distracting painful injuries.* Injuries that are severely painful may prevent the patient from giving reliable responses during the assessment.[8] Examples would include a fractured femur or a large burn (see Figure 9-12).
- *Communication barriers.* Communication problems include language barriers, deafness, very young patients, or patients who for any reason cannot communicate effectively.

The patient should be continually rechecked for reliability at all phases of an assessment. If at any time the patient exhibits these signs or symptoms, it should be assumed that the patient has a spinal injury, and full immobilization management techniques should be implemented.

In many situations the mechanism of injury is not indicative of neck injury (e.g., falling on outstretched hand and producing Colles' fracture). In these patients, in the presence of a normal examination and proper assessment, spinal immobilization is not indicated.

Management

The management for an unstable spine is to immobilize the patient in a supine position on a rigid long backboard in a neutral inline position. The head, neck, torso, and pelvis should each be immobilized in a neutral inline position to prevent any further movement of the unstable spine that could result in damage to the spinal cord. Spinal immobilization follows the common principle of fracture management: immobilizing the joint above and the joint below an injury. Because of the anatomy of the spinal column and the interaction caused by forces that affect any part of the spine, this principle simply needs to be extended to spinal immobilization. The joint above the spine means the head, and the joint below means the pelvis.

Moderate anterior flexion or extension of the arms may cause significant movement of the shoulder girdle. Any movement or angulation of the pelvis results in movement of the sacrum and of the vertebrae attached to it. For example, lateral movement of both legs together can result in angulation of the pelvis and lateral bending of the spine.

Fractures of one area of the spine are often associated with fractures of other areas of the spine.[26] Therefore the entire weight-bearing spine (cervical, thoracic, lumbar, and sacral) should be considered as one entity and the entire spine immobilized and supported to achieve proper immobilization. The supine position is the most stable position to ensure continued support during handling, carrying, and transporting a patient. It also provides the best access for further examination and additional resuscitation and management of a patient. When the patient is supine, the airway, mouth and nose, eyes, chest, and abdomen can be accessed simultaneously.

Patients usually present in one of four general postures: sitting, semiprone, supine, or standing. The patient's spine needs to be protected and stabilized immediately and continuously from the time the patient is discovered until the patient is mechanically secured to a long backboard. Techniques and equipment, such as manual stabilization, half-spine boards, immobilization vests, scoop stretchers, proper logroll methods, and rapid extrication with full manual stabilization, are interim techniques used to protect a patient's spine. These techniques allow for a patient's safe movement from the position in which the patient was found until full supine immobilization on a rigid long backboard can be implemented. A recent study suggests that one type of scoop stretcher currently manufactured may be as effective as a standard rigid long backboard.[28]

Often, too much focus is placed on particular immobilization devices without an understanding of the principles of immobilization and how to modify these principles to meet individual patient needs. Specific devices and immobilization methods can be safely used only with an understanding of the anatomic principles that are generic to all methods and equipment. Any inflexible, detailed method for using a device will not meet the varying conditions found in the field. Regardless of the specific equipment or method used, the management of any patient with an unstable spine should follow the general steps described in the next section.

General Method

When the decision is made to immobilize a trauma patient, follow these principles:

1. Move the patient's head into a proper neutral inline position (unless contraindicated; see next section). Continue manual support and inline stabilization without interruption.
2. Evaluate the patient in the primary survey, and provide any immediately required intervention.
3. Check the patient's motor ability, sensory response, and circulation in all four extremities, if the patient's condition allows.
4. Examine the patient's neck, and measure and apply a properly fitting, effective cervical collar.
5. Position the device on the patient, such as a shortboard or vest-type device, or place the patient on the device, such as a long backboard.
6. Immobilize the patient's torso to the device so that it cannot move up, down, left, or right.
7. Evaluate and pad behind the adult patient's head or pediatric patient chest as needed.
8. Immobilize the patient's head to the device, maintaining a neutral inline position.
9. Once the patient is on the long backboard (if a short device is used), immobilize the legs so that they cannot move anteriorly or laterally.
10. Fasten the patient's arms to the backboard.
11. Reevaluate the primary survey, and reassess the patient's motor ability, sensory response, and circulation in all four extremities, if the patient's condition allows.

Manual Inline Stabilization of the Head

Once it has been determined from the mechanism of injury that an injured spine potentially exists, the first step is to provide manual inline stabilization. The patient's head is grasped and carefully moved into a neutral inline position unless contraindicated (see below). A proper neutral inline position is maintained without any significant traction. Only enough pull should be exerted on a sitting or standing patient to cause *axial unweighting* (taking the weight of the head off the axis and the rest of the cervical spine). The head should be constantly maintained in the manually stabilized, neutral inline position until mechanical immobilization of the torso and head is completed or the examination reveals

no need for spinal immobilization. In this way the patient's head and neck are immediately immobilized and remain so until after examination at the hospital. Moving the head into a neutral inline position presents less risk than if the patient were carried and transported with the head left in an angulated position. In addition, both immobilization and transport of the patient are much simpler with the patient in a neutral position.

Movement of the patient's head into a neutral inline position is contraindicated in a few cases. If careful movement of the head and neck into a neutral inline position results in any of the following, *the movement must be stopped:*

- Resistance to movement is noted
- Neck muscle spasm
- Increased pain
- Commencement or increase of a neurologic deficit, such as numbness, tingling, or loss of motor ability
- Compromise of the airway or ventilation

Neutral inline movement should not be attempted if a patient's injuries are so severe that the head presents with such misalignment that it no longer appears to extend from the midline of the shoulders. In these situations the patient's head must be immobilized in the position in which it was initially found. Fortunately, such cases are rare.

Rigid Cervical Collars

Rigid cervical collars alone do not provide adequate immobilization; they simply aid in supporting the neck and promote a lack of movement. Rigid cervical collars limit flexion by about 90% and limit extension, lateral bending, and rotation by about 50%. A rigid cervical collar is an important adjunct to immobilization but must always be used with manual stabilization or mechanical immobilization provided by a suitable spine immobilization device. A soft cervical collar is of no use as an adjunct to spinal immobilization in the field.

The unique primary purpose of a cervical collar is to protect the cervical spine from compression. Prehospital methods of immobilization (using a vest, shortboard, or a long backboard device) still allow some slight movement because these devices only fasten externally to the patient, and the skin and muscle tissue move slightly on the skeletal frame even when the patient is extremely well immobilized. Most rescue situations involve movement when carrying and loading the patient. This type of movement also occurs when an ambulance accelerates and decelerates in normal driving conditions.

An effective cervical collar sits on the chest, posterior thoracic spine and clavicle, and trapezius muscles, where the tissue movement is at a minimum. This still allows movement at C6, C7, and T1 but prevents compression of

---

BOX 9-2   Guidelines for Rigid Cervical Collars

- Do not adequately immobilize by their use alone
- Must be properly sized for each patient
- Must not inhibit a patient's ability to open the mouth or the prehospital care provider's ability to open the patient's mouth if vomiting occurs
- Should not obstruct or hinder ventilation in any way

---

these vertebrae. The head is immobilized under the angle of the mandible and at the occiput of the skull. The rigid collar allows the unavoidable loading between the head and the torso to be transferred from the cervical spine to the collar, eliminating or minimizing the cervical compression that could otherwise result.

Even though it does not fully immobilize, a cervical collar aids in limiting head movement. The rigid anterior portion of the collar also provides a safe pathway for the lower head strap across the neck.

The collar must be the correct size for the patient. A collar that is too short will not be effective and will allow significant flexion. A collar that is too large will cause hyperextension or full motion if the chin is inside of it. A collar must be applied properly. A collar that is too loose will be ineffective in limiting head movement and can accidentally cover the anterior chin, mouth, and nose, obstructing the patient's airway. A collar that is too tight can compromise the veins of the neck.

A collar should be applied after bringing the patient's head into a neutral inline position. If the head cannot be returned to a neutral inline position, use of any collar is difficult and should not be considered. In this case the use of an improvised blanket or towel roll may assist in stabilization. A collar that does not allow the mandible to move down and the mouth to open without motion of the spine will produce aspiration of gastric contents into the lungs if the patient vomits and therefore should not be used. Alternative methods to immobilize a patient when a collar cannot be used may include use of such items as blankets, towels, and tape. In the prehospital setting the care provider may need to be creative when presented with these types of patients. Whatever method is used, the basic concepts of immobilization should be followed (Box 9-2).

Immobilization of Torso to the Device

Regardless of the specific device used, the patient must be immobilized so that the torso cannot move up, down, left, or right. The rigid device is strapped to the torso and the torso to the device. The device is secured to the patient's torso so that the head and neck will be supported and immobilized when affixed to it. The patient's torso and pelvis are immobilized to the device so that the thoracic, lumbar, and sacral sections of the spine are supported and cannot move. The torso should be immobilized to the device before the head is secured. In this way, any movement of the device that may occur when fastening the torso straps is prevented from angulating the cervical spine.

Many different methods exist for immobilizing the device to the torso. Protection against movement in any direction—up, down, left, or right—should be achieved at both the upper torso (shoulders or chest) and the lower torso (pelvis) to avoid compression and lateral movement of the vertebrae of the torso. Immobilization of the upper torso can be achieved with several specific methods; an understanding of the basic anatomic principles common to each method must be applied. Cephalad movement of the upper torso is prohibited by use of a strap on each side, fastened to the board inferior to the upper margin of each shoulder, which then passes over the shoulder and is fastened at a lower point. Caudad movement of the torso can be prohibited by use of straps that pass snugly around the pelvis.

In one method, two straps (one going from each side of the board over the shoulder, then across the upper chest and through the opposite armpit, to fasten to the board on the armpit side) produce an X, which stops any upward, downward, left, or right movement of the upper torso. The same immobilization can be achieved by fastening one strap to the board and passing it through one armpit, then across the upper chest and through the opposite armpit, to fasten to the second side of the board. A strap or cravat is then added to each side and passed over the shoulder to fasten it to the armpit strap, similar to a pair of suspenders.

Immobilization of the upper torso of a patient with a fractured clavicle is accomplished by placing backpack-type loops around each shoulder through the armpit and fastening the ends of each loop in the same handhold. The straps remain near the lateral edges of the upper torso and do not cross the clavicles. With any of these methods, the straps are over the upper third of the chest and can be fastened tightly without producing the ventilatory compromise typically produced by tight straps placed lower on the thorax.

Immobilization of the lower torso can be achieved by use of a single strap fastened tightly over the pelvis at the iliac crests. If the long backboard will have to be upended or carried on stairs or over a distance, a pair of groin loops will provide stronger immobilization than the single strap across the iliac crests.

Lateral movement or anterior movement away from the rigid device at the midtorso can be prevented by use of an additional strap around the midtorso. Any strap that surrounds the torso between the upper thorax and the iliac crests should be snug but not so tight that it inhibits chest excursion impairing ventilatory function or causes a significant increase in intraabdominal pressure.

A

B

FIGURE 9-13 A, In some patients, pulling the skull back to the level of the backboard can produce severe hyperextension. **B,** Padding is needed between the back of the head and the backboard to prevent such hyperextension.

A

B

FIGURE 9-14 A, The larger size of a child's head relative to body size, combined with the reduced development of the posterior thoracic muscles, produces hyperflexion of the head when a child is placed on a backboard. **B,** Padding beneath the shoulders and torso will prevent this hyperflexion.

Maintenance of Neutral Inline Position of the Head

In many patients, when the head is placed in a neutral inline position, the outer measurement of the occipital region at the back of the head is between $1/2$ and $3^1/2$ inches anterior of the posterior thoracic wall (Figure 9-13, *A*). Therefore, in most adults, a space exists between the back of the head and the device when the head is in a neutral inline position, so suitable padding should be added before securing the head to the device (Figure 9-13, *B*). To be effective, this padding must be made of a material that does not readily compress. Firm, semirigid pads designed for this purpose or folded towels can be used. The amount of padding needed must be individualized for each patient; a few individuals require none. If too little padding is inserted or if the padding is of an unsuitable spongy material, the head will be hyperextended when head straps are applied. If too much padding is inserted, the head will be moved into a flexed position. Both hyperextension and flexion of the head can increase spinal cord damage and are contraindicated.

The same anatomic relationship between the head and back applies when most people are supine, whether on the ground or on a backboard. When most adults are supine, the head falls back into a hyperextended position. On arrival, the head should be moved into a neutral inline position and manually maintained in that position, which in many adults will require holding the head up off the ground. Once the patient is placed on the long backboard and the head is about to be fastened to the board, proper padding (as described) should be inserted between the back of the head and the board to maintain the neutral position. These principles should be used with all patients, including athletes with shoulder pads and patients with abnormal curvature of the spine (see Box 9-4 in Specific Skills).

In small children, generally those with the body size of a 7-year-old or younger, the size of the head is much larger relative to the rest of the body than in adults, and the muscles of the back are less developed.[28] When a small child's head is in a neutral inline position, the back of the head usually extends 1 to 2 inches (2.5-5 cm) beyond the posterior plane of the back. Therefore, if a small child is placed directly on a rigid surface, the head will be moved into a position of flexion (Figure 9-14, A).

Placing small children on a standard long backboard results in unwanted flexion. The long backboard needs to be modified by either creating a recess in the board or inserting padding under the torso to maintain the head in a neutral position (Figure 9-14, B). The padding placed under the torso should be of the appropriate thickness so that the head lies on the board in a neutral position; too much will result in extension, too little in flexion. The padding under the torso must also be firm and evenly shaped. Use of irregularly shaped or insufficient padding, or placing it under only the shoulders, can result in movement and misalignment of the spine.

Completing Immobilization

Head

Once the patient's torso has been immobilized to the rigid device and appropriate padding inserted behind the head as needed, the head should be secured to the device (only after securing the torso). Because of its rounded shape, the head cannot be stabilized on a flat surface with only straps or tape. Use of these alone will still allow the head to rotate and move laterally. Also, because of the angle of the forehead and the slippery nature of moist skin and hair, a simple strap over the forehead is unreliable and can easily slide off. Although the human head weighs about the same as a bowling ball, it has a significantly different shape. The head is ovoid, being longer than it is wide and having almost completely flat lateral sides, resembling a bowling ball with about 2 inches (5 cm) cut off to form left and right sides. Adequate external immobilization of the head, regardless of method or device, can be achieved only by placing pads or rolled blankets on these flat sides and securing them with straps or tape. In the case of vest-type devices, this is accomplished with hinged side flaps that are part of the vest.

The sidepieces, whether they are preshaped foam blocks or rolled blankets, are placed on the flat lateral planes of the head. The sidepieces should extend to an area at least as wide as the opening of the patient's ears, or beyond, and stack at least as high as the level of the patient's eyes. Two straps or pieces of tape surrounding these headpieces draw the sides together. When it is packaged between the blocks or blankets, the head now has a flat posterior surface that can be realistically fixed to a flat board. The upper forehead strap is placed tightly across the front of the lower forehead (across the supraorbital ridge) to help prevent anterior movement of the head. This strap should be pulled tightly enough to indent the blocks or blankets and rest firmly on the forehead. Sandbags are not recommended for use as sidepieces because of the weight that may be placed on the head and neck when the immobilized patient is turned on his side.[30]

The use of chin cups or straps encircling the chin prevents opening of the mouth to vomit, so these devices should not be used. The device that holds the head, regardless of type, also requires a lower strap to help keep the sidepieces firmly pressed against the lower sides of the head and to anchor the device further and prevent anterior movement of the lower head and neck. The lower strap passes around the sidepieces and across the anterior rigid portion of the cervical collar. This strap should not place too much pressure on the front of the collar, which could produce an airway or venous return problem at the neck. Use of sandbags secured to the long backboard on the sides of the head and neck represents a dangerous practice. Regardless of how well they are secured, these heavy objects can shift and move. Should the need arise to rotate the patient and board to the side, the combined weight of the sandbags can produce localized lateral pressure against the cervical spine. Raising or lowering the head of the board when moving and loading the patient, or any sudden acceleration or deceleration of the ambulance, can also produce shifting of the bags and movement of the head and neck.

Legs

Significant outward rotation of the legs may result in anterior movement of the pelvis and movement of the lower spine; tying the feet together eliminates this possibility. Placing a rolled blanket or piece of padding between the legs will increase comfort for the patient.

The patient's legs are immobilized to the board with two or more straps: one strap proximal to the knees at about midthigh and one strap distal to the knees.

The average adult measures 14 to 20 inches (35-50 cm) from one side to the other at the hips and only 6 to 9 inches (15-23 cm) from one side to the other at the ankles. When the feet are placed together, a V shape is formed from the hips to the ankles. Because the ankles are considerably narrower than the board, a strap placed across the lower legs can prevent anterior movement but will not prevent the legs from moving laterally from one edge of the board to the other. If the board is angled or rotated, the legs will fall to the lower edge of the board, which can angulate the pelvis and produce movement of the spinal column.

One way to hold the patient's lower legs effectively in place is to encircle them several times with the strap before attaching it to the board. The legs can be kept in the middle of the board by placing blanket rolls between each leg and the edges of the board before strapping.

Arms

For safety, the patient's arms should be secured to the board or across the torso before moving the patient. One way to achieve this is with the arms placed at the sides on the board with the palms in, secured by a strap across the forearms and torso. This strap should be snug but not so tight as to compromise the circulation in the hands.

The patient's arms should not be included in the strap at the iliac crests or in the groin loops. If the straps are tight enough to provide adequate immobilization of the lower torso, they can compromise the circulation in the hands. If the straps are loose, they will not provide adequate immobilization of the torso or arms. Use of an additional strap exclusively to hold the arms allows the strap to be opened for taking a blood pressure measurement or starting an intravenous line once the patient is in the ambulance without compromising the immobilization. If the arm strap is also a torso strap, loosening it to free just an arm has the side effect of loosening the torso immobilization as well.

Most Common Mistakes

The following are the three most common immobilization errors:

1. *Inadequate immobilization.* The device can move significantly up or down on the torso, or the head can still move excessively.
2. *Immobilization with the head hyperextended.* The most common cause is a lack of appropriate padding behind the head.
3. *Readjusting the torso straps after the head has been secured.* This causes movement of the device on the torso, which results in movement of the head and cervical spine.

Complete spine immobilization is generally not a comfortable experience for the patient. As the degree and quality of the immobilization increase, the patient's comfort decreases. Spine immobilization is a balance between the need to protect and immobilize the spine completely and the need to make it tolerable for the patient. This is why proper evaluation of the need for spinal immobilization is indicated (Box 9-3).

Obese Patients

With the increasing size of the current U.S. population, care of the *bariatric* (overweight, obese) patient is becoming more common. Transport of a 400-lb (182-kg) patient is becoming an everyday occurrence, and special bariatric transport cots have been developed for this purpose. However, a review of commercially available backboards shows that most long backboards measure 16 × 72 inches, with

---

BOX 9-3   Criteria for Evaluating Immobilization Skills

Practice is needed using immobilization skills in hands-on sessions using mock patients before use with real patients. When practicing or when evaluating new methods or equipment, the following generic criteria will serve as good tools for measuring how effectively the "patient" has been immobilized:

1. Was manual inline stabilization initiated immediately, and was it maintained until it was replaced mechanically?
2. Was an effective, properly sized cervical collar applied appropriately?
3. Was the torso secured before the head?
4. Can the device move up or down the torso?
5. Can the device move left or right at the upper torso?
6. Can the device move left or right at the lower torso?
7. Can any part of the torso move anteriorly off the rigid device?
8. Does any tie crossing the chest inhibit chest excursion, resulting in ventilatory compromise?
9. Is the head effectively immobilized so that it cannot move in any direction, including rotation?
10. Was padding behind the head used, if necessary?
11. Is the head in a neutral inline position?
12. Does anything inhibit or prevent the mouth from being opened?
13. Are the legs immobilized so that they cannot move anteriorly, rotate, or move from side to side, even if the board and patient are rotated to the side?
14. Are the pelvis and legs in a neutral inline position?
15. Are the arms appropriately secured to the board or torso?
16. Have any ties or straps compromised distal circulation in any limb?
17. Was the patient bumped, jostled, or in any way moved in a manner that could compromise an unstable spine while the device was being applied?
18. Was the procedure completed within an appropriate time frame?

Many methods and variations can meet these objectives. The selection of a specific method and specific equipment will be based on the situation, the patient's condition, and available resources.

---

a few measuring 18 inches wide. The weight limit for these long backboards varies from 250 lb (113 kg) to 600 lb (272 kg). When using backboards on bariatric trauma patients, special care is needed to ensure that the safe operating limits are not exceeded. Also, additional personnel must be used to lift and extricate bariatric patients, without further injury to the patient or provider. This subgroup of trauma patients presents challenges of safe packaging and moving procedures balanced against short scene times normally recommended in the critically injured trauma patients.

Use of Steroids

A series of studies suggested that high doses of methylprednisolone improve the neurologic outcome of patients with acute spinal cord injuries resulting from blunt trauma, when started within 8 hours of the injury. In many centers, it has become common for patients with such injuries to receive a bolus of 30 mg/kg of methylprednisolone followed by an infusion of 5.4 mg/kg/hr for up to 48 hours, depending upon when the medication was initiated. Spinal cord injuries resulting from penetrating trauma were not studied and steroids are not indicated for neurologic deficits resulting from stab or gunshot wounds. Because steroids have known adverse effects, including suppression of adrenal glands and immune functioning, and because of concerns regarding the scientific validity of these studies, administration of steroids to patients with spinal cord injuries has become increasingly controversial.[31] The decision to administer steroids should be left to the trauma surgeons, orthopedic surgeons, or neurosurgeons ultimately caring for the patient. A recent position paper recommends against prehospital administration of steroids for patients with acute spinal cord injury.[32]

Prolonged Transport

As with other injuries, the prolonged transport of patients with suspected or confirmed spinal and spinal cord injuries presents special considerations. Keeping in mind the goal to move patients with a suspected spinal cord injury only once, care should be taken to pad a long backboard prior to securing the patient. Cervical spine stabilization and spinal movement precautions should be utilized as the patient is moved to the padded backboard. Such efforts should help reduce the risk for the development of pressure ulcers in a patient with spinal cord injury. Any areas where there could be pressure on the patient's body, especially over bony prominences, should be sufficiently padded.

Patients who are immobilized to long backboards are at risk for aspiration should they regurgitate. Suction should be kept near the head of the patient so it is readily accessible should vomiting occur. Insertion of a gastric tube (either nasogastric or orogastric) and the judicious use of antiemetic medications may help reduce this risk.

Patients with high spinal cord injuries may have involvement of their diaphragm and accessory respiratory muscles (i.e., intercostal muscles) predisposing them to respiratory failure. Impending respiratory failure may be aggravated and hastened by straps placed for spinal immobilization that further restrict respiration. Prior to initiating a prolonged transport, double check to make sure that the patient's torso is secured at the shoulder girdle and at the pelvis, and that any straps do not limit chest wall excursion.

As described in the text, patients with high spinal cord injuries may experience hypotension from loss of sympathetic tone (neurogenic "shock"). Although these patients rarely suffer from widespread hypoperfusion of their tissues, crystalloid boluses are generally sufficient to restore their blood pressure to normal. Vasopressors are rarely, if ever, necessary to treat neurogenic shock. Another hallmark of a high cervical spine injury is bradycardia. If associated with significant hypotension, bradycardia may be treated with intermittent doses of atropine, 0.5 to 1.0 mg administered intravenously.

The presence of tachycardia combined with hypotension should raise suspicion for the presence of hypovolemic, rather than neurogenic, shock. Careful assessment may pinpoint the source of hemorrhage, although intra-abdominal sources and pelvic fractures are most likely. Insertion of a urinary catheter will allow urine output to be used as another guide to tissue perfusion. In an adult, a urine output of greater than 30 to 50 mL per hour generally indicates satisfactory end-organ perfusion. The loss of sensation that accompanies a spinal cord injury may prevent a conscious patient from perceiving peritonitis or other injuries below the level of the sensory deficit.

Patients with spinal injuries may have significant back pain or pain from associated fractures. As described in Chapter 12, pain may be managed with small doses of intravenous narcotics titrated until pain is relieved. Narcotics may exaggerate the hypotension associated with neurogenic shock. Padding the backboard as described above may also provide some comfort for spinal fractures.

Patients with spinal cord injuries lose some ability to regulate body temperature, and this effect is more pronounced with higher injuries. Thus, these patients are sensitive to the development of hypothermia, especially when they are in a cold environment. Patients should be kept warm (normothermic), but remember that covering them with too many blankets may lead to hyperthermia.

Spine and spinal cord injuries are best managed at facilities that have excellent orthopedic or neurosurgical service and are experienced in the management of these injuries. All Level I and II trauma centers should be capable of managing the spinal cord injury and any associated injuries. Some facilities that specialize in the management of spine and spinal cord injuries may directly accept a patient who has suffered only a spinal cord injury (i.e., a shallow water diving injury no with evidence of aspiration).

SUMMARY

The vertebral column is composed of 24 separate vertebrae plus the sacrum and coccyx stacked on top of one another. Their major functions are to support the weight of the body and allow movement. The spinal cord is enclosed within the vertebral column and is vulnerable to injury from abnormal movement and positioning.

When support for the vertebral column has been lost as a result of injury to the vertebrae or to the muscles and ligaments that help hold the spinal column in place, injury to the spinal cord can occur. Because the cord does not regenerate, permanent injury, often involving paralysis, can result.

The presence of spinal trauma and the need to immobilize the patient may be indicated by other injuries that could occur only with sudden, violent forces acting on the body or by specific signs and symptoms of vertebral or spinal cord injury. Damage to the bones of the spinal column is not always evident. If an initial injury to the cord has not occurred, a neurologic deficit may not be present, even though the spinal column is unstable. If any of these indications is present, regardless of the absence of any of the others, the prehospital care provider needs to assume that an unstable spine exists and manage it accordingly.

Immobilization of spinal fractures, as with other fractures, requires immobilization of the joint above and the joint below the injury. For the spine, the joints above are the head and neck, and the joint below is the pelvis. The device selected should immobilize the head, chest, and pelvis areas in a neutral inline position without causing or allowing movement. Interim methods and devices to protect the spine can be used until the patient is immobilized in a supine position on a long backboard.

SCENARIO SOLUTION

This patient is exhibiting signs of neurogenic shock. Unopposed parasympathetic influence on the vascular system below the point of spinal injury results in an increased size of the vascular container and imposes a relative hypovolemia. The body's response to decreased tissue perfusion is normal above the point of spinal cord injury, resulting in typical signs of shock caused by sympathetic nervous system response. Patients with neurogenic shock, however, are bradycardic as opposed to tachycardic.

The first priorities of care are to continue to maintain a patent airway and oxygenation and assist ventilation to ensure an adequate minute volume while concurrently providing manual stabilization of the cervical spine. Immobilize the patient effectively and efficiently on a long backboard and transport the patient to an appropriate facility. Manage hypotension caused by neurogenic shock with intravenous fluids.

The goals of prehospital management for this patient are to prevent additional spinal cord trauma, maintain tissue perfusion, and care for extremity trauma en route, and transport without delay to a trauma center for definitive care. ■

References

1. DeVivo MJ: Causes and costs of spinal cord injury in the United States, *Spinal Cord* 35:809, 1997.

2. Jackson AB, Dijkers M, Devivo MJ, Poczatek RB: A demographic profile of new traumatic spinal cord injuries: change and stability over 30 years, *Arch Phys Med Rehabil* 85:1740, 2004.

3. Meldon SW, Moettus LN: Thoracolumbar spine fractures: clinical presentation and the effect of altered sensorium and major injury, *J Trauma* 38:1110, 1995.

4. Ross SE, O'Malley KF, DeLong WG, et al: Clinical predictors of unstable cervical spine injury in multiply injured patients, *Injury* 23:317, 1992.

5. Marion DW, Pryzybylski G: Injury to the vertebrae and spinal cord. In Mattox KL, Feliciano DV, Moore EE, editors: *Trauma*, New York, 2000, McGraw-Hill.

6. Tator CH, Fehlings MG: Review of the secondary injury theory of acute spinal cord trauma with special emphasis on vascular mechanisms, *J Neurosurg* 75:15, 1991.

7. Tator CH: Spinal cord syndromes: physiologic and anatomic correlations. In Menezes AH, Sonntag VKH, editors: *Principles of spinal surgery,* New York, 1995, McGraw-Hill.

8. Bilello JP, Davis JW, Cunningham MA, et al. Cervical spinal cord injury and the need for cardiovascular intervention, *Arch Surg* 138:1127, 2003.

9. Section on Disorders of the Spine and Peripheral Nerves of the American Association of Neurologic Surgeons/Congress of Neurologic Surgeons: Blood pressure management after acute spinal cord injury, *Neurosurgery* 50:S58, 2002.

10. Ullrich A, Hendey GW, Geiderman J, et al: Distracting painful injuries associated with cervical spinal injuries in blunt trauma, *Acad Emerg Med* 8:25, 2001.

11. Domeier RM, Evans RW, Swor RA, et al: Prospective validation of out-of-hospital spinal clearance criteria: a preliminary report, *Acad Emerg Med* 4:643, 1997.

12. Domeier RM, Swor RA, Evans RW, et al: Multicenter prospective validation of prehospital clinical spinal clearance criteria, *J Trauma* 53:744, 2002.

13. Hankins DG, Rivera-Rivera EJ, Ornato JP, et al: Spinal immobilization in the field: clinical clearance criteria and implementation, *Prehosp Emerg Care* 5:88, 2001.

14. Stroh G, Braude D: Can an out-of-hospital cervical spine clearance protocol identify all patients with injuries? An argument for selective immobilization, *Ann Emerg Med* 37:609, 2001.

15. Dunn TM, Dalton A, Dorfman T, Dunn WW: Are emergency medical technician-basics able to use a selective immobilization of the cervical spine protocol? A preliminary report, *Prehosp Emerg Care* 8:207, 2004.

16. Domeier RM, Frederiksen SM, Welch K: Prospective performance assessment of an out-of-hospital protocol for selective spine immobilization using clinical spine clearance criteria, *Ann Emerg Med* 46:123, 2005.

17. Domeier RM, National Association of EMS Physicians Standards and Practice Committee: Indications for prehospital spinal immobilization, *Prehosp Emerg Care* 3:251, 1997.

18. Kwan I, Bunn F: Effects of prehospital spinal immobilization: a systematic review of randomized trials on healthy subjects, *Prehosp Disast Med* 20:47, 2005.

19. Connell RA, Graham CA, Munro PT: Is spinal immobilization necessary for all patients sustaining isolated penetrating trauma? *Injury* 34:912, 2003.

20. Kennedy FR, Gonzales P, Beitler A, et al: Incidence of cervical spine injuries in patients with gunshot wounds to the head, *Southern Med J* 87:621, 1994.

21. Chong CL, Ware DN, Harris JH: Is cervical spine imaging indicated in gunshot wounds to the cranium? *J Trauma* 44:501, 1998.

22. Kaups KL, Davis JW: Patients with gunshot wounds to the head do not require cervical spine immobilization and evaluation, *J Trauma* 44:865, 1998.

23. Lanoix R, Gupta R, Leak L, Pierre J: C-spine injury associated with gunshot wounds to the head: retrospective study and literature review, *J Trauma* 49:860, 2000.

24. Barkana Y, Stein M, Scope A, et al: Prehospital stabilization of the cervical spine for penetrating injuries of the neck: is it necessary? *Injury* 34:912, 2003.

25. Cornwell EE, Chang, DC, Boner JP, et al: Thoracolumbar immobilization for trauma patients with torso gunshot wounds—is it necessary? *Arch Surg* 136:324, 2001.

26. American College of Surgeons Committee on Trauma: *Advanced trauma life support for doctors, student course manual,* ed 7, Chicago, 2004, American College of Surgeons.

27. Krell JM, McCoy MS, Sparto PJ, et al: Comparison of the Ferno Scoop stretcher with the long backboard for spinal immobilization, *Prehosp Emerg Care* 10:46, 2006.

28. DeBoer SL, Seaver M: Big head, little body syndrome: what EMS providers need to know, *Emerg Med Serv* 33:47, 2004.

29. Section on Disorders of the Spine and Peripheral Nerves of the American Association of Neurologic Surgeons/Congress of Neurologic Surgeons: Cervical spine immobilization before admission to the hospital, *Neurosurgery* 50:S7, 2002

30. Nesathurai S: Steroids and spinal cord injury: revisiting the NASCIS 2 and NASCIS 3 trials, *J Trauma* 45:1088, 1998.

31. Bledsoe BE, Wesley AK, Salomone JP: High-dose steroids for acute spinal cord injury in emergency medical services, *Prehosp Emerg Care* 8:313, 2004.

32. Donaldson WF, Lauerman WC, Heil B, et al: Helmet and shoulder pad removal from a player with suspected cervical spine injury: a cadaveric model, *Spine* 23:1729, 1998.

33. Gastel JA, Palumbo MA, Hulstyn MJ, et al: Emergency removal of football equipment: a cadaveric cervical spine injury model, *Ann Emerg Med* 32:411, 1998.

34. Kleiner DM, Almquist JL, Bailes J, et al: *Prehospital care of the spine-injured athlete.* Inter-Association Task Force for Appropriate Care of the Spine-Injured Athlete, Dallas, 2001, National Athletic Trainers' Association.

35. Palumbo MA, Hulstyn MJ: The effect of protective football equipment on the alignment of the injured cervical spine, *Am J Sports Med* 24:446, 1996.

36. Prinsen RKE, Syrotuik DG, Reid DC: Position of the cervical vertebrae during helmet removal and cervical collar application in football and hockey, *Clin J Sport Med* 5:155, 1995.

37. Swenson TM, Lauerman WC, Blanc RO, et al: Cervical spine alignment in the immobilized football player: radiographic analysis before and after helmet removal, *Am J Sports Med* 25:226, 1997.

38. Waninger KN: Management of the helmeted athlete with suspected cervical spine injury, *Am J Sports Med* 32:1331, 2004.
39. Waninger KN: On-field management of potential cervical spine injury in helmeted football players: leave the helmet on! *Clin J Sport Med* 8:124, 1998.

Suggested Reading

American College of Surgeons Committee on Trauma: *Advanced trauma life support for doctors, student course manual*, ed 7, Chicago, 2004, ACS.
Pennardt AM, Zehner WJ: Paramedic documentation of indicators for cervical spine injury, *Prehosp Disaster Med* 9:40, 1994.

Spine Management

Manual Inline Stabilization

Principle: To maintain the cervical spine in a neutral inline position until the patient is completely immobilized.

Behind

From behind the patient, the prehospital care provider places his or her hands over the patient's ears without moving the patient's head. The thumbs are placed against the posterior aspect of the patient's skull. The little fingers are placed just under the angle of the mandible. The remaining fingers are spread on the flat lateral planes of the patient's head. Pressure is applied in such a manner as to maintain the head in a stable position. If the head is not in a neutral inline position, the provider slowly moves the head until it is, unless contraindicated. The provider brings his or her arms in and rests them against the seat, headrest, or torso for additional support.

Side

Standing at the side of the patient, the prehospital care provider passes his or her arm over the patient's shoulder closest to the provider and cups the back of the patient's head with his or her hand, being careful not to move the patient's head. The thumb and first finger of one hand are placed on either side of the patient's face. The thumb and finger should rest in the notch formed where the patient's teeth and maxilla join. Enough pressure is supplied to support and stabilize the patient's head. If the patient's head is not in a neutral inline position, the provider slowly moves the head until it is, unless contraindicated. The provider braces his or her elbows on the patient's torso for additional support.

Front

Standing directly in front of the patient, the prehospital care provider places his or her hands on both sides of the patient's head as shown. The little fingers are placed at the posterior aspect of the patient's skull. One thumb is placed in the notch between the patient's upper teeth and the maxilla on each cheek. The remaining fingers are spread on the flat lateral planes of the patient's head. Pressure is applied in such a manner as to maintain the head in a stable position. If the patient's head is not in a neutral inline position, the provider slowly moves the head until it is, unless contraindicated. The provider brings his or her arms in and braces the elbows against the patient's torso for additional support.

Note: The provider can also use this method when kneeling alongside the thorax of a supine patient and facing toward the patient's head.

Supine Patient

The prehospital care provider positions himself or herself above the supine patient's head, either kneeling or lying. The hands are placed on either side of the patient's head, covering the patient's ears with the palms. The fingers are spread in a fashion to stabilize the patient's head with the fingers pointing toward the patient's feet (caudal). The fourth and fifth digits of each hand should wrap around the posterior portion of the patient's skull. The elbows and forearms can be rested on either the ground or the provider's knees for additional support.

Logroll

Principle: To turn a patient while maintaining manual stabilization with minimal movement of the spine. The logroll is indicated for (1) positioning a patient onto a long backboard or other device to facilitate movement of the patient and (2) turning a patient with suspected spinal trauma to examine the back.

Supine Patient

While one prehospital care provider maintains neutral inline stabilization at the patient's head, a second provider applies a properly sized cervical collar.

While one provider maintains neutral inline stabilization, a second provider kneels at the patient's midthorax, and a third provider kneels at the level of the patient's knees. The patient's arms are straightened and placed palms-in next to the torso while the patient's legs are brought into neutral alignment. The patient is grasped at the shoulder and hips in such a fashion as to maintain a neutral inline position of the lower extremities. The patient is "logrolled" slightly onto his or her side. The long backboard is placed with the foot end of the board positioned between the patient's knees and ankles (the head of the long backboard will extend beyond the patient's head).

The long backboard is held at an angle against the patient's back. The patient is logrolled onto the long backboard, and the board is lowered to the ground with the patient.

Once on the ground, the patient is grasped firmly by the shoulders, the pelvis, and the lower extremities.

The patient is moved upward and laterally onto the long backboard. Neutral inline stabilization is maintained without pulling on the patient's head and neck.

The patient is positioned onto the long backboard with the head at the top of the board and the body centered.

Prone or Semiprone Patient

When a patient presents in a prone or semiprone position, a stabilization method similar to that used for the supine patient can be used. The method incorporates the same initial alignment of the patient's limbs, the same positioning and hand placement of the prehospital care providers, and the same responsibilities for maintaining alignment.

The patient's arms are positioned in anticipation of the full rotation that will occur. With the semiprone logroll method, a cervical collar can be safely applied only after the patient is in an inline position and supine on the long backboard, not before.

Whenever possible, the patient should always be rolled away from the direction in which the patient's face initially points. One provider establishes inline manual stabilization of the patient's head and neck. Another provider kneels at the patient's thorax and grasps the patient's opposite shoulder and wrist and pelvis area. A third provider kneels at the patient's knees and grasps the patient's wrist and pelvis area and lower extremities. The long backboard is placed on the lateral edge with the foot of the board between the patient's knees and ankles.

The patient is logrolled onto his or her side. The patient's head rotates less than the torso, so by the time the patient is on his or her side (perpendicular to the ground), the head and torso have come into proper alignment.

Once the patient is supine on the long backboard, the patient is moved upward and toward the center of the board. The prehospital care providers should take care not to pull the patient but to maintain neutral inline stabilization. Once the patient is positioned properly on the long backboard, a properly sized cervical collar can be applied, and the patient can be secured to the backboard.

Long Backboard Immobilization

Principle: To fully immobilize a supine patient to a long backboard while maintaining the head and neck in a neutral position and minimizing the risk of additional injuries.

Long backboard immobilization is indicated when spinal immobilization is indicated (see Figure 9-12). This is not to be confused with transporting a trauma patient strapped to a long backboard for ease of movement when immobilization is *not* indicated.

Adult Patient

The patient's head and neck are moved into a neutral inline position (unless contraindicated; see p. 235), manual inline stabilization is maintained, and a properly sized cervical collar is applied. With an acceptable method, the patient is positioned on the long backboard.

While maintaining manual stabilization, the patient's upper torso is first secured to the backboard. The lower torso (pelvis) is then secured. The patient's body must be secured in such a fashion as not to allow any movement up, down, or laterally. Padding is inserted under the patient's head as needed to maintain a neutral inline position, and pads or rolled towels are placed on each side of the patient's head.

Note: When immobilizing the patient's head to the backboard, a strap is fastened tightly over the pads and the lower forehead. A second strap is placed over the pads and the rigid cervical collar and fastened snugly to the board.

The final step in immobilizing the patient to the board is to secure the lower extremities. Padding is placed between the patient's legs and on the outside of the legs to help prevent movement. The straps are placed distal to the patient's knees and just above the knees, and the patient's lower legs are secured with the toes pointing straight up.

Pediatric Patient

Two major adjustments from the adult method are necessary when immobilizing a small child to a long backboard. Because of the relatively large size of the child's head in comparison to the body, padding is needed under the torso to elevate it and maintain the spine in a neutral alignment. The accompanying photo shows prehospital care providers preparing a child for immobilization to a long backboard. Note that the padding extends from the patient's shoulders down to the top of the pelvis and to the lateral sides of the board.

Note: Small children are usually narrower than an adult-sized backboard. Padding should be placed between the child's sides and the sides of the board to prevent lateral movement. Pediatric-sized devices take these differences into account and are preferable if available.

Standing Long Backboard Application

Principle: To fully immobilize a standing patient to a long backboard while maintaining the head and neck in a neutral position and minimizing the risk of additional injury.

This application is indicated for spinal immobilization of a trauma patient who is ambulatory but is found to have an indication for spinal immobilization (see Figure 9-12).

Two general methods exist for immobilizing a standing patient to a long backboard. The first method involves securing the standing patient's torso and head to the board before lowering the board to the ground. This method causes some discomfort to the patient and may not allow the patient to be lowered to the ground without movement. The second method involves manual stabilization of the patient to the board while lowering the board and patient to the ground and then securing the patient to the board. This second method is the preferred method and can be accomplished with three rescuers.

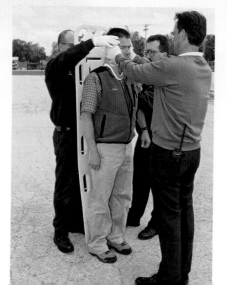

Three or More Providers

Prehospital care providers can apply manual inline stabilization from either behind the patient or in front of the patient. Once manual inline stabilization is applied, a properly sized rigid cervical collar can be applied. A long backboard is placed behind the patient from the side and pressed against the patient. Once the board is in place, manual inline stabilization is maintained until the patient is secured to the long backboard.

Two prehospital care providers stand on either side of the patient, turned slightly toward the patient. Each provider inserts the hand closest to the patient under the patient's armpit and grasps the nearest handhold of the backboard without moving the patient's shoulders. The other hand grasps a higher handhold on the board. While manual inline stabilization is maintained, the patient and backboard are lowered to the ground.

As the patient is lowered to the ground, manual stabilization is maintained through rotation of the hands. Once the patient and board are on the ground, the patient is secured to the long backboard.

Two Providers

When three or more prehospital care providers are not available, two providers can achieve immobilization. The two providers stand on each side of the patient, turned slightly toward the patient. Each provider places the hand closest to the patient under the patient's armpit and grasps the nearest handhold on the backboard. The other hand is placed with the palm surface (finger extended) against the lateral sides of the patient's head and pressed inward toward each other to maintain manual stabilization.

The patient is lowered, along with the backboard, to the ground. The prehospital care providers need to work together during this move to ensure maximum manual stabilization. Once the patient and backboard are on the ground, manual inline stabilization is maintained while a properly sized cervical collar is applied and the patient is secured to the long backboard.

Sitting Immobilization (Vest-Type Extrication Device)

Principle: To immobilize a trauma patient without critical injuries before moving the patient from a sitting position.

This type of immobilization is used when spinal stabilization is indicated for a sitting trauma patient without life-threatening conditions.

Several brands of vest-type extrication devices are available. Each model is slightly different in design, but any model can serve as a general example. The KED is used in this demonstration. The details (but not the general sequence) are modified when using a different model or brand of extrication device. Also, during this demonstration, the roof and windshield of the vehicle have been removed for clarification purposes. Once manual inline stabilization is initiated and a properly sized cervical collar applied, the patient is positioned in an upright seated position with an adequate amount of space between the patient's back and the vehicle seat.

Note: Before placing the vest-type device behind the patient, the two long straps (groin straps) are unfastened and placed behind the vest device. After placing the vest device behind the patient, the side flaps are placed around the patient and moved until the side flaps are touching the patient's armpits.

The torso straps are positioned and fastened, starting with the middle chest strap and followed by the lower chest strap. Each strap is tightened after attachment. Use of the upper chest strap at this time is optional. If the upper chest strap is used, the provider should ensure that it is not so tight that it impedes the patient's ventilations. The upper chest strap should be tightened just before moving the patient.

Each groin strap is positioned and fastened. Each strap is placed under the patient's leg and attached to the vest on the same side as the strap's origin. Using a back-and-forth motion, the strap is worked under the patient's thigh and buttock until it is in a straight line in the intergluteal fold from front to back. Once in place, each groin strap is tightened. The patient's genitalia should not be placed under the straps but to the side of each strap.

Note: The torso straps should be evaluated and readjusted as needed. Pads should be placed behind the patient's head as needed to maintain a neutral inline position. The head flaps will need to be positioned, which will involve careful changing of the hands supporting the patient's head. The patient's head is secured to the head flaps of the vest device. The provider should be careful not to seat the patient's mandible or obstruct the airway. All straps should be rechecked before moving the patient. If the upper chest strap has not been secured, it should be attached and tightened.

If possible, the ambulance cot with a long backboard should be brought to the opening of the vehicle door. The long backboard is placed under the patient's buttocks so that one end is securely supported on the vehicle seat and the other end on the ambulance cot. If the ambulance cot is not available or the terrain will not allow the placement of the cot, other prehospital care providers can hold the long backboard while the patient is rotated and lifted out of the vehicle.

While rotating the patient, the patient's lower extremities must be elevated onto the seat. If the vehicle has a center console, the patient's legs should be moved over the console one at a time.

Once the patient is rotated with his or her back to the center of the long backboard, the patient is lowered to the board while keeping the legs elevated. After placing the patient onto the long backboard, the two groin straps are released and the patient's legs are lowered. The patient is positioned by moving him or her up on the board with the vest device in place. The provider should consider releasing the upper chest strap at this time.

Once the patient is positioned on the long backboard, the vest device is left secured in place to continue to immobilize the patient's head, neck, and torso. The patient and vest device are secured to the long backboard. The patient's lower extremities are immobilized to the board, and the long backboard is secured to the ambulance cot.

Rapid Extrication

Principle: To manually stabilize a patient with critical injuries before and during movement from a sitting position.

Three or More Providers

Sitting patients with life-threatening conditions and indications for spinal immobilization (see Figure 9-12) can be rapidly extricated. Immobilization to an interim device before moving the patient provides more stable immobilization than when using only the manual (rapid extrication) method. However, it requires an additional 4 to 8 minutes to complete. The prehospital care provider will use the vest or halfboard methods in the following situations:

- When the scene and patient's condition are stable and time is not a primary concern.

or

- When a special rescue situation involving substantial lifting or technical rescue hoisting exists, and significant movement or carrying of the patient is involved before it is practical to complete the supine immobilization to a long backboard.

Rapid extrication is indicated in the following situations:

- When the patient has life-threatening conditions identified during the primary survey.
- When the scene is unsafe and clear danger to the prehospital care provider and patient exists, necessitating rapid removal to a safe location.
- When the patient needs to be moved quickly to access other, more seriously injured patients.

Note: Rapid extrication is only selected when life-threatening conditions are present and not on the basis of personal preference.

Once the decision is made to extricate a patient rapidly, manual inline stabilization of the patient's head and neck in a neutral position is initiated. This is best accomplished from behind the patient. If a provider is unable to get behind the patient, manual stabilization can be accomplished from the side. Whether from behind the patient or the side, the patient's head and neck are brought into a neutral alignment, a rapid assessment of the patient is performed, and a properly sized cervical collar is applied. An ambulance cot with a long backboard should be placed next to the open vehicle door.

While manual stabilization is maintained, the patient's upper torso and lower torso and legs are controlled. The patient is rotated in a series of short, controlled movements until control of manual stabilization can no longer be maintained.

A second prehospital care provider goes outside the vehicle and takes control of the manual stabilization. The provider in the backseat moves and takes control of the patient's lower torso and legs.

The rotation of the patient is continued until the patient can be lowered out of the vehicle door opening and onto the long backboard. The long backboard is placed with the foot end of the board onto the vehicle seat and the head end on the ambulance cot. If the cot cannot be placed next to the vehicle, other prehospital care providers can hold the long backboard while the patient is lowered onto the backboard.

Once the patient's torso is down on the board, the weight of the patient's chest is controlled while the patient's pelvis and lower legs are controlled. The patient is moved upward onto the long backboard. The prehospital care provider who is maintaining manual stabilization is careful not to pull the patient but to support the patient's head and neck.

After the patient is positioned onto the long backboard, the prehospital care providers can secure the patient to the board and the board to the ambulance cot. The patient's upper torso is secured first, then the lower torso and pelvis area, then the head. The patient's legs are secured last. If the scene is unsafe, the patient should be moved to a safe area before being secured to the board or cot.

Note: This represents only one example of rapid extrication. Because very few field situations are ideal, prehospital care providers may need to modify the steps for extrication for the particular patient and situation. The principle of rapid extrication should remain the same regardless of the situation: maintain manual stabilization throughout the extrication process without interruption, and maintain the entire spine in an inline position without unwanted movement. Any positioning of the prehospital care providers that works can be successful. However, numerous position changes and hand position takeovers should be avoided because they invite a lapse in manual stabilization.

The rapid extrication technique can effectively provide manual inline stabilization of the patient's head, neck, and torso throughout a patient's removal from a vehicle. The following are three key points of rapid extrication:

1. One prehospital care provider maintains stabilization of the patient's head and neck at all times, another rotates and stabilizes the patient's upper torso, and a third moves and controls the patient's lower torso, pelvis, and lower extremities.
2. Maintaining manual inline stabilization of the patient's head and neck is impossible if attempting to move the patient in one continuous motion. The prehospital care providers need to limit each movement, stopping to reposition and prepare for the next move. Undue haste will cause delay and may result in movement of the spine.
3. Each situation and patient may require adaptation of the principles of rapid extrication. This can only work effectively if the maneuvers are practiced. Each provider needs to know the actions and movements of the other providers.

Two Providers

In some situations an adequate number of providers may not be available to extricate a critical patient rapidly. In these situations a two-provider technique is useful.

One prehospital care provider initiates and maintains manual inline stabilization of the patient's head and neck. A second provider places a properly sized cervical collar on the patient and places a prerolled blanket around the patient. The center of the blanket roll is placed at the patient's midline on the rigid cervical collar. The ends of the blanket roll are wrapped around the cervical collar and placed under the patient's arms.

The patient is turned using the ends of the blanket roll and until the patient's back is centered on the door opening.

The first provider takes control of the blanket ends, moving them under the patient's shoulders, and moves the patient by the blanket while the second provider moves and controls the patient's lower torso, pelvis, and legs.

Helmet Removal

Principle: To remove a safety helmet while minimizing the risk of additional injury.

Patients who are wearing full-face helmets must have the helmet removed early in the assessment process (Box 9-4). This provides immediate access for the prehospital care provider to assess and manage a patient's airway and ventilatory status. Helmet removal ensures that hidden bleeding is not occurring into the posterior helmet and allows the provider to move the head (from the flexed position caused by large helmets) into neutral alignment. It also permits complete assessment of the head and neck in the secondary survey and facilitates spinal immobilization when indicated (see Figure 9-12). The prehospital care provider explains to the patient what will occur. If the patient verbalizes that the provider should not remove the helmet, the provider explains that properly trained personnel can remove it by protecting the patient's spine. Two providers are required for this maneuver.

One provider takes position above the patient's head. With palms pressed on the sides of the helmet and fingertips curled over the lower margin, the first provider stabilizes the helmet, head, and neck in as close to a neutral inline position as the helmet allows. A second provider kneels at the side of the patient, opens or removes the face shield if needed, and unfastens or cuts the chin strap.

The patient's mandible is grasped between the thumb and the first two fingers at the angle of the mandible. The other hand is placed under the patient's neck on the occiput of the skull to take control of manual stabilization. The provider's forearms should be resting on the floor or ground or on the provider's thighs for additional support.

The first provider pulls the sides of the helmet slightly apart, away from the patient's head, and rotates the helmet with up-and-down rocking motions while pulling it off of the patient's head. Movement of the helmet is slow and deliberate. The provider takes care as the helmet clears the patient's nose.

Once the helmet is removed, padding should be placed behind the patient's head to maintain a neutral inline position. Manual stabilization is maintained, and a properly sized cervical collar is placed on the patient.

Note: Two key elements are involved in helmet removal, as follows:

1. While one provider maintains manual stabilization of the patient's head and neck, the other provider moves. At no time should both providers be moving their hands.
2. The provider rotates the helmet in different directions, first to clear the patient's nose and then to clear the back of the patient's head.

BOX 9-4   Athletic Equipment Removal

A number of recent publications, including a position paper, have advocated the immobilization of helmeted athletes to a long backboard with the helmet in place.[32-39] A search of the medical literature for supporting evidence reveals that these recommendations are based on, at best, Class III research. Studies criticizing the practice of helmet removal have primarily been done in cadavers. These studies report that extreme hyperextension of the cervical spine occurs when the helmet alone is removed and the shoulder pads are left in place; however, all the studies were done without the placement of appropriate padding under the head to prevent it from falling back onto the backboard. Adherence to proper spinal precautions and application of treatment principles will best accomplish the task of spinal immobilization whether or not the helmet or shoulder pads are removed.

Athletic equipment should be removed by personnel trained and experienced in the removal of sports equipment. Historically, these trained and experienced personnel generally have been those individuals, usually athletic trainers, present at the athletic event site. Emergency medical services (EMS) responders, however, need to receive training in such removal, because access to the airway, if needed, can be accomplished only by appropriate access to the patient's face and head, which requires removal of the facemask at a minimum and the helmet in many cases. If the decision is made *not* to remove the equipment at the scene, someone knowledgeable in sports equipment removal should accompany the patient to the hospital.

While special care for helmeted athletes is needed, the general principles of spinal immobilization taught in Prehospital Trauma Life Support (PHTLS) courses are appropriate and need to be followed. Ideally, the helmet and shoulder pads should be removed as one unit. However, it is still possible to immobilize a player to a long backboard without causing hyperextension of the cervical spine when the helmet alone is removed. This is accomplished by the appropriate use of padding behind the head to maintain the head in neutral alignment with the rest of the spine if the shoulder pads are not removed. EMS responders must determine the specific medical needs for an injured athlete and take appropriate steps to meet those needs, which may often include immediate removal of the athletic equipment.

Padding to Maintain Neutral Inline Position

Failure to provide proper padding behind the patient's head can result in either hyperextension or hyperflexion of the patient's neck. This may result in excessive movement of the spine and or may compromise the airway.

Proper padding behind the head will place the head and neck in a neutral inline position. Each patient will require difference amounts of padding based on body type. Proper alignment will have the opening of the patient's ear in line with the point of the shoulder, with the patient's face centered on the midline.

Padding to Secure Patient to Long Backboard

When securing a patient to a long backboard, all voids between the sides of the patient and the sides of the long backboard need to be filled with padding. Filling the side voids with proper strapping will help prevent the patient from moving laterally on the board.

Chapter Objectives

At the completion of this chapter, the reader will be able to do the following:

✓ Discuss the normal anatomy and physiology of the thoracic organs.

✓ Describe the alterations in anatomy and physiology that result from thoracic injury.

✓ Discuss the relationships among the kinematics of trauma, thoracic anatomy and physiology, and various assessment findings, leading to an index of suspicion for various injuries.

✓ Differentiate between patients in need of rapid stabilization and transport and patients in whom further on-scene assessment and management is warranted or appropriate.

✓ Discuss the impact of an urban or suburban and rural or austere setting on assessment and management of thoracic injury.

✓ Describe the signs, symptoms, pathophysiology, and management of the following specific thoracic injuries:

> Rib fractures
> Flail chest
> Pulmonary contusion
> Pneumothorax (simple, open, and closed)
> Tension pneumothorax
> Hemothorax
> Blunt cardiac injury
> Cardiac tamponade
> Commotio cordis
> Traumatic aortic disruption
> Tracheobronchial disruption
> Traumatic asphyxia
> Diaphragmatic rupture

CHAPTER 10

Thoracic Trauma

SCENARIO

You are called to the scene of a motorcycle crash on the downtown freeway. You anticipate a 5- to 8-minute response time. While you are en route, the first responders radio a report that the incident involves a 37-year-old male who skidded on a patch of oil on the pavement. He spun out and struck the concrete wall on the righthand side of the road, coming to a halt with the motorcycle on top of his right lower extremity. When you arrive, the bike has been removed, the scene secured, and the patient is on a long backboard in the breakdown lane with a cervical collar in place.

As you begin your assessment, you ascertain that the patient is awake and having difficulty breathing. He complains of chest and right lower extremity pain. He is able to describe the incident but speaks in three- and four-word bursts between rapid, labored respirations. His skin is pale, cool, and moist. His pulse is rapid and full. His right pant leg is torn and bloody, and the foot appears to be abnormally rotated. Your partner applies oxygen as you continue the assessment. The trachea is midline, and there is no jugular venous distention. There is significant tenderness along the right lateral chest wall with crepitance, and the breath sounds are diminished on that side. Associated abrasions and bruising are present over the lateral chest. The abdomen is not distended or tender. The right lower extremity has a laceration over the midtibia with exposed bone.

Why is this patient in respiratory distress? Does he have life-threatening injuries? What interventions should you undertake in the field? What modality should be used to transport this patient? How would a different location (e.g., rural) impact your management and plans during prolonged transport? What other injuries do you suspect based on the above information? ■

As with other forms of injury, thoracic trauma can result from blunt or penetrating mechanisms. Blunt force applied to the thoracic cage in motor vehicle crashes, high falls, beatings, or crush injuries can cause disruption of the normal anatomy and physiology of the thoracic organs. Similarly, penetrating wounds from gunshots, knives, or impalement on objects such as rebar can injure the thorax. Definitive management of most thoracic injuries does not require *thoracotomy* (opening the chest cavity operatively). In fact, only 15% to 20% of all chest injuries require thoracotomy. The remaining 85% are well managed with relatively simple interventions, such as supplemental oxygen, ventilatory support, analgesia, and tube *thoracostomy* (chest tube placement) when necessary.[1-3]

Nevertheless, these injuries can be quite significant. The thoracic organs are intimately involved in the maintenance of oxygenation, ventilation, and oxygen delivery. Injury to the chest, especially if not promptly recognized and appropriately managed, can lead to significant morbidity. *Hypoxia* (inadequate amounts of oxygen in the blood), *hypercarbia* (excessive carbon dioxide in the blood), *acidosis* (excessive acid in the blood), and *shock* (inadequate amounts of oxygen reaching the body's organs and tissues) can result from inadequate management of chest injury in the short term and thereby contribute to late complications such as multisystem organ failure. This accounts for the 25% of trauma deaths that result from thoracic injury.[1-3]

Anatomy

The chest is roughly a hollow cylinder formed by its bony and muscular structures. There are 12 paired ribs. The upper 10 pairs attach to the spinal column in the back and either the sternum or the rib above in the front. The lower two pairs of ribs only attach in back to the spine. In the front they are free and thus referred to as "floating ribs." This bony cage provides a great deal of protection to the internal organs of the chest cavity. In fact, the lower ribs also shield the organs of the upper abdomen (most notably the spleen and liver). This bony cage is reinforced with muscle. The *intercostal muscles* lie between and connect the ribs to one another. A number of muscle groups move the upper extremity and are part of the chest wall, including the major and minor pectoral muscles, anterior and posterior serratus muscles, and latissimus dorsi muscles, along with the various muscles of the back. All this "padding" means that it takes a considerable amount of force to injure the internal organs.

There are also muscles involved in the process of breathing (ventilation), including the intercostal muscles; the *diaphragm*, which is a dome-shaped muscle attached around the lower aspect of the chest; and muscles in the neck that attach to upper ribs. An artery, vein, and nerve course along the lower edge of each rib, providing blood and stimulation to the intercostal muscles.

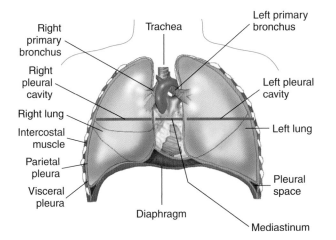

FIGURE 10-1 The thoracic cavity, including the ribs, intercostal muscles, diaphragm, mediastinum, lungs, heart, great vessels, bronchi, trachea, and esophagus.

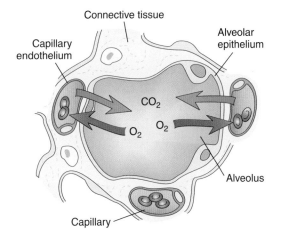

FIGURE 10-2 The capillaries and alveolus lie in close proximity; therefore, oxygen *(O₂)* can easily diffuse through the capillary, alveolar walls, capillary walls, and red blood cells. Carbon dioxide *(CO₂)* can diffuse back in the opposite direction.

Lining the cavity formed by these structures is a thin membrane called the *parietal pleura.* A matching thin membrane covers the other organs of the chest cavity, called the *visceral pleura.* There is normally no space between these two membranes. In fact, they are adhered to one another by a small amount of fluid between them that holds them together, much as a thin layer of water will hold two sheets of glass together. This pleural fluid creates a surface tension, which serves to oppose the elastic nature of the lungs, preventing their otherwise natural tendency to collapse.

The lungs occupy the right and left sides of the chest cavity (Figure 10-1). Between them and enveloped by them is a space called the *mediastinum,* which contains the trachea, the main bronchi, the heart, the major arteries and veins to and from the heart, as well as the esophagus.

Physiology

The two components of chest physiology that are most likely to be impacted by injury are *breathing* and *circulation.*[1-3] Both these processes need to be working properly for oxygen to reach the body's organs, tissues, and ultimately cells and to expel carbon dioxide. To best understand what happens to patients when their chests are injured, and how to manage their injuries, it is important to understand the physiology of these two processes.

Ventilation

The lay terms "breathing" and "respiration" actually refer to the physiologic process of ventilation. *Ventilation* is the mechanical act of drawing air through the mouth and nose into the trachea and bronchi and then into the lungs, where it arrives in small air sacs known as *alveoli.* The

process of drawing air in is called *inhalation.* Oxygen in that air is transported across the lining membrane of the alveoli, into adjacent small blood vessels known as *capillaries,* where it attaches to hemoglobin in the red blood cells for transport to the body. This process is known as *oxygenation.* Simultaneously, carbon dioxide (CO_2), which is dissolved in the blood, diffuses out into the air within the alveoli for expulsion when that air is blown out again in the process of *exhalation* (Figure 10-2). *Cellular respiration* is the use of oxygen by the cells to produce energy (see Chapter 7).

Inhalation is brought about by contraction of the muscles of respiration (primarily the intercostals and the diaphragm), which results in a lifting and separating of the ribs and downward motion of the diaphragm. This action increases the size of the thoracic cavity and creates a negative pressure within the chest cavity compared with the air pressure outside the body, resulting in flow of air into the lungs (Figures 10-3 and 10-4). *Expiration* is achieved by relaxing the intercostals and diaphragm, resulting in the return of the ribs and diaphragm to their resting positions. This return causes the pressure within the chest to exceed the pressure outside the body, and air from the lungs is emptied through the bronchi, trachea, mouth, and nose to the outside.

Control of ventilation is under the control of the respiratory center of the brainstem. There are two main pathways by which the brain controls ventilation. The primary method is through detection of the partial pressure of arterial carbon dioxide ($Paco_2$) by specialized cells in the respiratory center known as *chemoreceptors.* The "backup method" is by detection of oxygen by other chemoreceptors in the aorta and carotid arteries. $Paco_2$ reflects how much acid is in the blood. The body neutralizes acid with bicarbonate, which is then converted to CO_2. Carbon dioxide is eliminated through the lungs, as previously noted. If the chemoreceptors

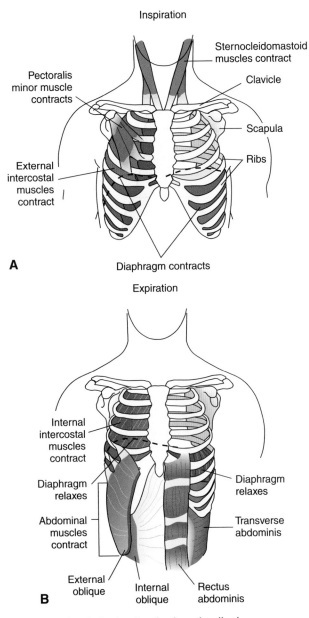

FIGURE 10-3 **A,** During inspiration, the diaphragm contracts and flattens. Accessory muscles of inspiration, such as the external intercostal, pectoralis minor, and sternocleidomastoid muscles, lift the ribs and sternum, which increases the diameter and volume of the thoracic cavity. **B,** In expiration during quiet breathing, the elasticity of the thoracic cavity causes the diaphragm and ribs to assume their resting positions, which decreases the volume of the thoracic cavity. In expiration during labored breathing, muscles of expiration, such as the internal intercostal and abdominal muscles, contract, causing the volume of the thoracic cavity to decrease more rapidly.

detect increased Pa_{CO_2}, they stimulate the respiratory center to increase the depth and frequency of breaths, eliminating more CO_2 and returning Pa_{CO_2} to normal (Figure 10-5). This process is very efficient and can increase the volume of air moved in and out of the lungs per minute by a factor of 10.

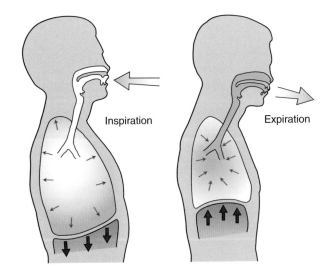

FIGURE 10-4 When the diaphragm is relaxed and the glottis is open, the pressure inside and outside the lungs is equal. When the chest cavity expands, the intrathoracic pressure decreases and air goes in the lungs.

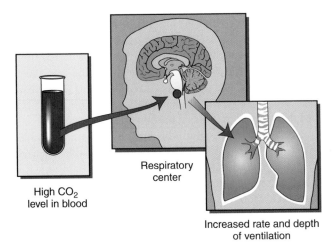

FIGURE 10-5 An increased level of carbon dioxide is detected by nerve cells sensitive to this change, which stimulates the lung to increase both depth and rate of ventilation.

In certain lung diseases, such as emphysema, or chronic obstructive pulmonary disease (COPD), the lungs are not able to eliminate CO_2 as effectively. This results in a chronic elevation of the CO_2 level in the blood. The chemoreceptors become insensitive to changes in Pa_{CO_2} in this case. In this situation the backup chemoreceptors in the aorta and carotid arteries stimulate breathing when the partial pressure of arterial oxygen (Pa_{O_2}) falls. Similar to when the brainstem chemoreceptors detect an increase in Pa_{CO_2} and stimulate increased respirations to lower the CO_2 level, the oxygen chemoreceptors stimulate the respiratory muscles to be more active, increasing the respiratory rate and depth to raise the Pa_{O_2} to more normal values (Figure 10-6).

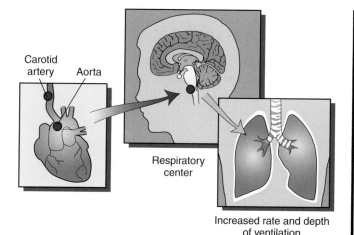

Carotid artery   Aorta

Respiratory center

Increased rate and depth of ventilation

FIGURE 10-6 Receptors located in the aorta and carotid arteries are sensitive to the oxygen level and will stimulate the lungs to increase air movement into and out of the alveolar sacs.

Box 10-1 defines several terms that are important in discussing and understanding the physiology of ventilation.[4]

Circulation

The other major physiologic process that may be affected after thoracic injury is circulation. Chapter 7 covers this topic more extensively, but the following discussion sets the stage for the pathophysiology of chest injury.

The heart, which lies in the center of the chest, within the mediastinum, functions as a biologic pump. For a pump to work, it must be primed with fluid. For the heart, this priming function is provided by the return of blood through two large veins, the *superior vena cava* (SVC) and the *inferior vena cava* (IVC). The heart then normally contracts 70 to 80 times per minute, ejecting blood out to the body through the aorta.

Processes that interfere with the return of blood to the heart through the SVC and IVC (e.g., loss of blood through hemorrhage, increased pressure in chest cavity from tension pneumothorax) cause the output of the heart and thus the blood pressure to decrease. Similarly, processes that injure the heart itself (e.g., cardiac contusion) may make the heart a less efficient pump, causing the same physiologic abnormalities. Just as chemoreceptors recognize changes in CO_2 or O_2 levels, *baroreceptors* recognize changes in blood pressure and direct the heart to change the rate and forcefulness of its beating to return to the blood pressure to normal.

Pathophysiology

As mentioned earlier, both blunt and penetrating mechanisms may disrupt the physiologic processes just described.

> **BOX 10-1   Pulmonary Volumes and Relationships**
>
> **Dead space:** Amount of air brought into the lungs that does not have the opportunity to exchange oxygen and carbon dioxide with the blood in the alveolar capillaries (e.g., air in trachea and bronchi).
>
> **Expiratory reserve volume (ERV):** Remaining air that can be forced out of the lungs after a normal exhalation (1.8-0.8 liters [L]).
>
> **Functional residual capacity (FRC):** Amount of air remaining in the lungs after a normal exhalation; also referred to as the *resting lung volume* (3.0-2.6 L).
>
> **Inspiratory capacity (IC):** Amount of air that can be inhaled after a normal exhalation (3.0-2.6 L).
>
> **Inspiratory reserve volume (IRV):** Amount of air that can additionally be inhaled after a normal inhalation (2.5-1.2 L).
>
> **Minute ventilation (V_E):** Total volume of air moved into and out of the lungs in 1 minute.
>
> **Residual volume (RV):** Amount of air remaining in the lungs after a maximal exhalation (1.8-1.2 L).
>
> **Tidal volume (V_T):** Amount of air that is inhaled then exhaled during a normal breath (0.5-0.4 L).
>
> **Total lung capacity (TLC):** Total volume the lungs contain when maximally inflated. This volume declines with age from 6.0 L in young adults to approximately 4.0 L in elderly persons.
>
> **Vital capacity (VC):** Amount of air that can be exhaled after a maximal inhalation (4.8-2.4 L).
>
> **Work of breathing:** Physical work or effort performed in moving the chest wall and diaphragm to breathe. This work increases with rapid breathing, increasing minute ventilation, and when the lungs are abnormally stiff.
>
> The relationships between these volumes and capacities can be further illustrated through the following equations:
>
> $$TLC = FVC + RV$$
> $$VC = IRV + V_T + ERV = IC + ERV$$
> $$TLC = FRC + IC$$
> $$FRC = ERV + RV$$
> $$IC = IRV + V_T$$

There are common elements in the disturbances created by these mechanisms.

Penetrating Injury

Conceptually, penetrating injuries are easier to understand. In these injuries, objects of varying size transgress the chest wall, enter the thoracic cavity, and lacerate the organs within the thorax. Normally, no space exists between the pleural membranes. However, when a penetrating wound creates a communication between the chest cavity and the outside world, air tends to rush into the pleural space through the wound with respiration, because the resistance to airflow through the wound is often less than that through the airways. Air in the pleural space *(pneumothorax)* disrupts the adherence between the pleural membranes created by the thin film of pleural fluid. All these processes together allow the lung to collapse, preventing effective ventilation. Wounds of the lung by a penetrating object also allow air to escape into the pleural space and result in collapse of the lung. In either case, the patient becomes short of breath. To make up for the lost ventilation capacity, the respiratory center will stimulate more rapid breathing. This increases the work of breathing. The patient may be able to tolerate the increased workload for a time, but if not recognized and treated, the patient is at risk for ventilatory failure, which will be manifested by increasing respiratory distress as the CO_2 levels in the blood rise and the O_2 levels fall.

If there is continued entry of air into the chest cavity without any exit, pressure will begin to build in the pleural space, leading to tension pneumothorax. This will further impede the patient's ability to ventilate. It also will begin to impact circulation negatively as venous return to the heart is reduced by the increasing intrathoracic pressure, with displacement of the mediastinal structures into the opposite side of the chest. Shock may then ensue.

Lacerated tissues bleed, and torn blood vessels certainly bleed. Penetrating wounds to the chest may result in bleeding into the pleural space *(hemothorax)* from the chest wall muscles, the intercostal vessels, and the lungs. Penetrating wounds to the major vessels in the chest result in catastrophic bleeding. Each pleural space can accommodate approximately 3000 mL of fluid. Thoracic bleeding into the pleural space may not be readily apparent externally, but it may be of sufficient magnitude to create a shock state. The presence of large volumes of blood in the pleural space will also impede the patient's ability to breathe; the blood in the pleural space prevents expansion of the lung on that side.

Wounds of the lung may also result in bleeding into the lung tissue itself. This blood floods the alveoli, preventing them from filling with air. Alveoli filled with blood cannot participate in gas exchange. The more alveoli that are flooded, the more compromised are the patient's ventilation and oxygenation.

Blunt Force Injury

Similar physiologic disturbances as in penetrating injury result from blunt trauma, although the pathway is less direct. Blunt force applied to the chest wall is transmitted through the chest wall to the thoracic organs, especially the lungs. This wave of energy can tear lung tissue and blood vessels, which may result in bleeding into the alveoli. In this setting the injury is called a *pulmonary contusion.* The impact on oxygenation and ventilation is the same as with penetrating injury.

If the force applied to the lung tissue also tears the parietal pleura, air may escape from the lung into the pleural space, creating a pneumothorax and the potential for a tension pneumothorax, as previously described. Blunt force trauma to the chest can also break ribs, which can then lacerate the lung, resulting in pneumothorax as well as hemothorax (both caused by bleeding from the broken ribs as well as from the torn lung and intercostal muscles). Blunt force injury may also cause shearing or rupture of the major blood vessels in the chest, particularly the aorta, leading to catastrophic hemorrhage. Finally, in some cases, blunt force can disrupt the chest wall, allowing air to enter the chest cavity through the wound, as in penetrating injury.

Energy and Injury

The ability of any mechanism to cause injury is related to the amount of energy that that mechanism delivers to a particular body part or organ. Penetration from knives and impalements carry little energy, and the organs are injured from direct laceration by the penetrating object. Gunshot wounds will transmit greater amounts of energy as the mass of the projectile and particularly its velocity increase. The greater the energy, the farther the zone of injury will be from the wound tract. Similarly, the higher the energy imparted in a blunt force injury, the greater is the risk for injury. Compare a low fall in which the chest strikes a coffee table, to an assault with a baseball bat, to a high-speed motor vehicle crash (MVC). The greater the energy, the greater is the prehospital care provider's suspicion that the injuries will interfere with ventilation, oxygenation, or circulation.

Blunt and penetrating mechanisms may also directly involve the heart, resulting in cardiac contusion or cardiac tamponade. These entities are described in the following sections.

Assessment

As in all aspects of medical care, assessment involves taking a history and performing a physical examination. In trauma situations, we speak of an *AMPLE history,* in which the patient's **a**ge, **m**edications, **p**ast history, time of the **l**ast meal, and the **e**vents surrounding the injury are elucidated.[5]

Besides the overall mechanism that resulted in injury, patients are asked about any symptoms they may be experiencing if they are conscious and able to communicate. Victims of chest trauma will likely be experiencing chest pain, which may be sharp, stabbing, or constricting.

Frequently the pain is worse with respiratory efforts or movement. The patient may report a sense of being short of breath or being unable to take in an adequate breath. The patient may feel apprehensive or lightheaded if shock is developing. It is important to remember that the absence of symptoms does not equate to the absence of injury.

The next step in assessment is the performance of a physical examination. There are four components to the physical examination: observation, palpation, percussion, and auscultation. The assessment should also include a determination of vital signs. Placement of a pulse oximeter to assess arterial oxygen saturation is a useful adjunct in the assessment of the injured patient.[5,6]

- **Observation.** The patient is observed for pallor of the skin and sweating, which may indicate the presence of shock. The patient may also appear apprehensive. The presence of *cyanosis* (bluish discoloration of skin, especially around mouth and lips) may be evident in advanced hypoxia. The frequency of respirations and whether the patient appears to be having trouble breathing (gasping, contractions of the accessory muscles of respiration in the neck, nasal flaring) should be noted. Is the trachea in the midline, or deviated to one side or the other? Are the jugular veins distended? The chest is examined for contusions, abrasions, lacerations, and whether the chest wall expands symmetrically with breathing. Does any portion of the chest wall move paradoxically with respiration (instead of moving out during inspiration, does it collapse inward, and vice versa, during exhalation)?
- **Auscultation.** The entire chest is evaluated. Decreased breath sounds on one side compared to the other may indicate pneumothorax or hemothorax on the examined side. Pulmonary contusions may result in rhonchi or rales.
- **Palpation.** Next, by gently pressing the chest wall with hands and fingers, assessment for the presence of tenderness, crepitance (either bony or subcutaneous emphysema), and instability of the chest wall is performed.
- **Percussion.** This examination technique is difficult to perform in the field because the environment is often noisy, making evaluation of the percussion note difficult. A finger is placed flat on the chest wall, then that finger is struck sharply with a finger of the opposite hand. This produces a sound wave in the percussed structure. A *dull* percussion note over the chest may indicate underlying pulmonary contusion or hemothorax. A *resonant* percussion note may indicate the presence of a pneumothorax.

Repeat determinations of the respiratory rate may be the most important assessment tool. As patients become hypoxic and compromised, an early clue to this change is a gradual increase in the respiratory rate.

Management of Specific Injuries

Rib Fractures

Despite the ribs being fairly well protected by overlying musculature, rib fractures are a common occurrence in thoracic trauma. The upper ribs are broad, thick, and particularly well protected by the shoulder girdle and muscles.[1-3] Because it requires great energy to fracture the upper ribs, this patient is at risk for harboring other significant injuries, such as traumatic disruption of the aorta. Rib fractures occur most often in ribs 4 to 8 laterally, where they are thin and have less overlying musculature. The broken ends of the ribs may tear muscle, lung, and blood vessels, with the possibility of an associated pulmonary contusion.[1,3,7] Simple rib fractures are rarely life threatening in adults. Fracture of the lower ribs[8-10] may be associated with injuries of the spleen and liver.[1,3,7] Compression of the lung may rupture the aveolae.

Assessment

Patients with simple rib fractures may have few symptoms. Most often they will complain of chest pain and perhaps shortness of breath. They may have labored respirations, chest wall tenderness, and crepitance. The prehospital care provider assesses vital signs, paying particular attention to the respiratory rate. Pulse oximetry also should be performed.[1,11,12]

Management

Pain relief is a primary goal in the initial management of patients with rib fractures. This may involve reassurance, immobilization with appropriate padding to minimize motion, and positioning of the patient's arms using a sling and swath. It is important to reassure and continuously reassess the patient, keeping in mind the potential for deterioration in ventilation and the development of shock. Establishing intravenous (IV) access should be considered, depending on the patient's condition and anticipated transport time. Administration of small doses of IV narcotic analgesics may be appropriate in some situations for advanced units with appropriate medical control. The patient is encouraged to take deep breaths and cough to prevent the collapse of the alveoli *(atelectasis)* and the potential for pneumonia and other complications. Rigid immobilization of the rib cage with tape or straps should be avoided because these interventions predispose to the development of atelectasis and pneumonia.[1,3] Administration of oxygen and ventilatory support may be necessary.

Flail Chest

Flail chest occurs when two or more adjacent ribs are fractured in more than one place along their length. This produces a segment of chest wall that is no longer in continuity with the remainder of the chest. The force necessary to produce such a lesion guarantees that the underlying lung will be contused. The patient thus has two sources of respiratory embarrassment: the flail segment and the underlying pulmonary contusion. Because the flail segment is not connected to the surrounding chest wall, it tends to move paradoxically during breathing. When the respiratory muscles contract to raise the ribs up and out and lower the diaphragm, the flail segment paradoxically moves inward in response to the negative pressure being created within the thoracic cavity (Figure 10-7). This so-called paradoxical motion of the flail segment makes ventilation inefficient. The degree of inefficiency is directly related to the size of the flail segment. As described earlier, the second embarrassment is the pulmonary contusion, which does not allow for gas exchange in the contused portion of the lung because of alveolar flooding.

Assessment

As with a simple rib fracture, assessment of flail chest will reveal a patient in pain. The pain is typically more severe, however, and the patient usually appears to be in distress. The respiratory rate is elevated, and the patient does not take deep breaths. Hypoxia may be present, as demonstrated by pulse oximetry or cyanosis. Paradoxical motion may or may not be evident or easily recognized. Initially, the intercostal muscles will be in spasm and tend to stabilize the flail segment. As these muscles fatigue, the paradoxical motion becomes evident. The patient will have tenderness and potentially bony crepitus over the injured segment. The instability of the segment may also be appreciated on palpation.

Management

Management of flail chest is directed toward pain relief, ventilatory support, and monitoring for deterioration. The respiratory rate may be the most important parameter to follow. Pulse oximetry, if available, is also useful to detect hypoxia.[6] Oxygen should be administered and IV access obtained, except in cases of extremely short transport times. Support of ventilation with bag-valve-mask (BVM) assistance or endotracheal intubation and positive-pressure ventilation may be necessary (particularly with prolonged transport times).[11] Efforts to stabilize the flail segment with sandbags or other means are contraindicated.[1]

Pulmonary Contusion

When lung tissue is lacerated or torn by blunt or penetrating mechanisms, bleeding into the alveolar air spaces can result in pulmonary contusion. The chief physiologic abnormality is prevention of gas exchange because no air enters these alveoli. Blood and edema fluid in the tissue between the alveoli further impedes gas exchange in the alveoli that are ventilated. As previously noted, pulmonary contusion is almost always present in the patient with a flail segment. Pulmonary contusion is a common and potentially lethal

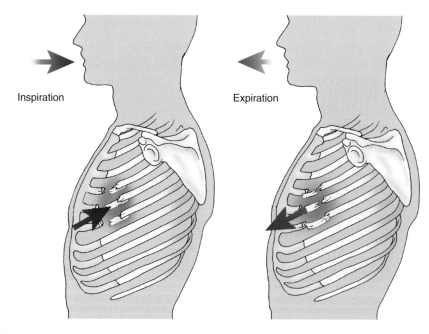

Inspiration

Expiration

FIGURE 10-7   Paradoxical motion. If stability of the chest wall has been lost by ribs fractured in two or more places, in which case intrathoracic pressure decreases during inspiration, the external air pressure forces the chest wall inward. When intrathoracic pressure increases during expiration, the chest wall is forced outward.

complication of thoracic injury.[3,7] Deterioration to the point of frank respiratory failure may occur over the first 24 hours after injury.

Assessment

Assessment findings of the patient are variable depending on the severity of the contusion (percentage of involved lung). Early assessment may reveal no respiratory embarrassment. A high index of suspicion is necessary, particularly in the presence of a flail segment.

Management

Management is directed toward support of ventilation. Supplemental oxygen should be administered. Meticulous reevaluation is necessary. The prehospital care provider repeatedly reassesses the respiratory rate and checks pulse oximetry (ensuring that it remains at least 95%) and the patient's degree of respiratory distress. Support of ventilation with BVM or endotracheal intubation may be necessary.[12] In the absence of hemodynamic compromise, IV fluid administration should be limited to keep the vein open because excess fluid may further increase edema and compromise ventilation and oxygenation.

Pneumothorax

Pneumothorax is present in up to 20% of severe chest injuries.[8] The three types of pneumothorax represent increasing levels of severity: simple, open, and tension.

Simple pneumothorax is the presence of air within the pleural space. As the amount of air in the pleural space increases, the lung on that side collapses (Figure 10-8). *Open pneumothorax* (also called "sucking chest wound") involves a pneumothorax associated with a defect in the chest wall that allows air to enter and exit the pleural space from the outside with ventilatory effort. *Tension pneumothorax* occurs when air continues to enter the pleural space but has no avenue for egress. This results in increasing pressure within the pleural space, compromising circulatory function.

Simple Pneumothorax

Assessment. Assessment in simple pneumothorax is likely to demonstrate findings similar to those in rib fracture. The patient frequently complains of pleuritic chest pain and may exhibit varying symptoms and signs of respiratory dysfunction. The classic findings are decreased breath sounds on the side of injury and a tympanitic percussion note. Any patient with respiratory distress and diminished breath sounds should be assumed to have a pneumothorax. Auscultation over the apices of the lungs is more likely to demonstrate decreased breath sounds than the midlung fields.

Management. A key point in management is the recognition that a simple pneumothorax may become a tension pneumothorax at any moment. The patient needs to be monitored closely for development of tension pneumothorax

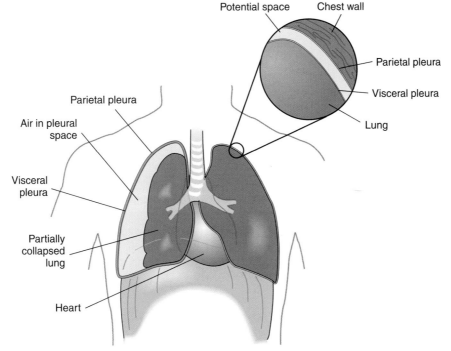

FIGURE 10-8   Air in the pleural space forces the lung in, decreasing the amount that can be ventilated and therefore decreasing oxygenation of the blood leaving the lung.

in case intervention is needed (see later discussion).[8-14] In addition to monitoring and being prepared to decompress a tension pneumothorax, the provider administers supplemental oxygen, obtains IV access, and is prepared to treat shock if it develops. If spinal immobilization is not necessary, the patient may be more comfortable in a semi-recumbent position. Rapid transport is essential.[9,12,13] If the provider is functioning at the basic level, rendezvous with an advanced life support (ALS) unit should be considered.

Open Pneumothorax

Open pneumothorax, as with simple pneumothorax, involves air entering the pleural space, causing the lung to collapse. In the open type, a defect in the chest wall results in a communication between the outside air and the pleural space. When the patient attempts to inhale, air crosses the wound and enters the pleural space because of the negative pressure created in the thoracic cavity as the muscles of respiration contract. In larger wounds, there may be free flow of air in and out of the pleural space with the different phases of respiration (Figure 10-9). This abnormal airflow through the chest wall may occur preferentially to the normal flow through the upper airways into the lung, because resistance to flow through the wound is often lower than that through the airway, particularly when the defect is large. Effective ventilation is then inhibited by collapse of the lung on the injured side, with preferential flow of air into the pleural space rather than into the lung. Some patients may have airflow into the pleural space with inspiration, but no flow out during expiration, creating a ball-valve effect. This sets the stage for the development of a tension pneumothorax.

Mechanisms leading to open pneumothorax include gunshot wounds, shotgun blasts, stabbings, impalements, and occasionally blunt trauma.

Assessment. Assessment of the patient with open pneumothorax generally reveals obvious respiratory distress. The patient will be anxious and tachypneic. The pulse rate will be elevated and potentially thready. Observation of the chest wall will reveal the wound, which may make audible sucking sounds during inspiration, with bubbling during expiration.

Management. Initial management of an open pneumothorax involves closing the defect in the chest wall and administering supplemental oxygen. Airflow through the wound usually can be stopped by application of an occlusive dressing to the wound, which is secured on three sides.[1] This prevents airflow into the chest cavity during inspiration while allowing air to escape through the loose side of the dressing during exhalation (Figure 10-10).

If these measures fail to support the patient adequately, endotracheal intubation and positive-pressure ventilation may be necessary.[11] If positive pressure is utilized, the provider needs to monitor the patient carefully for the development of tension pneumothorax. If signs of increasing respiratory distress develop, the dressing over the wound should be removed to allow for decompression of any accumulating tension. If this is ineffective, needle decompression and positive-pressure ventilation should be considered if not already employed.[10]

A patient with an open pneumothorax virtually always has an injury to the underlying lung. Thus, two sources can leak air into the pleural space: the hole in the chest wall and the hole in the lung. Even if an injury to the chest wall is sealed with an occlusive dressing, air leakage into the pleural space can continue from the injured lung, setting the stage for a tension pneumothorax (Figure 10-11). At least one commercially available device is marketed for management of open pneumothoraces (Asherman chest seal). No data has been published demonstrating that this device is equivalent or superior to a simple occlusive dressing (aluminum foil or Vaseline gauze). Thus, the added cost is probably not justified.

FIGURE 10-9   A gunshot or stab wound to the chest produces a hole in the chest wall through which air can flow both into and out of the pleural cavity.

FIGURE 10-10   Taping a piece of foil or plastic to the chest wall on three sides creates a flutter-valve effect, allowing air to escape from the pleural space but not enter into it.

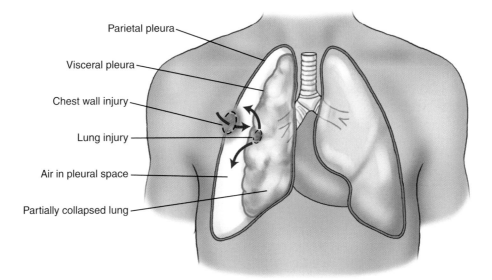

FIGURE 10-11   Because of the proximity of the chest wall to the lung, it would be extremely difficult for the chest wall to be injured by penetrating trauma and the lung not to be injured. Stopping the hole in the chest wall does not necessarily decrease air leakage into the pleural space; leakage can come from the lung just as easily.

Tension Pneumothorax

Tension pneumothorax is a life-threatening emergency. If air continues to enter the pleural space and does not vent, intrathoracic pressure builds up. This has two devastating consequences: respiratory embarrassment and shock. The increasing pressure on the injured side of the chest pushes the structures in the mediastinum to the other side of the chest (Figure 10-12). This distortion of anatomy impedes venous return to the heart through the kinked IVC and makes inflation of the lung on the uninjured side more difficult by restricting the space within which it may expand. The result may be uncompensated shock. Respiratory compromise results from the same processes. The shift of the mediastinal structures into the uninjured chest compresses the lung on that side, increasing the work necessary to fill it with air. At the same time, the lung on the injured side is collapsed and does not participate significantly in gas exchange. The end result can be hypoxia and frank respiratory failure.

Any patient with thoracic injury is at risk for development of tension pneumothorax. Patients at particular risk are those who likely have a pneumothorax (e.g., patient with signs of rib fracture), those who have a known pneumothorax (e.g., patient with a penetrating wound to the chest), and those with chest injury who are undergoing positive-pressure ventilation. Such patients must be closely monitored and transported to an appropriate facility as quickly as possible.

Assessment. Assessment findings depend on how much pressure has accumulated in the pleural space. Initially, patients will exhibit apprehension and discomfort. They will generally complain of chest pain and at least some

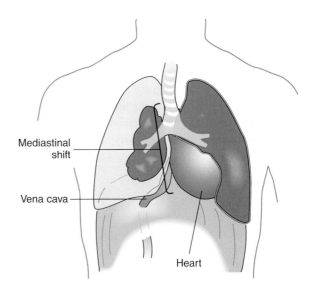

FIGURE 10-12   Tension pneumothorax. If the amount of air trapped in the pleural space continues to increase, not only is the lung on the affected side collapsed, but the mediastinum is also shifted to the opposite side. The lung on the opposite side then collapses and intrathoracic pressure increases, which decreases capillary blood flow and kinks the vena cava.

shortness of breath. As the tension worsens, they will exhibit increasing agitation and respiratory distress. In severe cases, cyanosis and apnea may occur. The classic findings are tracheal deviation away from the side of injury, diminished breath sounds on the side of injury, and a tympanitic percussion note. It is difficult enough to detect diminished breath sounds in the field environment. Constant practice in auscultation of all patients will hone the provider's

Although the following signs are frequently discussed with a tension pneumothorax, many may not be present or are difficult to identify in the field:

- *Tracheal deviation* is usually a late sign. In the neck, the trachea is bound to the cervical spine by fascial and other supporting structures; thus the deviation of the trachea is more of an intrathoracic phenomenon, although it may be felt if it is severe. Tracheal deviation is not often seen in the prehospital environment. Even when it is present, it can be difficult to diagnose by physical examination.
- *Distended neck veins* are described as a classic sign of tension pneumothorax. However, since a patient with a tension pneumothorax may also have lost a considerable amount of blood, distended neck veins may not be prominent. If the patient has a pneumatic antishock garment (PASG) applied, the neck veins may be distended by the device and not by a tension pneumothorax.
- *Cyanosis* is difficult to see in the field. Poor lighting, variation in skin color, and dirt and blood associated with trauma often render this sign unreliable.
- *Decreased breath sounds on the injured side.* The most helpful part of the physical examination is checking for decreased breath sounds on the side of the injury. However, to use this sign the prehospital care provider must be able to distinguish between normal and decreased sounds. Such differentiation requires a great deal of practice. Listening to breath sounds during every patient contact will help.
- *Percussion of the chest* is an excellent method for determining the status of the chest cavity in the relative quiet of a hospital. In the noisy prehospital environment this sound is much more difficult to detect. Given the difficulty in obtaining this sign and the time and environment necessary with which to perform it, it is not recommended for field diagnosis of tension pneumothorax.

FIGURE 10-13 Needle decompression of the thoracic cavity is most easily accomplished and produces the least chance for complication if it is done at the midclavicular line through the second intercostal space.

skill and make detection of this important finding more likely. Detection of a tympanitic percussion note in the field is basically impossible, but the finding is mentioned for the sake of completeness. Other physical findings that may be evident are jugular venous distention, chest wall crepitance, and cyanosis. Tachycardia and tachypnea become increasingly prominent as the intrathoracic pressure builds, culminating in hypotension and uncompensated shock.

Management. The first priority in management is to decompress the tension pneumothorax.[10] In the patient with an open pneumothorax, if an occluding dressing has been applied, it should be removed for several seconds. This should allow the tension pneumothorax to decompress through the wound with a rush of air. This procedure may need to be repeated periodically during transportation if symptoms of tension recur. If removing the dressing for several seconds is ineffective, or if there is no open wound, an ALS provider may proceed with needle thoracostomy (10- to 16-gauge) to decompress the tension pneumothorax (see Specific Skills section for complete description of the procedure). In general, chest tubes (tube thoracostomy) are not inserted in the prehospital setting because of concerns of infection, potential complications, and the need for maintenance of skill proficiency. Published complication rates with tube thoracostomy range from 2.8% to 21%.[15,16] Decompressive needle thoracostomy should be performed when three findings are present: (1) worsening respiratory distress or difficulty ventilating with a BVM device, (2) unilateral decreased or absent breath sounds, and (3) decompensated shock (systolic blood pressure <90 mm Hg).[10,14] If decompression is not an option, rapid transport to an appropriate facility while administering high-concentration (≥85%) oxygen is imperative.

Needle Decompression. Needle decompression is performed though the second or third intercostal space in the midclavicular line (Figure 10-13). This location is chosen because of ease of access for the prehospital care provider transporting a patient who likely has been "packaged for transport" on a backboard with cervical collar, with arms down along the sides (making access to the midaxillary line difficult, where chest tubes are usually placed). The decompressive catheter, once placed, is less likely to be displaced from the midclavicular line. The lung on the affected side is collapsed and shifted to the contralateral side; thus it is unlikely to be injured during the procedure. Decompression is performed with a large bore (10- to 16-gauge) intravenous needle. In some cases, needle decompression may not be effective, possibly because the needle is too short (<5 cm) to penetrate the chest wall, or because the catheter kinked after removal of the needle, blocking further air escape.[17,18] A pleural decompression needle/catheter is commercially available that has a large bore (8.5 French) and wire reinforcement of the catheter, lessening the likelihood of kinking (Emergency Pneumothorax Set-Prehospital, Cook Critical Care, Bloomington, Ind). The needle and catheter should be advanced until the return of a rush of air is achieved and advanced no farther. Once the decompression is achieved, the catheter is taped to the chest to prevent dislodgement. Improper placement (location of depth) may result in injuries to the lungs, heart, or great vessels.[19]

This procedure converts the tension pneumothorax into a negligible open pneumothorax. Usually, the relief to respiratory effort far outweighs the negative effect of the open pneumothorax. Continued provision of supplemental oxygen, as well as ventilatory support as needed, is appropriate.

As a general rule, bilateral tension pneumothorax is exceedingly rare in patients who are not intubated and ventilated with positive pressure. The first step in reassessing the patient is to confirm the location of the endotracheal (ET) tube, ensure that it has no kinks or bends causing compression of the tube, and ensure that the tube has not inadvertently moved down into a mainstem bronchus. Extreme caution should be exercised with bilateral needle decompression in patients who are not being ventilated with positive-pressure ventilation. If the provider's assessment is in error, the creation of bilateral pneumothoraces can cause severe respiratory distress.

The patient should be rapidly transported to an appropriate facility. Intravenous access should be obtained unless transport time is particularly short. The patient must be closely observed for deterioration. Repeat decompression and endotracheal intubation may become necessary.

Hemothorax

Hemothorax occurs when blood enters the pleural space. Because this space can accommodate between 2500 and 3000 mL, hemothorax can represent a source of significant blood loss. In fact, the loss of circulating blood volume from bleeding into the pleural space represents a greater physiologic insult to the patient with chest injury than the collapse of the lung that the hemothorax produces (Figure 10-14). It is rare that enough blood accumulates

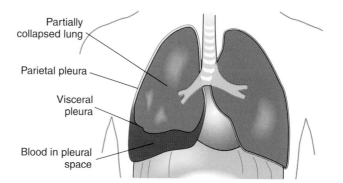

FIGURE 10-14 Hemothorax. The amount of blood that can accumulate in the thoracic cavity (leading to hypovolemia) is a much more severe condition than the amount of lung compressed by this blood loss.

to create a "tension hemothorax." The mechanisms resulting in hemothorax are the same as those causing the various types of pneumothorax. The bleeding may come from the chest wall musculature, the intercostal vessels, the lung parenchyma, pulmonary vessels, or the great vessels of the chest.

Assessment

Assessment reveals a patient in some distress. Chest pain and shortness of breath again are prominent features. The prehospital care provider should actively look for signs of shock: pallor, confusion, tachycardia, tachypnea, and hypotension. Breath sounds on the side of the injury are diminished, but the percussion note is dull. Pneumothorax may be present in conjunction with hemothorax, increasing the likelihood for cardiorespiratory compromise.

Management

Management includes serial observation to detect physiologic deterioration while providing appropriate support. High-concentration oxygen should be administered and ventilation supported if necessary with BVM or more advanced techniques, if available and indicated. Hemodynamic status is closely monitored and fluid therapy provided. Rapid transport to an appropriate facility capable of immediate surgical intervention completes the management algorithm for hemothorax.

Blunt Cardiac Injury

Cardiac injury most often results from application of force to the anterior chest, especially in a deceleration event such as an MVC with frontal impact.[1,20] An example would be the patient's chest impacting the steering wheel of the vehicle as the car crashes into a bridge abutment. The heart is then compressed between the sternum anteriorly and the spinal column posteriorly (Figure 10-15). This compression of the heart causes an abrupt increase in the pressure

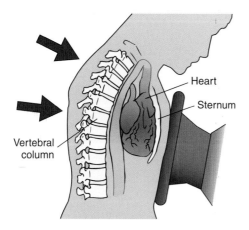

FIGURE 10-15 The heart can be compressed between the sternum (as the sternum stops against the steering column or dashboard) and the posterior thoracic wall (as the wall continues its forward motion). This can contuse the myocardium.

within the ventricles to several times normal, which results in cardiac contusion, sometimes valvular injury, and rarely cardiac rupture, as follows:

- *Cardiac contusion.* The most common result of cardiac compression is cardiac contusion; the heart muscle is bruised, with varying amounts of injury to the myocardial cells. This most often results in abnormal heart rhythms, such as sinus tachycardia.[20] Of greater concern but less common are premature ventricular contractions (PVCs) or nonperfusing rhythms such as ventricular tachycardia (VT) and ventricular fibrillation (VF). If the septal region of the heart is injured, the electrocardiogram (ECG) may demonstrate interventricular conduction abnormalities, such as right bundle branch block (RBBB). If a sufficient volume of myocardium is injured, the contractility of the heart may be impaired, and cardiac output falls, resulting in cardiogenic shock. Unlike the other forms of shock usually encountered in the trauma setting, this shock does not improve with fluid administration and may actually worsen.
- *Valvular rupture.* Rupture of the supporting structures of the heart valves or the valves themselves typically renders the valves incompetent. The patient will present in varying degrees of shock with symptoms and signs of congestive heart failure (CHF), such as tachypnea, rales, and new-onset heart murmur.
- *Blunt cardiac rupture.* A rare event, blunt cardiac rupture occurs in less than 1% of patients with blunt chest trauma.[20-22] Most of these patients will die at the scene from exsanguination or fatal cardiac tamponade. The surviving patients will present with cardiac tamponade, as discussed later.

Assessment

Assessment in the patient with blunt cardiac injury reveals a mechanism that imparted a frontal impact to the center of the patient's chest. A bent steering column accompanied by bruising over the sternum implies such a mechanism. As with other chest injuries, the patient is likely to complain of chest pain or shortness of breath. If a dysrhythmia is present, the patient may complain of palpitations. Physical findings of concern are bruising over the sternum, crepitance over the sternum, and sternal instability. With a floating sternum *(flail sternum),* the ribs on either side of the sternum are broken, allowing it to move paradoxically with respirations, similar to flail chest, as described earlier. If valvular disruption has occurred, a harsh murmur may be detectable over the precordium along with signs of acute CHF, such as hypotension, jugular venous distention, and rales. ECG monitoring may demonstrate tachycardia, PVCs, other rhythm disturbances, or ST-segment elevation.

Management

The key management strategy is correct assessment that blunt cardiac injury may have occurred and to transmit that concern along with the clinical findings to the receiving hospital. In the meantime, high-concentration oxygen is administered and IV access established for judicious fluid therapy. The patient should be placed on a cardiac monitor to detect arrhythmias and ST-segment elevations if present. If dysrhythmias are present and ALS providers are present, pharmacotherapy should be instituted. As always, ventilatory support measures should be implemented as indicated.

Cardiac Tamponade

Cardiac tamponade occurs when fluid acutely accumulates between the pericardial sac and the heart.[1,21] The pericardial sac is composed of a fibrous, inelastic tissue. Normally there is very little fluid in the pericardial sac, similar to the pleural space, as described earlier. Because the pericardium is inelastic, pressure begins to rise rapidly within the pericardial sac as fluid accumulates within it. This rising pericardial pressure impedes venous return to the heart and leads to diminished cardiac output and blood pressure. With each contraction of the heart, additional fluid may enter the pericardial sac, further impeding the ability of the heart to fill in preparation for the next contraction (Figure 10-16). This can become profound enough to precipitate *pulseless electrical activity* (PEA) and is a life-threatening injury requiring coordinated response by providers in all phases of care to achieve an optimal outcome. The normal adult pericardium may be able to accommodate as much as 300 mL of fluid before pulselessness occurs, but as little as 50 mL is usually enough to impede cardiac return and thus cardiac output.[1]

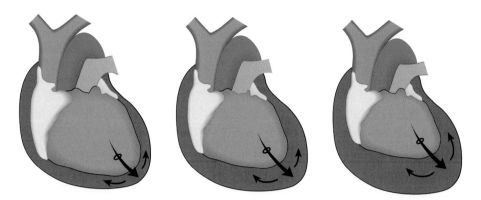

FIGURE 10-16 Cardiac tamponade. As blood courses from the cardiac lumen into the pericardial space, it limits expansion of the ventricle. Therefore the ventricle cannot fill completely. As more blood accumulates in the pericardial space, less ventricular space is available to accumulate blood, and cardiac output is reduced.

Most often, cardiac tamponade is caused by a stab wound to the heart. This may result in penetration into one of the cardiac chambers or just a laceration of the myocardium. In either event, bleeding into the pericardial sac occurs. The rising pressure within the pericardium results in the cardiac tamponade physiology. At the same time, the increased pressure within the pericardium may temporarily tamponade further bleeding from the cardiac wound, allowing for survival. In the case of gunshot wounds to the heart, the damage to the heart and pericardium is so severe that the pericardium cannot contain the hemorrhage, resulting in rapid exsanguination. The same is true in the case of impalements. Blunt rupture of a cardiac chamber can result in cardiac tamponade but more often causes exsanguinating hemorrhage.

Cardiac tamponade should be kept in mind as a possibility in evaluating any patient with a thoracic penetration. This index of suspicion should be raised to the level of "present until proven otherwise" posture when the penetrating injury is within a rectangle (the cardiac box) formed by drawing a horizontal line along the clavicles, vertical lines from the nipples to the costal margins, and a second horizontal line connecting the points of intersection between the vertical lines and the costal margin (Figure 10-17). The presence of such a wound should be communicated to the receiving institution as soon as it is recognized.

Assessment

Assessment involves quickly recognizing the presence of at-risk wounds, as previously described, in combination with an appreciation for the physical findings of pericardial tamponade. *Beck's triad* is a constellation of findings indicative of cardiac tamponade: (1) muffled heart sounds (the fluid around the heart makes it difficult to hear the sounds of the valves closing), (2) jugular venous distention (caused by the increasing pressure in the pericardial sac backing blood up into the neck veins), and (3) low blood pressure. Another physical finding described in cardiac tamponade

FIGURE 10-17 In a series of 46 patients with penetrating cardiac injuries, 40 had a wound within the "cardiac box." (Richardson JD, Flint LM: *Trauma: pathophysiology and clinical care*, Chicago, 1987, Yearbook Medical.

is paradoxical pulse. This is actually an accentuation of the normal, slight drop in systolic blood pressure (SBP) that occurs during inspiration. As the lungs expand, there is preferential filling and ejection of blood from the right side of the heart at the expense of the left side. Thus peripheral blood pressure falls. This decrease in SBP is usually less than 10 to 15 mm Hg. A greater decrease in SBP constitutes the so-called paradoxical pulse.

Detection of some of these signs is difficult in the field, especially muffled heart tones and paradoxical pulse. Thus the field provider needs to maintain a high index of suspicion, based on the location of the wounds and hypotension, and implement therapy accordingly.

Management

Management requires rapid, monitored transport to a facility that can perform immediate surgical repair.[9,12,23-27] The prehospital care provider first needs to recognize that cardiac tamponade likely exists and to inform the receiving facility so that preparations can be made for emergent surgical intervention. Oxygen in high concentration should be administered. Intravenous access should be obtained and fluid therapy initiated, because this can augment central venous pressure and thus improve cardiac filling for a time. The provider strongly considers endotracheal intubation and positive-pressure ventilation if the patient is hypotensive.[13,25,26]

Definitive therapy requires release of the tamponade and repair of the cardiac injury. Draining some of the pericardial fluid by needle pericardiocentesis is often an effective temporizing maneuver. In rare cases, resuscitative thoracotomy has been performed in the field by physicians in systems where they respond to field emergencies.[28,29] The use of the pneumatic antishock garment (PASG) has been demonstrated to be detrimental in these patients.[30]

Commotio Cordis

The term *commotio cordis* refers to the clinical situation in which an apparently innocuous blow to the anterior chest results in sudden cardiac arrest. Commotio cordis is believed to account for about 20 deaths per year in the United States, predominantly in children and adolescents (mean age about 13 years). Most experts theorize that commotio cordis results from a relatively minor, nonpenetrating blow to the precordium (area over the heart), occurring at an electrically vulnerable portion of the cardiac cycle, whereas some believe that coronary artery vasospasm may play a role in its development.

This condition most frequently occurs during amateur sporting events in which the victim is struck by a projectile, such as a baseball (most common), ice hockey puck, lacrosse ball, or softball. However, commotio cordis has also been reported after bodily impacts (e.g., karate blows), a low-velocity MVC, and the collision of two outfielders trying to catch a baseball. After the impact, victims have been known to walk a step or two, then drop to the ground and found to be in cardiac arrest. Typically, no injury is noted to the ribs, sternum, or heart at autopsy. Most victims have no known history of heart disease. The condition may be prevented through the use of chest wall protectors and other equipment, such as safety baseballs.

Assessment

Patients who have sustained commotio cordis are found to be in cardiopulmonary arrest. In some victims a minor bruise is noted over the sternum. Ventricular fibrillation (VF) is the most common rhythm, although complete heart block and left bundle branch block (LBBB) with ST-segment elevations have also been seen.

Management

Once cardiac arrest is confirmed, cardiopulmonary resuscitation (CPR) is initiated. Commotio cordis is managed in a manner similar to cardiac arrests resulting from myocardial infarction, rather than those resulting from trauma.

The cardiac rhythm should be determined as expeditiously as possible, with rapid defibrillation administered if VF is identified. Prognosis is poor, with chance of survival at 15% or less. Virtually all survivors of this condition received both rapid, bystander-initiated CPR and immediate defibrillation, often with an automatic external defibrillator (AED). Precordial thumps have not been shown to terminate VF. If immediate attempts at defibrillation are unsuccessful, the airway is secured and IV access initiated. Epinephrine and antidysrhythmics may be administered as outlined in cardiac arrest protocols.

Traumatic Aortic Disruption

Traumatic aortic disruption results from a deceleration/acceleration mechanism of significant force.[31] Examples include high-speed frontal-impact MVCs and high falls in which the patient lands flat.

The aorta arises from the upper portion of the heart in the mediastinum. The heart and the aortic arch are relatively mobile within the chest cavity. As the arch of the aorta becomes the descending aorta, the aorta becomes adherent to the vertebral column and is relatively immobile. When there is a sudden deceleration of the body, such as occurs in a high-speed frontal impact, the heart and aortic arch continue to move forward relative to the fixed (immobile) descending aorta. This produces shear forces in the aortic wall at the junction between these two segments of the aorta.[31] This shearing is augmented because this junction is also the point where the ligamentum arteriosum attaches to the aorta, further tethering it and promoting shear. This shear force can disrupt the wall of the aorta in varying degrees (Figure 10-18). When the tear extends through the full thickness of the aortic wall, the patient rapidly exsanguinates. However, if the tear is only partially through the wall, leaving the outer layer intact, the patient may survive for a variable length of time, making rapid identification and treatment essential for a successful outcome.[31]

Assessment

Assessment of aortic disruption hinges on index of suspicion. A high index should be maintained in situations involving high-energy deceleration/acceleration. Ironically, for such a devastating injury, there may be little external evidence of chest injury. Nevertheless, the prehospital care provider needs to assess the adequacy of the airway and breathing. Careful auscultation and palpation should be undertaken. The pulse quality may be different between the upper extremities or between the upper and lower extremities, suggesting the presence of aortic disruption.

Definitive diagnosis requires radiographic imaging in the hospital. Plain chest radiographs may demonstrate a variety of signs indicating the injury may be present. The most reliable of these is widening of the mediastinum. The injury can be definitively demonstrated with aortography,

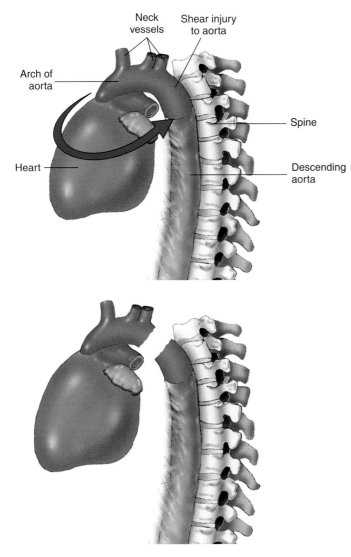

FIGURE 10-18 The descending aorta is tightly affixed to the thoracic vertebrae. The arch of the aorta and the heart are not attached to the vertebrae. Disruption from shear force usually occurs at the junction of the arch and the descending aorta.

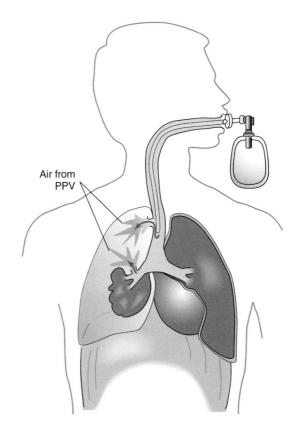

FIGURE 10-19 Tracheal or bronchial rupture. Positive-pressure ventilation *(PPV)* can directly force large amounts of air through the trachea or bronchus, rapidly producing a tension pneumothorax.

> ### BOX 10-2 Blood Pressure Maintenance
>
> *Caution:* When performing interhospital transfer of patients with suspected aortic disruption, it is important not to raise the patient's blood pressure aggressively because this may lead to exsanguinating hemorrhage (see Chapter 7). Many of these patients may be given medications, such as beta blockers (e.g., esmolol, metoprolol), to maintain the blood pressure at a lower level, typically a mean arterial pressure of 70 mm Hg or less.
>
> In many cases, nurses or physicians may accompany the patient to direct the ongoing pharmacologic management of the patient's blood pressure.

computed tomography (CT) of the chest, and transesophageal echocardiography.[31]

Management

Management of traumatic aortic disruption in the field is supportive. A high index of suspicion for its presence is maintained when the appropriate mechanism exists. Other thoracic injuries are looked for. High-concentration supplemental oxygen should be administered. Intravenous access should be obtained, except in cases of extremely short transport times. Communication with the receiving facility about the mechanism and suspicion for aortic disruption should occur at the earliest opportunity. Strict blood pressure control is imperative to the successful outcome of these injuries (Box 10-2).

Tracheobronchial Disruption

Tracheobronchial disruption is an uncommon but potentially highly lethal entity.[32] All lacerations of the lung involve disruption of airways. The intrathoracic portion of the trachea itself or one of the mainstem or secondary bronchi is disrupted. This results in high flow of air across the injury into the mediastinum or pleural space. Pressure rapidly accumulates, resulting in tension pneumothorax or even tension pneumomediastinum, which is similar to cardiac tamponade. Unlike the usual situation in tension pneumothorax, needle thoracostomy may result in continuous flow of air through the catheter and may fail to relieve the tension (Figure 10-19). This is caused by the ongoing high flow of air across these major airways into the pleural space. Respiratory function may be significantly impaired because of preferential airflow across the lesion as well as the pressure. Positive pressure may worsen the tension. Penetrating trauma is more likely to cause this injury than blunt trauma. However, blunt injury of high energy may also cause tracheobronchial disruption.[32]

Assessment

Assessment demonstrates a patient in obvious distress who may be pale and diaphoretic. The patient with tracheobronchial disruption will demonstrate signs of respiratory distress, such as use of accessory muscles of respiration, grunting, and nasal flaring. Subcutaneous emphysema in the neck and jugular venous distention or deviation of the trachea may be observed. Respiratory rate will be elevated, and oxygen saturation may be diminished. The patient may or may not be hypotensive and may cough up blood (hemoptysis). The hemorrhage associated with penetrating trauma may not be present in the blunt cases, but hemothorax is a possibility in both penetrating and blunt trauma.

Management

Successful management of tracheobronchial disruption requires administration of supplemental oxygen and judicious use of ventilatory assistance. If assisted ventilation makes the patient more uncomfortable, only oxygen is administered and the patient is transported as quickly as possible to an appropriate facility.

Traumatic Asphyxia

Traumatic asphyxia is so named because the victims physically resemble strangulation patients. They exhibit the same bluish discoloration of the face and neck (and in the case of traumatic asphyxia, upper chest) as patients who have been strangled. Unlike strangled patients, however, traumatic asphyxia patients do not suffer from true asphyxia (cessation of air and gas exchange). The similarity in appearance with strangulation patients results from the impaired venous return from the head and neck that is present in both groups of patients.

The mechanism for traumatic asphyxia is an abrupt, significant increase in thoracic pressure resulting from a crush to the torso (e.g., car falling off a jack onto the patient's chest). This results in blood being forced back out of the heart and up into the neck and head. Small capillaries

and venules may be ruptured. This may result in brain and eye dysfunction. Traumatic asphyxia is reported to be a marker for blunt cardiac rupture.[33]

Assessment

Assessment demonstrates a patient with the characteristic bluish discoloration ("plethora") above the level of the crush (Figure 10-20). The skin below the level of injury is normal. Because of the force applied to the chest necessary to cause this injury, many of the injuries already discussed in this chapter may be present and should be sought.

Management

Management is supportive. High-concentration oxygen (fraction of inspired oxygen [Fio_2] ≥0.85) is administered, IV access obtained, and judicious ventilatory support provided, if indicated. The reddish-purple discoloration typically fades within a week.

Diaphragmatic Rupture

Small lacerations of the diaphragm may occur in penetrating injuries to the thoracoabdominal region.[1] Because the diaphragm rises and falls with respiration, any penetration that is below the level of the nipples anteriorly or the level of the scapular tip posteriorly is at risk for having traversed the diaphragm. Generally, these lesions do not present any problems on their own acutely, but they should be repaired because of the risk for herniation and strangulation of abdominal contents through the defect in the future. Significant injuries to thoracic or abdominal organs may accompany these otherwise apparently innocuous injuries.

Blunt diaphragmatic injury results from sufficient force being applied to the abdomen to increase abdominal pressure acutely, abruptly, and sufficiently to disrupt the diaphragm. Unlike the small tears that usually accompany penetrating injury, the tears resulting from blunt mechanisms are frequently large and allow acute herniation of the abdominal viscera into the chest cavity.[1] Respiratory distress results from the pressure of the herniated organs on the lungs, preventing effective ventilation, as well as from contusion of the lungs. This impairment of ventilation may be life threatening (Figure 10-21). In addition to the ventilatory dysfunction, rib fractures, hemothorax, pneumothorax, and injury of intraabdominal organs may accompany the injury to the diaphragm. These patients are frequently in acute distress and require rapid intervention to recover.

Assessment

Assessment frequently reveals a patient in acute respiratory distress who may appear anxious, tachypneic, and pale. The patient may have contusions of the chest wall, bony crepitance, or subcutaneous emphysema. Breath sounds on the affected side may be diminished, or bowel sounds may be auscultated over the chest. The abdomen may be scaphoid

FIGURE 10-20   Traumatic asphyxia. **A,** The patient on admission to the hospital. **B,** The patient 3 weeks after injury.
(From Moore JD, Mayer JH, Gago O: Traumatic asphyxia, *Chest* 62(5), 1972.)

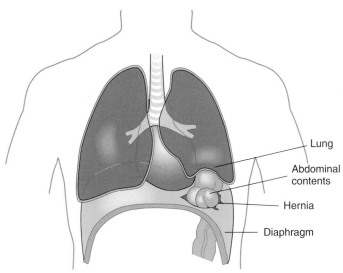

Lung
Abdominal contents
Hernia
Diaphragm

FIGURE 10-21   Diaphragmatic rupture may cause the bowel or other structures to herniate through the tear, causing partial compression of the lung and respiratory distress.

if enough of the abdominal contents have herniated into the chest.

Management

Prompt recognition that diaphragmatic rupture may be present is necessary. Supplemental oxygen in high concentration should be administered and ventilation supported as necessary. The patient should be rapidly transported to an appropriate facility. Use of a PASG is contraindicated

in patients with diaphragmatic rupture. These patients typically exhibit increased distress when the abdominal compartment of the PASG is inflated.[1]

Prolonged Transport

Priorities for managing patients with known or suspected thoracic injuries during prolonged transport remain fundamental, including managing the airway, supporting ventilation and oxygenation, controlling hemorrhage, and providing appropriate volume resuscitation. When faced with a prolonged transport, prehospital care personnel may have a lower threshold for securing the airway with endotracheal intubation. Indications for performing endotracheal intubation include increasing respiratory distress or impending respiratory failure (after exclusion or treatment of a tension pneumothorax), a flail chest, open pneumothorax, and multiple rib fractures. Oxygen should be provided to maintain oxygen saturation at 95% or greater.

Ventilations should be assisted as necessary. Pulmonary contusions worsen over time, and the use of positive end-expiratory pressure (PEEP) with a transport ventilator (or PEEP valves with BVM device) may facilitate oxygenation. Any patient with significant thoracic trauma may have a tension pneumothorax, and ongoing assessment should look for the hallmark signs. In the presence of decreased or absent breath sounds, worsening respiratory distress (or difficulty squeezing BVM device), and hypotension, pleural decompression should be performed. Tube thoracostomies ("chest tubes") may be done by authorized personnel, typically air medical flight crews, if the patient requires needle decompression or is found to have an open pneumothorax.

Intravenous access should be secured and IV fluids administered judiciously. Patients with suspected intrathoracic, intraabdominal, or retroperitoneal hemorrhage should be maintained with SBP in the range of 80 to 90 mm Hg. Overaggressive volume resuscitation may significantly worsen pulmonary contusions, as well as lead to recurrent internal hemorrhage (see Chapter 7). Patients with severe pain from multiple rib fractures may benefit from small doses of narcotics titrated intravenously. If narcotic administration results in hypotension and respiratory failure, volume resuscitation and ventilatory support should be provided.

Patients with cardiac dysrhythmias associated with blunt cardiac injury may benefit from the use of antidysrhythmic medications. Any interventions performed should be carefully documented on the patient care record (PCR) and the receiving facility made aware of the procedures.

SUMMARY

Chest injuries are particularly significant because of the potential for compromise of respiratory and circulatory function and because thoracic injuries are frequently associated with multisystem trauma. Patients with chest injury need to be managed aggressively and transported quickly to definitive care. Particular attention should be paid to the administration of oxygen and the need for ventilatory support in any patient suspected of having chest trauma. Signs of tension pneumothorax should be sought because, although quickly lethal if left untreated, a tension pneumothorax can be treated in the field with needle compression. Because of the high risk of multisystem trauma, especially in blunt chest trauma, spinal immobilization is considered and, as with any trauma patient, hemorrhage is controlled. Intravenous access should be obtained en route to the medical facility, and ECG monitoring may suggest blunt cardiac injury. Although many thoracic injuries can be managed nonsurgically, the patient with a chest injury must still be evaluated and managed at an appropriate medical facility.

SCENARIO SOLUTION

The scene report, patient complaints, and examination lead you to suspect that this patient harbors serious and potentially life-threatening injuries. He is awake and speaking coherently, indicating that he has a stable airway and is unlikely to harbor a severe head injury. He is experiencing severe respiratory distress. The crepitance, tenderness of the right chest wall, and decreased breath sounds indicate possible rib fractures and pneumothorax. Move quickly to provide the patient with supplemental oxygen and consider ventilatory assistance with a BVM device. You are also concerned about the possibility of intra-abdominal injury. The obviously fractured lower extremity needs to be splinted and dressed.

The first priorities in this scenario are to recognize the seriousness of the injuries, stabilize the patient, and initiate transfer to an appropriate facility. Given this patient's respiratory distress and multiple injuries, he is at significant risk for complications. Transportation to the closest trauma center is appropriate. Intravenous access should be obtained en route. There is some risk for respiratory deterioration, and the patient's ventilatory status needs to be monitored closely. If transport time will be extended, air transport should be considered. ■

References

1. American College of Surgeons: Thoracic trauma. In ACS Committee on Trauma: *Advanced trauma life support for doctors, student course manual,* Chicago, 2004, ACS.

2. Wall MJ, Huh J, Mattox KL: Thoracotomy. In Mattox KL, Feliciano DV, Moore EE: *Trauma,* ed 5, New York, 2004, McGraw-Hill.

3. Livingston DH, Hauser CJ: Trauma to the chest wall and lung. In Mattox KL, Feliciano DV, Moore EE: *Trauma,* ed 5, New York, 2004, McGraw-Hill.

4. Wilson RF: Pulmonary physiology. In Wilson RF: *Critical care manual: applied physiology and principles of therapy,* ed 2, Philadelphia, 1992, Davis.

5. American College of Surgeons (ACS): Initial assessment. In ACS Committee on Trauma: *Advanced trauma life support for doctors,* Chicago, 2004, ACS.

6. Silverston P: Pulse oximetry at the roadside: a study of pulse oximetry in immediate care, *BMJ* 298:711, 1989.

7. Richardson JD, Adams L, Flint LM: Selective management of flail chest and pulmonary contusion, *Ann Surg* 196:481, 1982.

8. Di Bartolomeo S, Sanson G, Nardi G, et al: A population-based study on pneumothorax in severely traumatized patients, *J Trauma* 51(4):677, 2001.

9. Regel G, Stalp M, Lehmann U, Seekamp A: Prehospital care: importance of early intervention outcome, *Acta Anaesthesiol Scand Suppl* 110:71, 1997.

10. Eckstein M, Suyehara DL: Needle thoracostomy in the prehospital setting, *Prehosp Emerg Care* 2:132, 1998.

11. Barone JE, Pizzi WF, Nealon TF, Richman H: Indications for intubation in blunt chest trauma, *J Trauma* 26:334, 1986.

12. Mattox KL: Prehospital care of the patient with an injured chest, *Surg Clin North Am* 69(1):21, 1989.

13. Cooper C, Militello P: The multi-injured patient: the Maryland Shock Trauma protocol approach, *Semin Thorac Cardiovasc Surg* 4(3):163, 1992.

14. Barton ED, Epperson M, Hoyt DB, et al: Prehospital needle aspiration and tube thoracostomy in trauma victims: a six year experience with aeromedical crews, *J Emerg Med* 13:155, 1995.

15. Davis DP, Pettit K, Rum CD, et al: The safety and efficacy of prehospital needle and tube thoracostomy by aeromedical personnel, *Prehosp Emerg Care* 9:191, 2005.

16. Etoch SW, Bar-Natan MF, Miller FB, et al: Tube thoracostomy: factors related to complications, *Arch Surg* 130:521, 1995.

17. Cullinane DC, Morris JA, Bass JG, Rutherford EJ: Needle thoracostomy may not be indicated in the trauma patient, *Injury* 32:749, 2001.

18. Givens ML, Ayotte K, Manifeld C: Needle thoracostomy: implications of computed tomography chest wall thickness, *J Acad Emerg Med* 11:211, 2004.

19. Butler KL, Best IM, Weaver WL, Bumpers HL: Pulmonary artery injury and cardiac tamponade after needle decompression of a suspected tension pneumothorax, *J Trauma* 54:610, 2003.

20. Newman PG, Feliciano DV: Blunt cardiac injury, *New Horizons* 7(1):26, 1999.

21. Ivatury RR: The injured heart. In Mattox KL, Feliciano DV, Moore EE: *Trauma,* ed 5, New York, 2004, McGraw-Hill, p 555.

22. Symbas NP, Bongiorno PF, Symbas PN: Blunt cardiac rupture: the utility of emergency department ultrasound, *Ann Thorac Surg* 67(5):1274, 1999.

23. Ivatury RR, Nallathambi MN, Roberge RJ, et al: Penetrating thoracic injuries: in-field stabilization vs. prompt transport, *J Trauma* 27:1066, 1987.

24. Bleetman A, Kasem H, Crawford R: Review of emergency thoracotomy for chest injuries in patients attending a UK Accident and Emergency department, *Injury* 27(2):129, 1996.

25. Durham LA III, Richardson RJ, Wall MJ Jr, et al: Emergency center thoracotomy: impact of prehospital resuscitation, *J Trauma* 32(6):775, 1992.

26. Honigman B, Rohweder K, Moore EE, et al: Prehospital advanced trauma life support for penetrating cardiac wounds, *Ann Emerg Med* 19(2):145, 1990.

27. Lerer LB, Knottenbelt JD: Preventable mortality following sharp penetrating chest trauma, *J Trauma* 37(1):9, 1994.

28. Wall MJ Jr, Pepe PE, Mattox KL: Successful roadside resuscitative thoracotomy: case report and literature review, *J Trauma* 36(1):131, 1994.

29. Coats TJ, Keogh S, Clark H, Neal M: Prehospital resuscitative thoracotomy for cardiac arrest after penetrating trauma: rationale and case series, *J Trauma* 50(4):670, 2001.

30. Honigman B, Lowenstein SR, Moore EE, et al: The role of the pneumatic antishock garment in penetrating cardiac wounds, *JAMA* 266:2398, 1991.

31. Mattox KL, Wall MJ, Lemaire SA: Injury to the thoracic great vessels. In Mattox KL, Feliciano DV, Moore EE: *Trauma,* ed 5, New York, 2004, McGraw-Hill.

32. Riley RD, Miller PR, Meredith JW: Injury to the esophagus, trachea, and bronchus. In Mattox KL, Feliciano DV, Moore EE: *Trauma,* ed 5, New York, 2004, McGraw-Hill.

33. Rogers FB, Leavitt BJ: Upper torso cyanosis: a marker for blunt cardiac rupture, *Am J Emerg Med* May 15(3):275, 1997.

Suggested Reading

Bowley DM, Boffard KD: Penetrating trauma of the trunk, *Unfallchirurg* 104(11):1032, 2001.

Brathwaite CE, Rodriguez A, Turney SZ, et al: Blunt traumatic cardiac rupture: a 5-year experience, *Ann Surg* 212(6):701, 1990.

Callaham M: Peridcardiocentesis in traumatic and nontraumatic cardiac tamponade, *Ann Emerg Med* 13:924, 1984.

Deakin CD: Morbidity in 624 patients requiring prehospital chest tube decompression, *J Trauma* 44(1):98, 1998.

Gervin AS, Fischer RF: The importance of prompt transport in salvage of patients with penetrating heart wounds, *J Trauma* 22:443, 1982.

Helm M, Schuster R, Hauke J: Tight control of prehospital ventilation by capnography in major trauma victims, *Br J Anaesth* 90(3):327, 2003.

Kulshrestha P, Das B, Iyer KS, et al: Cardiac injuries: a clinical and autopsy profile, *J Trauma* 30(2):203, 1990.

Lateef F: Commotio cordis: an underappreciated cause of sudden death in athletes, *Sports Med* 30:301, 2000.

Luna GK, Eddy AC, Copass M: The sensitivity of vital signs in identifying major thoracoabdominal hemorrhage, *Am J Surg* 157(5):512, 1989.

Papadopoulos IN, Bukis D, Karalas E, et al: Preventable prehospital trauma deaths in a Hellenic urban health region: an audit of prehospital trauma care, *J Trauma* 41(5):864, 1996.

Rozycki GS, Feliciano DV, Oschner MG, et al: The role of ultrasound in patients with possible penetrating cardiac wounds: a prospective multicenter study, *J Trauma* 46:542, 1999.

Ruchholtz S, Waydhas C, Ose C, et al: Prehospital intubation in severe thoracic trauma without respiratory insufficiency: a matched-pair analysis based on the Trauma Registry of the German Trauma Society, *J Trauma* 52(5):879, 2002.

Schmidt U, Stalp M, Gerich T, et al: Chest tube decompression of blunt chest injuries by physicians in the field: effectiveness and complications, *J Trauma* 44(1):98, 1998.

Streng M, Tikka S, Leppaniemi A: Assessing the severity of truncal gunshot wounds: a nation-wide analysis from Finland, *Ann Chir Gynaecol* 90(4):246, 2001.

SPECIFIC SKILLS

Thoracic Trauma Skills

Needle Chest Decompression

In patients with increasing intrathoracic pressure from a developing tension pneumothorax, the side of the thoracic cavity that has the increased pressure should be decompressed. If this pressure is not relieved, it will progressively limit the patient's ventilatory capacity and cause inadequate venous return, producing inadequate cardiac output and death.

In patients in whom an open pneumothorax has been treated by the use of an occlusive dressing and a tension pneumothorax develops, decompression can usually be achieved through the wound, which provides an existing opening into the thorax. Opening the occlusive dressing over the wound for a few seconds should initiate a rush of air out of the wound as increased pressure in the thorax is relieved.

Once this pressure has been released, the wound is resealed with the occlusive dressing to allow for proper alveolar ventilation and to stop air from "sucking" into the wound. The patient should be monitored carefully and, if any signs of tension recur, the dressing should be "burped" again to release the intrathoracic pressure.

Decompression in a closed tension pneumothorax is achieved by providing an opening—a thoracostomy— in the affected side of the chest. Different methods for performing a thoracostomy exist. Because needle thoracostomy is the most rapid method and does not require special equipment, it is the preferred method for use in the field.

Needle decompression carries minimal risk and can greatly benefit the patient by improving oxygenation and circulation. Needle decompression should be performed when the following three criteria are met:

1. Evidence of worsening respiratory distress or difficulty with a BVM device
2. Decreased or absent breath sounds
3. Decompensated shock (SBP <90 mm Hg)

Necessary equipment for needle chest decompression includes a needle, a syringe, $1/2$-inch adhesive tape, and alcohol swabs. The needles should be large-bore, over-the-needle IV catheters between 10 and 14 gauge. A 16-gauge catheter can be used if a larger bore is not available.

One prehospital care provider attaches the needle to the syringe while a second provider auscultates the patient's chest to confirm which side has the tension pneumothorax, which is indicated by absent or diminished breath sounds.

After confirmation of a tension pneumothorax, the anatomic landmarks are located on the affected side (midclavicular line, second or third intercostal space) and the site swabbed with an alcohol wipe. The skin is stretched over the site between the fingers of the nondominant hand. The needle is placed for entrance over the top of the rib. Once the needle enters the thoracic cavity, air will escape. The needle should not be advanced farther. The catheter should be left in place and the needle removed, being careful not to kink the catheter. As the needle is removed, a rush of air from the hub of the catheter should be heard. If no air escapes, the catheter should be left in place to indicate that needle decompression of the chest was attempted.

After the needle is removed, the catheter is taped in place with adhesive tape. After securing the catheter, the chest is auscultated to check for increased breath sounds. The patient is monitored and transported to an appropriate facility. The provider does not waste time applying a one-way valve.

Chapter Objectives

At the completion of this chapter, the reader
will be able to do the following:

✓ Analyze scene assessment data to determine the level of suspicion for abdominal trauma.

✓ Recognize the secondary survey assessment findings indicative of intraabdominal bleeding.

✓ Relate external signs of abdominal injury to the potential for specific abdominal organ injuries.

✓ Surmise the pathophysiologic effects of a blunt or penetrating injury to the abdomen based on assessment data obtainable by a prehospital care provider.

✓ Identify the indications for rapid intervention and transport in the context of abdominal trauma.

✓ Understand appropriate field management decisions for patients with suspected abdominal trauma, including those with impaled objects, evisceration, and external genital trauma.

✓ Describe the indications, contraindications, advantages, disadvantages, and limitations of the use of a pneumatic antishock garment (PASG) for abdominal and pelvic hemorrhage.

✓ Relate the anatomic and physiologic changes associated with pregnancy to the pathophysiology and management of trauma.

✓ Describe the effects of maternal trauma on the fetus and the priorities of management.

CHAPTER 11

Abdominal Trauma

SCENARIO

You have been dispatched for "an injured person from an MVC." En route to the scene, dispatch advises that the patient is a pregnant woman who was involved in a rollover crash. On arrival you find a 19-year-old female on the ground lying next to an upright vehicle. She is on her side with her knees drawn up. You observe obvious signs of significant damage to the vehicle, including a deployed air bag and a shattered windshield. The patient has a moderate amount of blood in her hair and on her face. Her eyes are closed, but as you kneel next to her and speak, she opens her eyes. In response to your question, the patient states that she "got out by herself." She is unable to give you the details of her pregnancy and is confused about the events of the incident. She is clutching her abdomen and repeatedly asks if her baby is okay.

In your assessment you find that the patient has a patent airway, a ventilatory rate of 28 breaths/min, a heart rate of 110 beats/min, and a blood pressure of 100/68 mm Hg. The patient has a scalp laceration; her pupils are equal, round, and reactive to light; her skin is pale but dry; palpation of her abdomen elicits tenderness of the lower left quadrant; and she has an obvious deformity of the right forearm. You notice marked ecchymosis across her lower abdomen, consistent with a "seat belt sign."

What are the priorities in the care of this patient? What modifications to patient management are necessary because of her pregnancy? What additional information is pertinent to the care of this patient? What are the effects of the patient's condition on the fetus? Are the priorities for care of the mother different because of the pregnancy? How is the interpretation of assessment findings affected by the anatomic and physiologic changes associated with pregnancy? ■

Unrecognized abdominal injury is one of the major causes of death in the trauma patient. Because of the limitations of prehospital assessment, patients with suspected abdominal injuries are best managed by prompt transportation to the closest appropriate facility.

Early deaths from severe abdominal trauma typically result from massive blood loss caused by either penetrating or blunt injuries. Complications and death may occur from liver, spleen, colon, small intestine, stomach, or pancreatic injuries that were not initially detected. The absence of local signs and symptoms does not rule out the possibility of abdominal trauma, especially in the patient whose level of consciousness is altered by alcohol, drugs, or traumatic brain injury. Consideration of the kinematics will raise the index of suspicion of the alert prehospital care provider to possible abdominal trauma and intraabdominal hemorrhage. A prehospital care provider should not be as concerned with pinpointing the exact extent of abdominal trauma as with treating the clinical findings.

Anatomy

The abdomen contains the major organs of the digestive, endocrine, and urogenital systems and major vessels of the circulatory system. The abdominal cavity is located below the diaphragm; its boundaries include the anterior abdominal wall, the pelvic bones, the vertebral column,

and the muscles of the abdomen and flanks. The abdominal cavity is divided into two regions. The *peritoneal cavity* (the "true" abdominal cavity) contains the spleen, liver, gallbladder, stomach, portions of the large intestine (transverse and sigmoid colon), most of the small intestines (primarily the jejunum and ileum), and female reproductive organs (uterus and ovaries) (Figure 11-1). The *retroperitoneal space* (potential space behind the "true" abdominal cavity) contains the kidneys, ureters, inferior vena cava, abdominal aorta, pancreas, much of the duodenum, the ascending and descending colon, and rectum (Figure 11-2). The urinary bladder and male reproductive organs (penis, testes, and prostate) lie inferior to the peritoneal cavity.

A significant portion of the abdomen lies in the lower thorax. This superior portion of the abdomen is protected in front and along the flanks by the ribs and in back by the vertebral column, and contains the liver, gallbladder, spleen, stomach, and diaphragm. Although any of these organs may sustain injury as a result of a rib fracture, the organs most often injured by the same forces that fracture ribs are the liver and the spleen.

The most inferior portion of the abdomen is protected on all sides by the pelvis. This area contains the rectum, a portion of the small intestine (especially when the patient is upright), the urinary bladder, and in the female, the reproductive organs. Retroperitoneal hemorrhage associated with a fractured pelvis is a major concern in this portion of the abdominal cavity. The abdomen between the rib cage and the pelvis is only protected by the abdominal muscles

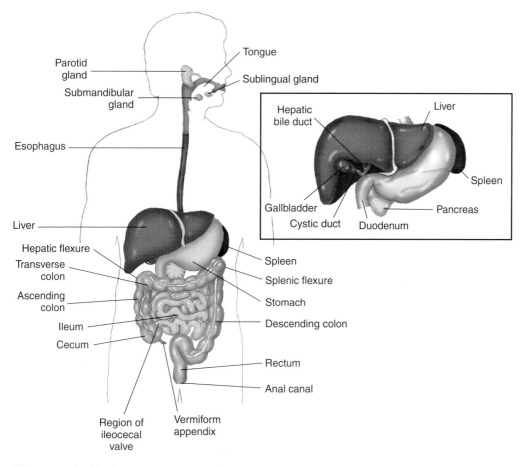

FIGURE 11-1   The organs inside the peritoneal cavity frequently produce peritonitis when injured. Organs in the peritoneal cavity include solid organs (spleen and liver), hollow organs of the gastrointestinal tract (stomach, small intestine, and colon), and the reproductive organs.

and other soft tissues anterior and laterally. Posteriorly, the lumbar vertebrae and the thick, strong paraspinous and psoas muscles provide more protection (Figure 11-3).

For purposes of patient assessment, the surface of the abdomen is divided into four quadrants. These quadrants are formed by drawing two lines: one in the middle from the tip of the xiphoid to the symphysis pubis and one perpendicular to this midline at the level of the umbilicus (Figure 11-4). Knowledge of anatomic landmarks is important because of the high correlation of organ location to pain response. The right upper quadrant (RUQ) includes the liver and gallbladder, the left upper quadrant (LUQ) contains the spleen and stomach, and the right lower quadrant (RLQ) and left lower quadrant (LLQ) contain primarily the intestines. A portion of the intestinal tract exists in all four quadrants. The urinary bladder is midline between the lower quadrants.

Pathophysiology

Dividing the abdominal organs into hollow, solid, and vascular (blood vessel) groups helps explain manifestations of injury to these structures. When injured, solid organs and blood vessels (liver, spleen, aorta, vena cava) bleed, whereas hollow organs (intestine, gallbladder, urinary bladder) primarily spill their contents into the peritoneal cavity or retroperitoneal space. Loss of blood into the abdominal cavity, regardless of its source, can contribute to or can be the primary cause of the development of hypovolemic shock. The release of acids, digestive enzymes, or bacteria from the gastrointestinal (GI) tract into the peritoneal cavity results in *peritonitis* (inflammation of the peritoneum or the lining of the abdominal cavity) and *sepsis* (massive infection) if not promptly treated by surgical intervention. Because urine and bile are generally sterile (do not contain bacteria) and do not contain digestive enzymes, perforation of the gallbladder or urinary bladder does not produce peritonitis as quickly as material spilled from the intestine. Similarly, because it also lacks acids, digestive enzymes, and bacteria, blood in the peritoneal cavity does not cause peritonitis for a number of hours. Bleeding from intestinal injury is typically minor, unless the larger blood vessels in the mesentery are damaged.

Injuries to the abdomen can be caused by either penetrating or blunt trauma. Penetrating trauma, such as a

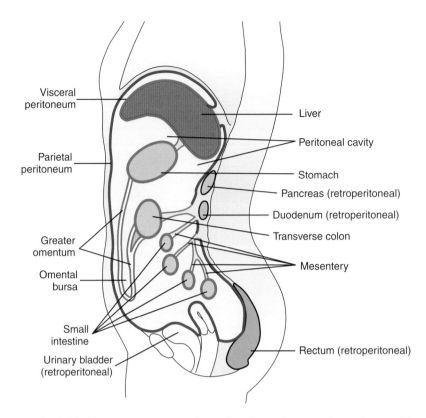

FIGURE 11-2   The abdomen is divided into two spaces: peritoneal cavity and retroperitoneal space. The retroperitoneal space includes the portion of the abdomen behind the peritoneum. Because the retroperitoneal organs are not within the peritoneal cavity, injury to these structures generally does not produce peritonitis.

FIGURE 11-3   This transverse section of the abdominal cavity provides an appreciation of the organs' positions in the anteroposterior direction.

FIGURE 11-4   As with any part of the body, the better the description of pain, tenderness, guarding, and other signs, the more accurate the diagnosis. The most common system of identification divides the abdomen into four quadrants: left upper, right upper, left lower, and right lower.

Lateral view of diaphragm position

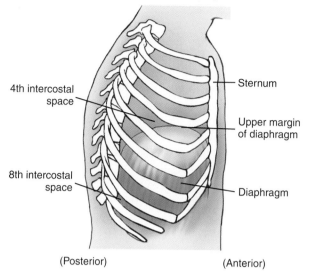

FIGURE 11-5   Lateral view of diaphragm position.

FIGURE 11-6   With increased pressure inside the abdomen, the diaphragm can rupture.

gunshot or stab wound, is more readily visible than blunt trauma. Multiple organ damage can occur in penetrating trauma, although it is less likely with a stab wound than with a gunshot wound. A mental visualization of the potential trajectory of a missile, such as a bullet or the path of a knife blade, can help identify possible injured internal organs.

The diaphragm extends superiorly to the fourth intercostal space anteriorly, the sixth intercostal space laterally, and the eighth intercostal space posteriorly during maximum expiration (Figure 11-5). Patients with penetrating injury to the thorax below this line may also have an abdominal injury. Penetrating wounds of the flanks and buttocks may involve organs in the abdominal cavity as well. These penetrating injuries may cause bleeding from a major vessel or solid organ and perforation of a segment of the intestine, the most frequently injured organ in penetrating trauma.

Blunt trauma often poses a greater threat to life because potential injuries are more challenging to diagnose than those caused by penetrating trauma. These injuries to abdominal organs result from either compression or shear forces. In *compression* incidents the organs of the abdomen are crushed between solid objects, such as between the steering wheel and spinal column. *Shear forces* create rupture of the solid organs or rupture of blood vessels in the cavity because of the tearing forces exerted against their supporting ligaments. The liver and spleen can shear and bleed easily, and blood loss can occur at a rapid rate. Increased intraabdominal pressure produced by compression can rupture the diaphragm, causing the abdominal organs to move upward into the pleural cavity (see Chapters 3 and 10). The intraabdominal contents forced into the chest cavity can compromise lung expansion and affect both respiratory and cardiac function (Figure 11-6). Although rupture of

each half of the diaphragm is now believed to occur equally, rupture of the left hemidiaphragm is diagnosed more often.

Pelvic fractures may be associated with the loss of large volumes of blood caused by damage to the many smaller arteries and veins adjacent to the pelvis. Other injuries associated with pelvic fractures include damage to the urinary bladder and the rectum, as well as injuries to the urethra in the male and the vagina in the female.

Assessment

The assessment of abdominal injury can be difficult, especially with the limited diagnostic capabilities of the prehospital setting. An index of suspicion for abdominal injury should develop from a variety of sources of information, including kinematics, findings from the physical examination, and input from the patient or bystanders (Box 11-1).

BOX 11-1   Signs of Abdominal Trauma*

- Mechanism of injury consistent with rapid deceleration or significant compression forces
- Bent steering wheel
- Soft tissue injuries to the abdomen, flank, or back
- Shock without an obvious cause
- Level of shock greater than explained by other injuries
- "Seat belt signs"
- Peritoneal signs

*Findings that raise the index of suspicion for abdominal trauma.

Kinematics

As with other types of trauma, knowledge of the mechanism of injury plays an important role in shaping the prehospital care provider's index of suspicion for abdominal trauma. Abdominal trauma may result from numerous types of trauma, including both penetrating and blunt forces. Overall, only about 15% of patients with stab wounds to the abdomen will require surgical intervention, whereas about 85% of patients with gunshot wounds will need surgery for definitive management of their abdominal injuries. Stab wounds are less likely to penetrate the peritoneal cavity than projectiles fired from a handgun, rifle, or shotgun. Even if it enters the abdominal cavity, a knife blade has lower propensity for causing injury to internal organs than a projectile because of its lower kinetic energy.

Numerous mechanisms lead to the compression and shear forces that may damage abdominal organs. Although these organs are most often injured in events associated with significant kinetic injury, such as those with rapid deceleration or severe compression, abdominal injuries may result from more innocuous-appearing mechanisms, such as assaults, falls down a flight of stairs, and sporting activities (e.g., being tackled in football). A patient may experience considerable deceleration or compression forces when involved in motor vehicle and motorcycle crashes, when struck or run over by a vehicle, or after falling from a significant height. Any protective devices or gear should be noted, including seat belts or sports padding.

History

History may be obtained from the patient, family, or bystanders and should be documented on the patient care report (PCR) and relayed to the receiving facility. In addition to the components of the AMPLE history (**a**llergies, **m**edications, **p**ast medical/surgical history, **l**ast meal, **e**vents preceding injury), other questions should be tailored to the type of injury. Those related to motor vehicle crashes (MVCs) include the following:

- Type of collision and position of patient in the vehicle
- Extent of vehicle damage, including compromise of the passenger compartment, steering wheel deformity, and requirement for prolonged extrication
- Use of safety devices, including seat belts, deployment of air bags, and presence of child safety seats

Questions related to penetrating injury include the following:

- Type of weapon (handgun vs. rifle, caliber, length of knife)
- Number of times the patient was shot or stabbed
- Amount of blood at the scene

Physical Examination

Primary Survey

Most severe abdominal injuries will present as abnormalities identified in the primary survey, primarily in the evaluation of breathing and circulation. Unless there are associated injuries, patients with abdominal trauma generally present with a patent airway. The alterations found in the breathing, circulation, and disability assessments generally correspond to the degree of shock present. Patients with early, compensated shock may have mild increases in their respiratory rate, whereas those with severe hypovolemic shock demonstrate marked tachypnea. Rupture of a hemidiaphragm often compromises respiratory function, and bowel sounds may be heard over the thorax when breath sounds are auscultated. Similarly, shock from intraabdominal hemorrhage may range from mild tachycardia, with few other findings, to severe tachycardia, marked hypotension and pale, cool, clammy skin.

The most reliable indicator of intraabdominal bleeding is the presence of hypovolemic shock from an unexplained source.[1] When assessing disability, the prehospital care provider may note only subtle signs, such as mild anxiety or agitation, in the patient with compensated shock from abdominal trauma, whereas patients with life-threatening hemorrhage may have serious depression in their mental status. When abnormalities are found in the assessment of these systems, the abdomen should be exposed and examined for evidence of trauma, such as bruising or penetrating wounds.

Secondary Survey

During the secondary survey the abdomen is examined in greater detail. This examination primarily involves inspection and palpation of the abdomen and should be approached systematically. Box 11-2 lists physical findings consistent with the presence of peritonitis.

Inspection. The abdomen is examined for soft tissue injuries and distention. Intraabdominal injury may be suspected when soft tissue trauma is noted over the abdomen, flanks, or back. Such injuries may include contusions, abrasions,

---

BOX 11-2 Peritoneal Signs*

- Significant abdominal tenderness on palpation or with coughing (either localized or generalized)
- Involuntary guarding
- Percussion tenderness
- Diminished or absent bowel sounds

*Findings from the physical examination that support a diagnosis of peritonitis.

FIGURE 11-7 An abdominal "seat belt sign" in an elderly patient, resulting from the patient decelerating against a lap belt.

stab or gunshot wounds, obvious bleeding, and unusual findings such as evisceration, impaled objects, or tire marks. *Grey-Turner's sign* (ecchymosis involving the flanks) and *Cullen's sign* (ecchymosis around the umbilicus) indicate retroperitoneal bleeding; however, these signs may not be seen in the first few hours after injury. The "seat belt" sign (ecchymosis or abrasion across the abdomen consistent with the pattern of a shoulder harness or lap belt) indicates that significant force was applied to the abdomen. Seat belt signs have been associated with intraabdominal injury, especially in children (Figure 11-7).

The contour of the abdomen should be noted, assessing if it is flat or distended. Distention of the abdomen may indicate significant internal hemorrhage; however, the adult peritoneal cavity can hold up to 1.5 liters of fluid before showing any signs of distention. Abdominal distention may also be the result of a stomach filled with air, as can occur during artificial ventilation with a bag-valve-mask (BVM) device. Although these signs may indicate intraabdominal injury, some patients with substantial internal injury may lack these findings.

Palpation. Palpation of the abdomen is undertaken to identify areas of tenderness. Ideally, palpation is begun in an area where the patient does not complain of pain. Then, each of the abdominal quadrants is palpated. While palpating a tender area, the provider may note that the patient "tenses up" the abdominal muscles in that area. This reaction, called *voluntary guarding*, serves to protect the patient from the pain resulting from palpation. *Involuntary guarding* represents rigidity or spasm of the abdominal wall muscles in a response to peritonitis. Unlike voluntary guarding, involuntary guarding remains when the patient is distracted (e.g., with conversation) or the abdomen is surreptitiously

palpated (e.g., with pressure on the stethoscope while appearing to auscultate bowel sounds). Although the presence of *rebound tenderness* has been long considered an important finding indicating peritonitis, many surgeons now consider that this maneuver—pressing deeply on the abdomen and then quickly releasing the pressure—causes excessive pain. If rebound tenderness is present, the patient will note more severe pain when the abdominal pressure is released.

Deep or aggressive palpation of an obviously injured abdomen should be avoided because palpation may dislodge blood clots and promote existing hemorrhage and may increase spillage of contents of the GI tract if perforations are present. Great care during palpation should also be exercised if there is an impaled object in the abdomen. Although tenderness is an important indicator of intra-abdominal injury, several factors may confound the assessment of tenderness. Patients with altered mental status, such as those with a traumatic brain injury (TBI) or under the influence of drugs or alcohol, may have an *unreliable* examination; that is, the patient may not report tenderness or respond to palpation even when significant internal injuries are present. Pediatric and geriatric patients are more likely to have unreliable abdominal examinations because of impaired pain responses. Conversely, patients with lower rib fractures or a pelvic fracture may have an *equivocal* examination, with tenderness resulting from either the associated fractures or internal injuries. If the patient has distracting pain from injuries, such as extremity or spinal fractures, abdominal pain may not be elicited on palpation.

The pelvis should be gently palpated for instability and tenderness. This is evaluated in three steps by (1) pressing posteriorly on the iliac crests, (2) pressing inward on the iliac crests, and (3) pressing posteriorly on the symphysis pubis. If instability is noted, no further palpation of the pelvis should take place.

Auscultation. Auscultation of bowel sounds is generally not a helpful prehospital assessment tool. Time should not be wasted trying to determine their presence or absence because this diagnostic sign will not alter the prehospital management of the patient. If bowel sounds are heard over the thorax during auscultation of breath sounds, however, the presence of a diaphragmatic rupture may be considered.

Percussion. Although percussion of the abdomen may reveal tympanitic or dull sounds, this information does not alter prehospital management of the trauma patient. Significant tenderness on percussion (e.g., pain on coughing) represents a key finding or peritonitis.

Special Examinations and Key Indicators

Surgical intervention remains a key need for most abdominal injuries; time should not be wasted in attempts to determine the exact details of injury. In many patients, identification of specific organ injury will not be revealed until the abdomen is further evaluated by computed tomography (CT) scanning or surgical exploration.

In the emergency department, ultrasound has become the primary bedside modality used to assess a trauma patient for intraabdominal hemorrhage.[1-3] The *focused assessment with sonography for trauma* (FAST) involves three views of the peritoneal cavity (of four views taken) to assess for the presence of fluid, presumably blood (Box 11-3). Because of ease of use and improved ultrasound technology, certain air medical services and military teams have explored use of FAST in the prehospital setting. The FAST exam has been shown to be feasible in the field, but no published data have demonstrated that use of this technology results in improved outcomes for patients with abdominal trauma.[4,5] Thus, use of FAST is not recommended for routine prehospital care.

BOX 11-3   Focused Assessment with Sonography for Trauma (FAST)*

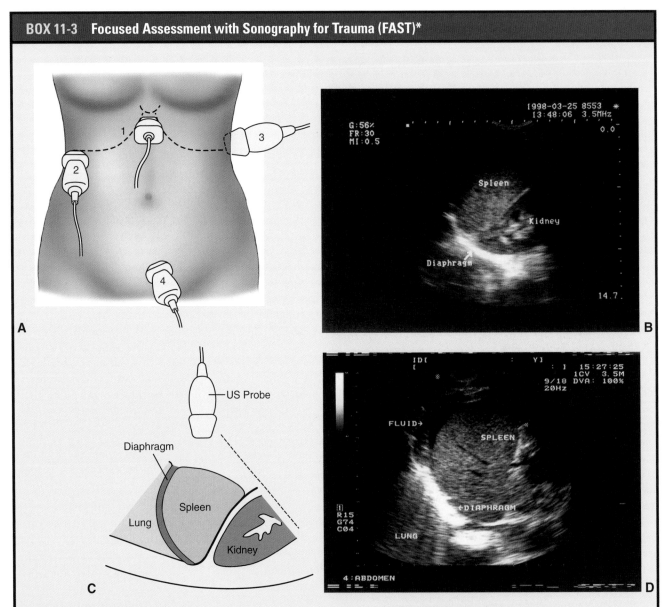

A, Four views constituting the FAST examination. **B,** Normal Splenorenal view. **C,** Normal Splenorenal view identifying organs. **D,** Abnormal view demonstrating the presence of blood (*black stripe* between spleen and kidney).

The FAST examination has value in the trauma patient because most significant intraabdominal injuries are associated with hemorrhage into the peritoneal cavity.

Although ultrasound cannot differentiate the type of fluid present, any fluid in the trauma patient is presumed to be blood.

Despite all these different components, the assessment of abdominal injury can be difficult. The following are key indicators for establishing the index of suspicion for abdominal injury (see Box 11-1):

- Obvious signs of trauma (e.g., soft tissue injuries, gunshot wounds)
- Signs of hypovolemic shock without an obvious cause
- Degree of shock greater than can be explained by other injuries (e.g., fractures, external hemorrhage)
- Presence of peritoneal signs
- Mechanism of injury (e.g., bent steering wheel)

Management

The key aspects of prehospital management of abdominal trauma are to recognize the presence of potential injury and initiate rapid transport to the closest facility that is capable of managing the patient. Abnormalities in vital functions identified in the primary survey are supported during transport. The following guidelines apply:

1. After ensuring scene safety, rapidly evaluate the scene and the patient.
2. Use appropriate airway management techniques, apply oxygen to maintain saturation at 95% or greater, and assist ventilations as needed.
3. Control external hemorrhage, and immobilize the patient on a long backboard.
4. Rapidly package and transport the patient to the closest appropriate facility. Because patients with abdominal trauma often require surgical intervention to control internal hemorrhage and repair injuries, patients with suspected abdominal trauma should be transported to a facility that has readily available surgeons (i.e., a trauma center). Transporting a patient with intraabdominal injuries to a facility that does not have an operating room (OR) and a surgical team immediately available defeats the purpose of rapid transportation. In a rural setting where there is no hospital with general surgeons on staff, consideration should be given to direct transfer to a trauma center, either by ground or air. Early surgical intervention is the key to survival of the unstable patient with abdominal trauma.
5. For patients with decompensated shock and suspected intraperitoneal or retroperitoneal hemorrhage or a pelvic fracture, apply and inflate the pneumatic antishock garment (PASG) (see Chapter 7). Inflation of the abdominal compartment is contraindicated in patients with obvious respiratory compromise, presence of an evisceration, or suspected diaphragmatic rupture and in pregnancy.
6. Initiate intravenous (IV) access and administer crystalloid fluid replacement en route to the receiving facility. As discussed in Chapter 7, aggressive administration of IV fluid in animal models of hypovolemic shock from intraabdominal hemorrhage resulted in recurrence of bleeding that had ceased because of blood clotting and hypotension. Thus, prehospital care providers must achieve a delicate balance: maintenance of a blood pressure that maintains perfusion to vital organs without restoring blood pressure to normal (which may reinitiate bleeding sites in the abdomen). In the absence of TBI, the target systolic blood pressure is 80 to 90 mm Hg (mean arterial pressure [MAP] of 60-65 mm Hg).

Special Considerations

Impaled Objects

Because removal of an impaled object may cause additional trauma and because the object's distal end may be actively controlling (tamponading) the bleeding, removal of an impaled object in the prehospital environment is contraindicated (Figure 11-8). The prehospital care provider should neither move nor remove an object impaled in a patient's abdomen. In the hospital these objects are not removed until their shape and location have been identified by radiographic evaluation and until blood replacement and a surgical team are present and ready. Often these objects are removed in the OR. A prehospital care provider may stabilize the impaled object, either manually or mechanically, to prevent any further movement in the field and during transport. If bleeding occurs around it, direct pressure should be applied around the object to the wound with the flat of the hand. Psychological support of the patient is important, especially if the impaled object is visible to the patient.

The abdomen should not be palpated or percussed in these patients because these actions may produce additional organ injury from the distal end of the object. Further examination is unnecessary because the presence of impaled objects indicates the need for management by a surgeon. Presence of an impaled object in the abdomen is a contraindication to inflating the abdominal compartment of the PASG.

Evisceration

In an abdominal evisceration, a section of intestine or other abdominal organ is displaced through an open wound and protrudes externally outside the abdominal cavity (Figure 11-9). The tissue most often visualized is the fatty omentum that lies over the intestines. Attempts should not be made to replace the protruding tissue in the abdominal cavity. The viscera should be left on the surface of the abdomen or protruding as found. Efforts should focus on protecting the protruding segment of intestine or other organ from further damage. Most of the abdominal contents require a moist environment. If the intestine or some of the other abdominal organs become dry, cell death will occur. Therefore the eviscerated abdominal contents should be covered with clean or sterile dressing that has been moistened with saline (normal saline IV fluid can be used). These dressings should be periodically remoistened with saline to prevent them from drying out. Wet dressings may be covered with a large, dry dressing to keep the patient warm.

Psychological support is extremely important for patients with an abdominal evisceration, and care should be taken to keep the patient calm. Any action that increases intraabdominal pressure, such as crying, screaming, or coughing, can force more of the organs outward. These patients should be expeditiously transported to a facility that has surgical capability.

Pregnancy

Anatomic and Physiologic Changes

Pregnancy causes both anatomic and physiologic changes to the body's systems. These changes affect the potential patterns of injuries and can make the assessment of a potentially injured patient especially challenging. The prehospital care provider is dealing with two or more patients and must be aware of the changes that have occurred to the mother's anatomy and physiology throughout the pregnancy.

FIGURE 11-8 Knife impaled in the abdomen.

FIGURE 11-9 Small bowel eviscerated through a wound in the abdominal wall.

A human pregnancy typically last about 40 weeks from conception to birth, and this period is divided into three sections, or trimesters. The first trimester ends about the 12th week of gestation, and the second trimester is slightly longer than the other two, ending about week 28.

Following conception and implantation of the fetus, the uterus continues to enlarge through the 38th week of pregnancy. Until about the 12th week, the growing uterus remains protected by the bony pelvis. By the 20th week of gestation, the top of the uterus (fundus) is at the umbilicus, and the fundus approaches the xiphoid process by the 38th week. This anatomic change makes the uterus and its contents more susceptible to both blunt and penetrating injury (Figure 11-10). Injury to the uterus can include rupture, penetration, abruptio placentae (when a portion of the placenta is pulled away from the uterine wall), and premature rupture of the membranes. The placenta and gravid uterus are highly vascular; injuries to these structures can result in profound hemorrhage. Because the hemorrhage can also be concealed inside the uterus or peritoneal cavity, it may not be externally visible.

Although a marked protuberance of the abdomen is obvious in late pregnancy, abdominal organs remain essentially unchanged, with the exception of the uterus. Intestine that is displaced superiorly is shielded by the uterus in the last two trimesters of pregnancy. The increased size and weight of the uterus alter the patient's center of gravity and increase the risk of falls. Because of its prominence, the gravid abdomen is often injured in a fall.

FIGURE 11-10 In the pregnant patient, as the uterus and fetus enlarge above the symphysis pubis, the fetus becomes more susceptible to both blunt and penetrating trauma.

Uterus

Symphysis pubis

In addition to these anatomic changes, physiologic changes also occur throughout pregnancy. The mother's heart rate normally increases throughout pregnancy by 15 to 20 beats/min above normal by the third trimester. This makes the interpretation of tachycardia more difficult. Systolic and diastolic blood pressures normally drop 5 to 15 mm Hg during the second trimester but often return to normal at term. By the 10th week of pregnancy, the mother's cardiac output increases by 1 to 1.5 L/min. By term, the mother's blood volume has increased by about 50%. *Because of these increases in cardiac output and blood volume, the pregnant patient may lose 30% to 35% of her blood volume before signs and symptoms of hypovolemia become apparent.*

Some women may have significant hypotension when supine. This supine hypotension of pregnancy typically occurs in the third trimester and is caused by the compression of the vena cava by the uterus. This dramatically decreases venous return to the heart, and because there is less filling, cardiac output and blood pressure fall. The following maneuvers may be used to relieve supine hypotension:

1. The woman may be placed on her left side (left lateral decubitus position), or if spinal immobilization is indicated, 4 to 6 inches (10 to 15 cm) of padding should be placed under the right side of the long backboard.
2. If the patient cannot be rotated, the patient's right leg should be elevated to displace the uterus to the left.
3. The uterus may be manually displaced toward the patient's left side.

These three maneuvers reduce compression on the vena cava, increasing venous return to the heart and improving cardiac output.

During the third trimester, the diaphragm is elevated and may be associated with mild dyspnea, especially when the patient is supine. Peristalsis (propulsive, muscular movements of intestines) is slower during pregnancy, so food may remain in the stomach many hours after eating. Therefore the pregnant patient is at greater risk for vomiting and subsequent aspiration.

Toxemia of pregnancy (also known as eclampsia) is a late complication of pregnancy. Whereas *preeclampsia* is characterized by edema and hypertension, *eclampsia* is characterized by mental status changes and seizures, thus mimicking TBI. A careful neurologic assessment and asking about complications of pregnancy and other medical conditions are important.[6,7]

Assessment

Pregnancy typically does not alter the mother's airway, but significant respiratory distress may occur when a patient in her third trimester is placed supine on a long backboard. The decrease in peristalsis of the GI tract makes vomiting and aspiration more likely. Airway patency and pulmonary function are assessed, including auscultation of breath sounds and monitoring of pulse oximetry.

As with hemoperitoneum from other sources, intra-abdominal bleeding associated with uterine injury may not produce peritonitis for hours. More likely, blood loss from any injury may be masked by the pregnant female's increased cardiac output and blood volume. Therefore, a high index of suspicion and assessment for subtle changes (e.g., skin color) may provide important clues. In general, the condition of the fetus often depends on the condition of the mother; however, the fetus may be in jeopardy while the mother's condition and vital signs appear hemodynamically normal. This occurs because the body shunts blood away from the uterus (and fetus) to the vital organs. Neurologic changes should be noted and documented, although the exact etiology may not be identifiable in the prehospital setting.

As with the nonpregnant patient, auscultation of bowel sounds is generally not helpful in the prehospital setting. Similarly, spending valuable minutes searching for fetal heart tones at the scene is also not useful; their presence or absence will not alter prehospital management. The external genitalia should be checked for evidence of vaginal bleeding, and the patient should be asked about the presence of contractions and fetal movement.

Management

With an injured pregnant patient, the survival of the fetus is best ensured by focus on the mother's condition. In essence, for the baby to survive, usually the mother needs to survive. It is wise to anticipate vomiting and have suction nearby. Priority is given to ensuring an adequate patent airway and supporting ventilatory function. Sufficient oxygen should be administered to maintain a pulse oximetry reading of 95% or higher. Ventilations may need to be assisted, especially in the later stages of pregnancy.

The goals of shock management are essentially the same as for any patient and include IV fluid administration, especially if evidence of decompensated shock is present. Any evidence of vaginal bleeding or a rigid, boardlike abdomen with external bleeding in the last trimester of pregnancy may indicate abruptio placentae or a ruptured uterus. These conditions threaten not only the life of the fetus, but also that of the mother because exsanguination can occur rapidly. No good data exist to define the best target blood pressure for an injured pregnant patient. However, restoration of normal systolic and mean blood pressures will most likely result in better fetal perfusion, despite the risk of promoting additional internal hemorrhage.

Transport of the pregnant trauma patient should not be delayed. Every pregnant trauma patient should be rapidly transported—even those who appear to have only minor injuries—to the closest appropriate facility. An ideal facility is one that has both surgical and obstetric capabilities immediately available. Adequate resuscitation of the mother is the key to survival of the mother and fetus.

Genitourinary Injuries

Injuries to the kidneys, ureters, and bladder most often present with hematuria. This sign will not be noted unless the patient has a urinary catheter inserted. Because the kidneys receive a significant portion of cardiac output, blunt or penetrating injuries to these organs may result in life-threatening retroperitoneal hemorrhage. Pelvic fractures may be associated with lacerations of the urinary bladder and either the vaginal or the rectal walls. Severe external hemorrhage may result.

Trauma to the external genitalia may occur from multiple mechanisms, although injuries resulting from ejection from a motorcycle or motor vehicle, an industrial accident, gunshot wounds, or sexual assault typically predominate. Because of the numerous nerve endings in these organs, such injuries are associated with significant pain and psychological concern. These organs also contain numerous blood vessels, and copious amounts of blood may be seen (Figure 11-11). In general, such bleeding can be controlled with direct pressure or a pressure dressing. Dressings should be inserted vaginally or in the urethra to control bleeding, particularly in pregnant women. If direct pressure is not required to control hemorrhage, these injuries should be covered with moist, clean, saline-soaked gauze. Any amputated parts should be managed as described in Chapter 12. Further evaluation of all genital injuries should occur at the hospital.

FIGURE 11-11 Gunshot wound through penis and into right thigh. Penile injuries may be associated with significant hemorrhage.

SUMMARY

The potential threat to life from intraabdominal injuries is extremely high. No other area of the body is more susceptible to major hemorrhage without apparent physical evidence of injury. A patient with an abdominal injury can deteriorate rapidly and without warning. Maintaining a high index of suspicion for abdominal injury is therefore crucial.

The extent of specific abdominal organ injury is seldom identifiable in the prehospital setting. Management of the patient with abdominal trauma includes rapid evaluation and preparation for transport, oxygenation, hemorrhage control, and support of circulation. A PASG is useful in the management of shock caused by abdominal and pelvic trauma, as long as no contraindications to its use exist. Definitive care of the patient with abdominal trauma is achieved only by transporting the patient to a facility with the capability to perform rapid surgical intervention.

Although the priorities for treatment are the same, some cases of abdominal trauma require special considerations. The patient with an abdominal impalement or evisceration also requires special handling to prevent further injury and complications. The key to optimal care of the patient with abdominal trauma is to maintain a high index of suspicion based on the mechanism of injury and shock in the absence of an obvious cause. The anatomic and physiologic changes of pregnancy have implications for the pattern of injury, presentation of signs and symptoms of trauma, and management of the trauma patient. Management of potential fetal compromise caused by trauma in the prehospital setting is accomplished only through effective management of maternal perfusion.

SCENARIO SOLUTION

The patient's vital signs may be explained by the physiologic changes of pregnancy or may be subtle indications of shock, but combined with the known mechanism of injury and the other assessment findings (seat belt sign), you maintain a high index of suspicion for internal injury. The patient's scalp laceration and disorientation to the event as well as the mechanism warrant spinal immobilization, which you need to modify to prevent compression of the vena cava. Because fetal oxygenation depends on maternal cardiorespiratory function, the administration of oxygen and circulatory support of the mother constitute the best treatment of the fetus. Additional information about the exact mechanisms of injury and information about the patient's obstetric history are pertinent to the patient's care. Because of the potential for placental abruption and internal injuries, transport to a trauma center with perinatal and surgical resources is ideal. ∎

References

1. American College of Surgeons Committee on Trauma: Abdominal trauma. In *Advanced trauma life support for doctors, student course manual,* ed 7, Chicago, 2004, ACS.

2. Rozycki GS, Ochsner MG, Jaffin JH, et al: Prospective evaluation of surgeons' use of ultrasound in the evaluation of trauma patients, *J Trauma Injury Infect Crit Care* 34(4):516, 1993.

3. Rozycki GS, Ochsner MG, Schmidt JA, et al: A prospective study of surgeon-performed ultrasound as the primary adjuvant modality for injured patient assessment, *J Trauma Injury Infect Crit Care* 39(3):492, 1995.

4. Rozycki GS, Ochsner MG, Feliciano DV, et al: Early detection of hemoperitoneum by ultrasound examination of the right upper quadrant: a multicenter study, *J Trauma Injury Infect Crit Care* 45(5):878, 1998.

5. Rozycki GS, Ballard RB, Feliciano DV, et al: Surgeon-performed ultrasound for the assessment of truncal injuries: lessons learned from 1540 patients, *Ann Surg* 228(4):557, 1998.

6. American College of Surgeons Committee on Trauma: Trauma in women. In *Advanced trauma life support for doctors, student course manual,* ed 7, Chicago, 2004, ACS.

7. Knudson MM, Rozycki GS, Paquin MM: Reproductive system trauma. In Moore EE, Feliciano DV, Mattox KL, editors: *Trauma,* ed 5, New York, 2004, McGraw-Hill.

8. Polk JD, Fallon WF Jr: The use of focused assessment with sonography for trauma (FAST) by a prehospital air medical team in the trauma arrest patient, *Prehosp Emerg Care* 4(1):82, 2000.

9. Melanson SW, McCarthy J, Stromski CJ, et al: Aeromedical trauma sonography by flight crews with a miniature ultrasound unit, *Prehosp Emerg Care* 5(4):399, 2001.

10. Walcher F, Kortum S, Kirschning T, et al: Optimized management of polytraumatized patients by prehospital ultrasound, *Unfallchirurg* 105(11):986, 2002.

11. Strode CA, Rubal BJ, Gerhardt RT, et al: Wireless and satellite transmission of prehospital focused abdominal sonography for trauma, *Prehosp Emerg Care* 7(3):375, 2003.

Suggested Reading

Berry MJ, McMurry RG, Katz VL: Pulmonary and ventilatory responses to pregnancy, immersion and exercise, *J Appl Physiol* 66(2):857, 1989.

Coburn M: Genitourinary trauma. In Moore EE, Feliciano DV, Mattox KL, editors: *Trauma,* ed 5, New York, 2004, McGraw-Hill, p 809.

Esposito TJ: Trauma during pregnancy, *Emerg Med Clin North Am* 12:167, 1994.

Frame SB, Timberlake GA, Rosh DS, et al: Penetrating injuries of the abdominal aorta, *Am Surg* 56(10):651, 1990.

Hill DA, Delaney LM, Duflou J: A population-based study of outcome after injury to car occupants and to pedestrians, *J Trauma* 40(3):351, 1996.

Pearlman MD, Tintinalli JE, Lorenz RP: Blunt trauma during pregnancy, *N Engl J Med* 323:1606, 1991.

Schoenfeld A, Ziv E, Stein L, et al: Seat belts in pregnancy and the obstetrician, *Obstet Gynecol Surv* 42(5):275, 1987.

Timberlake GA, McSwain NE Jr: Trauma in pregnancy: a 10-year perspective, *Am Surg* 55(3):151, 1989.

Tso EL, Beaver BL, Haller JA Jr: Abdominal injuries in restrained pediatric passengers, *J Pediatr Surg* 28(7):915, 1993.

Chapter Objectives

*At the completion of this chapter, the reader
will be able to do the following:*

✓ List the three categories used to classify patients with extremity injuries, and relate this classification to priority of care.

✓ Describe the primary and secondary surveys as related to extremity trauma.

✓ Discuss the significance of hemorrhage in both open and closed fractures of the long bones, pelvis, and ribs.

✓ List the five major pathophysiologic problems associated with extremity injuries that may require management in the prehospital setting.

✓ Explain the management of extremity trauma as an isolated injury and in the presence of multisystem trauma.

✓ Given a scenario involving an extremity injury, select an appropriate splint and splinting method.

✓ Describe the special considerations involved in femur fracture management.

✓ Describe the management of amputations.

CHAPTER 12

Musculoskeletal Trauma

SCENARIO

You and your partner are called to the scene of an elderly woman who has fallen down a flight of stairs. She is found supine at the bottom of stairs inside her house, awake and alert, complaining of pain to her left hip, thigh, and right upper arm. Vital signs are as follows: BP 108/64, HR 112, RR 20; her skin is warm to the touch, but it is slightly diaphoretic. Her left leg is obviously deformed.

How would you complete the assessment on this patient? What injuries would you expect to find? How does the mechanism of injury lead you to these expectations? What is your first priority in the care of this patient? What is your second priority in the care of this patient? On what body systems should you focus your treatment of this patient? ■

Extremity injury, although common in trauma patients, rarely poses an immediate life-threatening condition. Extremity trauma can be life threatening, however, when it produces severe blood loss (hemorrhage), either externally or from internal bleeding into the extremity.

When caring for a critical trauma patient, the prehospital care provider has three primary considerations with regard to extremity injuries, as follows:

1. Maintain assessment priorities. Do not be distracted by dramatic, non–life-threatening musculoskeletal injuries (Figure 12-1).
2. Recognize potentially life-threatening musculoskeletal injuries.
3. Recognize the kinematics of injury that created the musculoskeletal injuries and the potential for other life-threatening injuries caused by that energy transfer.

If a life-threatening or potentially life-threatening condition is discovered anywhere in the body during the primary survey (initial assessment), the secondary survey (detailed history and physical examination) should not be started. Any problems found during the primary survey should be corrected in ABC order before moving to the secondary survey (see later discussion). This may mean delaying the secondary survey until the patient is en route or even until arrival at the emergency department (ED).

Each critical trauma patient with suspected fractures is secured to a long backboard in the supine position, with as much normal anatomic positioning as possible, to allow for resuscitation. This positioning is called *anatomic splinting*. Securing the patient to the long backboard can effectively support and splint every bone and joint. If this can be done in an efficient manner, it will not detract from focusing on critical conditions. The prehospital care provider is not responsible for differentiating every type of musculoskeletal injury, but for identifying and treating life-threatening injuries and, if time permits, identifying and stabilizing extremity injuries.

FIGURE 12-1 Some extremity injuries, although dramatic in appearance, are not life threatening.

Anatomy and Physiology

Understanding the gross anatomy and physiology of the human body is an important piece of the prehospital care provider's fund of knowledge. Anatomy and physiology is the foundation on which assessment and management are based. Without a good grasp of the structures of the bones and muscles, one will not be able to relate mechanism of injury (MOI) and superficial injuries to injuries that are internal. Although this textbook does not discuss all the anatomy and physiology of the musculoskeletal system, it reviews some of the basics.

The mature human body has approximately 206 bones separated into categories by shape: long, short, flat, sutural, and sesamoid. *Long* bones include the femur, humerus, ulna, radius, tibia, and fibula. *Short* bones include metacarpals, metatarsals, and phalanges. *Flat* bones are usually thin and compact, such as the sternum, ribs, and scapulae. *Sutural* bones are part of the skull and are located between the joints of certain cranial bones. *Sesamoid* bones are bones located within tendons; the patella is the largest sesamoid bone (Figure 12-2).

The human body has more than 700 individual muscles, which are categorized by function. The muscles that are specific to this chapter are the voluntary, or skeletal, muscles. They are termed *skeletal* because they move the skeletal system. Muscles in this category voluntarily move the structures of the body (Figure 12-3).

Other important structures discussed in this chapter are tendons and ligaments. A *tendon* is a band of tough, inelastic, fibrous tissue that connects a muscle to bone. It is the white part at the end of a muscle that directly attaches a muscle to the bone that it will move. A *ligament* is a band of tough, fibrous tissue connecting bone to bone; its function is to hold joints together.

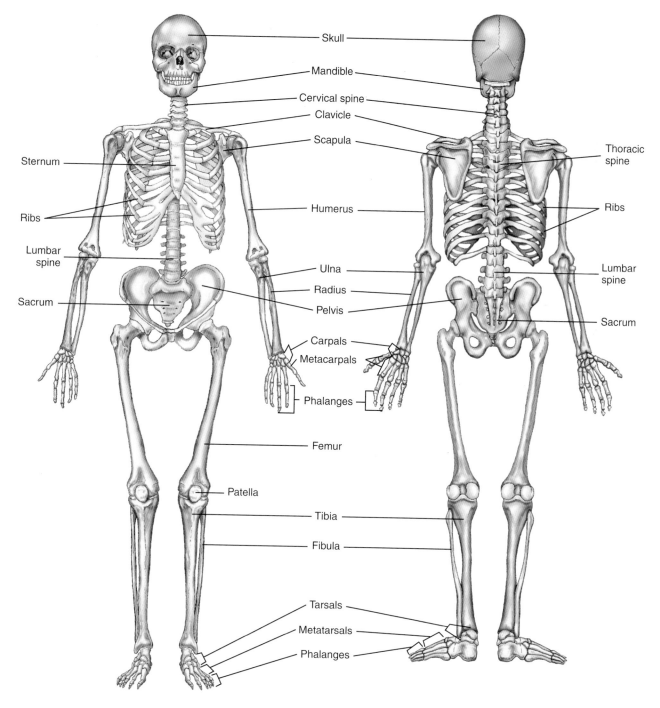

FIGURE 12-2 The human skeleton.

FIGURE 12-3 Major muscles of the human body.

Assessment

Within the scope of triage, musculoskeletal trauma can be categorized into the following three main types:

1. Isolated non–life-threatening musculoskeletal trauma (isolated limb fractures)
2. Non–life-threatening musculoskeletal trauma, but with multisystem life-threatening trauma (life-threatening injuries and limb fractures)
3. Definite musculoskeletal life-threatening injuries (pelvic and femur fractures with life-threatening blood loss)

The purpose of the primary survey is to identify and treat life-threatening injuries. The presence of a non–

life-threatening musculoskeletal injury can be an indicator of possible multisystem trauma and should not distract the prehospital care provider from performing a complete primary assessment. The prehospital care provider asks the following questions in this situation:

- If enough lateral force was delivered to fracture a humerus, a bone covered by thick muscle, can there also be damage to the chest and lungs?
- Could a potentially life-threatening injury exist in the thorax or the organs of the upper abdomen with a simple rib fracture?
- Could a potentially life-threatening injury occur with multiple lacerations to the face and fractures to the underlying bony structures of the maxilla, mandible, and frontal bones of the face?

The answer to all these questions is "yes." Although the presence of musculoskeletal trauma should not distract from the care of more life-threatening conditions, recognition of these injuries as possible indicators of the presence of life-threatening injuries is necessary for good patient care. This action may delay or even prevent a potentially life-threatening injury from becoming life threatening.

Mechanism of Injury

Determining the MOI is one of the most important functions of the assessment and management of a trauma patient. Rapidly determining the MOI and low-energy versus high-energy transference (e.g., falling from a bike vs. being thrown from a motorcycle) will lead the prehospital care provider to the recognition of most critical injuries. The best source for the MOI is directly from the patient. If the patient is unresponsive, details of the injury mechanism can be obtained from witnesses. Often a "best guess" approach to the events based on injuries can be used if no one was present at the incident. This information should be reported to the receiving facility and documented on the run report.

Based on the history of the MOI obtained, a high index of suspicion is provided as to the injuries that a patient might have sustained. Primary injuries are the most obvious based on the MOI; however, from a musculoskeletal perspective, these injuries are not life threatening and can be treated with splints unless there is associated blood loss. Secondary injuries are not as obvious but are located on the "path of injury." The following examples further illustrate the difference between primary and secondary injuries:

- If a patient jumps out of a window feet first, the primary injury suspicion would be fractures of the calcaneus, tibia, fibula, femur, pelvis, and spine and aortic shear injuries. However, secondary injuries might include abdominal injury or head injury from tumbling forward after hitting the ground.
- If a patient is involved in a motorcycle collision with a telephone pole and hits the head on the pole, primary injuries will include head, cervical spine, and thoracic injury. A secondary injury might include a femur fracture from "striking" the femur on the handlebars.

Another example involves a patient riding in the passenger side of a vehicle that sustains a side-impact collision. As discussed in Chapter 3, Newton's first law of motion states that a body in motion will stay in motion until acted on by an equal but opposite force. The vehicle is the moving object until acted on by the other vehicle. The door of the target vehicle is pushed against the upper arm, which can then be pushed into the chest wall, producing rib fractures, lung contusion, and possibly a fractured humerus. Given the kinematics of this crash, primary suspicion for musculoskeletal injury would include humerus, pelvis, and femur fractures. Secondary injury suspicion would include rib fractures, chest wall muscle injury, and lung and heart injuries. Another secondary injury to consider is abrasion from a deployed air bag.

Another possible secondary injury from a side-impact collision results from an unrestrained passenger becoming a missile (object) inside the vehicle. The other vehicle striking the passenger side sets the passenger in motion until he or she is stopped by another object, such as the driver. However, near-side injuries are more severe than far-side injuries. In this case the MOI for the driver is the unrestrained passenger's body.

Appropriately visualizing the incident from the first object set in motion until the last possible object that could be set in motion is the crux of truly understanding MOI and its importance.

Primary and Secondary Surveys

The first step of any assessment is to ensure scene safety and assess the situation. Once the scene is safe, patient care can be provided. The primary survey addresses the immediately life-threatening conditions that are identified. Treating an amputated leg injury is unimportant if the patient is not breathing. Airway, breathing, and circulation (ABC) remain the most important part of assessment. Gross hemorrhage is included in the primary survey and must be controlled when deemed life threatening.

If the patient has no life-threatening injuries, the prehospital care provider proceeds to the secondary survey. In the secondary survey the provider should perform the following:

- Remove any clothing that was not removed during the primary survey.
- If the patient is conscious, question the patient about the MOI, sensation, pain, and weakness.
- Visually assess the patient for swelling, lacerations, abrasions, hematomas, color, movement, capillary refilling time, and deformity.
- Palpate for pulses, temperature, and crepitus.
- Test for sensation in several locations on the hands and fingers and feet and toes. Three nerves provide sensation to the hand and two nerves supply the foot. Sensation can be spotty. Also, evaluate gross motor functions: opening and closing a fist, grip strength, and wiggling toes. Voluntary movement of the extremities tests for neurologic and muscular function at the same time.
- Check pulses, movement, and sensation before and after splinting.
- Immobilize all suspected fractures or dislocations.

Lacerations can present with minor or major bleeding. Hemorrhage contained within soft tissue will produce swelling and ecchymosis (bruising). Hematomas and deformity may indicate a closed fracture or a significant injury to a major blood vessel. Most patients with significant musculoskeletal injuries have pain, unless a nerve injury is present.

Pulses, movement, and sensation are an important part of assessment. Although loss of motor and sensory function usually indicates a neurologic (nerve) injury, these findings in conjunction with a loss of pulses typically represent a serious arterial injury. The primary survey is performed to identify life-threatening injuries and establish a baseline. Reassessment of the patient on multiple occasions is important to identify changes from the initial baseline assessment.

Crepitus is the feeling that bones make when the fractured ends rub against one another. Crepitus can be elicited by palpating the site of injury and by movement of the extremity. Crepitus sounds like a "snap, crackle, and pop" or the popping of plastic "bubble wrap" used for packing. This feeling of bones grating against one another during the assessment of a patient can produce further injury, and therefore, once the crepitus is noted, no additional or repetitive steps should be taken to produce it. Crepitus is a distinct feeling that is not easily forgotten.

Specific Musculoskeletal Injuries

Injuries to the extremities result in two primary problems that require management in the prehospital setting: hemorrhage and instability (fractures and dislocations).

Hemorrhage

Bleeding can be dramatic or subtle. Whether it is the capillary ooze of a large abrasion, the dark-red blood flowing from a superficial laceration, or the bright-red spurting of an open artery, the amount of blood lost and the rate of its loss will determine the patient's ability to compensate or descend into shock. A good rule to remember is, "No bleeding is minor; every red blood cell counts." Even a small trickle of blood can add up to substantial blood loss if it is ignored for a long period.

External arterial bleeding should be identified during the primary survey. Generally, this type of bleeding is easily recognized, but assessment can be difficult when blood is hidden under a patient or in heavy or dark clothing. Ideally, obvious hemorrhage is controlled while the patient's airway and breathing are being managed, if sufficient assistance is present; otherwise, it is controlled when identified during assessment of circulation or when the patient's clothing is removed. Estimation of external blood loss is

TABLE 12-1 Approximate Internal Blood Loss Associated with Fractures

Bone fractured	Internal blood loss (mL)
Rib	125
Radius or ulna	250-500
Humerus	500-750
Tibia or fibula	500-1000
Femur	1000-2000
Pelvis	1000-massive

extremely difficult. While less experienced individuals tend to overestimate the amount of external hemorrhage, underestimation is also possible as overt signs of external blood loss may not always be apparent. The patient may have been moved from the site of injury, or lost blood may have been absorbed by clothing or soil or washed away in water or by rain.

Internal hemorrhage is also common with musculoskeletal trauma. It may result from damage to major blood vessels, from disrupted muscle, and from the bone marrow of fractured bones. Continued swelling of an extremity or a cold, pale, pulseless extremity could indicate internal hemorrhage from major arteries or veins. Significant internal blood loss can be associated with fractures (Table 12-1). The prehospital care provider considers both the potential internal and the external blood loss associated with extremity trauma. This will help the provider anticipate decreased perfusion and shock and will prepare the provider for the possibility of systemic deterioration and to intervene appropriately to minimize its occurrence.

Management

The initial management of external hemorrhage involves the application of direct pressure. As discussed in Chapter 7, elevation of an extremity has not been shown to slow hemorrhage, and in musculoskeletal trauma, it may aggravate injuries that are present. If hemorrhage is not controlled with direct pressure, a tourniquet should be applied, following the principles described in Chapter 7. Commercially available topical hemostatic agents have not been sufficiently studied in civilian emergency medical services (EMS) systems and should be reserved for prolonged-transport situations.

After controlling bleeding in patients with life-threatening hemorrhage from an extremity, prehospital care providers can reassess the primary survey and focus on resuscitation and rapid transport to the facility that can best treat the condition. During transport, administration of oxygen and initiation of intravenous (IV) fluid resuscitation for patients with Class II, III, or IV shock can be begun. For patients with more minor bleeding and no signs of shock or other life-threatening problems, bleeding can be controlled with direct pressure and the secondary survey performed.

Instability (Fractures and Dislocations)

Tears of the supporting structures of a joint, fracture of a bone, and major muscle or tendon injury affect the ability of an extremity to support itself. The two injuries that cause instability of bones or joints are fractures and dislocations.

Fractures

If a bone is fractured, immobilizing it will reduce the potential for further injury and pain. Movement of the sharp ends of the fractured bone may damage blood vessels, resulting in internal and external hemorrhage. Additionally, fractures can damage muscle tissue and nerves.

In general, fractures are classified as either closed or open. In a *closed fracture* the skin is not punctured by the bone ends, whereas in an *open fracture* the integrity of the skin has been interrupted (Figure 12-4, *A*). Orthopedic surgeons may classify fractures by their pattern (e.g., greenstick, comminuted), but these types cannot be differentiated without an x-ray film, and knowledge of the fracture pattern really does not alter field management.

Closed fractures are fractures in which the bone has been broken but the patient has no loss of skin integrity (i.e., the skin is not broken) (Figure 12-4, *B*). Signs of a closed fracture include tenderness, deformity, hematomas, and crepitus, although in some patients, tenderness may be the only finding. Pulses, skin color, and motor and sensory function should be assessed distal to the suspected fracture site. Asking a patient to move the fractured extremity could

FIGURE 12-4   A, Open versus closed fracture. **B,** Closed fracture of the femur. **C,** Open fracture of the tibia.

result in an open fracture. It is not always true that an extremity is not fractured because the patient can voluntarily move it; adrenaline from a traumatic event may motivate patients to do things they normally would not tolerate. Additionally, some patients have a remarkably high pain tolerance.

Open fractures usually occur when a sharp bone end penetrates the skin from the inside or an injury lacerates the skin and muscle down to a fracture site (Figure 12-4, C). When a bone punctures the skin, the end can be contaminated with bacteria from the skin or environment. This serious complication of an open fracture is a bone infection (osteomyelitis), which can interfere with healing of the fracture. Although the skin wound associated with an open fracture often is not associated with significant hemorrhage, persistent bleeding may come from the marrow cavity of the bone or may arise as a hematoma deep inside the tissue decompresses through the skin opening. The prehospital care provider needs to consider any open wound near a possible fracture to be an open fracture and treat it as such. The provider will not try to replace a protruding bone or bone end; however, the bones occasionally return to a near-normal position when realigned or by the muscle spasms that usually occur with fractures. Inadequate splinting or rough handling of a fractured extremity may convert a closed fracture into an open one. Open fractures may be easy to locate on a trauma patient.

As noted earlier, fractures may result in significant internal hemorrhage into the tissue planes surrounding the fracture. The two most common fractures associated with the greatest hemorrhage are femur and pelvic fractures. An adult can lose 1000 to 2000 mL of blood per thigh. Thus, internal hemorrhage associated with bilateral femur fractures may be sufficient to result in death from hypovolemic shock.

Pelvic fractures also are a common cause of significant hemorrhage (Figure 12-5). Multiple small arteries and veins lie adjacent to the pelvis and may be torn by bone ends or as the sacroiliac joints fracture or open up. Overaggressive palpation or manipulation of the pelvis (pelvic rock) can significantly increase blood loss when an unstable pelvic fracture is present. To assess the pelvis, gentle palpation is acceptable but should only be performed once. Gentle manual pressure anterior to posterior and from the sides may identify crepitus or instability. The area around the pelvis is a "potential space" because it can expand and accommodate a huge amount of blood. Because of the amount of space in the pelvic cavity, hemorrhage may occur with few external signs of compromise. Open fractures of the pelvis, often resulting when a pedestrian is struck by a car or when an occupant is ejected from a motor vehicle, are particularly deadly. Often, massive external rather than internal hemorrhage results, and bone ends may lacerate the rectum or vagina, resulting in severe pelvic infection (Box 12-1).

FIGURE 12-5 Radiograph of a severe anterior-posterior compression fracture of the pelvis. There is marked widening of the symphysis pubis, disruption of the sacroiliac joint, and fractures of the pubic rami.

Management

Open and Closed Fractures. The first consideration in managing fractures is to control hemorrhage and treat for shock. Direct pressure and pressure dressings will control virtually all external hemorrhage encountered in the field. Open wounds or exposed bone ends should be covered with a sterile dressing. Internal hemorrhage is primarily controlled by immobilization, which has the added benefit of providing pain relief. If the bone ends retract into the wound during splinting, this information must be documented on the run report and reported to ED personnel. There is little to be gained from administering IV antibiotics to patients with open fractures in the field, especially in the urban or suburban setting.

An injured extremity should be moved as little as possible. The primary objective of splinting is to prevent movement of the body part. This will help decrease the patient's pain and prevent further soft tissue damage and hemorrhage. To immobilize any long bone in an extremity effectively, the entire limb should be immobilized. To do this, the injured site should be supported manually while the joint and bone above (proximal to) and the joint and bone below (distal to) the injury site are immobilized. Numerous types of splints are available, and most can be used with both open and closed fractures (Box 12-2). With virtually all splinting techniques, further inspection of the extremity is limited, and a thorough assessment should be performed before splinting.

In general, most fractures are splinted in the position in which they are found. Exceptions include fractures in patients with pulseless extremities and patients with

BOX 12-1 Pelvic Fractures

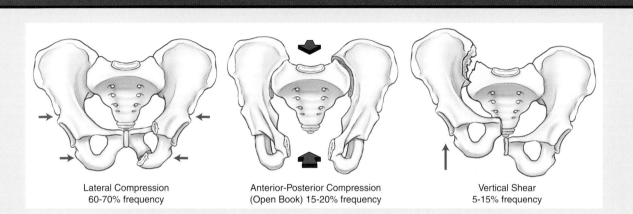

| Lateral Compression 60-70% frequency | Anterior-Posterior Compression (Open Book) 15-20% frequency | Vertical Shear 5-15% frequency |

Pelvic fractures can range from minor, relatively insignificant fractures to complex injuries associated with massive internal and external hemorrhage. Fractures of the **pelvic ring** are associated with overall mortality of 6%, whereas mortality from open fractures may exceed 50%. Blood loss accounts for the leading cause of death in patients with pelvic fractures; the remaining deaths are from traumatic brain injury (TBI) and multiple organ failure. Because the pelvis is a strong bone and difficult to fracture, patients with pelvic fractures frequently have associated injuries, including TBIs (51%), long-bone fractures (48%), thoracic injuries (20%), urethral disruption in men (15%), splenic trauma (10%), and liver and kidney trauma (7% each).

TYPES OF PELVIC FRACTURES:

- **Rami fractures.** Isolated fractures of the inferior or superior rami are generally minor and do not require surgical stabilization. Individuals who fall forcibly on their perineum may fracture all four rami ("straddle" injury). These fractures typically are not associated with significant internal hemorrhage.
- **Acetabular fractures.** These fractures occur when the head of the femur is driven into the acetabulum of the pelvis. Surgical intervention is generally needed to optimize normal hip function. These injuries may be associated with significant internal hemorrhage.
- **Pelvic ring fractures.** Fractures of the pelvic ring are typically classified into three categories. Life-threatening

hemorrhage is probably most common with vertical shear fractures, but it may be associated with each type of pelvic ring fracture. The prehospital care provider may palpate crepitus and note bony instability with each of these ring fractures.

1. **Lateral compression fractures** account for the majority of pelvic ring fractures. These injuries may occur when forces are applied to the lateral aspects of the pelvis (e.g., pedestrian is struck by a car). The volume of the pelvis is decreased in these fractures.
2. **Anterior-posterior compression fractures** account for about 15% of pelvic ring fractures. These injuries occur when forces are applied in an anteroposterior direction (e.g., person pinned between a vehicle and wall). These injuries are also known as "open book" pelvic fractures because usually the symphysis is separated and the volume of the pelvis greatly increased.
3. **Vertical shear fractures** account for the smallest proportion of pelvic ring fractures but tend to cause the highest mortality. They occur when a vertical force is applied to the hemipelvis (e.g., fall from a height, landing on one leg first). Because one half of the pelvis is sheared off the remaining portion, blood vessels are often torn, resulting in severe internal hemorrhage.

---

extremity trauma who cannot be transported because of the extremity's unusual position. In these situations the prehospital care provider may attempt to straighten the extremity gently, returning it to a normal anatomic position. If one or two attempts do not restore circulation, continued attempts will not likely prove successful. Attempts at straightening an extremity should be abandoned if the patient complains of significant pain or if resistance to movement

is felt. Returning the extremity to a normal position will facilitate splinting and improve circulation.

Four additional points are important to remember when applying any type of splint, as follows:

1. Pad rigid splints to prevent movement of the extremity inside the splint, to help increase the patient's comfort, and to prevent pressure sores.

BOX 12-2 Types of Splints

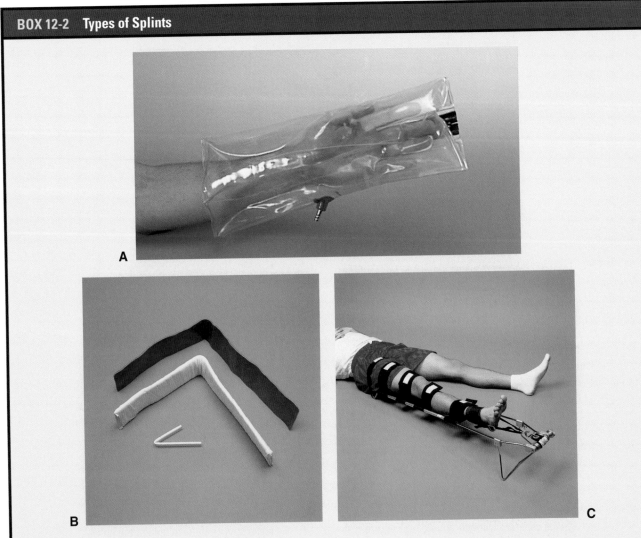

A, Rigid splint. **B,** Formable splint. **C,** Traction splint.
(*A* from McSwain NE, Paturas J: *The basic EMT: comprehensive prehospital patient care,* ed 2, St Louis, 2001, Mosby; *B* and *C* from Sanders MJ: *Mosby's paramedic textbook,* ed 3, St Louis, 2006, Mosby.)

Various splints and splinting materials are available, including the following:

■ **Rigid splints** cannot be changed in shape (see **A** figure). They require that the body part be positioned to fit the splint's shape. Examples of rigid splints include board splints (wood, plastic, or metal) and inflatable "air splints." This group of splints also includes the long backboard. Rigid splints are best used for long-bone injuries.

■ **Formable splints** can be molded into various shapes and combinations to accommodate the shape of the injured extremity (see **B** figure). Examples of formable splints include vacuum splints, pillows, blankets, cardboard splints, wire ladder splints, and foam-covered moldable metal splints. Formable splints are best used for ankle, wrist, and long-bone injuries.

■ **Traction splints** are designed to maintain mechanical inline traction to help realign fractures (see **C** figure). Traction splints are most often used to stabilize femur fractures.

2. Remove jewelry and watches so that these objects will not inhibit circulation as additional swelling occurs. Lubrication with lotion or a lubricating jelly may facilitate removal of tight rings.

3. Assess neurovascular functions distal to the injury site before and after applying any splint and periodically thereafter. A pulseless extremity indicates either a vascular injury or a compartment syndrome, and rapid

transport to an appropriate facility becomes even more of a priority.

4. After splinting, consider elevating the extremity, if possible, to decrease edema and throbbing. Ice or cold packs can also be used to decrease pain and swelling and may be placed on the splinted extremity near the suspected fracture site.

Femur Fractures. Femur fractures represent a unique splinting situation because of the musculature of the thigh. In addition to providing key structural support for the lower extremity, the femur also provides resistance to the powerful thigh muscles, keeping them out to length. When the femur is fractured in the midshaft area, this resistance to contraction is removed. As these muscles contract, the sharp bone ends tear through muscle tissue, producing additional internal hemorrhage and pain and predisposing the patient to an open fracture. In the absence of life-threatening conditions, a *traction splint* should be applied to stabilize suspected midshaft femoral fractures. The application of traction, both manually and by the use of a mechanical device, will help decrease internal bleeding as well as decrease the patient's pain. One study of prehospital use of traction splints documented that almost 40% of the patients had an injury that either complicated or contraindicated use of a traction splint.[1] Contraindications to the use of a traction splint include the following:

- Suspected pelvic fracture
- Suspected femoral neck (hip) fracture
- Avulsion or amputation of the ankle and foot
- Suspected fractures adjacent to the knee (A traction splint may be used as a rigid splint in this situation, but traction should not be applied.)

When midshaft femoral fractures are encountered in a patient with additional injuries that are life threatening, time should not be taken to apply a traction splint. Instead, attention should be focused on the critical problems, and the suspect lower extremity fractures will be sufficiently stabilized when the patient is immobilized to a long backboard. If used for decompensated (Class III or IV) shock, a pneumatic antishock garment (PASG) may also offer stabilization to a femur fracture.

Pelvic Fractures. Severe pelvic fractures present two challenging problems for prehospital care providers. The greatest concern is internal hemorrhage, which can be very difficult to manage. Some data suggest that a PASG can be very useful in compressing the pelvis and presumably tamponading internal hemorrhage.[2,3] It should only be applied and inflated when a patient with a suspected pelvic fracture has decompensated (Class III or IV) hemorrhage. If a PASG is unavailable, consideration should be given to wrapping a bedsheet tightly around the lower aspect of the pelvis and tying it as a sling. The lower extremities should also be adducted and internally rotated and secured in that position. Several companies manufacture "pelvic binders," designed to stabilize certain types of pelvic fractures. No convincing evidence has yet been published supporting the use and expense of these devices during transport of patients with suspected pelvic fractures from the scene to the trauma center or hospital (Box 12-3).

A second and related concern is that patients with grossly unstable pelvic fractures may be difficult to move, and even turning using a modified logroll procedure can shift bone fragments, causing additional hemorrhage. The best way to move a patient with an unstable fracture identified on palpation may be with a scoop stretcher. If a scoop stretcher is not available, the patient should be turned using a modified logroll procedure only enough to slide a long backboard under the patient. This action should be carried out expeditiously.

Dislocations

Joints are held together by ligaments. The bones are attached to muscles by tendons. Movement of an extremity is accomplished by muscles contracting (shortening). This reduction of muscle length pulls the tendons that are attached to a bone and moves the extremity at a joint. A *dislocation* is a separation of two bones at the joint, resulting from significant disruption to the ligaments that normally provide stability at a joint (Figures 12-6 and 12-7). A dislocation, similar to a fracture, produces an area of instability that the prehospital care provider needs to secure. Dislocations can produce great pain. A dislocation can be difficult to distinguish from a fracture and may be associated with fractures as well (fracture-dislocation). Individuals with prior dislocations have more lax ligaments and may be prone to more frequent dislocations unless the problem is corrected surgically. Unlike those sustaining a dislocation for the first time, these patients are often familiar with their injury and can help in assessment and stabilization.

FIGURE 12-6 A dislocation is a separation of a bone from a joint.
(From McSwain NE Jr, Paturas JL: *The basic EMT: comprehensive prehospital patient care,* ed 2, St Louis, 2001, Mosby.)

BOX 12-3 Pelvic Binders

As noted in the text, at least three pelvic binders are commercially available: Pelvic Binder (Pelvic Binder, Dallas); Sam Sling (Sam Products, Newport, Ore); and TPOD (BioCybernetics International, LaVerne, Calif).

RATIONALE

Some pelvic ring fractures are associated with an increase in the pelvic volume (e.g., anteroposterior [AP] compression fracture), permitting large amounts of third-space hemorrhage. Because the volume is increased, there is less tissue surrounding the pelvis to tamponade bleeding. Before the development of pelvic binders, patients with these injuries and hemodynamic instability (shock) would undergo external fixation of the pelvis to decrease the pelvic volume and increase the likelihood of tamponading hemorrhage. Although external fixation seemed to decrease blood requirements, minimal published data exist to suggest external fixation lowered mortality from these fractures.

PROBLEMS

Several potential problems exist with the use of pelvic binders in the prehospital setting.

1. Pelvic fractures are difficult to diagnose in the absence of an x-ray film. No published data show that prehospital care personnel can reliably diagnose a pelvic fracture based on clinical examination. Furthermore, not all pelvic fractures benefit from compression. Although AP compression fractures may benefit, lateral compression fractures already have a decreased pelvic volume.

2. Limited data exist on efficacy. Only a few retrospective case series have reported on patients with in-hospital use of pelvic binders. Although some demonstrate that the pelvic volume is significantly decreased, few address transfusion requirements, and none has shown a decrease in mortality in those treated with a pelvic binder.

3. No published research exists on the use of pelvic binders in the prehospital setting, and therefore no data show improved outcome.

4. There is significant cost for this single-use device.

POTENTIAL USE

One conceivable use for the pelvic binder in the out-of-hospital setting would be the interfacility transfer of a patient with an AP compression fracture, confirmed by x-ray film, and associated Class II, III, or IV shock. In these patients the device could be applied before transfer, especially to those in decompensated shock. The decision to use the device should be made in conjunction with medical control.

FIGURE 12-7 Right anterior knee dislocation with overriding tibia on the femur.
(From Ferrera PC, Colucciello SA, Marx JA, et al: *Trauma management: an emergency medicine approach*, St Louis, 2001, Mosby.)

Management. As a general rule, suspected dislocations should be splinted in the position found. Gentle manipulation of the joint can be done to try to return blood flow when the pulse is absent or weak. When faced with a brief transport time to the hospital, however, the better decision may be to initiate transport rather than attempt manipulation. This manipulation will cause the patient great pain, so the patient should be prepared before moving the extremity. A splint should be used to immobilize the injury. Documentation of how the injury was found and of the presence of pulses, movement, sensation, and color before and after splinting is important. During transport, ice or cold packs can be used to decrease pain and swelling. Analgesia should also be provided to reduce pain.

The National Association of EMS Physicians (NAEMSP) recommends reduction of dislocations when transport time is prolonged.[4] Their rationale is that joints are more difficult to reduce if they are left in a dislocated position for a prolonged period; therefore the prehospital care provider can attempt reduction in the field. Before attempting reduction of dislocation in the prehospital setting, the provider should be properly trained in appropriate techniques. Attempted reduction should only be undertaken when permitted by written protocols or online medical control. The procedures should be properly documented.

Special Considerations

Critical Multisystem Trauma Patient

Adherence to the primary assessment priorities in patients with multisystem trauma that includes injured extremities does not imply that extremity injuries should be ignored or that injured extremities should not be protected from further harm. Rather, it means that when faced with a critically injured trauma patient with extremity injuries that are not bleeding, *life takes precedence over limb*. The focus should be on maintaining vital functions through resuscitation, and only limited measures should be taken to address the extremity injuries, regardless of how dramatic the injuries appear. By properly immobilizing a patient to a long backboard, all extremities are essentially splinted in an anatomic position. A secondary survey need not be completed if the life-threatening problems identified in the primary survey require ongoing interventions and if transport time is short. If a secondary survey is deferred for this reason, the prehospital care provider can simply document the findings that precluded performing the secondary survey.

Pain Management

NAEMSP recommends that analgesia be considered in patients with isolated extremity trauma and hip fractures.[5] Basic interventions should be attempted first (i.e., immobilization, ice packs, elevation), as well as good communication skills with the patient to decrease anxiety. Protocols for analgesia use should be in place with clear indications and contraindications. Examples of acceptable pharmaceutical intervention include morphine sulfate, fentanyl, meperidine, hydromorphone, nitrous oxide, and nonsteroidal antiinflammatory drugs. The patient must be monitored with proper documentation before and after administration of the analgesic. Monitoring includes continuous pulse oximetry and serial vital signs, including pulse, respiratory rate, and blood pressure. Continuous capnography may provide early warning signs that a patient is becoming overmedicated ("narcotized").[6]

Analgesics are recommended for isolated joint and limb injuries but are generally not advocated in multisystem trauma patients. Once the fracture or dislocation is stabilized and splinted, the patient should experience a great reduction in pain. Stabilizing the affected extremity decreases the amount of movement of the area, thus decreasing the amount of discomfort. The patient should be observed for signs of alcohol or drug use if he or she does not appear to be in much pain with significant injuries.

Pain medications should be used judiciously and as tolerated by the patient. Analgesics should not be administered when (1) the patient presents or develops signs and symptoms of shock, (2) pain is significantly relieved with stabilization and splinting, or (3) the patient appears under the influence of drugs or alcohol. Medication should not be administered without understanding the potential complications.

Treating pain in trauma patients involves both the physical pain and the anxiety about the pain and the situation in which patients find themselves. Analgesics manage the pain, and sedatives address the anxiety. Benzodiazepines such as diazepam (Valium), midazolam (Versed), lorazepam (Ativan), and alprazolam (Xanax) are the best known and have the added benefit of antegrade amnesia. The patients often will not remember details of what happened after the drug is administered. Extreme caution must be used when administering simultaneous doses of both a benzodiazepine and a narcotic.

Severe pain is frequently treated with narcotics (opiates). Morphine, fentanyl, meperidine (Demerol), butorphanol (Stadol), and nalbuphine (Nubain) are frequently used narcotics. Respiratory depression, even apnea, is the greatest concern of the possible detrimental effects of narcotics. Another worrisome adverse effect is that narcotics are vasodilators. This is of particular concern for trauma patients because patients who are in a compensated state of shock (Class II) may have their hypovolemia "unmasked" by the narcotic, and profound hypotension may occur. In patients with potential compensated shock, the lowest possible dose should be administered, intravenously (IV), and slowly titrated upward until satisfactory pain relief is noted. Narcotics are best given IV in trauma patients because intramuscular (IM) doses may be absorbed erratically if hypoperfusion is present. Other possible adverse reactions for all narcotics include nausea and emesis, dizziness, sedation, and euphoria. For this reason, these agents should be used with caution in patients with head injuries because intracranial hypertension may be exaggerated. Data suggest that the analgesic and adverse affects of morphine and fentanyl are comparable.[7]

Morphine

Morphine is for use in patients with moderate to severe pain. Dosage should be titrated to the patient's response to the pain and physiologic status. It can be given IV, IM, or subcutaneously (SQ). Adult IV dosage is typically 2.5 to 15 mg administered slowly over several minutes while monitoring the patient for relief and complications. For IM or subcutaneous (SQ) administration, the adult dose is 10 mg/70 kg body weight.

Fentanyl

Fentanyl has properties that make it attractive for prehospital trauma patients. Fentanyl has rapid onset and does not cause an increase in the release of histamine (as morphine does), which can exacerbate hypotension in hypovolemic patients. As with all narcotics, the dose should be titrated to patient relief and overall physiologic status. Typical adult dose is 50 to 100 µg; 1 to 2 µg/kg is the typical dose for children. The adverse effects are similar to morphine, but specific contraindications include allergy to fentanyl, traumatic brain injury (TBI) with possible increased intracranial pressure (ICP), respiratory depression, and loss of airway control.

Meperidine

Meperidine is typically used for mild to severe chronic pain. The usual dose is 50 to 150 mg IM or SQ and should be titrated to patient response and overall physiologic status. Meperidine has a dose-dependent depression of cardiac output, particularly in doses exceeding 5 mg/kg. As the liver breaks it down, meperidine is converted into metabolites that can cause hallucinations and seizures. The typical prehospital single-dose administration is unlikely to cause these effects. Meperidine should be used with caution in patients taking other central nervous system (CNS) depressants or alcohol. As with the other opiates, meperidine may cause respiratory depression. The dose in elderly patients is 1 to 2 mg/kg IM, IV, or SQ. When given IV, it should be diluted and administered slowly. Rapid administration increases the possibility of adverse effects. Patients with atrial flutter or supraventricular tachycardia should receive meperidine with caution. Meperidine is contraindicated in patients who are allergic to the drug or if they have taken monoamine oxidase (MAO) inhibitors in the last 2 weeks.

Amputations

When tissue has been totally separated from an extremity, the tissue is completely without nutrition and oxygenation. This type of injury is termed amputation or avulsion. An *amputation* is the loss of part or all of a limb, and an *avulsion* involves the tearing away of soft tissue. Initially, bleeding may be severe with these injuries; however, vessels at the injured site may constrict, and clotting may combine to diminish the blood loss. Movement may disrupt the blood clot, and bleeding can recur. Partial amputations may be accompanied by significant bleeding.

Amputations are often evident on the scene (Figure 12-8). This type of injury receives great attention from bystanders, and the patient may or may not know that the extremity is missing. Psychologically, the prehospital care provider needs to deal with this injury cautiously. The patient may not be ready to confront the loss of a limb and should be told after being assessed and treated. The missing extremity should be located for possible reattachment. Even if it is not possible to regain complete function of the extremity, the patient may regain partial function. The primary survey should be performed before looking for a missing extremity. The appearance of an amputation may

FIGURE 12-8 Near-complete amputation of the left leg after it became entangled in machinery. Black material is fiber produced by the machinery that is entangled with the leg.

be horrifying, but if the patient is not breathing, the loss of the limb is secondary.

Amputations are often very painful. Pain management should be employed once life-threatening problems have been excluded in the primary survey. In some circumstances the patient may complain of pain distal to the amputation. This *phantom pain* is the sensation that pain exists in a missing extremity. The reason for phantom pain is not understood completely, but the brain may not realize that the extremity is not present. This is usually not present at the time of the initial injury.

Principles of managing an amputated part include the following[8]:

1. Clean the amputated part by gentle rinsing with lactated Ringer's (LR) solution.
2. Wrap the part in sterile gauze moistened with LR solution, and place it in a plastic bag or container.
3. After labeling the bag or container, place it in an outer container filled with crushed ice.
4. *Do not* freeze the part by placing it directly on the ice or by adding another coolant such as dry ice.
5. Transport the part along with the patient to the closest appropriate facility.

The longer the amputated portion is without oxygen, the less likely that it can be replaced successfully. Cooling the amputated body part, without freezing it, will reduce the metabolic rate and prolong this critical time. However, replantation is not a guarantee. Because lower extremity prostheses generally allow the patient to resume a near-normal life, lower extremities are rarely considered for replantation. Furthermore, only cleanly separated amputations in otherwise healthy, nonsmoking young individuals are usually considered for replantation. Patients who are candidates for replantation of fingers or a hand/forearm should be transported to a Level I trauma center because

Level II and III facilities are not required to have specialists capable of repairing small blood vessels (microvascular surgery).

Transport of a patient should not be delayed to locate a missing amputated part. If the amputated part is not readily found, law enforcement officials or other responders should remain at the scene to search for it. When the amputated part is being transported in a separate vehicle from the patient, the prehospital care provider ensures that the transporters of the amputated part understand clearly where the patient is being transported and how to handle the part once located. The receiving facility should be notified as soon as the part is located, and transportation of the part should be initiated as soon as possible.

On rare occasions, a patient has an entrapped extremity in which a field amputation may be the only reasonable option. In general, many entrapped extremities can be released with additional extrication expertise. If the patient has the extremity entangled in a machine, an often-overlooked expert is the maintenance person who repairs the machine. This person often has the technical knowledge for expeditiously removing parts from a machine, thereby facilitating extrication. If an amputation is necessary, ideally a surgeon should perform it. Significant sedation may need to be administered for the procedure.

Compartment Syndrome

Compartment syndrome refers to a limb-threatening condition in which blood supply to an extremity is compromised by increased pressure in that limb. The muscles of extremities are enveloped by dense connective tissue called *fascia.* This fascia forms numerous compartments in the extremities in which the muscles are contained. The forearm has three compartments, and the lower leg (calf) has four. Muscle fascia has minimal stretch, and any force that increases the pressure inside the compartments may result in a compartment syndrome. The two most common causes of compartment syndrome are hemorrhage from a fracture or vascular injury and third-space edema that forms when ischemic muscle tissue is reperfused after a period of diminished or absent blood flow. However, a splint or cast that is applied too tightly may also produce a compartment syndrome. As the pressure in the compartment increases beyond that of capillary pressure (about 30 mm Hg), flow is impaired to the capillaries. The tissue served by these vessels then becomes ischemic. The pressure may continue to build to the point that even arterial flow is compromised by compression in the arteries.

The signs of a compartment syndrome can be recalled by thinking of the "five Ps": pain, paresthesias, pulselessness, pallor, and paralysis. The two earliest signs of a developing compartment syndrome are pain and paresthesias. Pain is often described as out of proportion to the injury. This pain may be dramatically increased on passive movement of a finger or toe in that extremity. Nerves are extremely sensitive to their blood supply, and any compromised blood flow soon manifests as paresthesias. Because these symptoms may be normally associated with a fracture, this underscores the need for baseline circulatory, motor, and sensory examinations and repeated serial examinations so that the prehospital care provider can identify changes.

The other three signs—pulselessness, pallor, and paralysis—are late findings and indicate a clear compartment syndrome and a limb in jeopardy of muscle death (necrosis). Compartments may also be extremely tense and firm to palpation, although it is difficult to judge the compartment pressures by physical examination alone. In the hospital, compartment pressures are measured in extremities where compartment syndrome is suspected.

Compartment syndrome can be definitively managed only in the hospital. Only basic maneuvers can be attempted in the field. Elevating a limb in question may help reduce edema and decrease the risk of developing a compartment syndrome. Any tightly applied splint or dressings should be removed and distal perfusion reassessed. Because compartment syndrome may develop during a long-distance transfer, serial examinations are essential for early identification of this problem. In the hospital, compartment syndrome is managed with surgical intervention (fasciotomy), with an incision through the skin into the affected compartments.

Crush Syndrome

Crush syndrome, also known as *traumatic rhabdomyolysis,* is a clinical entity characterized by renal failure and death after severe muscle trauma. Crush syndrome was first described in World War I in German soldiers rescued from collapsed trenches, then again in World War II in patients of the London Blitz. In World War II, crush syndrome had a mortality rate in excess of 90%. During the Korean War, mortality was 84%, but after the advent of hemodialysis, mortality decreased to 53%. In the Vietnam War the mortality rate was approximately the same, at 50%.

The importance of crush syndrome, however, should not be limited to historical or military interest. Approximately 3% to 20% of the survivors of earthquakes have sustained a crush injury, and approximately 40% of survivors from collapsed buildings will have crush injuries.[9,10] In 1978 an earthquake near Beijing, China, injured more than 350,000 persons, with 242,769 deaths. More than 48,000 of these people died from crush syndrome.

Crush syndrome occurs when destruction of muscle releases the molecule known as myoglobin. *Myoglobin* is a protein found in muscle that is responsible for giving meat its characteristic red color. The function of myoglobin in muscle tissue is to serve as an intracellular storage site for oxygen. When myoglobin is released from damaged muscle, however, it is capable of causing damage to the kidneys and acute renal failure (ARF).

Patients with crush syndrome are identified by the following:

- Prolonged entrapment
- Traumatic injury to muscle mass
- Compromised circulation to the injured area

Traumatic injury to the muscle causes release of not only myoglobin but also potassium. Once the patient has been extricated, the affected limb becomes reperfused with new blood, but the old blood with elevated levels of myoglobin and potassium is washed out of the injured area and into the rest of the body. Elevated potassium can result in life-threatening cardiac arrhythmias, and free myoglobin will produce tea- or cola-colored urine and will eventually result in renal failure.

The key in improving outcomes in crush syndrome is early and aggressive fluid resuscitation. It is important for the prehospital care provider to remember that toxins are accumulating within the entrapped limb during the extrication. On freeing the entrapped limb, the accumulated toxins wash into the central circulation, similar to a bolus of poison. Therefore, success will depend on minimizing the toxic effects of accumulated myoglobin and potassium before release of the limb. Resuscitation needs to occur before extrication.[11] Some authors have advocated that final extrication be delayed until the patient has been adequately resuscitated.[12] A delay in fluid resuscitation will result in renal failure in 50% of the patients, and a delay of 12 hours or more produces renal failure in almost 100% of the patients. A poorly resuscitated patient may go into cardiac arrest during extrication.[13] Fluid resuscitation should proceed with normal saline at a rate of up to 1500 mL per hour. LR solution is avoided because of the presence of potassium.

Once the blood pressure is stabilized and volume status restored, attention is turned toward prophylaxis against hyperkalemia and the toxic effects of serum myoglobin. Alkalinization of the urine will provide some degree of protection to the kidneys. Addition of one ampule (50 mEq) of sodium bicarbonate and 10 g of mannitol to each liter of fluid used during the extrication period may help decrease the incidence of renal failure. Once the patient has been extricated, the normal saline fluids can be slowed to 500 mL per hour, alternating with 5% dextrose in water (D5W), with one ampule of sodium bicarbonate per liter.[14]

Mangled Extremity

A "mangled extremity" refers to a complex injury resulting from high energy transfer in which significant injury occurs to two or more of the following: (1) skin and muscle, (2) tendons, (3) bone, (4) blood vessels, and (5) nerves (Figure 12-9). Common mechanisms producing mangled extremities include motorcycle crashes, ejection from a motor vehicle crash (MVC), and a pedestrian struck by an automobile. When encountered, patients may be in shock from either external blood loss or hemorrhage from associated injuries, which are common because of the high-energy mechanism. Most mangled extremities involve severe open fractures, and amputation may be necessary in 50% to 75% of patients. Limb salvage is possible in some patients, typically involving six to eight procedures, and success often depends on the experience of the trauma and orthopedic surgeons.

Even with a mangled extremity, the focus is still on the primary survey to rule out or address life-threatening conditions. Hemorrhage control, including the use of a tourniquet, may be required. The mangled extremity should be splinted, if the patient's condition allows. These patients are probably best cared for at high-volume, Level I trauma centers.

Sprains

A *sprain* is an injury in which ligaments are stretched or torn. Sprains are caused by a sudden twisting of the joint beyond its normal range of motion. They are characterized by significant pain, swelling, and possible hematoma. Externally, sprains may resemble a fracture or dislocation. Definitive differentiation between a sprain and a fracture is accomplished only through a radiographic study. In the prehospital setting, it is reasonable to splint a suspected sprain in case it turns out to be a fracture or dislocation. An ice or cold pack may help relieve pain, as well as use of narcotic pain medication.

FIGURE 12-9 Mangled extremity resulting from crushing injury between two vehicles. The patient has fractures, transection of the popliteal artery and vein, and extensive soft tissue injury. An external fixator has been placed.

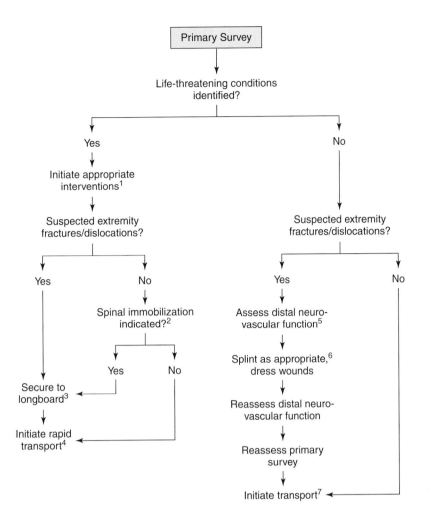

[1] Airway management, ventilatory support, shock therapy.

[2] See Indications for Spinal Immobilization algorithm (p. 235).

[3] Injured extremities are immobilized in anatomic position by securing to longboard.

[4] Transport to closest appropriate facility (trauma center, if available); assess distal neurovascular function and apply traction splint (if suspected femur fracture) as time permits.

[5] Assess perfusion (pulses and capillary refilling) and neurologic function (motor and sensory) distal to the suspected fracture or dislocation.

[6] Use appropriate splinting technique to immobilize suspected fracture or dislocation; if suspected midshaft femur fracture, apply traction splint.

[7] Transport to closest appropriate facility.

The general management for suspected extremity injury includes the following steps:

1. Complete and treat any and all life-threatening injuries found in the primary assessment.
2. Stop any bleeding, and treat the patient for shock.
3. Evaluate for distal neurovascular function.
4. Support the area of injury.
5. Immobilize the injured extremity, including the joint above and the joint below the injury site.
6. Reevaluate the injured extremity after immobilization for changes in distal neurovascular function.
7. Provide pain management as appropriate.

Prolonged Transport

Patients with extremity trauma often have coexisting injuries. Ongoing internal blood loss may be from abdominal or thoracic injuries, and during a prolonged transport the prehospital care provider will need to assess the primary survey frequently to ensure that all life-threatening conditions are identified and no new ones have emerged. Vital signs should be obtained at regular intervals. Intravenous crystalloid solutions should be administered at a rate to maintain normal vital signs, unless significant internal hemorrhage is suspected in the pelvis, abdomen, or thorax.

During long transports, the prehospital care provider needs to focus greater attention on extremity perfusion. In limbs with compromised vascular supply, the provider can attempt to restore normal, anatomic positioning to optimize the chance for improved blood flow. Similarly, dislocation with impaired distal circulation should be considered for reduction in the field. Distal perfusion, including pulses, color, and temperature, as well as motor and sensory function, should be examined in a serial manner. Compartments should be palpated for the development of potential compartment syndromes.

Measures to ensure patient comfort should be taken. Splinting devices should be comfortable and well padded. The limbs should be assessed for any potential points inside the splint where pressure could contribute to the creation of an ulcer, especially in an extremity with compromised perfusion. Parenteral narcotic analgesia should be given at regular intervals, with monitoring of respiratory rate, blood pressure, pulse oximetry, and capnography, if available. If properly trained personnel are present, nerve blocks may be particularly comforting to the patient, such as a femoral nerve block for a midshaft femoral fracture.

Contaminated wounds should be flushed with normal saline irrigation so that gross particulate matter (e.g., soil, grass) is removed. If the transport will take longer than 120 minutes, antibiotics may be administered for patients with open fractures. A first-generation cephalosporin, cefazolin, is sufficient for minor open fractures, whereas a broader-spectrum agent, such as cefoxitin, might be administered for a more serious open fracture. If a body part has been amputated, it should also be periodically assessed so that it remains cool but does not freeze or become macerated by soaking in water.

SUMMARY

The management of patients with extremity trauma varies based on an evaluation of the priority of the patient's extremity injuries compared with the patient's other injuries and conditions. In patients with multisystem trauma, the prehospital care provider directs attention toward the primary survey and the identification and management of all life-threatening injuries, including internal or external hemorrhage in the extremities. These patients should be rapidly secured to a long backboard in a normal, supine, anatomic position to stabilize all injured extremities efficiently and allow the provider to address the patient's critical needs. The prehospital care provider cannot treat non–life-threatening injuries in multisystem trauma patients until the patient's systemic condition is stabilized. The provider is careful not to be distracted from addressing life-threatening conditions by the gross, dramatic appearance of any noncritical injuries or by the patient's request for their management.

Patients with noncritical, isolated injuries represent another category. The initial priority is to establish that the patient does not have life-threatening injuries. Only after the prehospital care provider has fully assessed the patient and found only isolated injuries without systemic implication can the patient be managed in the normally prescribed way. When the mechanism of injury indicates sudden, violent changes in motion, multisystem trauma, or spinal trauma, the prehospital care provider needs to anticipate potential systemic decline and to include the patient's age, physical condition, and medical history in the evaluation.

SCENARIO SOLUTION

After completion of the primary survey, focus attention on the possible fracture sites. Three possible fractures exist in this scenario: left hip, left thigh, and right humerus. The first priority after primary assessment and treatment is to decrease the amount of movement of the fractures and manually stabilize the cervical spine. The proper way to immobilize all fractures simultaneously is with the long backboard. At this time, although vital signs are stable, the patient's diaphoretic skin is a clue that she may soon be in trouble. With the probability of fracture to her hip and femur, the index of suspicion for internal bleeding and shock should be high. Focus of treatment should be on stabilization of all fractures and the spine and initiation of IV access en route to a trauma center. Careful monitoring of vital signs is mandatory because shock may be present. ∎

References

1. Wood SP, Vrahas M, Wedel S: Femur fracture immobilization with traction splints in multisystem trauma patients, *Prehosp Emerg Care* 7:241, 2003.
2. Flint LM, Brown A, Richardson JD, et al: Definitive control of bleeding from severe pelvic fractures, *Ann Surg* 189:709, 1979.
3. Flint L, Babikian G, Anders M, et al: Definitive control of mortality from severe pelvic fracture, *Ann Surg* 211:703, 1999.
4. Goth P, Garnett G: Clinical guidelines for delayed or prolonged transport: II. Dislocations. Rural Affairs Committee, National Association of Emergency Medical Services Physicians, *Prehosp Disaster Med* 8(1):77, 1993.
5. Alonso-Serra HM, Wesley K: Prehospital pain management, *Prehosp Emerg Care* 7:842, 2003.
6. Hatlestad D: Capnography in sedation and pain management, *J Emerg Med Serv,* 34:65, 2005.
7. Galinski M, Dolveck F, Borron SW, et al: A randomized, double blind study comparing morphine with fentanyl in prehospital analgesia, *Am J Emerg Med* 23:114, 2005.
8. Seyfer AE: *Guidelines for management of amputated parts,* Chicago, 1996, American College of Surgeons Committee on Trauma.
9. Pepe E, Mosesso VN, Falk JL: Prehospital fluid resuscitation of the patient with major trauma, *Prehosp Emerg Care* 6:81, 2002.
10. Better OS: Management of shock and acute renal failure in casualties suffering from crush syndrome, *Ren Fail* 19:647, 1997.
11. Michaelson M, Taitelman U, Bshouty Z, et al: Crush syndrome: experience from the Lebanon war, 1982, *Isr J Med Sci* 20:305, 1984.
12. Pretto EA, Angus D, Abrams J, et al: An analysis of prehospital mortality in an earthquake, *Prehosp Disaster Med* 9:107, 1994.
13. Collins AJ, Burzstein S: Renal failure in disasters, *Crit Care Clin* 7:421, 1991.
14. Sever MS, Vanholder R, Lameire N: Management of crush-related injuries after disasters, *N Engl J Med* 354:1052, 2006.

Suggested Reading

Ashkenazi I, Isakovich B, Kluger Y, et al: Prehospital management of earthquake casualties buried under rubble, *Prehosp Disast Med* 20:122, 2005.

American College of Surgeons Committee on Trauma: Musculo-skeletal trauma. In *Advanced trauma life support,* Chicago, 2005, ACS.

Coppola PT, Coppola M: Emergency department evaluation and treatment of pelvic fractures, *Emerg Med Clin North Am* 18(1):1, 2003.

Gregory RT, Gould RJ, Peclet M, et al: The mangled extremity syndrome: a severity grading system for multisystem injury of the extremity, *J Trauma* 25:1147, 1985.

Howe HR, Poole GV, Hansen KJ, et al: Salvage of lower extremities following combined orthopedic and vascular trauma: a predictive salvage index, *Am Surg* 53:205, 1987.

McSwain NE Jr, Paturas JL, editors: *The basic EMT: comprehensive prehospital patient care,* ed 2, St Louis, 2001, Mosby.

Roessler MS, Wisner DH, Holcroft JW: The mangled extremity: when to amputate? *Arch Surg* 126:1243, 1991.

Chapter Objectives

*At the completion of this chapter, the reader
will be able to do the following:*

✓ Define various depths of burns.

✓ Define the zones of burn injuries.

✓ Understand how ice can deepen the depth of burns.

✓ Estimate burn size using the "rule of nines."

✓ Calculate fluid resuscitation using the Parkland formula.

✓ Define the additional fluid needs in children with burns.

✓ Describe appropriate burn dressings for prehospital care.

✓ Discuss the unique concerns of electrical injuries.

✓ Discuss the management concerns in patients with circumferential
   burns.

✓ Discuss the three elements of smoke inhalation.

✓ Apply principles of various zones in hazardous material (hazmat)
   scenes.

✓ Discuss criteria for the transfer of patients to burn centers.

CHAPTER 13

Burn Trauma

SCENARIO

Your unit is initially dispatched to a residential structure fire for standby purposes. While en route, you are informed by the fireground commander that two adults have initially escaped the fire. According to neighbors, one male subject reentered the building in an attempt to rescue two children entrapped on the second floor. On your arrival, fire crews are administering care to three fire victims on the front lawn.

Victim 1:

A 34-year-old male who is coughing and wheezing. Large portions of his clothing have been burned away. His breathing is spontaneous but labored. His heart rate is 118 beats/min, blood pressure 148/94 mm Hg, respirations 22 breaths/min, and pulse oximeter reading 92%. The patient appears to have suffered partial- and full-thickness burns involving his face, both arms and hands, and anterior trunk.

Victim 2:

An 11-year-old female who is unresponsive with shallow respirations. Her heart rate is 140 beats/min, blood pressure 88/48 mm Hg, respirations 26 breaths/min, and pulse oximeter reading 92%. She has full-thickness burns on her entire right arm and some small areas of her left arm. First responders have placed her on oxygen by nonrebreather facemask.

Victim 3:

A 2-year-old female patient. The child is covered with soot and does not appear to have any obvious burns. The child is in cardiopulmonary arrest, and first responders have initiated cardiopulmonary resuscitation.

What is the extent of burns for each patient? What are the initial steps for managing these patients? How does the prehospital care provider recognize an inhalation injury? ■

Many people consider burns to be the most frightening and dreaded of all injuries. Almost everyone has suffered a burn of some degree and experienced the intense pain and anxiety associated with even a small burn. Burns are common in industrialized and agricultural cultures and in civilian and military settings. Burns can range from small to catastrophic injuries covering large regions of the body.

A common misconception is that burn injuries are isolated to the skin. On the contrary, large burns can be extensive, multisystem injuries capable of life-threatening effects to the heart, lungs, kidneys, gastrointestinal (GI) tract, and immune system. The most common cause of death in a fire victim is not from the direct complications of the burn wound, but from complications of respiratory failure.

Although considered a form of trauma, burns have some significant differences that merit consideration. After a trauma, such as a motor vehicle crash (MVC) or a fall, the victim's physiologic response is to initiate several adaptive mechanisms to preserve life. These responses can include the shunting of blood, increase in cardiac output, and increase in production of various protective serum proteins. By contrast, after a burn the patient's body essentially attempts to shut down, go into shock, and die. A substantial portion of initial burn care is directed at reversal of this initial shock.

Consideration of the etiology of burns will prevent the rescuer from sustaining unnecessary injury, as well as provide optimal care for the victim. Prehospital care providers also need to consider the circumstances in which the burn occurred, because a large percentage of burns in both children and adults result from an intentional injury.

Smoke inhalation is a dangerous and life-threatening injury that is often more dangerous than a burn injury. Inhalation of toxic fumes from smoke is a greater predictor of burn mortality than the age of the patient or the size of the burn.[1] A victim need not inhale a large quantity of smoke to predispose the patient to a severe injury, and often life-threatening complications may not manifest for several days.

Approximately 20% of all burn victims are children, and 20% of these children are the victims of intentional injury or child abuse.[2a,2b] Most health care providers are surprised to learn that intentional burn injury is second only to beating in the forms of physical violence inflicted on children. Burns as a form of abuse are not limited to children. It is common to see women burned in cases of domestic violence, as well as elderly persons in cases of elder abuse.

Anatomy

The skin covers about 1.5 to 2.0 square meters in the average adult. The skin is made up of two layers, the epidermis and the dermis. The *epidermis* is about 0.05 mm thick in areas such as the eyelids and can be thick as 1 mm on the sole of the foot. The deeper *dermis* is on average 10 times thicker that the epidermis.

The skin of males is thicker than skin of females, and the skin of children and elderly persons is thinner than that of the average adult. These facts explain how an individual can suffer burns of varying depths when exposed to a singular burning agent, and how a child might experience a deep burn while an adult with the same exposure has only a superficial injury.

The skin serves several complex functions, including protection from the external environment, regulation of fluids, thermoregulation, sensation, and metabolic adaptation.

Burn Characteristics

The creation of a burn is analogous to frying an egg. When one breaks an egg into a hot skillet, the egg is initially liquid and transparent. As the egg is exposed to the high temperatures, it rapidly becomes opaque and solidifies. A virtually identical process occurs when a patient is burned. In the case of the egg, the proteins of the egg change shape and are destroyed in a process known as *denaturation.* When a burn occurs to a patient, the elevated or freezing temperature, radiation, or chemical agent causes the proteins in the skin to be severely damaged, resulting in protein denaturation.

A full-thickness burn has three zones of tissue injury[3] (Figure 13-1). The central zone is known as the *zone of coagulation,* and this is the region of greatest tissue destruction. This zone is necrotic and is not capable of tissue repair.

Adjacent to the zone of necrosis is a region of lesser injury, the *zone of stasis.* The cells in this zone are injured but not irreversibly. If deprived of their delivery of oxygen or blood flow, these viable cells will die and become necrotic. This zone is referred to as the zone of stasis because immediately after injury, the blood flow to this region is stagnant. Timely and appropriate burn care will preserve blood flow and oxygen delivery to these injured cells. Resuscitation of the patient will eliminate this stasis and reestablish delivery of oxygen to the injured and susceptible cells. Failure to resuscitate the patient appropriately results in death of the cells in the injured tissue, and a partial-thickness burn then converts to a full-thickness burn. A common error that results in damage to this area is the application of ice by a well-meaning bystander or provider.

FIGURE 13-1   Three zones of burn injury.

When ice is used to stop the burning process, the ice causes vasoconstriction, preventing reestablishment of blood flow. It is now argued that when ice is applied to a burn, the patient will experience some reduction in pain; however, the analgesia will be at the expense of additional tissue destruction. For these reasons, the burning should be arrested with the use of ambient or room-temperature water, and analgesia should be provided with oral or parenteral medications.

The outermost zone is known as the *zone of hyperemia.* This zone has minimal cellular injury and is characterized by increased blood flow secondary to an inflammatory reaction initiated by the burn injury.

Burn Depth

Estimation of burn depth can be deceptively difficult. Often, a burn that appears to be second degree will prove to be third degree in 24 to 48 hours. The surface of a burn may appear to be a first- or second-degree burn at first glance, but on debridement, the superficial epidermis separates off, revealing a white, third-degree burn eschar. Therefore it is often wise to withhold final judgment of burn depth for up to 48 hours after injury. Often it is best simply to tell patients that the injury is either superficial or deep and that time is required to determine ultimate burn depth.

First-Degree Burns

First-degree burns involve only the epidermis and are characterized as being red and painful (Figure 13-2). These are rarely clinically significant, with the exception of large areas of sunburn, where the patient will have significant pain and risks dehydration without attention to appropriate oral hydration. These wounds heal typically within a week, and the patient will not scar.

Second-Degree Burns

Second-degree burns, also known as *partial-thickness burns,* are those that involve the epidermis and varying portions of the underlying dermis (Figure 13-3). Second-degree burns can be further classified as either *superficial* or *deep.* These wounds blister and are painful. Second-degree

FIGURE 13-2   First-degree burn.

FIGURE 13-3   Second-degree burn.

FIGURE 13-4   Third-degree burn.

FIGURE 13-5   This patient has suffered from a full-thickness (third-degree) burn characterized as white and leathery in appearance.

burns will appear as blisters or as denuded, burned areas with a glistening or wet-appearing base. These wounds will be painful. Because remnants of the dermis survive, these burns are often capable of healing in 2 to 3 weeks. In partial-thickness burns the zone of coagulation involves the entire epidermis and varying depths of the superficial dermis. If not well cared for, the zone of stasis in these injuries can progress to necrosis, making these burns larger and perhaps converting the wound to a third-degree burn. A superficial second-degree burn will heal with vigilant wound care. Deep second-degree burns often require surgical correction.

Third-Degree Burns

Third-degree burns may have several appearances (Figure 13-4). Most often these wounds will appear as thick, dry, white, leathery burns, regardless of race or skin color (Figure 13-5). In severe cases the skin will have a charred appearance with visible thrombosis of blood vessels (Figure 13-6). Most patients will have pain because areas of third-degree burn are usually surrounded by second-degree burns. Burns of this depth can be disabling and life threatening. Prompt surgical excision and intensive rehabilitation at a specialized center will be required.

Fourth-Degree Burns

Fourth-degree burns are those that not only burn all layers of the skin, but also burn underlying fat, muscles, bone, or internal organs (Figure 13-7).

Blisters

Much discussion has been generated about blisters, including whether or not to debride them and how to approach the blister associated with partial-thickness burn. A blister occurs when the epidermis separates off of the underlying dermis and fluid that is leaking from nearby vessels fills the blister. The presence of osmotically active proteins in

FIGURE 13-6 Example of deep full-thickness burn with charring of the skin and visible thrombosis of blood vessels.

the blister fluid draws additional fluid into the blister space, causing the blister to continue to enlarge. As the blister enlarges, it creates pressure on the injured tissue of the wound bed, which increases the patient's pain. Many think that the skin of the blister acts as a dressing and prevents contamination of the wound. On the contrary, the skin of the blister is not normal and therefore cannot serve as a protective barrier. Additionally, maintaining the blister intact prevents one from applying topical antibiotics directly on the injury. For these reasons, blisters should be opened and debrided, but not in the field.[4]

Burn Size Estimation

Estimation of burn size is necessary to resuscitate the patient appropriately and prevent the complications associated with hypovolemic shock from burn injury. The most widely applied method is known is the "rule of nines." This method applies the principle that major regions of the body in adults are considered to be 9% of the total body surface area (Figure 13-8). The perineum or genital area represents 1%. The palm of the hand, not including the extended digits, also represents 1%.

Children have different proportions than adults. Children's heads are proportionally larger than adults, and their legs are shorter in proportion than adults. Because of this the rule of nines is modified for pediatric patients.

The *Lund-Browder chart* is a diagram that takes into account age-related changes in children. Using these charts, a provider maps the burn and then determines burn size based on an accompanying reference table (Figure 13-9).

A new method of determining burn size as well as fluid resuscitation has been developed that is easily applied in the prehospital setting. An alternative to the rule of nines, this method uses what the author refers to as the "rule of ones" and the "burn size score."

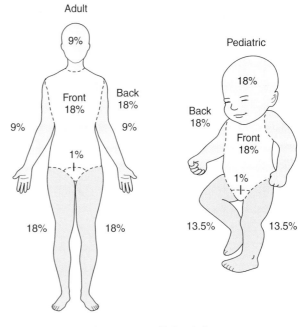

FIGURE 13-7 Fourth-degree burns to the arm, with burns not only to the skin but also to the subcutaneous fat, muscle, and bone.

FIGURE 13-8 Rule of nines.

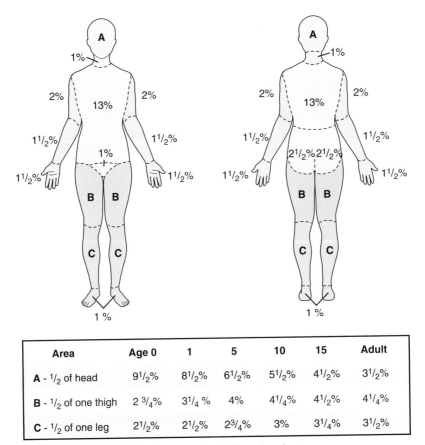

Area	Age 0	1	5	10	15	Adult
A - $1/2$ of head	$9^1/_2$%	$8^1/_2$%	$6^1/_2$%	$5^1/_2$%	$4^1/_2$%	$3^1/_2$%
B - $1/2$ of one thigh	$2^3/_4$%	$3^1/_4$%	4%	$4^1/_4$%	$4^1/_2$%	$4^1/_4$%
C - $1/2$ of one leg	$2^1/_2$%	$2^1/_2$%	$2^3/_4$%	3%	$3^1/_4$%	$3^1/_2$%

FIGURE 13-9. Lund-Browder chart.

Using the traditional methods, the burn size is estimated using the rule of nines, followed by mathematical calculation of a fluid resuscitation rate. Completion of this calculation requires two multiplication and two division operations. In an often chaotic environment while caring for a critically injured patient, this is a low priority.

By comparison, the rule of ones uses a resuscitation index with reference to a table to complete determination of fluid needs in a more simplified operation.[5] Fluid resuscitation needs are determined quickly by adding a few numbers (Figure 13-10) and referring to a simple table (Table 13-1).

The first step is using the *burn size score* (BSS). Using the same anatomic regions as the rule of nines, assign a score of one if more than 50% of that region is burned, and use a score of one-half if a region is burned less than 50%. Add all the points to obtain the BSS, and round up the total. Cross-reference the patient's weight and BSS to determine the fluid rate.

Consider the following example:

A 70-kg victim with burns to both legs, anterior chest, and abdomen and half the left arm. First, calculate the BSS:

Right leg, 2
Left leg, 2
Anterior abdomen, 1

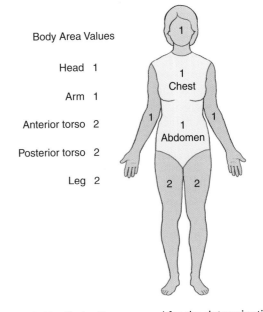

Body Area Values

Head   1

Arm   1

Anterior torso   2

Posterior torso   2

Leg   2

FIGURE 13-10 Body diagram used for the determination of burn index.

Anterior chest, 1
Half the left arm, 0.5

BSS = 2 + 2 + 1 + 1 + 0.5 = 6.5 (round up to BSS of 7)

TABLE 13-1   Determination of Fluid Resuscitation Using Burn Resuscitation Index

Patient weight		Initial intravenous resuscitation rate (Lactated Ringer's, mL/hr)										
		Burn size score (BSS)										
lb	kg	1	2	3	4	5	6	7	8	9	10	11
88	40	90	180	270	360	450	540	630	720	810	900	990
110	50	113	225	338	450	563	675	788	900	1013	1125	1238
132	60	135	270	405	540	675	810	945	1080	1215	1350	1485
154	70	158	315	473	630	788	945	1103	1260	1418	1575	1733
176	80	180	360	540	720	900	1080	1260	1440	1620	1800	1980
198	90	203	405	608	810	1013	1215	1418	1620	1823	2025	2228
220	100	225	450	675	900	1125	1350	1575	1800	2025	2250	2475
242	110	248	495	743	990	1238	1485	1733	1980	2228	2475	2723
264	120	270	540	810	1080	1350	1620	1890	2160	2430	2700	2970
286	130	293	585	878	1170	1463	1755	2048	2340	2633	2925	3218
308	140	315	630	945	1260	1575	1890	2205	2520	2835	3150	3465
330	150	338	675	1013	1350	1688	2025	2363	2700	3038	3375	3713

On Table 13-1, look at the 70-kg row and then the BSS column of 7. On the chart, you determine the fluid rate of 1103 mL/hr. A similar chart is available for pediatric patients.

Fluid Resuscitation

Administration of large amounts of intravenous (IV) fluids is needed to prevent a burn patient from going into hypovolemic shock. After a burn, the victim loses a substantial amount of intravascular fluid in the form of obligatory whole-body edema, as well as evaporative losses at the site of the burn. Massive fluid shifts will occur, even though total body water may remain unchanged. Evaporative losses can be enormous.

The resuscitation of burn shock is aimed at not only restoration of the loss of intravascular volume, but also replacement of anticipated intravascular losses at a rate that mimics those losses as they occur (Box 13-1). In trauma patients it may be necessary to replace the volume that the patient has already lost from hemorrhage from an open fracture or bleeding viscera. In contrast, when treating the burn patient, the objective is to calculate and replace the fluids that it is anticipated the patient will lose over the first 24 hours after the burn injury.

The use of IV fluids, especially lactated Ringer's (LR) solution, is the best way initially to manage a burn patient. The amount of fluids administered in the first 24 hours after injury is typically 2 to 4 mL/kg/% burn. The *Parkland formula* delivers 4 mL/kg/% burn. Half this fluid

---

BOX 13-1   Resuscitating a Burn Patient

Resuscitating a burn patient can be compared to filling a leaking bucket. The bucket is leaking water at a constant rate. The bucket has a line drawn in the inside near the top of the bucket. Your objective is to keep that water at the level of the line. Initially, when one comes to the bucket, the water depth will be very low. The longer the bucket has been unattended, the lower the water level, and the greater the amount of fluid that will need to be replaced. The container will continue to leak, so once the bucket has been filled to an appropriate level, fluids will need to be continuously added at a constant rate to maintain the desired level.

The longer the burn patient is not resuscitated or underresuscitated, the more hypovolemic the patient becomes. Therefore, greater amounts of fluids are required to establish a "level" of homeostasis. Once the patient has been resuscitated, the vascular space continues to leak in the same manner as the bucket. To maintain equilibrium with this homeostatic point, additional fluids need to be provided to replace the ongoing losses.

---

needs to be administered in the first 8 hours after injury, and the remaining half of the volume from hour 8 to 24. Importantly, the first half is administered within 8 hours from the time the patient was *injured,* not from the point the provider started to resuscitate the patient. This is especially important in frontier or military settings, where there may be an initial delay in treatment. If the patient presents for emergency care 3 hours after the injury with no or little fluid administration, the first half of the calculated total needs to be administered over 5 hours. In this way, the patient will be at the target volume by hour 8 after injury.

Pediatric Patient

Children require larger volumes of IV fluids than adults with similar-size burns. Also, children have less metabolic reserves of glycogen in their livers to maintain adequate blood glucose during the periods of burn resuscitation. For these reasons, children should receive 5% dextrose containing IV fluids (D5LR) at a standard maintenance rate in addition to burn resuscitation fluids.

Smoke Inhalation

The patient with both thermal burns and smoke inhalation will require significantly more fluid than the burn patient without smoke inhalation.[6] Smoke inhalation produces a chemical burn to the lungs. Less fluid than calculated is often administered in an attempt to "protect the lungs." Witholding fluids actually increases the severity of the pulmonary injury.

Initial Burn Care

The initial step in the care of a burn patient is to stop the burning process. *Stop the burning* does not mean *cool the burn.* These are two separate actions. The most effective and appropriate method of terminating the burning is irrigation with copious volumes of room-temperature water. Use of cold water or ice is contraindicated. As previously mentioned, the application of ice will stop the burning and provide analgesia, but it also will increase the extent of tissue damage in the zone of stasis. Remove all clothing and jewelry; these items maintain residual heat and will continue to burn the patient.

Effective wound care to the recent burn is the simple application of dry, sterile, nonadherent dressings. Cover the area with a dry, clean sheet. If a sheet is not readily available, substitute with a sterile surgical gown, drapes, or towels. The dry dressing will prevent ongoing environmental contamination while preventing the patient experiencing pain from air flowing over the exposed nerve endings (Box 13-2).

Prehospital providers have often been dissatisfied and frustrated with the simple application of sterile sheets to a burn. However, topical ointments and conventional topical antibiotics should *not* be applied because they prevent a direct inspection of the burn. Protection with only dry, sterile dressing is the first step. Such topical ointments and

---

> ### BOX 13-2   Prevent Airflow over Patient's Burn
>
> Most people have experienced the pain associated with a dental cavity. The pain is intensified when we inhale air over the exposed nerve. With a partial-thickness burn, thousands of the nerves are exposed, and the air currents in the environment produce pain in the patient when the currents come into contact with the exposed nerves of the wound bed. Therefore, by keeping burns covered, the patient will experience less pain.

FIGURE 13-11   Acticoat dressing.
(Courtesy Smith & Nephew Wound Management.)

antibiotics are removed on admission to the burn center to allow direct visualization of the burn and determination of burn severity. Also, some topical medications may complicate the application of tissue-engineered products used to aid wound healing.

High-concentration antimicrobial-coated dressings have become the mainstay of wound care in burn centers (Acticoat) (Figure 13-11). These dressings are sputter-coated with silver, which is time-released over several days when applied to an open burn wound. The released silver provides rapid antimicrobial coverage of the common organisms contaminating and infecting wounds. Recently, these dressings have been adapted from burn center use to prehospital applications. These large antimicrobial sheets can be rapidly applied to the burn and can eradicate any contaminating organisms. This method of wound care allows application of a nonpharmaceutical device that greatly reduces burn wound contamination within 30 minutes after application.[7-9] An advantage of these dressings in frontier and military application is their compact size and light weight. An entire adult can be covered with antibiotic dressings that can be stored in the volume of a manila envelope with minimal weight.

Primary Survey and Resuscitation

The goal of the primary assessment is to systematically evaluate and treat life-threatening disorders in order of importance to preserve life. The ABCDE method of trauma care applies to the management of the burn patient, although burn patients provide unique challenges in every step of the resuscitation.

Airway

Preservation of the patency of the airway is the highest priority in caring for a burn victim. The heat from the fire can cause edema of the airway above the level of the vocal cords and can occlude the airway. Therefore, careful and continuous evaluation is required. To avoid catastrophic airway occlusion, early control of the airway is prudent. Intubation of these patients is often difficult and hazardous. The airway should be managed by the most experienced personnel available. Often, patients are the best individuals suited to manage their own airway. Pharmacologic interventions will suppress the patient's ability to manage the airway, necessitating airway intervention and maintenance by the providers.

If the patient is intubated, special precautions must be taken in securing the endotracheal (ET) tube and preventing inadvertent dislodgement or extubation. With face burns, adhesive tapes are not suitable for securing the ET tube. The tube can be secured using two umbilical tapes or pieces of IV tubing wrapped around the head. One piece should be draped over the ear and the second under the ear. Commercially available cloth and Velcro devices are also suitable.

Breathing

As with any trauma patient, breathing can be adversely affected by such problems as broken ribs, pneumothoraces, and open chest wounds. In the event of circumferential chest wall burns, pulmonary compliance progressively decreases to such an extent that it inhibits the patient's ability to inhale. In such cases, prompt escharotomies of the chest wall will allow reestablishment of ventilation.

Circulation

Evaluation of circulation includes the determination of blood pressure, evaluation of circumferential burns, and establishment of IV catheters. Accurate measurement of blood pressure becomes difficult or impossible with burns to the extremities, and if blood pressure can be obtained it may not correctly reflect systemic arterial blood pressure because of full-thickness burns and edema to the extremities. Even if the patient has adequate arterial blood pressure, distal limb perfusions may be critically reduced because of circumferential injuries. Burned extremities should be elevated during transport to reduce the degree of swelling in the affected limb.

Establishment of two large-caliber IV catheters capable of the rapid flow rate needed in large-volume resuscitation is a requirement for burns that cover more than 20% of the total body surface area. Ideally, the IV catheters should not be placed through or adjacent to burned tissue; however, placement through the burn is appropriate if no alternative

sites are available. When the catheter is placed in or near a burn, special measures must be taken to ensure the catheter does not inadvertently fall out. Adhesive tapes and dressings typically used to secure IV catheters will be ineffective when applied on or adjacent to burned tissue. Alternative means to secure the lines include wrapping the site with Kerlix or Coban rolls. If prolonged transport is anticipated, the IV catheter can be sutured in place.

Disability

Burn patients are trauma patients and may have sustained injuries other than the thermal injuries. Burns are obvious and sometimes intimidating injuries, but it is vital to assess for other, less obvious internal injuries that may be more immediately life threatening than the burn injuries. In attempts to escape being burned, patients will leap from the windows of buildings; elements of the burning structure may collapse and fall on the patient; and the victim may be trapped in the burning wreckage of an MVC. Evaluate the patient for neurologic and motor deficits. Identify and splint fractures of long bones. Perform spinal immobilization if you suspect a potential spine injury.

Exposure/Environment

The next priority is to expose the patient completely. Every square inch of the patient should be exposed and inspected. All clothing and jewelry should be promptly removed; as noted earlier, these items may continue to injure the patient. A careful examination of all body surfaces may reveal injuries that were not previously apparent.

Controlling the environment is critical. Burn patients are not able to retain their own body heat and are extremely susceptible to hypothermia. Make every effort to preserve body temperature. Apply several layers of blankets. Keep the passenger compartment of the ambulance or fuselage of the aircraft warm, regardless of the time of year. As a general rule, if you as a prehospital care provider are not uncomfortable, the ambient temperature is not warm enough.

Secondary Survey

After completing the primary assessment, the next objective is completion of the secondary assessment. The secondary assessment of a burn patient is no different than that in any other trauma patient. The provider should complete a head-to-toe evaluation, attempting to identify additional injuries or medical conditions.

Dressings

Before transportation, the wounds should be dressed. The goal of the dressings is to prevent ongoing contamination and prevent airflow over the wounds.

Dry sterile dressings in the form of a sterile sheet or towel are sufficient before transporting the patient. Several layers of blankets are then placed over the sterile burn sheets. Topical antibiotics should not be applied until the patient has been evaluated by the burn center, as discussed earlier.

Transportation

Patients with burns who have multiple injuries should first be transported to a trauma center, where immediately life-threatening injuries can be identified and surgically treated, if necessary. Once stabilized at a trauma center, the patient with burns should be transported to a burn center for definitive burn care and rehabilitation. The American Burn Association and the American College of Surgeons have identified criteria for transfer of burn patients to a burn center, as outlined in Box 13-3.

BOX 13-3   Injuries Requiring Burn Unit Care

Patients with serious burns should receive care at centers that have special expertise and resources. Initial transport or early transfer to a burn unit should result in a lower mortality rate and fewer complications. A burn unit may treat adults, children, or both. The Committee on Trauma of the American College of Surgeons recommends referral to a burn unit for patients with burn injuries who meet the following criteria:

1. Inhalation injury
2. Partial-thickness burns over greater than 10% of the total body surface area (TBSA)
3. Full-thickness (third-degree) burns in any age group
4. Burns that involve the face, hands, feet, genitalia, perineum, or major joints
5. Electrical burns, including lightning injury
6. Chemical burns
7. Burn injury in patients with preexisting medical disorders that could complicate management, prolong recovery, or affect mortality
8. Any patients with burns and concomitant trauma (e.g., fractures) in which the burn injury poses the greatest risk of morbidity or mortality; if trauma poses the greater immediate risk, the patient may be initially stabilized in a trauma center before transfer to a burn unit
9. Burned children in hospitals without qualified personnel or equipment for the care of children
10. Burn injury in patients who will require special social, emotional, or long-term rehabilitative intervention

From the American College of Surgeons Committee on Trauma: *Resources for optimal care of the injured patient: 2006,* Chicago, 2006, ACS.

Fluid Resuscitation

Determination of fluid needs and initiation of the fluid resuscitation process are important to prevent the patient from going into hypovolemic shock. Burn size is estimated using the rule of nines or an alternative method.

As previously discussed, total 24-hour fluid amount and hourly rate are determined using the Parkland formula. Different centers will use a variety of resuscitation algorithms, but the Parkland formula is the most universally accept method of burn resuscitation. To determine resuscitation fluid rate, the provider needs to know size of the burn, weight of the patient in kilograms, and time elapsed since the patient was injured. The amount of fluids given in the first 24 hours after a burn should total 4 mL/kg/% surface area burned. Half this fluid is given in the first 8 hours from injury, and the second half is given in the remaining 16 hours.

For example, consider that an 80-kg man has sustained 30% third-degree burns, and you arrive on scene shortly after the injury. The resuscitation rate would be calculated as follows:

$$\text{24-hour fluid total} = 4 \text{ mL/kg/\% TBSA burn}$$
$$= 4 \times 80 \times 30$$
$$= 9600 \text{ mL}$$

Once you have the 24-hour total, divide that number by 2:

Fluid given from injury to hour 8 = 9600 mL/2 = 4800 mL

To determine the hourly rate for the first 8 hours, divide this total by 8:

Fluid rate for the first 8 hours =
4800 mL/8 hr = 600 mL/hr
Fluid rate for hours 8 to 24 = 9600 mL/2 = 4800 mL

To determine the hourly rate for the final 16 hours, divide this total by 16:

Fluid rate for final 16 hours =
4800 mL/16 hours = 300 mL/hr

Special Considerations

Electrical Burns

Electrical injuries are devastating injuries that prehospital care providers can easily underappreciate. In many cases the extent of apparent tissue damage does not accurately reflect the magnitude of the injury. Tissue destruction and necrosis are excessive compared with the apparent trauma

FIGURE 13-12 Patient after electrical injury from high-tension wires.

FIGURE 13-13 Urine of patient after electrical injury from high-tension wires. The patient has myoglobinuria after extensive muscle destruction.

because most of the destruction occurs internally as the electricity is conducted through the patient. The patient will have external burns at the points of contact with the electrical source as well as grounding points. As the electricity courses through the patient's body, deep layers of tissue are destroyed despite seemingly minor injuries on the surface (Figure 13-12).

Electrical and crush injuries share many similarities. In both injuries there is massive destruction of large muscle groups with resultant release of both potassium and myoglobin (see Chapter 12). The release of muscle *potassium* causes a significant increase in the serum level, which can result in cardiac arrhythmias. Elevated potassium levels can make use of the depolarizing muscle relaxant succinylcholine prohibitively dangerous. *Myoglobin* is a molecule found in the muscle that assists the muscle tissue in transportation of oxygen. When released into the bloodstream in considerable amounts, the myoglobin is toxic to the kidneys and can cause kidney failure. This condition, *myoglobinuria,* is evidenced by tea- or cola-colored urine (Figure 13-13).

In military situations or interhospital transfers, a victim of an electrical injury in whom a urinary catheter has been placed may need to be transported. These patients require

an aggressive urine output of greater than 100 mL/hr in adults or 1 mL/kg in children to avoid renal failure. Sodium bicarbonate is administered in some cases to make the myoglobin more soluble in urine and reduce the likelihood of renal injury.

The electrical burn patient may have associated injuries as well. Tympanic membranes may rupture, resulting in hearing difficulties. Intense and sustained muscle contraction *(tetany)* can result in fractures of multiple levels of the spine as well as long bones. Patients with electrical injury should have their spine immobilized. Long-bone fractures should be splinted when detected or suspected. Intracranial bleeds and cardiac arrhythmias may also occur.

Electrical flash burns are the result of superheated air. Nevertheless, because of the catastrophic and occult nature of conduction injuries, it is imperative that providers maintain a high index of suspicion for the presence of a transmission type of injury.

FIGURE 13-14 Escharotomies are performed to release the constricting effect of circumferential burns.

Circumferential Burns

Circumferential burns of the trunk or limbs are capable of producing a life- or limb-threatening condition. Circumferential burns create a tourniquet-like effect that can render an arm or leg pulseless. Circumferential burns of the chest can constrict the chest wall to such a degree that the patient suffocates from inability to take a breath. Therefore, all circumferential burns should be handled as an emergency and patients transported to a burn center. *Escharotomies* are surgical incisions made through the burn eschar to allow expansion of the deeper tissues and decompression of previously compressed and often occluded vascular structures (Figure 13-14).

Smoke Inhalation

The leading cause of death in fires is not thermal injuries but the inhalation of toxic smoke. Any patient with a history of exposure of smoke in a closed space should be considered at risk of having an inhalation injury. Any patient with burns to the face or soot in the sputum is clearly at risk for a smoke inhalation injury; however, the absence of these signs should not exclude the diagnosis of a toxic inhalation. Maintaining a high index of suspicion is vitally important because signs and symptoms may not manifest for days after the exposure.

The three elements of smoke inhalation are thermal injury, asphyxiation, and delayed–toxin-induced lung injury. Dry air is a poor conductor of heat; the inhalation of heated air associated with a structure fire rarely induces thermal injury to the airways below the level of the vocal cords. The large surface area of the nasopharynx acts effectively as a heat exchanger and cools the inhaled, heated air to about body temperature by the time the air reaches the level of the vocal cords. When heated dry air at 300° C is inhaled, the air is cooled to 50° C by the time it is at the level of

the trachea.[10] The vocal cords provide additional protection by reflexively moving into an adduction position.[11] The exception to this is the inhalation of steam. Steam has 4000 times the heat-carrying capacity of dry heat and is capable of burning the distal airways and bronchioles.[10] Fortunately, steam injuries are rare.

Asphyxiants

Two gaseous products that are clinically important as asphyxiants are *carbon monoxide* (CO) and *cyanide gas* (CN). Both molecules are classified as asphyxiants and thus cause cell death by cellular hypoxia or asphyxia. Patients with asphyxia from smoke containing one or both of these compounds will have inadequate delivery of oxygen to tissues despite an adequate blood pressure or pulse oximeter reading. CO binds to hemoglobin with greater affinity than oxygen. The symptoms of CO inhalation depend on the duration or severity and resultant serum levels. Symptoms can range from headache to coma.

Treatment of CO toxicity is removal from the source and administration of oxygen. When breathing room air (21% oxygen), the body will eliminate half the CO in 250 minutes.[12] When the patient is placed on 100% oxygen, the half-life of the CO-hemoglobin complex is reduced to 40 to 60 minutes.[13]

Cyanide gas is produced from the burning of plastics or polyurethane. Cyanide poisons cellular machinery, preventing the body's cells from using oxygen. The patient can die from asphyxia despite having adequate oxygen in the blood. Symptoms of cyanide toxicity include altered level of consciousness, dizziness, headache, and tachycardia or tachypnea. The treatment of cyanide poisoning is rapid transport to an emergency center capable of providing the patient with the antidote therapy. A commercially available antidote kit is available. The goal of the antidote therapy is to induce the formation of a second poison in the patient's blood. This second, therapeutically induced poison binds with the cyanide and allows the body to slowly detoxify the cyanide. Extreme caution is needed when administering the antidote.[14-16]

The "Lilly kit" is the antidote kit used for cyanide toxicity in the United States. This method of treating cyanide poisoning was developed in the 1930s and found to be effective in detoxifying animals poisoned with 21 times the lethal dose of cyanide.[17] This kit contains several agents. The first medications administered are amyl nitrate and sodium nitrite. *Amyl nitrite* is inhaled, and *sodium nitrite* is given intravenously. The nitrite medications cause changes in the patient's hemoglobin to create *methemoglobin*. Cyanide exerts its toxic effects by binding a molecule in the cellular machinery responsible for energy, *cytochrome aa3*. The cyanide molecule is more attracted to methemoglobin than to cytochrome aa3. Therefore, cyanide floats from cytochrome aa3 and binds to the methemoglobin molecule.

Once the cytochrome aa3 is free of cyanide, the cell can resume normal energy production. However, methemoglobin does not deliver oxygen to the peripheral tissues as well as hemoglobin. Decreased oxygen delivery from the induced methemoglobinemia can have harmful effects in patients with elevated blood CO levels or anemia from acute blood loss.[18] The third agent in the cyanide antidote kit is thiosulfate. *Thiosulfate* works by assisting the metabolism of cyanide to the less toxic thiocyanate, which can be excreted in the urine. Treatment using this kit can actually aggravate cellular hypoxia in patients with CO toxicity.

An alternative antidote for cyanide poisoning is the use of medications that directly bind to the cyanide molecule, rendering it harmless. *Cyanocobalamin* is widely used in Europe but is not currently available in the United States. The only U.S. form of cyanocobalamin is a dilute form of vitamin B_{12} preparation. Use of the U.S. preparation requires an infusion volume of approximately 5 liters.[19,20] A second chelating agent that has been used for cyanide poisoning is *dicobalt edetate.* If this medication is administered in the absence of cyanide poisoning, however, cobalt toxicity is a risk.

Toxin-Induced Lung Injury

The thermal and asphyxiant components of an inhalation injury are usually apparent at the time of the rescue. In contrast, the signs and symptoms of toxin-induced lung injury may not manifest for several days. The first several days after a smoke inhalation injury are often described as the "honeymoon period." During this period the patient may appear deceptively stable with little or no pulmonary dysfunction. The severity of this lung injury is largely dependent on two factors: the components of the smoke and the duration of exposure.[21]

In simplified terms, smoke is the product of incomplete combustion, that is, chemical dust. The chemicals in the smoke react with the lining of the trachea and lungs and damage the cells lining the airways and lungs.[22-24] Compounds such as ammonia, hydrogen chloride, and sulfur dioxide form corrosive acids and alkalies when inhaled.[25]

Prehospital Management

The initial and most important element of caring for a patient with smoke exposure is determining the need for orotracheal intubation. If the patency of the patient's airway is in doubt, the airway can be secured using orotracheal intubation.[26,27] Continuous reevaluation of airway patency is required. Change in the character of the voice, difficulty handling secretions, or drooling are signs of pending airway occlusion.

Patients should be transported to burn centers even in the absence of surface burns. Burn centers treat a greater volume of patients with smoke inhalation and offer unique modes of mechanical ventilation.

FIGURE 13-15 Stocking-type scald of child's foot indicative of intentional immersion burn injury consistent with child abuse.

Child Abuse

Approximately 20% of all child abuse is the result of intentional burning. The majority of the children intentionally burned are 1 to 3 years of age.[28]

The most common form of burn child abuse is forcible immersion. These injuries typically occur when an adult places a child in hot water, often as a punishment related to toilet training. Factors that determine the severity of injury include age of the patient, temperature of the water, and duration of exposure. The child may sustain deep second- or third-degree burns of the hands or feet in a glovelike or stockinglike pattern. This is especially suspicious when the burns are symmetric and lack splash patterns[29] (Figures 13-15 and 13-16). In cases of intentional scalding, the child will tightly flex the arms and legs into a defensive posture because of fear or pain. The resultant burn pattern will spare the flexion creases of the popliteal fossa, the antecubital fossa, and the groin. Sharp lines of demarcation will also be seen between burned and unburned tissue, essentially indicating a dip[30,31] (Figure 13-17).

In accidental scald injuries, the burns will have variable burn depth, irregular margins, and smaller burns remote from the large burns, indicating splash.[32]

FIGURE 13-16 The straight lines of the burn pattern and absence of splash marks indicate that this burn is the result of abuse.

FIGURE 13-17 The sparing of the areas of flexion and the sharp lines of demarcation between burned and unburned skin indicate that this child was in a tightly flexed, defensive position before injury. Such a posture indicates that the scald is not accidental.

Contact Burns

Contact burns are the second most common mechanism of burn injury in children, whether accidental or intentional. All body surfaces have some degree of curvature. When an accidental contact burn occurs, the burning agent makes contact with the curved body surface area. The burning instrument is deflected off the curved surface, or the victim of the burn withdraws. The resultant injury has an irregular burn edge and depth. When a child receives an intentional contact burn, the inflicting implement is pressed to the child's skin. The resultant injury has sharp lines of demarcation between burned and unburned tissue and uniform depth.[31]

Many jurisdictions require health care providers to report such cases of suspected child abuse.

Radiation Burns

The severity of burns produced from various forms of radiation is a product of the amount of energy absorbed by the target tissue. The various forms of radiation include electromagnetic, x-rays, gamma rays, and particulate radiation. The different forms of radiation are able to transfer varying degrees of energy to tissue. Additionally, some forms of radiation (e.g., electromagnetic) can pass through tissue or an individual, resulting in no damage. In contrast, other forms of radiation (e.g., neutron exposure) are absorbed by the target tissue and result in significant injury. It is the absorption of the radiation that results in damage to the absorbing tissue. The absorption capacity of the radiation is more damaging than the actual dose of radiation. Equivalent doses of different forms of radiation will have dramatically different effects on an individual.

The typical exposure to radiation occurs in the setting of an industrial or occupational incident. However, with the increasing threat of global terrorism, the detonation of a small, hybrid, nuclear device (i.e., "dirty nuke") is a real possibility.

The detonation of a nuclear weapon in a metropolitan area would injure and kill by three mechanisms: thermal burns from the initial firestorm, supersonic destructive blast, and production of radiation. Mortality from a combination of thermal and radiation burns is greater than that from thermal or radiation burns of equal magnitude. The combination of thermal and radiation burns has a synergistic effect on mortality.[33]

A nuclear attack would result in massive loss of life and casualties capable of overwhelming medical providers and facilities. An attack on a population center would destroy medical facilities, kill medical providers, and cripple supply lines. Prehospital providers would likely be required to care for victims over a long period.

Radiation is a hazardous material, and many of the initial priorities are the same as in the care of the patient with a chemical exposure. The initial priorities are to remove the patient from the source of contamination, remove contaminated clothing, and irrigate the patient with water. Any removed clothing should be considered contaminated and should be handled with caution. Irrigation is done carefully to remove any radioactive debris or particles from contaminated areas without spreading the injury to uncontaminated body surfaces. Irrigation is continued until contamination has been minimized to a steady state, as determined by a Geiger counter.[34] Patients with burns should undergo fluid resuscitation similar to any burn patient. Irradiated patients may experience vomiting and diarrhea, which will necessitate an increase in resuscitation fluids.

The physiologic consequences of whole-body radiation are termed *acute radiation syndrome* (ARS). The initial symptoms of ARS typically appear within hours of exposure. The cells of the body that are most sensitive to the effects of radiation are those that typically undergo rapid division. These rapidly dividing cells are found in the skin, GI tract, and bone marrow; therefore, these tissues manifest the first signs of ARS. Within a few hours after radiation exposure, the patient will experience nausea, vomiting, and cramping abdominal pain. Aggressive fluid management is required to prevent the development of renal failure. Over the following days, the patient may develop bloody diarrhea, ischemia of the bowel, and overwhelming infection and may die. The bone marrow is extremely sensitive to the effects of radiation. The bone marrow will stop production of white blood cells needed to fight infections and platelets needed to make blood clots. The resultant infections and bleeding complications are often fatal.

After a nuclear event, IV supplies, infusion pumps, and receiving medical facilities may be in short supply. If unable to provide the patient with IV resuscitation, the prehospital care provider can resuscitate the patient with oral fluids. A cooperative patient should be encouraged to drink a balanced salt solution to maintain a large urine output; alternatively, fluids can be delivered by nasogastric or nasoenteric tubes. Oral balanced salt solutions include Moyer's solution (5 mL sodium chloride and 1 tsp sodium bicarbonate in 1 L water) and World Health Organization oral rehydration solution (WHO ORS). Animal research has shown encouraging results with such resuscitation strategies in patients with burns as large as 40% total body surface area. Administration of balanced salt solution to the GI tract at a rate of 20 mL/kg provided resuscitation equivalent to standard IV fluid resuscitation.[35]

Chemical Burns

Regardless of practice location or type, all prehospital providers need to be familiar with the basics of treating chemical injuries. Providers in urban settings may be called to a chemical incident at an industrial setting, whereas a rural provider may be summoned to an occurrence with agents used in agriculture. Tons of hazardous materials are transported through urban and rural settings daily by both highways and rail systems. Military providers may treat casualties of chemical burns caused by weapons, incendiary devices, chemicals used to fuel or maintain equipment, or chemical spills after damage to civilian installations.

Injuries from chemicals are often the result of prolonged exposure to the offending agent. This is contrasted with thermal injuries, where the duration of exposure is usually very brief. The severity of chemical injury is determined by four factors: nature of the chemical, concentration of the chemical, duration of contact, and mechanism of action of the chemical.

Chemical agents are classified as acid, base, organic, or inorganic. *Acids* are chemicals with a pH between 7 (neutral) and 0 (strong acid). *Bases* are agents with a pH between 7 and 14. Acids damage tissue by a process called *coagulative necrosis;* this tissue transforms into a barrier that prevents deeper penetration of the acid. In contrast, alkali burns destroy the tissue by *liquefaction necrosis;* the base liquefies the tissue, which allows the tissue to penetrate more deeply and cause increasingly deeper damage.

The prehospital care provider may need to treat injuries to the eye caused by exposure to alkali. A small exposure to the eye can result in a vision-threatening injury. The eyes should be irrigated with large amounts of irrigation fluid. If possible, ocular decontamination with continuous irrigation using a Morgan lens is performed. Application of an ophthalmic local anesthetic such as proparacaine will simplify the patient's care for the provider (Figure 13-18).

Treatment

The greatest priority in the care of a chemically exposed patient, as in any emergency, is personal and scene safety. Always protect yourself first. If there is any question of a chemical hazard, ensure scene safety and determine if any special garment or breathing apparatus is required. Avoid contamination of equipment and emergency vehicles; a contaminated vehicle creates a risk of exposure to other, unsuspecting individuals wherever that vehicle travels. Attempt to obtain identification of the offending agent as soon as possible.

Remove all of the patient's clothing. Clothing will be contaminated with either liquid or powder chemical. The contaminated clothing needs to be discarded with care. If any particulate substance is on the skin, it should be brushed away. Next, lavage the patient with copious amounts of water. Lavage will dilute the concentration of the injurious

FIGURE 13-18 Eyes that have sustained a chemical injury require prompt irrigation with copious amounts of saline. A Morgan lens can be placed on the eye to provide appropriate ocular irrigation.

agent and wash away any unreacted reagent. The key to lavage is to use large amounts of water. A common practice is to rinse 1 or 2 L of water across the patient, then stop the lavage process once the water starts to pool and accumulate on the floor. When lavaged with only small amounts of fluid, the offending agent is only spread across the patient's surface area and not flushed away.[36,37] Failure to provide adequate runoff and drainage of lavage fluid may cause injury to previously unexposed and uninjured areas

of the body as the contaminated lavage accumulates. One simple way of promoting runoff in a prehospital setting is to place the patient on a long backboard and then tilt it with cribbing or other means to elevate an end. At the lower end of the board, tuck a large plastic garbage bag to contain the contaminated runoff.

Neutralizing agents for chemical burns are typically avoided. Often in the neutralizing process the agents give off heat in an exothermic reaction. Therefore a well-meaning provider may create a thermal burn in addition to the chemical burn. Most commercially available decontamination solutions are made for the purpose of decontaminating equipment, not people.

Specific Chemical Exposures

Cement is an alkali that may be retained on the clothing of individuals. The powdered cement will react with the victim's sweat in a reaction that gives off heat and excessively dries, or *desiccates,* the skin. These injuries typically present with a burn injury hours or the day after contact with the cement.

Fuels such as gasoline and kerosene can cause contact burns after prolonged exposure. These organic hydrocarbons can dissolve cell membranes, resulting in skin necrosis.[38] An exposure of sufficient duration or severity also may result in systemic toxicity. Decontamination of the patient covered with fuel is accomplished by irrigation with large volumes of water.

Hydrofluoric acid is a dangerous substance widely used in domestic, industrial, and military settings. The real danger of this chemical is the fluoride ion, which produces profound alterations in the exposed electrolytes, especially calcium and magnesium.[39] Left untreated, hydrofluoric acid will liquefy tissues and leach the calcium from bones. Initial treatment for hydrofluoric acid exposure is irrigation with water, followed by application of calcium gluconate gel at an emergency center. Patients with hydrofluoric acid burns should be promptly transferred to a burn center for additional treatment.

Injuries from phosphorus are often seen in military settings. *White phosphorus* (WP) is a powerful incendiary agent used in the production of munitions. WP burns violently when exposed to air, producing brilliant flames. WP will continue to burn until all agent has burned or is deprived of oxygen. The initial treatment is to deprive the WP of access to oxygen. All the clothing needs to be rapidly removed because it may contain some retained phosphorus particles that could ignite the clothing. Affected areas are immersed in water or saline-soaked dressings, and the dressings are remoistened during transport. If the dressings dry out, any retained WP will reignite and could ignite the dressings and continue to burn the patient.

Hypochlorite solutions are often used to produce household bleaches and industrial cleaners. These solutions are strong alkalies; commonly available solutions are 4% to 6%

and are not usually lethal unless large areas of the body are involved. In greater concentrations, however, small volumes are potentially lethal. About 30 mL of a 15% solution is considered a life-threatening exposure.

Sulfur and nitrogen mustards are compounds that are classified as *vesicants.* These agents have been used as chemical weapons and are recognized as a threat in chemical terrorism. These chemicals will burn and blister skin on exposure. These agents not only are irritants to the skin but also cause irritation to the lungs and the eyes. After exposure, patients will complain of a burning sensation of the throat and eyes. The skin involvement develops several hours later as redness is followed by blistering in the axillae and groins. After intense exposure, the victims will develop full-thickness necrosis and respiratory failure.[40-42] The principal treatment required from the prehospital care provider is decontamination.

In caring for victims of vesicant exposure, providers must wear appropriate gloves, garments, and breathing equipment. The patients must be decontaminated and irrigated with water or saline. Other agents used to decontaminate victims, used by specially trained personnel, include dilute hypochlorite solution and Fuller's earth powder. Additional specialized treatment is required when the patient arrives at a specialty center.

Tear gas and similar chemicals are known as "riot control agents." These agents will rapidly and briefly disable those exposed by causing irritation to the skin, lungs, and eyes. The extent of the injury is determined by the magnitude of exposure to the agent. The duration of the irritation typically lasts 30 to 60 minutes. Treatment consists of removing those exposed from the source of the exposure, removing contaminated clothing, and irrigating the skin and eyes.

Control of Contamination

Exposure to chemical contaminants poses a significant hazard to responders and care providers. As discussed in Chapter 4, the Environmental Protection Agency (EPA) and National Institute of Occupational Safety and Health (NIOSH) have developed and advocated the use of control zones with the specific goal of minimizing the risk of spreading contamination and exposing responders to dangerous chemical or radiologic agents. No one enters the hot zone without appropriate personal protective equipment (PPE). Contaminated patients should be decontaminated as they transition from the hot zone through the warm zone. In the cold zone, the outermost circle of the control zones, treatment can be provided by responders without the need for PPE.

The same considerations are applicable to care provided in the hospital. A patient who has been exposed to chemical or radiologic material but has not yet been decontaminated can be considered to be a mobile "hot zone." If such a

patient presents to a hospital or aid station with symptoms and complaints related to possible contamination, and the individual has not already been decontaminated, the receiving staff must perform decontamination using PPE appropriate to the situation before the patient is allowed to enter the treatment facility. It should never be assumed that a patient with exposure to chemical or radiologic material has been adequately decontaminated without confirming that appropriate measures were taken. The delivery of a contaminated patient to an emergency department results in disastrous consequences. Everyone in that area, including other patients and healthcare workers, will need to be decontaminated, causing a significant disruption in care. Unless exceptional circumstances exist, patients should be decontaminated prior to transport.

Prolonged Transport

The prolonged transport of burn victims presents numerous challenges for prehospital care providers. Of greatest concern is ongoing monitoring for the development of symptoms of airway burns. Virtually any patient with thermal injury, and especially those with burns to their head and neck or a history of being trapped in an enclosed space, is at risk for suffering burns to the airway and inhalation injury. Prior to initiating a prolonged transport, those at greatest risk for airway burns and those with impending ventilatory failure should be considered for preemptive endotracheal intubation. If rapid sequence intubation is performed, succinylcholine is generally regarded as relatively contraindicated in burn patients. Succinylcholine can be used in patients without muscle destruction and resultant hyperkalemia, but often this may be difficult for the prehospital care provider to determine.

In the absence of a method to detect carbon monoxide toxicity, patients should be maintained on 100% oxygen until a carbon monoxide level can be measured. Once an elevated carboxyhemoglobin level has been ruled out, burn patients should receive supplemental oxygen to maintain $Spo_2 \geq 95\%$, and ventilations should be assisted as needed. The patency status of the airway is a potentially constantly changing problem after a burn injury. Following thermal injury, the mucosa of the upper airway will swell both with time and fluid resuscitation. Therefore, an airway that is widely patent can develop obstruction during the transport. The key to successful management is early, aggressive care based on clinical suspicion.

Patients with chemical burns and exposure to hazardous materials should undergo decontamination prior to transportation. Failure to provide adequate decontamination will result in ongoing injury as well as potential injury to the provider. Fumes emanating from a poorly decontaminated patient can contaminate the patient compartment of an ambulance that poses a risk of toxicity to the prehospital care providers and creates potential for a crash. Those patients believed to be suffering from cyanide poisoning should be considered for therapy with a commercially available cyanide kit, if permitted by medical control. All burn injuries should be covered with dry, sterile dressings. Burned patients lose their ability to regulate their body temperature (thermoregulation), so assure that the patient is kept warm.

Patients with burn injury may have concomitant injuries, and a thorough assessment is performed looking for additional injuries. These problems are prioritized and managed as time permits. Ongoing assessment includes circulatory assessments on all injured limbs, especially those with circumferential burns. If authorized by medical control and trained personnel is present, escharotomies may be considered if ventilatory compromise or limb compromise is noted. In hospitals, bleeding from escharotomies is controlled with electrocautery; this is clearly not an option in the prehospital environment. The risk of

bleeding needs to be considered in the risk-benefit ratio of performing the procedure. Escharotomies of the chest wall impairing ventilations clearly have a higher priority than circumferential extremity burns that may wait several hours prior to being released. Patients with suspected spinal injury should be immobilized to a padded long backboard.

Appropriate fluid resuscitation is essential for the management of patients with significant thermal injury. Volume requirements should be calculated and intravenous replacement initiated. Calculated volumes serve as only a guide to replacement, and these rates should be adjusted based on vital signs and urinary output. As such, placement of a urinary catheter is invaluable. A target urine output is 0.5 to 1.0 mL/kg. Red-pigmented urine often indicates the release of myoglobin from burned skeletal muscle. In the event of pigmented urine, a urine output of greater than 100 mL/hr should be the target. Pain management should be provided to burn victims, and small doses of narcotics should be titrated intravenously. Vital signs and ventilatory effort are monitored for potential adverse effects.

SUMMARY

All burns are serious, regardless of their size. Some burns are larger than others, but there are no minor burns. Potentially life-threatening burns include large thermal burns, electrical injuries, and chemical burns. Unlike in mechanical trauma (e.g., penetrating, blunt), the body has few to no adaptive mechanisms to survive a burn injury. Burn injuries are not isolated to the skin; these are systemic injuries of unparalleled magnitude. Patients with major burn injury will experience dysfunction of the cardiovascular, pulmonary, GI, renal, and immune systems. In contrast to the body's response after blunt or penetrating trauma, the patient with a life-threatening burn often experiences a hypodynamic state of shock, and most of the body's systems attempt to shut down. In this initial period, aggressive and appropriate resuscitation is required. Failure to provide appropriate fluid resuscitation will lead to refractory shock, multiorgan dysfunction, and even deepening of the burns. The role of the prehospital care provider is therefore crucial in optimizing survival after a burn injury. Early and appropriate prehospital care often determines the patient's resuscitation for the following days to weeks.

Although complicated and dangerous, burns are rarely rapidly fatal. A patient with severe smoke inhalation and large thermal burns may take several hours to die. Burn patients also are likely to have other mechanical trauma. Dramatic burns may focus the prehospital provider's attention away from other, potentially life-threatening injuries. Performing primary and secondary assessments will reduce

the likelihood of missing these injuries (e.g., pneumothorax, pericardial tamponade, splenic rupture).

Another important factor in caring for burn patients is constant vigilance to avoid becoming a victim oneself. In prehospital care of a burn patient (thermal, smoke, electrical, or chemical), often the injuring agent still poses a risk for injuring the providers (e.g., four large breaths of smoke from a structure fire can produce a potentially life-threatening case of smoke inhalation injury).

Even small burns in areas of high function (hands, face, joints, perineum) may result in long-term impairment from scar formation. To maximize the patient's outcome, this potential needs to be recognized. Burn centers are not solely for patients with large, life-threatening injuries. Familiarity with burn center transport criteria will help ensure that all patients can achieve maximal function recovery after burn injury.

The leading cause of death in burn patients is complications from smoke inhalation: asphyxiation, thermal injury, and delayed toxic-induced lung injury. Frequently, patients do not develop symptoms of respiratory failure for 48 hours or longer. Even without burns to the skin, victims of smoke inhalation should be transported to burn centers.

Hazardous material (hazmat) threats exist in all communities, both urban and rural. Familiarity with responding to, extrication of, and decontamination of victims from such hazmat scenes is mandatory in our modern chemical world. Also, techniques required for hazmat treatment are used in responding to a potential weapon of mass destruction.

SCENARIO SOLUTION

Victim 1:

This patient has labored respiration and a pulse oximeter reading of 92%. With the clothes burned away and the large burn areas, consider that this patient has inhaled a large dose of smoke. Maintain a high index of suspicion for airway edema and an inhalation injury. Airway patency needs to be a concern; however, the patient currently is managing his own airway. Keeping in mind that often the best person to manage an airway is the patient, balance the time required to transport the patient with the difficulties of airway management in a patient with an edematous airway. If transport will be prolonged or delayed, secure the airway by tracheal intubation. The patient clearly needs 100% oxygen given the exposure to smoke and concerns about asphyxiants. If this patient is intubated be careful to secure the endotracheal tube. Anchor the tube with two pieces of umbilical tape or IV tubing placed above and below the ears.

The patient is burned on the face, both upper extremities, and the anterior trunk. Each limb is approximately 9% of total body surface area (TBSA), the anterior trunk 9%, and the face approximately 4%. Therefore the estimated burn surface area is approximately 31%. The patient weighs approximately 80 kg. Estimate the patient's fluid needs using the Parkland formula, as follows:

31% TBSA burn × 80 kg × 4 mL/kg/TBSA burn =
9920 mL to be administered in first 24 hours

Half this fluid total is administered in the first 8 hours after injury. Therefore the hourly rate for the first 8 hours is:

9920 mL/2 = 4960 mL to be administered in first 8 hours

Calculate the hourly fluid rate:

4960 mL/8 = 620 mL per hour for hours 0 to 8

Victim 2:

This child may have an inhalation injury. Given her altered mental status, immediately place the child on oxygen and work toward intubation. Burns of one entire arm and small areas of the other arm translate to a burn size of approximately 10%. With a burn of this size, the child requires attention at a burn center but does not require placement on a resuscitation protocol.

Victim 3:

This child likely went to hide from the fire in a closet or under a bed. She is in cardiac arrest from hypoxia and toxic asphyxiation from carbon monoxide and perhaps hydrogen cyanide. The likelihood of successful resuscitation is negligible. ∎

References

1. Tredget EE, Shankowsky HA, Taerum TV, et al: The role of inhalation injury in burn trauma: a Canadian experience, *Ann Surg* 212:720, 1990.

2a. Herndon D, Rutan R, Rutan T: Management of the pediatric patient with burns, *J Burn Care Rehabil* 14(1):3, 1993.

2b. Rossignal A, Locke J, Burke J: Pediatric burn injuries in New England, USA, *Burns* 16(1):41, 1990.

3. Robinson MC, Del Becarro EJ: Increasing dermal perfusion after burning by decreasing thromboxane production, *J Trauma* 20:722, 1980.

4. Heggers JP, Ko F, Robson MC, et al: Evaluation of burn blister fluid, *Plast Reconstr Surg* 65:798, 1980.

5. Lentz CW, Younan DS, Reid DJ: Burn resuscitation index: a tool for initiating fluid resuscitation, *J Burn Care Rehabil* 25:S49, 2004.

6. Navar PD, Saffle JR, Warden GD: Effect of inhalation injury on fluid resuscitation requirements after thermal injury, *Am J Surg* 150:716, 1985.

7. Dunn K, Edwards-Jones VT: The role of Acticoat with nanocrystalline silver in the management of burns, *Burns* 30(suppl):S1, 2004.

8. Wright JB, Lam K, Burrell RE: Wound management in an era of increasing bacterial antibiotic resistance: a role for topical silver treatments, *Am J Infect Control* 26:572, 1998.

9. Yin HQ, Langford R, Burrell RE: Comparative evaluation of the antimicrobial activity of Acticoat antimicrobial dressing, *J Burn Care Rehabil* 20:195, 1999.

10. Moritz AR, Henriques FC, McClean R: The effects of inhaled heat on the air passages and lungs, *Am J Pathol* 21:311, 1945.

11. Peters WJ: Inhalation injury caused by the products of combustion, *Can Med Assoc J* 125:249, 1981.

12. Forbes WH, Sargent F, Roughton FJW: The rate of carbon monoxide uptake by normal men, *Am J Physiol* 143:594, 1945.

13. Mellins RB, Park S: Respiratory complications of smoke inhalation in victims of fires, *J Pediatr* 87:1, 1975.

14. Feldstein M, Klendshoj NJ: The determination of cyanide in biological fluids by microdiffusion analysis, *J Lab Clin Med* 44:166, 1954.

15. Norris JC, Moore SJ, Hume AS: Synergistic lethality induced by the combination of carbon monoxide and cyanide, *Toxicology* 40:121, 1986.

16. Vogel SN, Sultan TR: Cyanide poisoning, *Clin Toxicol* 18:367, 1981.

17. Chen KK, Rose CL, Clowes GH: Comparative values of several antidotes in cyanide poisoning, *Am J Med Sci* 188:767, 1934.

18. Langford RM, Armstrong RF: Algorithm for managing injury from smoke inhalation, *BMJ* 299:902, 1989.

19. Houeto P, Borron SW, Sandouk P, et al: Pharmacokinetics of hydroxocobalamin in smoke inhalation victims, *J Toxicol Clin Toxicol* 34:397, 1996.

20. Sauer SW, Keim ME: Hydroxocobalamin: improved public health readiness for cyanide disasters, *Ann Emerg Med* 37:635, 2001.

21. Crapo R: Smoke inhalation injuries, *JAMA* 246:1694, 1981.

22. Herndon DN, Traber DL, Niehaus GD, et al: The pathophysiology of smoke inhalation in a sheep model, *J Trauma* 24:1044, 1984.

23. Till GO, Johnson KJ, Kunkel R, et al: Intravascular activation of complement and acute lung injury, *J Clin Invest* 69:1126, 1982.

24. Thommasen HV, Martin BA, Wiggs BR, et al: Effect of pulmonary blood flow on leukocyte uptake and release by dog lung, *J Appl Physiol Respir Environ Exerc Physiol* 56:966, 1984.

25. Trunkey DD: Inhalation injury, *Surg Clin North Am* 58:1133, 1978.

26. Haponik E, Summer W: Respiratory complications in the burned patient: diagnosis and management of inhalation injury, *J Crit Care* 2:121, 1987.

27. Cahalane M, Demling R: Early respiratory abnormalities from smoke inhalation, *JAMA* 251:771, 1984.

28. Hight DW, Bakalar HR, Lloyd JR: Inflicted burns in children: recognition and treatment, *JAMA* 242:517, 1979.

29. Chadwick DL: The diagnosis of inflicted injury in infants and young children, *Pediatr Ann* 21:477, 1992.

30. Adronicus M, Oates RK, Peat J, et al: Non-accidental burns in children, *Burns* 24:552, 1998.

31. Purdue GF, Hunt JL, Prescott PR: Child abuse by burning: an index of suspicion, *J Trauma* 28:221, 1988.

32. Lenoski EF, Hunter KA: Specific patterns of inflicted burn injuries, *J Trauma* 17:842, 1977.

33. Brooks JW, Evans EI, Ham WT, Reid JD: The influence of external body radiation on mortality from thermal burns, *Ann Surg* 136:533, 1953.

34. Association AB: Radiation injury. In *Advanced burn life support course,* 1999, American Burn Association.

35. Michell MW, Oliveira HM, Vaid SU, et al: Enteral resuscitation of burn shock using intestinal infusion of World Health Organization oral rehydration solution (WHO ORS): a potential treatment for mass casualty care, *J Burn Care Rehabil* 25:S48, 2004.

36. Bromberg BF, Song IC, Walden RH: Hydrotherapy of chemical burns, *Plast Reconstr Surg* 35:85, 1965.

37. Leonard LG, Scheulen JJ, Munster AM: Chemical burns: effect of prompt first aid, *J Trauma* 22:420, 1982.

38. Mozingo DW, Smith AD, McManus WF, et al: Chemical burns, *J Trauma* 28:642, 1998.

39. Mistry D, Wainwright D: Hydrofluoric acid burns, *Am Fam Physician* 45:1748, 1992.

40. Willems JL: Clinical management of mustard gas casualties, *Ann Med Milit Belg* 3S:1, 1989.

41. Papirmeister B, Feister AJ, Robinson SI, et al: The sulfur mustard injury: description of lesions and resulting incapacitation. In *Medical defense against mustard gas,* Boca Raton, Fla, 1990, CRC.

42. Sidell FR, Takafuji ET, Franz DR: *Medical aspects of chemical and biological warfare,* Washington, DC, 1997, Office of the Surgeon General.

Chapter Objectives

*At the completion of this chapter, the reader
will be able to do the following:*

✓ Identify the unique differences in injury patterns for children.

✓ Demonstrate an understanding of the special importance of
managing the airway and restoring adequate tissue oxygenation in
pediatric patients.

✓ Identify the quantitative vital signs for children.

✓ Demonstrate an understanding of management techniques for the
various injuries found in pediatric patients.

✓ Calculate the Pediatric Trauma Score.

✓ Identify the signs of pediatric trauma suggestive of child
maltreatment.

CHAPTER 14

Pediatric Trauma

SCENARIO

You are called to the scene of a motor vehicle crash involving a pedestrian. A child has been struck by a sport utility vehicle (SUV) after running into a busy intersection chasing after a ball. You know that the posted speed limit in this area is 45 miles per hour (72 km/hr). No weather-related factors are involved on this average spring afternoon.

On arrival at the scene, you see that the police have secured and blocked traffic from the area around the child. As you approach the patient, you see a young boy, approximately 6 years of age, lying on his back with his left leg angulated in a dramatic outward position. You also note that despite numerous abrasions about the face and neck, the child appears very calm.

Your primary and secondary surveys reveal a 6-year-old boy who can tell you only that his name is Scott. He has central and distal pulses at a rate of 130 beats/min, with the radial pulse weaker than the carotid; his blood pressure is 75 mm Hg by palpation; and his ventilatory rate is 16 breaths/min, slightly irregular, but without abnormal sounds. As you talk with Scott, you also note that, despite having an obvious angulated left femur, he is not complaining of significant pain, and he appears to be resting comfortably. As you continue to talk with him, you note that he has an altered awareness of his surroundings and what happened to him. You also note that his pupils are slightly dilated, and his skin is pale and sweaty. A woman who identifies herself as a friend of the family tells you that Scott's mother is en route and that you should wait for her. ■

What are the management priorities for this patient? What are the most likely injuries in this child? Where is the most appropriate destination for this child?

Injury is the most common cause of death of American children. More than 20,000 children die annually as a result of injuries, and more than 120,000 are permanently disabled. Tragically, as many as 80% of these deaths may be preventable, either by protective strategies that prevent the injury or by ensuring proper care.[1] As with all aspects of pediatric care, proper assessment and management of an injured child requires a thorough understanding of not only the unique characteristics of childhood growth and development, especially their immature anatomy and developing physiology, but also their unique mechanisms of injury.

Thus, good pediatric care is much more than a simple application of adult principles to a smaller person. Children have common and distinct patterns of injury, different physiologic responses, and special treatment needs, based on their physical and psychosocial development.

This chapter first describes the special characteristics of the pediatric trauma patient, then reviews optimal trauma management and its rationale. Although the unique characteristics of pediatric injury are important for the prehospital care provider to understand, the fundamental basic and advanced life support treatment approach using the primary and secondary surveys are the same for every patient, regardless of age or size.

The Child as Trauma Patient

Demographics of Pediatric Trauma

Many unique characteristics should be addressed when considering the child as a trauma patient. The incidence of blunt (vs. penetrating) trauma is highest in the pediatric population. As did its predecessor, the National Pediatric Trauma Registry (NPTR), the National Trauma Data Bank (NTDB) of the American College of Surgeons (ACS) continues to identify blunt trauma as the most common mechanism of injury, with penetrating injury accounting for only 10% of cases. The consequences of penetrating trauma are relatively predictable, but blunt trauma mechanisms have a greater potential for multisystem injury.

Falls are the most common cause of pediatric injury and occur most frequently in children younger than 10 years of age. Trauma to pedestrians struck by vehicles is the next most common mechanism and usually occurs in the 6- to 10-year-old child. In children over 12 years of age, the most common mechanism of injury is as passenger or driver of a motor vehicle. According to statistics, injury is "unintentional" in 87% of cases, sports related in 4%, and the result of assault in 5%. Multisystem involvement is the rule rather than the exception in major pediatric trauma. Therefore, prehospital care providers need to assume that all organ systems are injured until proved otherwise. Although minimal external evidence of injury may be present, the presence of potentially significant internal derangement of every major organ should be assumed until ruled out by definitive assessment or careful follow-up evaluation.

Kinematics of Pediatric Trauma

A child's size produces a smaller target to which linear forces from fenders, bumpers, and falls are applied. Because of minimal cushioning body fat, increased elasticity of connective tissue, and proximity of multiple organs to the surface of the body, these forces are not dissipated as well as in the adult and therefore disperse more energy to multiple organs. Because the skeleton of a child is incompletely calcified and contains multiple active growth centers, it is more resilient than that of an adult. However, the skeleton of a child is less able than that of an adult to absorb the kinetic forces applied during a traumatic event and may allow significant force to be transmitted to underlying organs, resulting in major internal derangement despite minor external injury. For example, although rib fractures are uncommon, pulmonary contusion is common.

Common Patterns of Injury

The unique anatomic and physiologic characteristics of the pediatric patient combine with the different mechanisms of injury to produce distinct patterns of injury (Table 14-1). Being familiar with these patterns will assist the initial responder in determining optimum management for the

injured child. For example, most blunt pediatric trauma involves closed head injury, and as a result, apnea, hypoventilation, and hypoxia are much more common than hypovolemia and hypotension. Therefore, pediatric trauma management protocols include greater emphasis on aggressive management of the airway and breathing (Box 14-1).

Thermal Homeostasis

The ratio between a child's body surface area (BSA) and body mass is highest at birth and diminishes throughout infancy and childhood. This means that relatively more surface area exists through which heat can be lost quickly. As a result, thermal energy loss becomes a significant risk factor in a smaller child. Although this may not be life threatening by itself, it frequently provides additional stress to the child, who may be hypotensive and in severe pain. Severe hypothermia results in severe coagulopathy and potentially irreversible cardiovascular collapse. In addition, many of the clinical signs of hypothermia are the same as those of impending shock, thereby potentially complicating the clinical assessment.

Psychosocial Issues

The psychological ramifications of caring for an injured child can also present a major challenge. Particularly with a very young child, regressive psychological behavior may result when stress, pain, or other perceived threats intervene in a child's environment. A child's ability to interact with unfamiliar individuals in strange surroundings is usually limited and makes history taking and cooperative manipulation extremely difficult. An understanding of these characteristics and a willingness to cajole and soothe

TABLE 14-1   Common Patterns of Injury Associated with Pediatric Trauma

Type of trauma	Patterns of injury
Motor vehicle crash (child is passenger)	*Unrestrained:* Multiple trauma, head and neck injuries, scalp and facial lacerations *Restrained:* Chest and abdomen injuries, lower spine fractures *Side impact:* Head, neck, and chest injuries; extremity fracture *Deployed air bag:* Head, face, chest injuries; upper extremity fractures
Motor vehicle crash (child is pedestrian)	*Low speed:* Lower extremity fractures *High speed:* Multiple trauma, head and neck injuries, lower extremity fractures
Fall from a height	*Low:* Upper extremity fractures *Medium:* Head and neck injuries, upper and lower extremity fractures *High:* Multiple trauma, head and neck injuries, upper and lower extremity fractures
Fall from bicycle	*Without helmet:* Head and neck lacerations, scalp and facial lacerations, upper extremity fractures *With helmet:* Upper extremity fractures *Striking handlebar:* Internal abdominal injuries

Modified from American College of Surgeons Committee on Trauma: Extremes of age: pediatric trauma. In *Advanced trauma life support for doctors, student course manual*, ed 7, Chicago, 2004, ACS.

BOX 14-1   Pediatric Injuries Associated with Seat Belts and Air Bags

Despite laws in all 50 states requiring the use of car safety seats or child restraint devices for young children, in almost half of motor vehicle crashes (MVCs) the child is not restrained or is improperly restrained.[3] If a child is the front-seat occupant in a vehicle with a passenger-side air bag, the child is just as likely to sustain serious injury whether appropriately restrained or not.[4] A child exposed to a passenger-side air bag is twice as likely to sustain significant injury as a front-seat passenger without an air bag.[5]

The American Academy of Pediatrics has defined *optimal restraint* for children in motor vehicles. Children should always ride in the rear seat. Children should be in child safety seats until 4 years of age (rear facing, up to 1 year), then graduate into a belt-positioning booster seat until they are 8 to 10 years old. At that time the standard three-point (never lap belt alone) adult restraint can be used. *Suboptimal restraint* is defined as the use of a seat belt alone in anyone under age 8 years, and use of a lap belt over age 8 years.[6] In a recent review, when these guidelines were observed, the risk of abdominal injury was 3.5 times less than in the suboptimally restrained pediatric population.[7] The protective benefit of the rear-seat position is such that risk of death is decreased by at least 30% even if restrained with a lap belt only in the rear seat versus three-point restraint in the front seat.[8]

Children with lap belt or inappropriate seat belt placement are thought to be at increased risk for bowel injury in MVCs. The incidence is difficult to determine. In one study, 20% of injured children had a visible seat belt bruise, and 50% of those had significant intraabdominal injuries; almost 25% of those had intestinal perforation.[9] Others have shown an increased risk, but not to this extent, with only 5% of injured children having an abdominal wall bruise from the seat belt, and only 13% of those with bruising having intestinal injury.[10] It is reasonable to assume that any child found restrained by a lap belt with abdominal wall bruising has an intraabdominal injury until proved otherwise.

Approximately 1% of all MVCs involving children also involved exposure of the children to a deployed passenger air bag. Of these children, 14% suffered serious injury, compared with 7.5% of restrained front-seat passengers not exposed. Overall risk of any injury was 86% versus 55% in the controls.[5] Minor air bag injury included minor upper torso and facial burns and lacerations. Major air bag injury consisted of significant chest, neck, face, and upper extremity injury.[11] There has been documented decapitation of a child injured by a passenger air bag.[4]

an injured child are frequently the most effective means of achieving good rapport and obtaining a more comprehensive assessment of the child's physiologic state.

The child's caregivers or parents also frequently have needs and issues that must be addressed to allow the prehospital care provider to care for the child successfully. Whenever a child is sick or injured, the caregivers are also affected and should be considered your patients as well. Treatment of these "parent-patients" consists of compassion, patience, and good communication skills. It is important to meet the needs of the caregivers so that they can act as functional members of their child's emergency care team.

Recovery and Rehabilitation

Another problem unique to the pediatric trauma patient is the effect that injury may have on subsequent growth and development. Unlike an anatomically mature adult, a child must not only recover from the injury but also continue the normal growing process. The effect of injury on this process—especially in terms of long-term disability, growth deformity, or abnormal subsequent development—cannot be overestimated. Children sustaining even minor injury may have prolonged disability in cerebral function, psychological adjustment, or an organ system. As many as 60% of children with severe multiple trauma have personality changes, and 50% are left with subtle cognitive or physical handicaps. In addition, pediatric trauma can substantially affect siblings and parents, resulting in a high incidence of family dysfunction, including divorce. The cost of correcting these problems can be staggering and lifelong.

The effect of inadequate or inappropriate care in the immediate posttraumatic period may have consequences not only on the child's survival but also, perhaps more importantly, on the quality of the child's life for many years. Major organ injury may exist with minimal external signs. A high index of suspicion and clinical common sense should prompt transport of the child to an appropriate facility for a more thorough evaluation when any possibility of severe injury exists.

Pathophysiology

The ultimate result of care for the injured child may be determined by the quality of care rendered in the first moments after injury. During these critical minutes, a systematized primary survey is the best defense against overlooking an injury that may be fatal or that may cause unnecessary morbidity. As in the adult, the three most common causes of immediate death in the child are hypoxia, massive hemorrhage, and overwhelming central nervous system (CNS) trauma. Lack of expedient triage and transport to the most appropriate center for treatment can compound these problems.

Hypoxia

The first priority in prehospital care is always the establishment of a patent airway. Confirming that a child has an open and functioning airway does not preclude the need for supplemental oxygen and assisted ventilation, especially when CNS injury, hypoventilation, or hypoperfusion is present. Injured children can rapidly deteriorate from labored breathing and tachypnea to a state of total exhaustion and apnea. Once an airway is established, the rate and depth of ventilation should be evaluated to confirm adequate alveolar ventilation. If alveolar ventilation is not adequate, merely providing an excessive concentration of oxygen will not prevent ongoing cellular hypoxia.

Adequate cerebral oxygenation is especially critical to the initial care of the patient with traumatic brain injury (TBI). A child may have significant alteration in level of consciousness (LOC) but have an excellent potential for good functional recovery if cerebral hypoxia is avoided. Patients who require advanced airway management should be preoxygenated before intubation. This basic maneuver may be sufficient to begin reversal of hypoxia and improve the margin of safety when intubation is performed. A prolonged period of hypoxia during multiple intubation attempts may be more detrimental to the child than immediate bag-valve-mask ventilation and transport.[12,14,15]

Hemorrhage

Most pediatric injuries do not cause immediate exsanguination. Unfortunately, children who sustain injuries with major blood loss die within moments or are dead on arrival at the receiving facility. Many injured children who require emergency care have multiple organ injuries with at least one injury associated with blood loss. This hemorrhage maybe minor (e.g., laceration, contusion) or potentially life threatening (e.g., ruptured spleen, lacerated liver, avulsed kidney).

As in adults, the injured child compensates for hemorrhage by increasing systemic vascular resistance (SVR) at the expense of peripheral perfusion. In fact, children can do this much better than adults, who often have peripheral vascular disease that limits vasoconstriction. Blood pressure alone is an inadequate sign of shock. Ineffective organ perfusion is a more appropriate indicator of shock and is evidenced by a decreased LOC, diminished skin perfusion (decreased temperature, poor color, delayed capillary refill), and decreased urine output over time. Unlike the adult, the early signs of hemorrhage in the child may be subtle and difficult to identify, leading to a deceptive presentation of shock. Tachycardia may be caused by hypovolemia or

may be the result of fear or pain. Moreover, the normal heart rate of a child varies with age. Poor peripheral perfusion may result from hypotension, hypothermia, or both. If the prehospital care provider misses the subtle early signs, a child may lose so much circulating blood volume that compensatory mechanisms fail. In this case, cardiac output plummets, organ perfusion decreases, and the child plunges into decompensated and usually fatal shock. Therefore, every child who sustains blunt trauma should be carefully monitored to detect the subtle signs that might indicate early shock in addition to changes in vital signs.

A major reason for the rapid transition to decompensated shock is the loss of red blood cell (RBC) mass. Restoration of shed blood with crystalloid solutions will provide a transient increase in blood pressure, but circulating volume will dissipate as the fluid leaks across capillary membranes. It is generally considered that isotonic crystalloid solutions must be administered at three times the volume of whole-blood loss to compensate for the tendency of crystalloids to leak out of the blood vessels. As RBCs are lost through bleeding and intravascular volume is replaced with crystalloids, the remaining RBCs are diluted in the bloodstream, reducing the blood's ability to carry oxygen to the tissues. Therefore, it should be assumed that any child who requires more than one 20-mL/kg bolus of crystalloid solution may be rapidly deteriorating and needs not only intravascular volume but also RBCs so that oxygen delivery capacity is restored.

There is a tendency to overresuscitate an injured child who is not in obvious shock, once vascular access has been secured. In the child with moderate bleeding and normal vital signs, fluid resuscitation should be limited to no more than one or two boluses of 20 mL/kg. The intravascular component of one bolus represents approximately 25% of a child's blood volume. More than this in the absence of bleeding can artificially dilute the hematocrit (packed cell volume of RBCs in total blood volume).

Given the high incidence of TBI with associated blunt trauma and the relatively low incidence of severe hemorrhagic shock, it was once thought that aggressive fluid resuscitation of a child with a TBI might actually worsen evolving cerebral edema. Currently, no evidence supports withholding fluid from a child with TBI to reduce cerebral edema.[16] In fact, there is more evidence in the literature to support aggressive resuscitation to prevent hypotension, a known and preventable secondary insult to head injury.[17,18] Cerebral perfusion must be adequate to deliver oxygen effectively to the brain. If the blood is hyperoxygenated but does not reach the brain because of low blood pressure, hypoxic brain damage can still occur. Careful assessment of the child's vital signs and evaluation of the therapeutic intervention are the primary considerations immediately after the injury.

Isotonic crystalloid solutions should be used for resuscitation of the injured brain, because *hypotonic* crystalloid solutions (e.g., dextrose in water) are known to increase cerebral edema. Although *hypertonic* crystalloid solutions (e.g., hypertonic saline) may be useful for treatment of cerebral edema in the pediatric intensive care unit, no evidence yet shows that they improve the outcome of pediatric trauma patients when administered in the field.

Brain Injury

The pathophysiologic changes after CNS trauma begin within minutes. Early and adequate resuscitation is the key to increased survival of children with CNS trauma. Although a certain percentage of CNS injuries are overwhelmingly massive and fatal, many children present with recoverable CNS injuries that may be exacerbated by subsequent hypoperfusion, hypoventilation, hyperventilation, or ischemia. Adequate ventilation and oxygenation (while avoiding excessive hyperventilation) are as critical in the management of TBIs as the avoidance of hypotension.[18] Even densely comatose children may recover if they do not develop cerebral hypoxia.

For given degrees of injury severity, children have lower mortality and a higher potential for survival than their adult counterparts. However, the addition of injuries outside the brain lessens the child's chances of survival. This illustrates the potentially negative effect of associated injury and shock from CNS trauma on outcome.

Children with TBI frequently present with mild obtundation (sensory dullness), and they may have sustained a period of unconsciousness not recorded during the initial evaluation. A history of loss of consciousness is one of the most important prognostic indicators of potential CNS injury, and this is investigated and recorded for every case. Similarly, complete documentation of baseline neurologic status is important, including the following:

1. Glasgow Coma Scale score
2. Pupillary reaction
3. Response to sensory stimulation
4. Motor function

These are essential steps in initial pediatric trauma assessment. CNS injury is a pathophysiologic continuum that begins as an initial depolarization of the intracranial neurons and proceeds along a recognizable course of secondary edema and hypoperfusion. The absence of adequate baseline assessment makes ongoing follow-up and evaluation of intervention extremely imprecise and difficult.

Attention to detailed history taking is especially important in patients with possible cervical spine injury. A child's skeleton is incompletely calcified and has multiple active growth centers, so minimal if any radiographic evidence may exist of a mechanism causing a stretch or contusion of the spinal cord (spinal cord injury without radiographic abnormality, or SCIWORA). A transient neurologic deficit may be the only indicator of a potentially significant spinal cord injury.

Assessment

Primary (Initial) Survey

The small and variable size of the pediatric patient (Table 14-2), the diminished caliber and size of the blood vessels and circulating volume, and the unique anatomic characteristics of the airway frequently make the standard procedures used in basic life support extremely challenging and technically difficult. The immediate availability of appropriately sized equipment is essential for successful initial management of an injured child. Attempting to place an overly large intravenous cannula or an inappropriately sized endotracheal (ET) tube can do more harm than good because of not only potential physical damage to the patient but also prolongation of out-of-hospital time. For this reason, a color-coded, length-based resuscitation tape was devised that allows for rapid identification of a patient's height with a correlated estimation of weight, size of equipment to be used, and appropriate dosages of potential resuscitative drugs.[19] Effective pediatric trauma resuscitation

TABLE 14-2 Height and Weight Range for Pediatric Patients

| Group | Age | Range of mean norms | |
		Average height (cm)	Average weight (kg)
Newborn	Birth-6 wk	51-63	4-5
Infant	7 wk-1 yr	56-80	4-11
Toddler	1-2 yr	77-91	11-14
Preschool	2-6 yr	91-122	14-25
School age	6-13 yr	122-165	25-63
Adolescent	13-16 yr	165-182	62-80

mandates the availability of appropriately sized laryngoscope blades, ET tubes, nasogastric tubes, blood pressure cuffs, oxygen masks, bag-valve-mask resuscitators, and associated equipment.

Airway

As in the adult, the immediate priority and focus in the child is on airway management. The relatively large tongue and more anterior position of the airway predispose small children to more risk of airway obstruction than adults. The smaller the child, the greater is the disproportion between the size of the cranium and midface. The relatively large occiput forces passive flexion on the cervical spine, leading to compromise of the pharynx. In the absence of trauma, the pediatric patient's airway is best protected by a slightly superior-anterior position of the midface, known as the *sniffing position*. In the presence of trauma, however, the *neutral position* best protects the cervical spine while ensuring adequate airway opening. Thus, in the pediatric trauma patient, the neck should be kept immobilized to prevent the hyperflexion at the fifth and sixth cervical vertebrae (C5-C6) and the hyperextension at C1-C2 that occurs with the sniffing position. Placing a pad or blanket of 2 to 3 cm in thickness under the child's torso will lessen the acute flexion of the neck and help keep the airway patent (Figure 14-1). Manual stabilization of the cervical spine is done during airway management and maintained until the child is immobilized on a long backboard.

Bag-valve-mask (BVM) ventilation with 100% oxygen (fraction of inspired oxygen [Fio_2] of 1.0) probably represents the best choice when the injured child requires assisted ventilation, whether for respiratory distress, decompensated shock, or traumatic coma.[12] If the child is unconscious, an oropharyngeal airway (OPA) may be safely placed, but it is likely to cause vomiting in the child with an intact gag reflex. This is also true of the laryngeal mask airway

FIGURE 14-1 Compared to an adult, a child has a larger occiput and more shoulder musculature. When placed on a flat surface, these factors result in flexion of the neck.

(LMA), which is an acceptable alternative airway for use in pediatric trauma patients. Tracheal intubation is therefore reserved for children in whom BVM ventilation is ineffective or results in excessive gastric distention. However, the child's larynx is smaller than that of an adult, has a slightly more anterior and cephalad location (forward and toward the head), making it more difficult to visualize for direct cannulation (Figure 14-2). Despite these characteristics, the most reliable means of ventilation in the child with airway compromise for whom BVM ventilation is not effective is direct orotracheal intubation. Nasotracheal intubation should only be attempted as a last resort in the child because it requires blind passage around a relatively acute posterior nasopharyngeal angle and can cause severe bleeding or even inadvertent penetration of the cranial vault. A child

Large tongue
High glottis
Cricoid area narrow

FIGURE 14-2 Comparison of the adult and child airways.

with craniofacial injuries that cause upper airway obstruction should be considered for immediate percutaneous transtracheal ventilation with a large angiocatheter. This is only a temporary measure, and a more definitive airway should be established as soon as safely possible.

Breathing

As in all trauma patients, a significantly traumatized child typically needs an oxygen concentration of 85% to 100% (Fio_2 of 0.85-1.0). This is accomplished by use of supplemental oxygen and an appropriately sized, *clear plastic, pediatric* mask. When hypoxia occurs in the small child, the body compensates by increasing the ventilatory rate (tachypnea) and by a strenuous increase in ventilatory effort, including increased thoracic excursion efforts and the use of accessory muscles in the neck and abdomen. This increased effort can produce severe fatigue, resulting in ventilatory failure. Ventilatory distress can rapidly progress from a compensated ventilatory effort to ventilatory failure, then respiratory arrest, and ultimately cardiac arrest secondary to the respiratory problem.

Evaluation of the child's level of ventilation with early recognition of distress and the provision of ventilatory assistance are key elements in the management of the pediatric trauma patient. The normal ventilatory rate of infants and children younger than 4 years is two to three times that of adults (Table 14-3).

Tachypnea with signs of increased effort or difficulty may be the first manifestation of respiratory distress and shock. As distress increases, additional signs and symptoms include shallow breathing with minimal chest movement. Breath sounds may be weak or infrequent, and air exchange at the nose or mouth may be reduced or minimal. Ventilatory effort becomes more labored and may include the following:

- Head bobbing with each breath
- Gasping or grunting
- Flared nostrils

- Stridor or snoring
- Suprasternal, supraclavicular, subcostal, and intercostal retractions
- Use of accessory muscles of neck and abdominal wall muscles
- Distention of the abdomen when the chest falls (seesaw effect between the chest and abdomen)

The effectiveness of a child's ventilation should be evaluated using the following indicators:

- Rate and depth (minute volume) and effort indicate adequacy of ventilation
- Breath sounds confirm the depth of exchange
- Wheezing, rales, or rhonchi indicate inefficient alveolar oxygenation
- Pink skin indicates adequate ventilation
- Dusky, gray, cyanotic, or mottled skin indicates insufficient oxygenation and perfusion
- Anxiety, restlessness, and combativeness are possible early signs of hypoxia
- Lethargy, lowered LOC, and unconsciousness are probably advanced signs of hypoxia

A rapid evaluation of ventilation includes assessment of the patient's ventilatory rate (particularly tachypnea), ventilatory effort (degree of labor, nostril flaring, accessory muscle use, retraction, seesaw movement), auscultation (air exchange, bilateral symmetry, pathologic sounds), skin color, and mental status. Central (rather than peripheral) cyanosis is a fairly late and often inconsistent sign of respiratory failure.

In the child initially presenting with tachypnea and increased ventilatory effort, a decreasing ventilatory rate and apparent lessening in effort may indicate exhaustion and should not be misinterpreted as a sign of improvement. Ventilatory assistance should be given to children with diminished air exchange or those in acute ventilatory distress. Because the main problem is one of inspired volume rather than concentration of oxygen, assisted ventilation

TABLE 14-3   Ventilatory Rates for Pediatric Patients

Group	Age	Ventilatory rate (breaths/min)	Ventilatory rate (breaths/min) that indicates possible decrease in minute volume and need for ventilatory assistance with bag-valve-mask
Newborn	Birth-6 wk	30-50	<30 or >50
Infant	7 wk-1 yr	20-30	<20 or >30
Toddler	1-2 yr	20-30	<20 or >30
Preschool	2-6 yr	20-30	<20 or >30
School age	6-13 yr	(12-20)-30	<20 or >30
Adolescent	13-16 yr	12-20	<12 or >20

TABLE 14-4   Pulse Rate for Pediatric Patients

Group	Age	Pulse rate (beats/min)	Pulse rate (beats/min) that indicates a possible serious problem*
Newborn	Birth-6 wk	120-160	<100 or >160
Infant	7 wk-1 yr	80-140	<80 or >150
Toddler	1-2 yr	80-130	<60 or >140
Preschool	2-6 yr	80-120	<60 or >130
School age	6-13 yr	(60-80)-100	<60 or >120
Adolescent	13-16 yr	60-100	<60 or >100

*Bradycardia or tachycardia.

is best given by use of a BVM device, supplemented with an oxygen reservoir attached to high-concentration oxygen (Fio_2 of 0.85-1.0). Because a child's airway is so small, initial and periodic suctioning may be necessary. In infants, who are obligate nose breathers, the nostrils should also be suctioned.

When obtaining a mask seal in infants, caution should be exercised to avoid compressing the soft tissues underneath the chin because this pushes the tongue against the soft palate and risks occluding the airway. Pressure on the uncalcified soft trachea should also be avoided. One or two hands can be used to obtain a mask seal.

Use of the correct mask size is essential for obtaining a proper mask seal, providing the proper tidal volume, and ensuring that the risks of hyperinflation (resulting in gastric distention) and barotrauma (resulting in tension pneumothorax) are minimized. *Gastric distention* can result in regurgitation and aspiration and can prevent adequate ventilation by limiting diaphragmatic excursion. *Tension pneumothorax* can result in both severe respiratory distress and sudden cardiovascular collapse, because infants and children have a much more mobile mediastinum than adults. This protects the mediastinum from aortic injuries but increases the susceptibility to tension pneumothorax. The more mobile mediastinum shifts more easily, allowing for earlier respiratory compromise and cardiovascular collapse than in an adult.

Changes in a child's ventilatory status can be subtle, and ventilatory effort can rapidly deteriorate until ventilation is inadequate and hypoxia occurs. The patient's breathing should be evaluated as part of the primary survey and carefully rechecked periodically to ensure its continued adequacy. Pulse oximetry should be monitored, and efforts should be made to keep oxygen saturation (Spo_2) at greater than 95%.

Circulation

The survival rate from immediate exsanguinating injury is low in the pediatric population. Fortunately, the incidence

TABLE 14-5   Blood Pressure (BP) for Pediatric Patients

Group	Age	Expected BP range (mm Hg)*	Lower limit of systolic BP (mm Hg)
Newborn	Birth-6 wk	74-100 50-68	<60
Infant	7 wk-1 yr	84-106 56-70	<70
Toddler	1-2 yr	98-106 50-70	<70
Preschool	2-6 yr	98-112 64-70	<75
School age	6-13 yr	104-124 64-80	<80
Adolescent	13-16 yr	118-132 70-82	<90

*Top numbers represent systolic range; bottom numbers represent diastolic range.

of this type of injury is also low. External hemorrhage should be identified and controlled by direct manual pressure during the primary survey. Injured children usually present with at least some circulating blood volume and respond appropriately to volume replacement. As in the assessment of the airway, a single measurement of heart rate (HR) or blood pressure (BP) does not equate with physiologic stability. Serial measurements and changing trends of vital signs are critical in gauging a child's hemodynamic state. Close monitoring of vital signs is absolutely essential to preventing hypotension and shock. Tables 14-4 and 14-5 provide the normal ranges for pulse rate and BP, respectively, for different pediatric age groups.

If the primary survey suggests hypotension, the most likely cause is blood loss through a major external wound that is readily observable (large scalp laceration, open femur fracture), an intrathoracic wound (identifiable by diminished ventilatory mechanics and auscultatory findings), or a major intraabdominal injury. Because blood is not a compressible medium, blood loss from a major intraabdominal injury can produce abdominal distention and increasing abdominal girth. However, increased abdominal girth in the young pediatric trauma patient is more likely to be caused by gastric distention from crying and air swallowing. Gastric decompression through a nasogastric or orogastric tube can help to distinguish between these causes of distention, although it is best to assume that a distended abdomen is a sign of potentially significant abdominal injury.

A major consideration in the assessment of a pediatric patient is compensated shock. Because of their increased physiologic reserve, children with hemorrhagic injury frequently present with only slightly abnormal vital signs. Initial tachycardia may be not only the result of hypovolemia but also the effect of psychologic stress, pain, and fear. All injured children should have their HR, ventilatory rate, and overall CNS status monitored closely. An accurate BP reading may be difficult to obtain in the prehospital setting, and focus should be placed on other signs of perfusion. If measured, a small patient may have a systolic BP that, although considered alarmingly low for an adult, may be within the normal range for a healthy child.

A child with hemorrhagic injury can maintain adequate circulating volume by increasing peripheral vascular resistance (PVR) to maintain mean arterial pressure (MAP). Clinical evidence of this compensatory mechanism includes prolonged capillary refill, peripheral skin pallor or mottling, cool peripheral skin temperature, and decreased intensity of the peripheral pulses. In the child, signs of significant hypotension develop with the loss of approximately 30% of the circulating volume. If initial resuscitation is inadequate, circulating volume will eventually diminish to a point below which increased PVR cannot maintain arterial pressure. The concept of evolving shock must be of paramount concern in the initial management of an injured child and is a major indication for transport to an appropriate facility for expeditious evaluation and treatment.

Disability

After assessment of airway, breathing, and circulation, the primary survey must include an assessment of neurologic status. Although the *AVPU scale* (**a**lert, responds to **v**erbal stimulus, responds to **p**ainful stimulus, **u**nresponsive) remains a rapid screening tool for assessment of LOC, it should be combined with a careful examination of the pupils to determine whether they are equal, round, and reactive to light. As in adults, the Glasgow Coma Scale (GCS) provides a more thorough assessment of neurologic status and should be calculated for each pediatric trauma victim. The scoring for the verbal section for children under 4 years of age must be modified because of limited communication skills

TABLE 14-6 Pediatric Verbal Score

Verbal response	Verbal score
Appropriate words or social smile; fixes and follows	5
Crying but consolable	4
Persistently irritable	3
Restless, agitated	2
No response	1

in this age group, and the child's behavior should be observed carefully (Table 14-6).

The GCS score should be repeated frequently and used to document progression or improvement of neurologic status during the postinjury period (refer to Chapters 5 and 8 for a review of the GCS). A more thorough assessment of motor and sensory function should be performed in the secondary survey if time permits.

Expose/Environment

Children should be examined for other potentially life-threatening injuries; however, they may be frightened at attempts to remove their clothes. Because children are more prone to developing hypothermia, once the examination to identify other injuries is complete, the patient should be covered to preserve body heat.

Pediatric Trauma Score

The decision as to which child requires what level of care must proceed from a careful and rapid evaluation of the entire child. Overlooking potential organ system injury and inadequately managing the patient are two common problems. For this reason, the Pediatric Trauma Score (PTS) has been developed to provide a reliable and simple protocol for assessment that is predictive of outcome (Figure 14-3). Six components of pediatric injury are graded and then added together to produce a score predictive of injury severity and potential for mortality. The system is based on an analysis of pediatric injury patterns and is designed to provide a protocol checklist to ensure that all the major injury factors related to injury outcome are considered in the initial evaluation of the child. The PTS is different than the Revised Trauma Score (RTS), which only considers the BP, ventilatory rate, and GCS score.

Size is the first component because it is readily observed and is a major consideration in the infant/toddler group. The airway is assessed next, because the functional status and the type of care required to provide adequate ventilation and oxygenation must be considered.

The most important factor in initial assessment of the CNS is LOC. Because children frequently sustain transient

Component	+2	+1	−1
Size	Child/adolescent >20 kg	Toddler 11-20 kg	Infant <10 kg
Airway	Normal	Assisted: O₂ mask, cannula	Intubated: ETT, cricothyroidotomy
Consciousness	Awake	Obtunded, lost consciousness	Coma, unresponsive
Systolic blood pressure	90 mm Hg Good peripheral pulses, perfusion	51-90 mm Hg Carotid, femoral pulse palpable	<50 mm Hg Weak or no pulses
Fracture	None seen or suspected	Single closed fracture anywhere	Open or multiple fractures
Cutaneous	No visible injury	Contusion, abrasion, laceration <7 cm not through fascia	Tissue loss, any gun shot wound or stab through fascia

FIGURE 14-3 Pediatric Trauma Score (PTS) is primarily designed to function as a checklist. Each component can be assessed by basic physical examination. Airway evaluation is designed to reflect intervention required for effective care. An open fracture is graded −1 for fracture and −1 for cutaneous injury. As clinical observation and diagnostic evaluation continue, further definition and reassessment will establish a trend that predicts severity of injury and potential outcome.

loss of consciousness during an injury, the obtunded grade (+1) is applied to any child with loss of consciousness, no matter how fleeting. This grade identifies children at higher risk of developing potentially fatal yet frequently treatable intracranial injuries that may lead to brain injury.

Systolic blood pressure (SBP) is used to identify children in whom evolving preventable shock may occur (SBP 51-90 mm Hg; +1). Regardless of size, a child whose SBP is less than 50 mm Hg (−1) is in obvious jeopardy (Box 14-2). A child whose SBP exceeds 90 mm Hg (+2) falls into a better outcome category. If the appropriately sized BP cuff is not available, SBP is assessed as +2 if the radial or pedal pulse is palpable, +1 if only the carotid or femoral pulse is palpable, and −1 if no pulse is palpable.

Because of the high incidence of skeletal injury in the pediatric population and its potential contribution to mortality and disability, the presence of a long-bone fracture is included in the PTS as a component. Finally, the skin is assessed for open wounds and penetrating injury.

By nature of its design, the PTS serves as a straightforward checklist that ensures all components necessary to identify a critically injured child are considered. As a predictor of injury, the PTS has a statistically significant, direct linear relationship with the Injury Severity Score (ISS) and an inverse linear relationship with patient mortality. There is a threshold score of 8, below which injured children should be taken to an appropriate pediatric trauma center, because they have the greatest potential for preventable mortality and morbidity. Although research has shown that other scores, such as the RTS, the unresponsive element (U) of the AVPU score, and a best motor response of "1" from the GCS, predict mortality at least as well as the PTS, the PTS remains the only score that includes size, skeletal injury, and open wounds. Although the PTS is a readily available assessment and triage tool, it has not been universally accepted. Other methods of triage may be used in many areas.

Secondary Survey (Detailed Physical Examination)

The secondary survey of the child should follow the primary survey only after life-threatening conditions have been identified and managed. The head and neck should be examined for obvious abrasions, lacerations, and deformity. The thorax should be reexamined. Potential pulmonary contusions may become evident after volume resuscitation, manifested by respiratory distress or abnormal lung sounds. Trauma patients frequently have full stomachs, so insertion of a nasogastric or orogastric tube may be needed. This is especially true for children who are obtunded or who have posttraumatic seizure activity.

Although rib fractures are rare in childhood, they are associated with a high risk of intrathoracic injury. Crepitance may be appreciated on examination and may be a sign of pneumothorax. The risk of mortality increases with the number of ribs fractured.

Examination of the abdomen should focus on distention, tenderness, discoloration, ecchymoses, and presence of a mass. Careful palpation of the iliac crests may suggest an unstable pelvic fracture and increase suspicion for possible retroperitoneal or urogenital injury as well as increased risk for hidden blood loss.

Each extremity should be inspected and palpated to rule out tenderness, deformity, diminished vascular supply, and neurologic deficit. A child's incompletely calcified skeleton with its multiple growth centers increases the possibility of epiphyseal (growth plate) disruption. Accordingly, any area of edema, pain, tenderness, or diminished range of motion should be carefully evaluated and suspected as being fractured until ruled out by radiographic examination. In children as in adults, a missed orthopedic injury in an extremity has little effect on mortality but may lead to long-term deformity and disability.

BOX 14-2   Pediatric Vital Signs and Quantitative Norms

The term *pediatric* or *child* includes a vast range of physical development, emotional maturity, and body sizes. The approach to the patient and the implications of many injuries vary greatly between an infant and an adolescent.

In most anatomic and therapeutic dosage considerations, a child's weight (or specific height or length) serves as a more accurate indicator than does exact chronologic age.[19] Table 14-2 lists the average height and weight for healthy children of varying ages.

The acceptable ranges of quantitative vital signs vary for the different ages within the pediatric population. Adult norms cannot be used as guidelines in smaller children. An adult ventilatory rate of 30 breaths/min is tachypneic, and an adult heart rate of 120 beats/min is tachycardic. Both are considered alarmingly high in an adult and are significant pathologic findings. However, the same findings in an infant may be within the normal ranges.

Normal ranges of vital signs for different age groups may not be consistent across all pediatric references. In an injured child without a previous history of normal vital signs, borderline vital signs may be viewed as pathologic, even though in that individual child the signs may be physiologically acceptable. The guidelines in Tables 14-3,

14-4, and 14-5 can aid in evaluating vital signs. These tables present statistically common ranges into which most children in these age groups will fall.

Several commercially available items serve as rapid references for pediatric vital signs and equipment size. These include the length-based resuscitation tape (Broselow tape) and several slide-rule–type plastic scales. The following guideline formulas can also be used to estimate the expected finding for any age:

Weight (kg) = 8 + (2 × Child's age [years])
***Lowest acceptable* systolic blood pressure (mm Hg) =**
70 + (2 × Child's age [years])
Total vascular blood volume (mL) =
80 mL × Child's weight (kg)

Quantitative vital signs in children, although important, are only an additional piece of information in making an assessment. A child can rapidly deteriorate into either critical ventilatory difficulty or decompensated shock. Vital signs should be considered along with mechanism of injury and other clinical findings.

Management

The keys to pediatric trauma survival are rapid cardiopulmonary assessment, appropriate aggressive management, and transport to a facility capable of managing pediatric trauma.

Airway

Ventilation, oxygenation, and perfusion are as essential to an injured child as an adult. Thus the primary goal of the initial resuscitation of an injured child is restoration of adequate tissue oxygenation as quickly as possible. The first priority of assessment and resuscitation is the establishment of a patent airway.

A patent airway should be ensured and maintained with suctioning, manual maneuvers, and airway adjuncts. As in the adult, initial management includes cervical spine stabilization. Adequate padding (2-3 cm) should be placed under the torso of the small child so that the cervical spine is maintained in a straight line rather than forced into slight flexion because of the disproportionately large occiput (Figure 14-4). When adjusting and maintaining airway positioning, compressing the soft tissues of the neck and trachea

should be avoided. Once manual control of the airway is achieved, an oropharyngeal airway can be placed if no gag reflex is present. The device should be inserted carefully and gently, parallel to the course of the tongue rather than turned 90 or 180 degrees in the posterior oropharynx as in

FIGURE 14-4   Provide adequate padding under the child's torso.

the adult. Use of a tongue blade to depress the tongue is helpful. Visualized orotracheal intubation is the preferred method of definitive airway control during long transports. One study suggests, however, that there is no improved survival or neurologic outcome in pediatric trauma patients intubated early in the field versus those who underwent BVM ventilation during short transports.[12] A more recent study in a rural setting found that multiple prehospital intubation attempts were associated with significant complications.[13]

Breathing

The patient's minute volume and ventilatory effort should be evaluated carefully. Because of the potential for rapid deterioration from hypoxia to ventilatory arrest, ventilation should be assisted if dyspnea and increased ventilatory effort are observed. A properly sized BVM with a reservoir and high-flow oxygen to provide an oxygen concentration of between 85% and 100% (Fio_2 of 0.85-1.0) should be used. Continuous pulse oximetry serves as an adjunct for ongoing assessment of airway and breathing. The Spo_2 should be kept at greater than 95%. In the intubated child with closed head injury, end-tidal carbon dioxide ($ETco_2$) monitoring should be used to document continuing appropriate endotracheal tube placement and avoid extremes of hypercarbia and hypocarbia, both of which can be just as detrimental to recovery from a closed head injury as hypoxia (Boxes 14-3 and 14-4). $ETco_2$ should be targeted at 30 to 40 mm Hg.[15]

Children are more susceptible than adults to acute cardiovascular collapse from a tension pneumothorax. Most children with tension pneumothorax will present with acute cardiac decompensation secondary to decreased venous return before any detectable changes in oxygenation and ventilation have occurred. Any child who acutely decompensates, especially after initiation of positive-pressure ventilation by BVM or endotracheal intubation, should urgently be assessed for tension pneumothorax. Jugular venous distention and tracheal shift are late signs and may be difficult to determine because an extrication collar has been applied on the short neck. In this child, decreased breath sounds on the right are an indication for emergency needle decompression. Diminished sounds on the left may indicate the need for right mainstem intubation, but when associated with acute cardiac decompensation, these sounds likely represent tension pneumothorax. Needle decompression is performed using the same landmarks as in the adult but is often more immediately effective in the child because the mediastinum rapidly shifts back to normal position.

Circulation

Once the patient's external hemorrhage is controlled, perfusion should be evaluated. Controlling external hemorrhage involves applying direct manual pressure on the bleeding point, not just covering it with layer after layer of absorbent

---

> **BOX 14-3   Pediatric Endotracheal Intubation**
>
> Endotracheal intubation of a child should include careful attention to the cervical spine. One person should maintain the patient's spine in a neutral position while another person intubates. The narrowest portion of the pediatric airway is the cricoid ring, so uncuffed tracheal tubes should always be used in children less than 8 years of age. The appropriately sized tracheal tube can be estimated by using the diameter of the child's fifth finger or external nares, or by using the formula (16 + Age)/4. A slight amount of cricoid pressure frequently brings the anterior structures of the child's larynx into better view and will passively obstruct the esophagus, thus diminishing gastric insufflation. Pharmacologically assisted intubation, or rapid-sequence intubation (RSI), should include the use of atropine sulfate to prevent bradycardia. Heart rate is a major determinant of perfusion in pediatric patients.
>
> A common error that occurs during intubation of children under emergency circumstances is an aggressive advancement of the tracheal tube into the right mainstem bronchus. The tube should never be advanced more than three times the tube size in centimeters. The chest should always be auscultated after the tracheal tube is placed. Tube placement should be frequently reassessed, especially after any movement of the patient. In addition to confirming endotracheal tube placement, auscultation may rule out the possibility of other pulmonary injury. The child with a compromised airway and a pulmonary injury who has been successfully intubated may be in greater jeopardy for the development of a tension pneumothorax as a result of more efficient delivery of tidal volume to the lungs.

dressing. The pediatric vascular system is usually able to maintain a normal BP until severe collapse occurs, at which point it is often unresponsive to resuscitation. Therefore, fluid resuscitation should be started whenever signs of compensated hypovolemic shock are present and *must* be started in patients who present with decompensated shock. Lactated Ringer's (LR) or normal saline (NS) solution in 20-mL/kg boluses should be used. For pediatric trauma patients who display any signs of hemorrhagic shock or hypovolemia, key factors to survival are volume resuscitation and rapid initiation of transport to a suitable facility. Transportation should not be delayed to obtain vascular access or administer intravenous (IV) fluid.

Vascular Access

Fluid replacement in a child with severe hypotension or signs of shock must deliver adequate fluid volume to

BOX 14-4   Prehospital Pediatric Intubation: the Great Debate

It would almost seem intuitive that providing a tracheal tube as early as possible in the management of the child with traumatic brain injury (TBI) would be of benefit. A retrospective review showed improved survival in adult patients with TBI intubated before arrival.[20] Subsequent studies evaluated rapid-sequence intubation (RSI), demonstrating its improved efficiency and success rate in intubation of adults and children.[21,22] However, many retrospective and prospective case-control studies found that prehospital intubation compared with BVM ventilation did not improve survival or neurologic outcome and even might have been detrimental.[14,23,24] A prospective randomized trial in children comparing endotracheal intubation versus BVM ventilation in an urban area with short transport times demonstrated no difference in survival or neurologic outcome between the two groups but an increased incidence of complications in the intubated group.[12]

Prolonged periods of hypoxia are often associated with the intubation process, as well as periods of overaggressive ventilation in patients en route to the trauma center.[15]

Data supporting prehospital pediatric tracheal intubation are limited and ambiguous. In the spontaneously breathing child, intubation with or without pharmacologic assistance should be initiated with extreme caution. EMS programs that justify pediatric prehospital intubation should include at least the following[25]:

1. Close medical direction and supervision
2. Training and continuing education, including hands-on operating room (OR) experience
3. Resources for patient monitoring, drug storage, and tube placement confirmation
4. Standardized RSI protocols
5. Availability of backup rescue airway
6. Continuing quality assurance/quality control and performance review

The Combitube has been a proven rescue airway device for adult trauma victims;[26] however, its large size and lack of smaller sizes makes it inadequate as a rescue device for small children. The laryngeal mask airway (LMA) has been shown to provide a safe rescue airway in children and may be the optimum choice as a rescue device in EMS systems providing pediatric prehospital intubation.[27]

BOX 14-5   Pediatric Intraosseous Infusion

Intraosseous (IO) infusion can provide an excellent alternative site for blood drawing and volume replacement in injured children of all ages. This is an effective route for infusion of medications, blood, or high-volume fluid resuscitation.

The most accessible site for IO infusion is the anterior tibia just below the tibial tuberosity. After preparing the skin antiseptically and securing the leg adequately, a site is chosen on the anterior portion of the tibia, 1 to 2 cm distal and medial to the tibial tuberosity. Specially manufactured IO infusion needles are optimal for the procedure, but spinal or bone marrow needles may also be used. Spinal needles that are 18 to 20 gauge work well because they have a trocar to prevent the needle from being obstructed as it passes through the bony cortex into the marrow. Any 14- to 20-gauge needle can be used in an emergency. The needle is placed at a 90-degree angle to the bone and advanced firmly through the cortex into the marrow. Evidence that the needle is adequately within the marrow includes the following:

1. A soft "pop" and lack of resistance after the needle has passed through the cortex
2. Aspiration of bone marrow into the needle
3. Free flow of fluid into the marrow without evidence of subcutaneous infiltration

IO infusion should be considered during initial resuscitation if percutaneous venous cannulation has been unsuccessful. Because the flow rate is limited, the IO route alone will seldom be sufficient after initial resuscitation.

the right atrium to avoid further reduction in cardiac preload. The most appropriate initial sites for IV access are the antecubital fossa and the saphenous vein at the ankle. Access through the external jugular vein is a possibility, but airway management and spinal immobilization make the neck poorly accessible for cannulation.

In the unstable or potentially unstable patient, attempts at peripheral access should be limited to two in 90 seconds. If peripheral access is unsuccessful, intraosseous access should be considered in the young child (Box 14-5), whereas femoral access by experienced providers may be considered in the older child if allowed by protocol.

If the child is older than 6 years, an intraosseous line or cannulation of the femoral vein is a short-term alternative until the child is transported to the definitive care setting. The femoral vein is readily accessible in the absence of severe pelvic trauma and less risky than using the subclavian or internal jugular vein.[28] Placement of a subclavian or internal jugular catheter in an injured child should be performed only under the most controlled circumstances within the hospital; this should not be attempted in the prehospital environment.

The determination of which pediatric patients should have intravascular access depends on transport times and other factors. If uncertainty exists as to which patients need intravascular access, or if fluid replacement is needed during transport, online medical direction should be obtained.

Fluid Therapy

Lactated Ringer's solution, or NS solution if LR solution is unavailable, is the initial resuscitation fluid of choice for a hypovolemic child. Because the time that a crystalloid fluid remains in the vascular system is short, a 3:1 ratio of crystalloid fluid to blood lost is used. An initial resuscitative bolus should equal approximately 25% of the normal circulating blood volume of the child, which is approximately 20 mL/kg. Considering the 3:1 ratio, as much as 60 mL/kg may be required to achieve adequate and rapid initial replacement in response to significant volume loss. Specific to trauma care, any child who does not show at least a minor improvement in hemodynamic status with the first 20-mL/kg fluid bolus and stabilization after the second 20-mL/kg bolus should receive a blood transfusion. The crystalloid bolus may temporarily restore cardiovascular stability as it transiently fills and then leaks from the circulatory system. However, until RBCs are replaced and oxygen transport is restored, the basic process of cellular hypoxia will continue.

Specific Injuries

Traumatic Brain Injury

Traumatic brain injury (TBI) is the most common cause of death in the pediatric population. Of the fatalities included in the first 40,000 patients in the NPTR, 89% had a CNS injury as either the primary or the secondary contributor to mortality. Although many of the most severe injuries are treatable only by prevention, initial resuscitative measures may at least lessen the serious consequences of the child's injury. Adequate ventilation, oxygenation, and perfusion are needed to prevent secondary morbidity. The outcome of children sustaining severe TBI is typically better than in adults. However, the outcome of children younger than 3 years is worse than that of older children.

The results of the initial neurologic assessment are useful for prognosis. Even with a normal initial neurologic evaluation, however, any child who sustains a head injury

may be susceptible to cerebral edema and hypoperfusion. These conditions can result even from a mechanism that appears minor.

A baseline GCS score should be assessed and repeated during transport. Supplemental oxygen should be administered, and if possible, pulse oximetry should be monitored. Although vomiting is common after a concussion, persistent vomiting is of concern and requires further evaluation.

As with hypoxia, hypovolemia may dramatically worsen the original TBI. External hemorrhage must be controlled and the patient's fractured extremities immobilized to limit internal blood loss associated with fractures. An attempt should be made to keep these children in a euvolemic state with IV volume resuscitation. On rare occasions, infants less than about 6 months of age may become hypovolemic as a result of intracranial bleeding because they have open cranial sutures and fontanelles. The infant with an open fontanelle may better tolerate an expanding intracranial hematoma but may not become symptomatic until rapid decompensation occurs. An infant with a bulging fontanelle should be considered to have a more severe TBI.

Children with a GCS score of 8 or less may benefit from tracheal intubation. However, prolonged attempts at securing an endotracheal airway may increase periods of hypoxia and also delay transport to an appropriate facility. Adequate oxygenation and ventilation should be the goal at all times, not the placement of an ET tube. The *best* airway for a child is the one that is both safest and most effective. Ventilation with a BVM device while being prepared to suction emesis, should it occur, may be safer than intubation and is often the best airway for the child with TBI.[12,14,15]

A child with signs and symptoms of intracranial hypertension, or increased intracranial pressure (ICP), such as a sluggishly reactive or nonreactive pupil, systemic hypertension, bradycardia, and abnormal breathing patterns, may benefit from hyperventilation to lower ICP transiently. However, hyperventilation also decreases overall oxygen delivery to the CNS and may aggravate hypoxic injury.[29] It is strongly recommended that this strategy not be used unless the child is exhibiting signs of herniation or lateralizing signs. ET_{CO_2} monitoring should guide management in the intubated child, with the target range about 35 mm Hg, Hyperventilation to an ET_{CO_2} of less than 25 mm Hg has been associated with worse neurologic outcome.[15] If capnography is not available, a ventilation rate of 30 breaths/min for children and 35 breaths/min for infants should be used.[16]

During prolonged transports, small doses of mannitol (0.5-1 g/kg body weight) may benefit children with evidence of intracranial hypertension. However, use of mannitol may result in hypovolemia with insufficient volume resuscitation. Mannitol should not be given in the field without discussing this option with the receiving physician or hospital, unless permitted by standing orders or protocol. Brief seizures may occur soon after TBI and often do not require treatment by prehospital care personnel. However, recurrent seizure activity is worrisome and may require IV boluses of a benzodiazepine, such as diazepam (0.1-0.2 mg/kg/dose). Depending on protocol, midazolam or lorazepam may also be used, but all benzodiazepines should be used with extreme caution because of the potential side effects of ventilatory depression and hypotension.

Spinal Trauma

The indication for spinal immobilization in a pediatric patient is based on the mechanism of injury and physical findings; the presence of other injuries that suggest violent or sudden movement of the head, neck, or torso; or the presence of specific signs of spine injury, such as deformity, pain, or neurologic deficit. As with adult patients, the correct prehospital management of a suspected unstable spine is manual stabilization followed by the use of a properly fitting cervical collar and immobilization of the patient to a long backboard so that the head, neck, torso, pelvis, and legs are maintained in a neutral inline position. This should be achieved without inhibiting the patient's ventilation, ability to open the mouth, or any other resuscitative efforts. The threshold for performing spinal immobilization is lower in young children because of their inability to communicate or otherwise participate in their own assessment. The same immaturity also contributes to children's fear and lack of cooperation with immobilization. A child who strongly fights attempts at immobilization may actually be at increased risk of worsening any existing spinal injuries. It may be valid to decide not to restrain such a patient if the child can be persuaded to lie quietly without restraints. Any decision to stop immobilization attempts in the interest of patient safety must be supported by thorough documentation of the reason as well as serial assessment of neurologic status during and immediately after transport.

When most small children are placed on a rigid surface, the relatively larger size of the child's occiput will result in neck flexion. Sufficient padding (2-3 cm) should be placed under the patient's torso to elevate it and allow the head to be in a neutral position. The padding should be continuous and flat from the shoulders to the pelvis and extend to the lateral margins of the torso to ensure that the thoracic, lumbar, and sacral spine are on a flat, continuous, stable platform without movement. Padding should also be placed between the lateral sides of the child and the edges of the board to ensure that no lateral movement occurs when the board is moved or if the patient and board need to be rotated to the side to avoid aspiration of vomitus.

Various new pediatric immobilization devices are available. The prehospital care provider needs to practice and be familiar with any specialized equipment used in the provider's system, as well as the required adjustments when immobilizing a child with adult-sized equipment. If a vest-type device is used on a child, the prehospital care provider

ensures adequate immobilization to prevent respiratory compromise. The provider also needs to be familiar with the techniques of immobilizing a young child in a car safety seat.[30,31]

Thoracic Injuries

The extremely resilient rib cage of a child results in less injury to the bony structure of the thorax but more risk for parenchymal injury, such as pulmonary contusion, pneumothorax, and hemothorax. A high index of suspicion is the key to identifying these injuries. Every child who sustains trauma to the chest and torso should be carefully monitored for signs of respiratory distress and shock. Carefully monitor any child with abrasions or contusions over the torso after blunt force trauma; these may be the only clues to an increased risk of intrathoracic injury.

When transporting a child who has sustained a high-impact blunt thoracic injury, the patient's cardiac rhythm should be monitored once the child is en route to a medical facility. In other cases the key items in managing thoracic trauma also involve careful attention to ventilation and oxygenation and timely transport to an appropriate facility.

Abdominal Injuries

The presence of blunt trauma to the abdomen; an unstable pelvis; posttraumatic abdominal distention, rigidity, or tenderness; or otherwise unexplained shock can be associated with possible intraabdominal hemorrhage. A seat belt mark across the abdomen of a child is often a marker of serious internal injuries (Figure 14-5). The key prehospital elements in management of abdominal injuries include fluid resuscitation, supplemental high-concentration oxygen, and rapid transport to an appropriate facility with continued

FIGURE 14-5 "Seat belt sign" in a 6-year-old patient who was found to have a ruptured spleen. Seat belt signs are often associated with serious intraabdominal injuries.

careful monitoring en route. If time permits and there are no obvious midfacial fractures, an orogastric or nasogastric tube may be placed to decompress the stomach.

Extremity Trauma

Compared with the adult skeleton, the child's skeleton is actively growing and consists of a large proportion of cartilaginous tissue and metabolically active growth plates. The collateral ligaments that hold the skeleton together are frequently stronger and better able to withstand mechanical disruption than the bones to which they are attached. As a result, children with skeletal trauma frequently sustain major traumatic forces before developing deformed long-bone fractures or dislocations. Incomplete ("greenstick") fractures are common and may be indicated only by bony tenderness and pain on use of the affected extremity.

Primary joint disruption from injury other than penetrating injury is uncommon compared with disruption of the diaphyseal or epiphyseal segments of bone. Fractures that involve the growth plate must be carefully identified and managed in a manner that will not only ensure adequate healing but also prevent subsequent displacement or deformity as the child grows. The association of vascular injuries with orthopedic injuries in children should always be considered, and the distal pulse should be evaluated carefully. Often the presence of a potentially debilitating injury can be determined only by radiologic study or, when the slightest suggestion of a decrease in distal perfusion exists, by arteriography.

The apparent gross deformity sometimes associated with extremity injury should not distract focus from potentially life-threatening injuries. Uncontrolled hemorrhage represents the sole life-threatening condition associated with extremity trauma. In multisystem pediatric and adult trauma patients alike, the initiation of transport to an appropriate facility without delay after completion of the primary survey, resuscitation, and rapid packaging remains paramount in reducing mortality. If basic splinting can be provided en route without detracting from the child's resuscitation, it will help to minimize bleeding and pain from long-bone fractures.

Burns

Following motor vehicle crashes and drowning, burns rate third as the cause of pediatric trauma deaths.[32] Caring for an injured child always poses significant physical and emotional challenges to the prehospital care provider, and these difficulties are only amplified when caring for the burned child. The burned child may have an edematous airway; IV access may be complicated by burns of the extremity; and the child may be hysterical from pain.

The ABCDEs of trauma care should be followed in pediatric trauma, but every step of the primary assessment may be more complicated than in a nonthermally injured child. Most deaths related to structure fires are not directly related to soft tissue burns but are secondary to smoke inhalation. When children are trapped in a structure fire, they often hide from the fire under beds or in closets. These children frequently die, and their recovered bodies often have no burns; they die from carbon monoxide or hydrogen cyanide toxicity and hypoxia. More than 50% of children less than 9 years old in structure fires have some degree of smoke inhalation injury.

Thermally induced edema of the airway is always a concern in burn patients, but especially in children. The smaller diameter of the pediatric trachea means that 1 mm of edema will produce a greater magnitude of airway obstruction than in an adult with a larger-diameter airway. Early control of the airway with endotracheal intubation should be done before the child develops signs or respiratory compromise. A child with an edematous airway may be sitting forward and drooling. Once an ET tube is placed, it needs to be protected against inadvertent dislodgement or removal. If the patient accidentally becomes extubated, the provider may not be able to intubate the child a second time; the results could be disastrous. Securing an ET tube in a child who has peeling facial skin and moist wounds is difficult. Securing the ET tube to the face with adhesive tape should not be attempted in children with facial burns. The ET tube should be secured with two pieces of umbilical tape, with one piece draped above the ear and the second piece placed below the ear. An effective alternative to umbilical tape is IV tubing.

Rapid establishment of intravascular access is vital to prevent the development of shock. Delayed fluid resuscitation in children has been associated with significantly worse clinical outcomes and an increased mortality, especially in burned infants.

Excessive fluids can result in respiratory complications as well as excessive edema, which is harmful to the burned areas. After securing an airway and providing adequate ventilation, it is critical that venous access is obtained quickly. Children have a small intravascular volume, and a delay in fluid resuscitation may lead to the development of hypovolemic shock. To provide the large volumes of IV fluids required in critical burns, such patients require two peripheral IV catheters to achieve the IV flow rates usually required. The insertion of a single large-bore IV catheter is often challenging enough, let alone two IV catheters. Burns on the extremities may make it difficult to impossible to establish enough access for an appropriate fluid resuscitation. In pediatric burn patients, a delay in IV initiation of even 30 minutes can result in hypovolemic shock. Once peripheral IV access has been obtained, provisions must be made to ensure that the IV line is not inadvertently removed or dislodged. Usual techniques used to secure IV lines are often ineffective when a line is placed in or adjacent to a burn because adhesive tape and dressings may adhere to burned tissue. If possible, the IV line is secured with a Kerlex dressing suture.

When peripheral venous access cannot be obtained, intraosseous catheters should be used. Although previously advocated only for children less than 3 years of age, intraosseous infusions are now used in older children as well as adults. If transporting a child with a Foley catheter, the fluids should be titrated to ensure a urine output of 1 mL/kg/hr. If the urine output is not adequate, a fluid bolus of 20 mL/kg is administered and the rate of administration of the resuscitative fluids is increased. The amount of fluids typically given to a burn patient is estimated using the "rule of nines," a rapid and imprecise method of estimating resuscitative fluid needs in *adult* battlefield casualties. The premise of this method of burn size estimation is that major regions of the adult body (e.g., head, arm, anterior torso) each comprise 9% of the total body surface area (TBSA). Children's anatomic regions are proportionally different than those in adults; children have larger heads and smaller limbs. Therefore, estimation of pediatric burn size should use diagrams that are age specific and not the rule of nines.

Based on the burn size, the IV volume is determined (see Chapter 13). Two important pediatric considerations merit mention. First, small children have a limited reserve of glycogen. *Glycogen* is a molecule used for carbohydrate storage that is mobilized in times of stress. If glycogen stores become depleted, the child may develop hypoglycemia. Second, children have a large volume/surface area ratio; the general shape of an adult is a cylinder, whereas children resemble a sphere. The clinical implication is that a child will require more IV fluids. To address both these issues, in addition to the calculated resuscitative fluids, maintenance fluids containing 5% dextrose are also administered.

Each year approximately 1.5 million children are abused by burning, accounting for 20% of all child abuse.[33-35] Approximately 20% to 25% of children admitted to a pediatric burn center are victims of child abuse.[36,37] An increased awareness of this problem among prehospital providers can improve detection and prosecution of the offenders.

The two mechanisms by which these children receive burns are scalds and contact burns. Scalds are the most common source of abuse burns. Scalding injuries typically are inflicted on children of toilet-training age. The usual scenario is that children soil themselves and are immersed in a tub of scalding water. These scald burns are characterized by a pattern of sharp demarcation between burned and unburned tissue and sparing of flexion creases.

Contact burns are the second most common mechanism of abuse burns. Common items used to inflict contact burns are curling irons, clothing irons, and cigarettes. Cigarette burns appear as round wounds measuring slightly over 1 cm in diameter (typically 1.3 cm). To conceal these injuries, the abuser may place these in areas usually covered by clothing, above the hairline in the scalp, or even in the axillae. Accidental contact burns will have irregular borders and a heterogenous depth. In contrast, intentional contact burns will have regular borders and a uniform depth. All the surfaces of the human body have some degree of curvature. Therefore, a hot item that falls onto any body surface will have an initial point of contact, and then the hot item will deflect from the point of contact. The resultant injury is one with irregular borders and depth. When a hot item is deliberately used to burn someone, the item is pressed onto the region of the body. The burn will then have a pattern with a sharp outline and uniform burn depth (see Chapter 13).

A high index of suspicion for abuse is important and all cases of suspected abuse should be reported. Make meticulous observations of the surroundings, such as the position of various pieces of furniture, curling irons, and depth of bath water. Record the names of individuals present at the scene. Any child suspected of being abused by burns, regardless of the size of the burns, needs to be cared for at a center experienced in pediatric burn care.

Pain Management

As with adults, pain management should be considered for children in the prehospital setting. Indications for analgesia include isolated limb injury and suspected spinal fracture. Small doses of a narcotic injected intravenously and appropriately titrated should not compromise the neurologic or abdominal examination. Both morphine and fentanyl are acceptable choices, but they should be administered only according to written protocol or with orders from medical control. Because of the side effects of hypotension and hypoventilation, all patients receiving IV narcotics should be monitored with pulse oximetry and serial vital signs. In general, benzodiazepines should not be administered in combination with narcotics because of possible respiratory arrest.

Transport

Because timely arrival at an appropriate facility may be the key element in the patient's survival, *triage* is an important consideration of management.

The tragedy of preventable pediatric traumatic death has been documented in multiple studies reported over the past three decades. It is estimated that as many as 80% of pediatric trauma deaths can be classified as preventable or potentially preventable. These statistics have been one of the primary motivations for the development of regionalized pediatric trauma centers, where continuous high-quality, sophisticated care can be provided.

Many urban areas have both pediatric trauma centers and adult trauma centers. If the patient experiences only a small delay in arrival, the pediatric multisystem trauma patient may benefit from the initial resuscitation capability and definitive care available at a slightly distant facility specialized in treating traumatized children. For many locations, however, the nearest specialized pediatric trauma center is hours away. In these cases the seriously traumatized child should be transported to the nearest adult trauma center, because early resuscitation and evaluation before transport to a pediatric facility may improve survival.[38] In areas where no specialized pediatric trauma center is nearby, personnel working in adult trauma centers should be experienced in the resuscitation and treatment of both adult and pediatric trauma patients. In areas where neither facility is readily close, the seriously injured child should be transported to the nearest appropriate hospital (for trauma victims) according to local protocols. Aeromedical transport should be considered in rural areas to expedite transport. There is little evidence that aeromedical transport provides any benefit in urban areas where ground transport to a pediatric trauma center is almost as quick.[39]

Review of more than 15,000 records in the NPTR indicates that 25% of children are injured severely enough to require triage to a designated pediatric trauma center. Use of the PTS will help with appropriate triage. Many emergency medical services (EMS) and trauma systems use other pediatric triage criteria, which may be dictated by state, regional, or local protocols. All prehospital care providers need to be familiar with the triage protocols in place within their own systems.

Prolonged Transport

Occasionally a situation arises as a result of triage or environmental considerations in which transport will be delayed and prehospital personnel need to manage the initial resuscitation of an injured child. Even though this may be suboptimal because of the lack of field resources (e.g., blood) and the inability to perform diagnostic and therapeutic interventions, by applying the principles discussed in this chapter in an organized fashion, the child can be safely managed until arrival at a trauma center. If radio or cellular contact with the receiving facility is possible, constant communication and feedback are crucial for both prehospital and hospital-based members of the trauma team.

Management should consist of continued serial evaluation of the ABCDEs. The child should be securely stabilized on a backboard with spine precautions. The board should be padded as well as possible. Because it will not delay transport to intubate the child, if the airway is questionable and the crew is trained in pediatric intubation with or without rapid-sequence intubation (RSI), endotracheal intubation should be performed. Pulse oximetry should be monitored, and preferably $ETCO_2$ as well, especially in the child with a head injury. If signs of shock exist, 20-mL/kg boluses of LR or NS solution are given until the signs are corrected or the child is transferred. GCS is calculated and followed serially. Assessment for other injuries continues, and all efforts to keep the child normothermic are initiated. Fractures should be splinted and stabilized with serial neurovascular assessments. This cycle of continued assessment of the primary survey should be repeated until the child can be safely transported.

Any change or decompensation in the child requires immediate reassessment of the ABCDEs. Is the tracheal tube still secure and in the airway? If so, has the child developed a tension pneumothorax, or is the tube now in the right mainstem bronchus? If the child has received what was thought to be sufficient fluid and is still in shock, is there now cardiac tamponade, severe cardiac contusion, or perhaps an occult source of bleeding, such as intraabdominal injury or missed scalp laceration? Has the GCS changed? Are there now lateralizing signs suggesting progressive head injury and requiring more aggressive ventilation or mannitol? Are the extremities still neurovascularly intact, and is the child normothermic? If radio contact is available, continued advice and guidance should be sought throughout the resuscitation.

By paying attention to the basics and continually reassessing the ABCDEs, adequate resuscitation can be performed until the child can be transferred to a definitive care center.

Pediatric Disaster Triage: JumpSTART

Many, if not most, mass-casualty (or multiple-casualty) incidents (MCIs) include children among the victims. Responders face not only the stress and potential chaos of having to deal quickly with multiple patients, but also the need to work effectively under the additional stress of caring for one or more potentially seriously injured children. In such a challenging environment, objective triage guidelines for patients of *all* ages can help ensure that the greatest good is done for the greatest number. In the primary disaster triage setting, no patient takes precedence over any other, regardless of age or social status. MCI triage must come from the head, not the heart. If pediatric victims receive preferential treatment at an MCI because of responder anxiety, lack of confidence, simple compassion, or good intention, resources may be assigned to children who do not need them or will not benefit from them, rather than to the adults who may benefit from these resources.

The START triage tool is the most common, objective MCI primary triage system in the United States and many other countries. Unfortunately, it is not well suited for children, especially younger children with normal vital sign ranges different from those of adults. To address the need for a pediatric-specific primary disaster triage tool, Dr. Lou Romig, a pediatric emergency and EMS physician in Florida, developed the JumpSTART triage tool in 1995. JumpSTART parallels the structure of START and can be used simultaneously with START during the primary triage of an MCI with both adult and pediatric victims. Patients are assigned to the same four categories of acuity (red/immediate, yellow/delayed, green/minor, and black/dead or expectant), and each victim is approached with the same structured assessment scheme. Decision points within the structured assessment are adjusted to suit the apparent age of each victim.

"Apparent age" is a key term when dealing with children. Children often look older or younger than their true age. Triage guidelines based on absolute age falter when the responder is forced to guess a child's age. The developers of START specify that their tool should be used on patients weighing 100 lb (45 kg) or more; this is obviously a difficult parameter to assess in the field. Because side-by-side comparisons of START and JumpSTART show a large degree of agreement for children in the teenage years, Dr. Romig suggests the following guidelines for applying START versus JumpSTART:

- If the patient appears to be a child, use JumpSTART.
- If the patient appears to be a young adult or older, use START.

Primary Triage

Primary triage using JumpSTART commences the same as with START, with the order for all ambulatory victims to move to a designated area to await secondary triage (Figure 14-6). Responders must be aware that (1) adults may carry children with them to the "green" triage area, and (2) some child victims may not be developmentally capable of walking. Therefore the ability to walk is not sufficient to screen some children who may have only minor injuries. The JumpSTART tool includes an adaptation for the assessment of children who are not ambulatory at their baseline because of age, developmental delay, or physical disability, as explained later. Ambulatory adults may carry children to the green area. These children have not yet been triaged, and therefore they should be the first patients assessed by responders performing secondary triage in the green area. JumpSTART should be used in the green area to perform primary triage on these children. Any child meeting red or yellow criteria should be moved to the appropriate treatment area.

For those victims remaining untriaged, JumpSTART and START proceed in the same manner, with responders triaging victims as they encounter them (Figure 14-7). If the victim is breathing spontaneously, the respiratory rate is assessed. If the victim is not breathing, the responder opens the airway and reassesses for spontaneous breathing. In both

triage schemes, if patients start breathing, they are tagged "red." At this point, START dictates that if the patient does not start to breathe with upper airway opening, no further assessment is performed, and the victim is tagged "black."

JumpSTART offers an additional pathway for apneic children. Children are more likely than adults to have a respiratory arrest but still have some circulation until the heart becomes irreversibly anoxic. Romig refers to this as the "window of salvageability." Adults are more likely to have a primary cardiac or circulatory arrest, which then triggers apnea. Although not proved scientifically, it is theoretically possible that a child in early respiratory arrest who still has some circulation may not progress to full cardiorespiratory arrest if breathing is restored. This is perhaps the most critical physiologic difference between children and adults in the triage setting. JumpSTART addresses this difference by having the responder check the victim for a pulse. If a pulse is found (using the pulse location most familiar to the responder), the responder gives the child five rescue breaths via a protective barrier device, thus opening the lower airways and possibly triggering spontaneous breathing. Note that this does *not* mean a BVM, which would be too awkward for a triage officer to carry around. A simple barrier device such as a keyring-style, folding cardiopulmonary resuscitation (CPR) shield is sufficient. If this lower airway–opening maneuver (the "jumpstart") triggers spontaneous breathing, the rescuer does not continue to ventilate the child but tags him or her as "red" and moves on. If sufficient rescuers are available, one might be assigned to watch the child and monitor the airway, but the triage responder must finish the task. If apnea persists after the five breaths, it must be assumed that circulatory and then full arrest will soon follow unless intensive resources are immediately applied; such resources are rarely available at an MCI, and therefore the patient must be tagged "black," and the triage officer moves on.

The remainder of the algorithm parallels the START tool, with decision points modified to match the range of pediatric norms. The JumpSTART respiratory rates that trigger red classification are less than 15 breaths/min and greater than 45 breaths/min. Note that JumpSTART includes a threshold for respirations that are too low, a situation more dangerous than tachypnea. The combined START/JumpSTART respiratory threshold numbers are then 15-30-45, an intentional effort to promote ease of recall.

Children with respiratory rates of 15 to 45 are assessed for perfusion by the presence or absence of pulses. Capillary refill is not used because this measure of peripheral perfusion is easily affected by the environment and can be difficult to assess in poor lighting. START also lists presence or absence of pulses as an alternative measure of perfusion. Again, rescuers should seek the pediatric pulse most familiar to them. If the pulse is easily palpable, mental status is assessed. If a pulse is not palpable, the patient is tagged "red."

JumpSTART Pediatric MCI Triage©

FIGURE 14-6 JumpSTART algorithm.
(Courtesy Dr. Lou Romig.)

START uses the ability to obey simple commands as a measure of adequate mental status. Because some children with normal mental status may not obey commands due to developmental status, fear, or misunderstanding, JumpSTART uses the AVPU system for neurologic assess-

ment. If the child is alert, not alert but responds to voice, or responds appropriately to painful stimulus, neurologic status is probably not dangerously compromised, and the child is tagged "yellow." Appropriate response to painful stimulus means the ability to localize pain and then

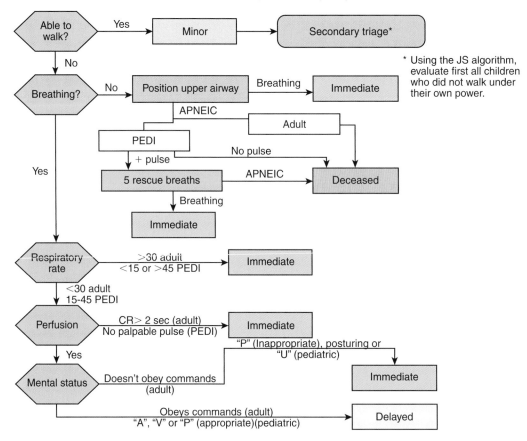

Combined START/JumpSTART Triage Algorithm

FIGURE 14-7 Combined START and JumpSTART algorithm.
(Courtesy Dr. Lou Romig.)

purposefully withdraw from the stimulus or push it away. Children who do not localize the painful stimulus and respond with generalized movement or meaningless sounds, who exhibit decorticate or decerebrate posturing, or who are truly unresponsive, are tagged "red." Note that children in the yellow category probably have sufficient neurologic status to have an intact gag reflex. Children in the red category are less likely to be able to protect their own airway using the gag reflex.

In brief, children who cannot walk (acutely) but who have spontaneous respirations between 15 and 45 breaths/min, who have palpable pulses, and who are appropriately responsive to pain (or better) on an AVPU assessment are tagged "yellow." Children who are apneic but have a pulse and respond to the five-breath ventilatory trial, who have respirations slower than 15/min or faster than 45/min, who lack a palpable pulse, or who respond inappropriately, with posturing, or not at all to a painful stimulus are tagged "red."

As previously mentioned, not all children have the basic ability to walk because of developmental reasons or disability. This does not mean that they cannot be assigned to the green primary triage category. For children who cannot walk as a baseline, take the child through the JumpSTART

algorithm. If the patient meets any red criteria, tag the child "red." If the patient meets yellow criteria, examine the child quickly for external signs of significant injury, including significant burns, penetrating wounds or tissue losses, uncontrollable bleeding, or abdominal distention. If the patient has significant external signs, tag the child "yellow." (Remember, it has already been determined that the child meets no physiologic red criteria.) If the patient has no external signs of significant injury, tag the child "green."

Under many circumstances, it is difficult to separate children from their guardians. If a guardian refuses to leave a child, triage both patients and send them to the treatment area corresponding to the most seriously injured patient. Whenever possible, do not spend time trying to overcome a family's insistence on staying together, although family members must be split up at certain times so that the best specialty care can be provided for each victim.

Secondary Triage

Primary triage, using JumpSTART and START or any other tool, is only the beginning of a dynamic process. All victims must be reassessed as often as possible to detect significant improvement or deterioration. Secondary triage is similar to a secondary survey, where physiology is reassessed, anatomic disruptions are identified, and when possible, treatment is initiated. Patients may be "up-triaged" or "down-triaged" during the secondary triage process. In general, transport priorities and destinations are determined in this stage.

There is no widely accepted MCI secondary triage tool or scheme. In general, patients requiring emergent treatment only available in the hospital setting (e.g., blood transfusion, lifesaving surgery) have the highest transport priority. Once primary triage has been completed and secondary triage and treatment for the most urgent patients have commenced, if sufficient field personnel are available, all black-category patients should be reassessed for signs of life. Resuscitation should be attempted *only* if more salvageable patients do not need the personnel and resources, and if the apparent injuries and the time frame dictate that there is a chance for survival. Palliative care may be provided to black-category patients who are still alive but have injuries that are not survivable with or without the extensive application of sophisticated resources.

Summary and Benefits

The JumpSTART Pediatric Field MCI Triage Tool works well as an adjunct to START or any other objective adult MCI triage tool for the primary triage of children in MCIs. In JumpSTART the physiologic decision points have been adjusted to account for the variations in normal physiology among children of different ages. JumpSTART recognizes that the primary pathway to death among most acutely injured children is respiratory failure/arrest and adds additional steps to identify victims in the "window of salvageability." The JumpSTART ventilatory trial opens the lower airways of apneic children with a pulse in an effort to stimulate spontaneous respiration. In addition, JumpSTART includes an adaptation for immature children or those with special needs who cannot satisfy green criteria by walking.

An objective triage system for children in MCIs benefits both victims and responders. By following an objective, precisely limited assessment scheme, responders can focus on a stressful, time-pressured task in a chaotic and emotion-laden setting. The triage *system* specifies treatment priorities. In this way, the triage responder may feel less of the responsibility for making difficult life-or-death decisions about children and may find some comfort in knowing that he or she played a significant role in providing the right care for the greatest number of patients.

Readers can obtain more information about JumpSTART at www.jumpstarttriage.com.

The Abused and Neglected Child

Child abuse (or maltreatment) is a significant cause of childhood injury. Almost 20% of all pediatric burns involve either child abuse or child neglect. Prehospital care providers

A

B

C

D

E

F

FIGURE 14-8 Indicators of possible child abuse. **A,** "Raccoon eyes," or periorbital bruising, a possible indication of anterior fossa skull fracture. **B,** Fresh cigarette burn to palm. **C,** Fresh abrasions of restraint injury. **D,** Human bites. **E,** "Dunking" burns to the feet. **F,** Welts and abrasions to legs as a result of abuse with an electric cord.
(From Sanders M: *Mosby's paramedic textbook,* ed 2, St Louis, 2001, Mosby.)

must consider the possibility of child abuse when circumstances warrant.

In many jurisdictions, prehospital care providers are legally mandated reporters if they identify potential child abuse. Generally, providers-reporters who act in good faith are protected from legal action by the reported party.

Prehospital care providers should suspect abuse or neglect if they note any of the following scenarios:

- Discrepancy between the history and the degree of physical injury, or the history changes frequently.
- Inappropriate response from the family.
- Prolonged interval between time of injury and arrival for medical care.
- History of the injury inconsistent with the developmental level of the child. For example, a history indicating that a newborn rolled off a bed would be suspect because newborns are developmentally unable to roll over.

Certain injury types also suggest abuse, such as the following (Figure 14-8):

- Multiple bruises in varying stages of resolution (excluding the palms, forearms, tibial areas, and the forehead, which are frequently injured in normal falls). Normal bruises usually occur over bony prominences.
- Bizarre injuries such as bites, cigarette burns, rope marks, or any pattern injury.
- Sharply demarcated burns or scald injuries in unusual areas (see Chapter 13).

Reporting procedures vary, so prehospital care providers should be familiar with the appropriate agencies that handle child abuse cases in their location. The need to report abuse is emphasized by data suggesting that up to 50% of maltreated children are released back to their abusers because abuse was not suspected or reported (Box 14-6).

BOX 14-6   Documenting Child Abuse

Emergency medical technicians (EMTs) may be the only responders to a potential crime scene involving child abuse. While recognizing that EMTs are under intense pressure at an emergency scene, they are in a unique position to collect items of evidentiary importance that may assist in determining the mechanism of injury and the identification of the abuser. EMTs should ideally document 10 fundamental items when responding to a "child in need of assistance" call:

1. Document all adults and children present.
2. Document all statements and the demeanor of all persons present. As recorders of "scene" statements, EMTs must be familiar with the general requirements that allow certain statements to be used in court.
   a. Identify and document the maker of the statement.
   b. Record all statements in the official report.
   c. Record verbatim content.
   d. Document the time when the statement was made.
   e. Record the speaker's demeanor.
   f. Explain your job.
   g. Ask probing follow-up questions.
   h. Record the question. The content of an answer can often be understood only by knowing the question.
   i. List all persons present who heard the statement.
3. Document the environment. EMTs may arrive before caregivers clean up, modify, or destroy evidence.
4. Collect significant items. Preserving the potential mechanism of injury is vital to verifying a suspect history.

5. Identify and record the child's age and developmental stage.
6. Know the signs of abuse and neglect.
   a. Signs of physical abuse: unexplained fractures, bruises, black eyes, cuts, burns, and welts; pattern injuries and bite marks; antisocial behavior; fear of adults; signs of apathy, depression, hostility, or stress; eating disorders.
   b. Signs of sexual abuse: difficulty walking or sitting, overcompliance, excessive aggressiveness, nightmares, bed-wetting, drastic change in appetite, inappropriate interest or knowledge of sexual acts, fear of a particular person.
   c. Signs of neglect: unsuitable clothing; unbathed/dirty; severe body odor; severe diaper rash; underweight; lack of food, formula, or toys; parent or child use of drugs or alcohol; apparent lack of supervision; unsuitable living conditions.
7. Assess children present at unrelated calls.
8. Evaluate children and adults with disabilities.
9. Adhere to mandatory reporting requirements and procedures.
10. Interact with the multidisciplinary team (MDT).

Child abuse and neglect cases are wrought with difficult issues. Holding abusers responsible for their acts requires meticulous documentation, evenhanded investigations, and teamwork. EMTs are uniquely positioned to observe and document vital information when assessing the possibility of child abuse.

Modified from Rogers LL: Emergency medical professionals: assisting in identifying and documenting child abuse and neglect, *NCPCA Update Newslett* 17(7):1, 2004.

SUMMARY

The initial and continuing prehospital care of the injured child requires application of standard trauma life support principles modified by the unique characteristics of children. Traumatic brain injury is the leading cause of death from trauma, as well as the most common injury for which the child requires airway management. Children have the ability to compensate for volume loss longer than adults, but when they exceed their ability to compensate, children deteriorate suddenly and severely. Significant underlying organ and vascular injury can occur without apparent external injury or with only mild external signs and symptoms. Children with trauma and the following signs are unstable and should be transported without delay to an appropriate facility:

- Difficulty breathing
- Signs of shock or circulatory instability
- Any period of postinjury unconsciousness
- Significant blunt trauma to the thorax or abdomen
- Fractured ribs
- Pelvic fracture

If possible, children with multisystem trauma and a PTS of less than 8 should be transported to a pediatric trauma center.

SCENARIO SOLUTION

You correctly identify this child as a victim of multisystem trauma who is in shock. Because of the mechanism of injury, you decide that Scott is critically injured. Because of the probable femur fracture combined with the change in mentation, you have to determine the greatest threat to his survivability: the brain injury, the potential volume loss from the femur, or other injuries not yet identified. You correctly identify hypotension and tachycardia, which you assume are related to hypovolemic shock, probably the result of an unrecognized intraabdominal injury, because a femur fracture by itself rarely causes hypotension in a child. Initially, Scott's breathing is supported with high-concentration oxygen through a nonrebreather mask. You realize that his respiratory rate is low for a child of his age and are prepared to provide more aggressive airway con-

trol if his condition deteriorates. As you consider options for airway management, you ask a partner to hold manual stabilization of the head and neck. You may consider rapid-sequence intubation (RSI) if it is appropriate and you are properly trained.

Because of the nature of the child's injuries, you consult with medical control, who agrees that helicopter transport to a more distant pediatric trauma center is more appropriate than ground transport to a nearby community hospital that has no pediatric critical care, neurosurgical, or orthopedic resources. Brief efforts at peripheral venous access are unsuccessful. You begin crystalloid infusion through an intraosseous line. The patient's mother arrives just as you are transferring care to the helicopter crew. ∎

References

1. Gaines BA, Ford HR: Abdominal and pelvic trauma in children, *Crit Care Med* 30(11 suppl):S416, 2002.
2. American College of Surgeons Committee on Trauma: Extremes of age: pediatric trauma. In *Advanced trauma life support for doctors, student course manual*, ed 7, Chicago, 2004, ACS.
3. Winston FK, Durbin DR, Kallan MJ, Moll EK: The danger of premature graduation to seat belts for young children, *Pediatrics* 105(6):1179, 2000.
4. Grisoni ER, Pillai SB, Volsko TA, et al: Pediatric airbag injuries: the Ohio experience, *J Pediatr Surg* 35(2):160, 2000.
5. Durbin DR, Kallan M, Elliott M, et al: Risk of injury to restrained children from passenger air bags, *Traffic Injury Prev* 4(1):58, 2003.
6. American Academy of Pediatrics Committee on Injury and Poison Prevention: Selecting and using the most appropriate car safety seats for growing children: guidelines for counseling parents, *Pediatrics* 109(3):550, 2002.
7. Nance ML, Lutz N, Arbogast KB, et al: Optimal restraint reduces the risk of abdominal injury in children involved in motor vehicle crashes, *Ann Surg* 239(1):127, 2004.
8. Braver ER, Whitfield R, Ferguson SA: Seating positions and children's risk of dying in motor vehicle crashes, *Injury Prev* 4(3):181, 1998.
9. Bensard DD, Beaver BL, Besner GE, Cooney DR: Small bowel injury in children after blunt abdominal trauma: is diagnostic delay important? *J Trauma Injury Infect Crit Care* 41(3):476, 1996.
10. Allen GS, Moore FA, Cox CS Jr, et al: Hollow visceral injury and blunt trauma, *J Trauma Injury Infect Crit Care* 45(1):69, 1998.
11. Durbin DR, Kallan M, Elliott M, et al: Risk of injury to restrained children from passenger airbags, *Annu Proc Assoc Adv Auto Med* 46:15, 2002.
12. Gausche M, Lewis RJ, Stratton SJ, et al: Effect of out-of-hospital pediatric endotracheal intubation on survival and neurological outcome: a controlled clinical trial, *JAMA* 283(6):783, 2000.
13. Ehrlich PF, Seidman PS, Atallah D, et al: Endotracheal intubation in rural pediatric trauma patients, *J Pediatr Surg* 39:1376, 2004.
14. Davis DP, Hoyt DB, Ochs M, et al: The effect of paramedic rapid sequence intubation on outcome in patients with severe traumatic brain injury, *J Trauma Injury Infec Crit Care* 54(3):444, 2003.
15. Davis DP, Dunford JV, Poste JC, et al: The impact of hypoxia and hyperventilation on outcome after paramedic rapid sequence intubation of severely head-injured patients, *J Trauma Injury Infect Crit Care* 57(1):1, 2004.
16. Adelson PD, Bratton SL, Carney NA, et al: Guidelines for the acute medical management of severe traumatic brain injury in infants, children, and adolescents. Chapter 4. Resuscitation of blood pressure and oxygenation and prehospital brain-specific therapies for the severe pediatric traumatic brain injury patient, *Pediatr Crit Care Med* 4(3 suppl):S12, 2003.
17. York J, Arrillaga A, Graham R, Miller R: Fluid resuscitation of patients with multiple injuries and severe closed head injury: experience with an aggressive fluid resuscitation strategy, *J Trauma Injury Infect Crit Care* 48(3):376, 2000.
18. Manley G, Knudson MM, Morabito D, et al: Hypotension, hypoxia, and head injury: frequency, duration, and consequences, *Arch Surg* 136(10):1118, 2001.
19. Luten R: Error and time delay in pediatric trauma resuscitation: addressing the problem with color-coded resuscitation aids, *Surg Clin North Am* 82(2):303, 2002.
20. Winchell RJ, Hoyt DB: Endotracheal intubation in the field improves survival in patients with severe head injury, *Arch Surg* 132(6):592, 1997.

21. Davis DP, Ochs M, Hoyt DB, et al: Paramedic-administered neuromuscular blockade improves prehospital intubation success in severely head-injured patients, *J Trauma Injury Infect Crit Care* 55(4):713, 2003.

22. Pearson S: Comparison of intubation attempts and completion times before and after the initiation of a rapid sequence intubation protocol in an air medical transport program, *Air Med J* 22(6):28, 2003.

23. Stockinger ZT, McSwain NE Jr: Prehospital endotracheal intubation for trauma does not improve survival over bag-valve-mask ventilation, *J Trauma Injury Infect Crit Care* 56(3):531, 2004.

24. Murray JA, Demetriades D, Berne TV, et al: Prehospital intubation in patients with severe head injury, *J Trauma Injury Infect Crit Care* 49(6):1065, 2000.

25. Davis BD, Fowler R, Kupas DF, Roppolo LP: Role of rapid sequence induction for intubation in the prehospital setting: helpful or harmful? *Curr Opin Crit Care* 8(6):571, 2002.

26. Davis DP, Valentine C, Ochs M, et al: The Combitube as a salvage airway device for paramedic rapid sequence intubation, *Ann Emerg Med* 42(5):697, 2003.

27. Martin SE, Ochsner MG, Jarman RH, et al: Use of the laryngeal mask airway in air transport when intubation fails, *J Trauma Injury Infect Crit Care* 47(2):352, 1999.

28. Venkataraman ST, Thompson AE, Orr RA: Femoral vascular catheterization in critically ill infants and children, *Clin Pediatr* 36(6):311, 1997.

29. Carmona Suazo JA, Maas AI, van den Brink WA, et al: CO_2 reactivity and brain oxygen pressure monitoring in severe head injury, *Crit Care Med* 28(9):3268, 2000.

30. De Lorenzo RA: A review of spinal immobilization techniques, *J Emerg Med* 14(5):603, 1996.

31. Valadie LL: Child safety seats and the emergency responder, *Emerg Med Serv* 33(7):68, 2004.

32. National Vital Statistics System, Centers for Disease Control and Prevention: Deaths: final data for 1997, *MMWR* 47 (19):1, 1999.

33. Heins M: The "battered child" revisited, *JAMA* 251:3295, 1984.

34. Weimer CL, Goldfarb IW, Slater H: Multidisciplinary approach to working with burn victims of child abuse, *J Burn Care Rehabil* 9:79, 1988.

35. Hight DW, Bakalar HR, Lloyd JR: Inflicted burns in children: recognition and treatment, *JAMA* 242:517, 1979.

36. Feldman KW, Schaller RT, Feldman JA, McMillon M: Tap water scald burns in children, *Pediatrics* 62:1, 1978.

37. Montrey JS, Barcia PJ: Nonaccidental burns in child abuse, *South Med J* 78:1324, 1985.

38. Larson JT, Dietrich AM, Abdessalam SF, Werman HA: Effective use of the air ambulance for pediatric trauma, *J Trauma Injury Infect Crit Care* 56(1):89, 2004.

39. Eckstein M, Jantos T, Kelly N, Cardillo A: Helicopter transport of pediatric trauma patients in an urban emergency medical services system: a critical analysis, *J Trauma Injury Infect Crit Care* 53(2):340, 2002.

Suggested Reading

Anonymous: EMSC Partnership for Children/National Association of EMS Physicians model pediatric protocols: 2003 revision, *Prehosp Emerg Care* 8(4):343, 2004.

Chapter Objectives

*At the completion of this chapter, the reader
will be able to do the following:*

✓ Discuss the epidemiology of trauma in the elderly population.

✓ Discuss the anatomic and physiologic effects of aging as a factor in
causes of geriatric trauma and as a factor in the pathophysiology of
trauma.

✓ Explain the interaction of various preexisting medical problems with
traumatic injuries in elderly patients to produce differences in the
pathophysiology and manifestations of trauma.

✓ Explain the physiologic effects of specific common classes of
medications on the pathophysiology and manifestations of geriatric
trauma.

✓ Compare and contrast the assessment techniques and
considerations used in the elderly population with those used in
younger populations.

✓ Demonstrate modifications in spinal immobilization techniques for
safe and effective spinal immobilization of the elderly patient with
the highest degree of comfort possible.

✓ Compare and contrast the management of the elderly trauma patient
with that of the younger trauma patient.

✓ Assess the scene and elderly patients for signs and symptoms of
abuse and neglect.

CHAPTER 15

Geriatric Trauma

SCENARIO

Your unit is dispatched to the scene of a "man down." On initial scene assessment, you note that a senior citizen is lying prone on the side of the road. Bystanders indicate that the gentleman was walking erratically before he fell. While maintaining appropriate inline stabilization of the spine, you and your partner place the patient in the supine position. The patient has a laceration on his forehead and a large skin tear on his right forearm that are both bleeding freely. The patient has extensive contusions of the face and periorbital ecchymosis. He has sonorous agonal breathing. He is wearing a Medic Alert bracelet that indicates that he takes "blood thinners."

Was the injury the primary event or secondary to a medical event? Did the fall cause the significant injuries, or was there an antecedent event? How does the information that the patient is on anticoagulant therapy affect your level of suspicion for traumatic brain injury and for occult intrathoracic or intraabdominal hemorrhage? How do the patient's age, medical history, and medications interact with the injuries received to make the pathophysiology and manifestations different from those in younger patients? What potential medical problems would require chronic anticoagulant use? How will you modify your approach to the management of this patient, especially in terms of stabilizing his airway? Should advanced age alone be used as an additional criterion for transport to a trauma center?

The elderly population represents the fastest-growing age group in the United States. Gerontologists (medical specialists who study and care for elderly patients) divide the term *elderly* into three specific categories, as follows:

- *Middle age:* 50 to 64 years of age
- *Late age:* 65 to 79 years of age
- *Older age:* 80 years of age and older

Although such definitions are important for epidemiologic data, it is also important to recognize that the physiologic changes of aging occur along the entire age spectrum and vary among individuals. Recovery from closed head injury starts to decline in the mid-20s age group, and overall survival from trauma starts to decline in the late 30s. In addition, age is often associated with multiple preexisting medical conditions. The approach to the elderly patient includes recognition of this fact, although younger patients with comorbidities may share similar attributes.

More than 34 million Americans (12% of the U.S. population) are 65 years of age or older, and the size of this group has risen dramatically during the last 100 years. At the same time, fertility rates have dropped, meaning that there will be fewer people under 65 years of age to support the costs of health care and living expenses of those over 65 years of age. By the year 2050, nearly 25% of Americans will be eligible for Medicare, and the population over 85 years of age will grow from 4 million to 19 million.[1]

The injured elderly present unique challenges in prehospital care management, second only to those encountered with infants. The sudden illness and trauma in elderly patients present a different prehospital care dimension than

in younger patients. Some of the earliest data looking at the effect of age on outcome is from the Major Trauma Outcome Study by the American College of Surgeons Committee on Trauma.[2] Data from more than 3800 patients age 65 and older were compared to almost 43,000 patients less than age 65. Mortality increased over ages 45 to 55 and doubled by age 75 years. The age-adjusted risk occurs across the spectrum of injury severity, suggesting that injuries that could be easily tolerated by younger patients may result in mortality in those of advanced age.

Because older persons are more susceptible to critical illness and trauma than the rest of the population, a wider range of complications in patient assessment and management needs to be considered. Because elderly patients access medical care through emergency systems (e.g., 911), rendering care is different than for younger patients. The range of disabilities experienced by elderly patients is enormous, and field assessment may take longer than with younger patients. Difficulties in assessment can be expected as a result of sensory deficits in hearing and vision, senility, and physiologic changes.

Advances in medicine and an increasing awareness of healthier lifestyles during the last several decades have resulted in a significant increase in the percentage of the population over 65 years of age. Although trauma occurs most frequently in young people and geriatric emergencies are most often medical problems, a growing number of geriatric calls result from or include trauma. Trauma is the fifth leading cause of death in the elderly population, before diabetes mellitus, influenza, and Alzheimer's disease. Approximately 15% of injury-related deaths in elderly patients are classified as homicide. Trauma deaths in this age group account for 25% of all trauma deaths nationwide.[3]

Specific patterns of injury are also unique to the geriatric population.[4] Although motor vehicle crashes (MVCs) are the leading cause of death from trauma overall, falls are the predominant cause of traumatic death in patients over age 75. As with small children (age <5 years), scald injuries account for a greater percentage of burns in those over 65.

Progress in recent years has not only increased adult life expectancy but has also affected the quality of life and therefore the range of physical activities performed at older ages. As more people live longer and enjoy better health in their older years, more of them travel, drive, and continue active physical pursuits that can result in an associated increase in geriatric trauma. Many who could retire continue to work despite a health problem or advancing age.

Recent social changes have increased the number of older people living in independent housing, retirement communities, and other assisted-living facilities over those in nursing homes or other, more guarded and limited environments. This suggests a probable increase in the incidence of simple household trauma, such as falls, in elderly persons. The past few years have also seen an increase in geriatric victims of crime in the home and on the streets. Older people are often singled out as "easy marks" and can sustain substantial trauma from crimes of seemingly limited violence, such as purse snatching, when they are struck, are knocked down, or fall.

With the growing awareness of this expanding population at risk, the prehospital care provider must understand the unique needs of an elderly trauma patient. Specifically, the aging process and the effects of coexisting medical problems on an elderly patient's response to trauma and trauma management must be understood. The special considerations outlined in this chapter should be included in the assessment and management of any trauma patient who is 65 years of age or older, physically appears elderly, or is a middle-aged adult who has any of the significant medical problems typically associated with the elderly population.

Anatomy and Physiology of Aging

The aging process causes changes in physical structure, body composition, and organ function, and it can create unique problems during prehospital care. The aging process does influence mortality and morbidity rates.

Aging, or *senescence,* is a natural biologic process and is sometimes referred to as a process of "biologic reversal" that begins during the years of early adulthood. At this time, organ systems have achieved maturation, and a turning point in physiologic growth has been reached. The body gradually loses its ability to maintain homeostasis (the state of relative constancy of the body's internal environment), and viability declines over a period of years until death occurs.

The fundamental process of aging occurs at the cellular level and is reflected in both anatomic structure and physiologic function. The period of "old age" is generally characterized by frailty, slower cognitive processes, impairment of psychological functions, diminished energy, the appearance of chronic and degenerative diseases, and a decline in sensory acuity. Functional abilities are lessened, and the well-known external signs and symptoms of older age appear, such as skin wrinkling, changes in hair color and quantity, osteoarthritis, and slowness in reaction time and reflexes (Figure 15-1).

Influence of Chronic Medical Problems

As people age, they experience the normal physiologic changes of aging and can also experience more medical problems. Although some individuals can reach an advanced age without any serious medical problems, statistically an older person is more likely to have one or more significant medical conditions. Seniors presently consume more than one third of health care resources in the United States.[5] Usually, proper medical care can control these conditions, avoiding or minimizing exacerbation into repeated acute and often life-threatening episodes. Some older individuals have reached advanced age with minimal medical problems, whereas others may live with chronic illnesses and depend on modern medical means. This latter group can deteriorate more rapidly in an emergency situation.

Repeated acute episodes or even the single occurrence of a significant episode can result in chronic residual effects on the body. A patient who has previously had an acute myocardial infarction sustains permanent heart damage. The resultant reduced cardiac capacity continues for the rest of the patient's life, affecting the heart and, because of the ensuing chronic decline in circulation, other organs as well.

As a person's age advances, additional medical problems can occur. None is truly isolated because the influence on the body is cumulative. The total influence on the body usually is greater than the sum of each individual effect. As this condition progresses and reduces the quality of the body's vital functions, the individual's ability to withstand even modest anatomic or physiologic insults is greatly diminished.

Regardless of whether the patient is pediatric, middle-aged, or elderly, the priorities, intervention needs, and life-threatening conditions that usually result from serious trauma are the same. However, often because of preexisting physical conditions, elderly patients can also die from less severe injuries and die sooner than younger patients. Data support that preexisting conditions play a role in the survival of an elderly trauma patient (Table 15-1), and that

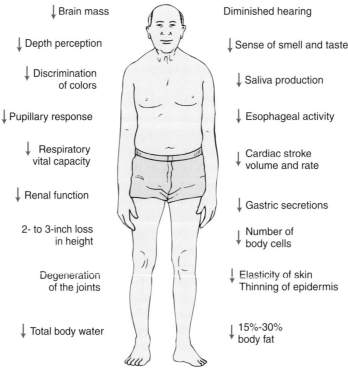

FIGURE 15-1　Changes caused by aging.

TABLE 15-1　Percentage of Patients with Preexisting Disease (PED)

Age (years)	PED (%)
15-24	2.8
25-34	8
35-44	17
45-54	30.8
55-64	44.1
65-74	50
>75	64.9

Modified from Milzman DP, Boulanger BR, Rodriguez A, et al: *J Trauma* 32:236, 1992.

TABLE 15-2　Number of Preexisting Diseases (PEDs) and Patient Outcome

Number of PEDs	Survived	Died	Mortality rate (%)
0	6341	211	3.2
1	868	56	6.1
2	197	36	15.5
3 or more	67	22	24.7

Modified from Milzman DP, Boulanger BR, Rodriguez A, et al: *J Trauma* 32:236, 1992.

the more conditions a trauma patient has, the higher his or her mortality rate (Table 15-2). Certain conditions are associated with a higher mortality rate because of the way in which they interfere with an elderly patient's ability to respond to trauma (Table 15-3).[6]

Ears, Nose, and Throat

Tooth decay, gum disease, and injury to teeth result in the need for various dental prostheses. The brittle nature of capped teeth, fixed bridges, or loose, removable bridges and dentures poses a special problem of foreign bodies that can be aspirated and obstruct the airway.

Changes in the contours of the face result from resorption of the mandible, in part because of absence of teeth *(edentulism)*. The characteristic look is an infolding and shrinking of the mouth. These changes can affect the ability to create an effective seal with a bag-valve-mask (BVM) device and sufficient visualization of the airway during endotracheal intubation. The nasopharyngeal tissues become increasingly fragile; in addition to the risk this quality poses to the initial trauma, interventions such as nasopharyngeal tubes may induce profuse bleeding if not placed with care.

Respiratory System

Changes in the airway and lungs of elderly persons may not always be related to senescence alone. Cumulative chronic exposure to environmental toxins over the course

TABLE 15-3   Prevalence of Preexisting Diseases (PEDs) and Associated Mortality Rates

PED	Number of patients	PED present (%)	Total (%)	Mortality rate (%)
Hypertension	597	47.9	7.7	10.2
Pulmonary disease	286	23	3.7	8.4
Cardiac disease	223	17.9	2.9	18.4
Diabetes	198	15.9	2.5	12.1
Obesity	167	13.4	2.1	4.8
Malignancy	80	6.4	1	20
Neurologic disorder	45	3.6	0.6	13.3
Renal disease	40	3.2	0.5	37.5
Hepatic disease	41	3.3	0.5	12.2

Modified from Milzman DP, Boulander BR, Rodriguez A, et al: *J Trauma* 32:236, 1992.

of their lives may be caused by occupational hazards or tobacco smoke. Also, innate changes may be expected to occur regardless of the effect of any toxins. Ventilatory function declines in the elderly person partly as a result of the inability of the chest cage to expand and contract and partly from stiffening of the airway. The increased stiffness in the chest wall is associated with a reduction in the ability to expand the chest wall and a stiffening of cartilaginous connections of the ribs. As a result of these changes, the chest cage is less pliable. With declines in the efficiency of the respiratory system, the elderly person requires more exertion to carry out daily activities.

The alveolar surface area decreases with age; it is estimated to decrease by 4% for each decade after 30 years of age. A 70-year-old person, for example, would have a 16% reduction in alveolar surface area. Any alteration of the already-reduced alveolar surface decreases oxygen uptake. Additionally, as the body ages, its ability to saturate hemoglobin with oxygen decreases, leading to lower baseline oxygen saturation as normal and less reserve available.[7] Because of impaired mechanical ventilation and diminished surface for gas exchange, the elderly trauma patient is less capable of compensating for physiologic losses associated with trauma.

Impaired cough and gag reflexes, along with poor cough strength and diminished esophageal sphincter tone, result in an increased risk of aspiration pneumonitis. A reduction in the number of *cilia* (hairlike processes that propel foreign particles and mucus from the bronchi) predisposes the elderly person to problems caused by inhaled particulate matter.

Another factor that affects the respiratory system is a change to the spinal curvature. Curvature changes accompanied by an anteroposterior hump (as seen in osteoporosis patients) often lead to additional ventilatory difficulty (Figure 15-2). Changes that affect the diaphragm can also contribute to ventilatory problems. Stiffening of the rib cage

can cause more reliance on diaphragmatic activity to breathe. This increased reliance on the diaphragm makes an older person especially sensitive to changes in intraabdominal pressure. Thus a supine position or a full stomach from a large meal can provoke ventilatory insufficiency. Obesity can also play a part in diaphragm restriction, especially when fat distribution tends to be central.

Cardiovascular System

Diseases of the cardiovascular system are the primary cause of death in the elderly population. Cardiovascular disease accounts for more than 3000 deaths per 100,000 persons over 65 years of age. In 2002, myocardial infarction accounted for 29% of deaths in the United States, with an additional 7% caused by stroke.[7]

Age-related decreases in arterial elasticity lead to increased peripheral vascular resistance. The myocardium and blood vessels rely on their elastic, contractile, and distensible properties to function properly. With aging, these properties decline, and the cardiovascular system becomes less efficient at moving circulatory fluids around the body. The cardiac output diminishes by approximately 50% from 20 to 80 years of age. As many as 10% of those over 75 years of age will have some degree of overt (asymptomatic) congestive heart failure.

Atherosclerosis is a narrowing of the blood vessels, a condition in which the inner layer of the artery wall thickens while fatty deposits build up within the artery. These deposits, called *plaque,* protrude above the surface of the inner layer and decrease the diameter of the internal channel of the vessel. The same luminal narrowing occurs in the coronary vessels. Almost 50% of the U.S. population have coronary artery stenosis by age 65 years.[8]

One result of this narrowing is *hypertension,* a condition that affects one of six adults in the United States. The calcification of the arterial wall reduces the ability of the

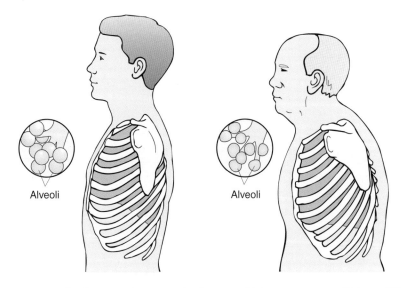

FIGURE 15-2 Spinal curvature can lead to an anteroposterior hump, which can cause ventilatory difficulties. Reduction in the alveolar surface area can also reduce the amount of oxygen that is exchanged in the lungs.

vessels to change size in response to endocrine and central nervous system stimuli. The lowered circulation can adversely affect any of the vital organs and is a common cause of heart disease. Of particular concern is that the baseline normal blood pressure of the elderly trauma patient may be higher than in younger patients. What would otherwise be accepted as normotension may indicate profound hypovolemic shock in the patient with preexisting hypertension.[9]

With age, the heart itself shows an increase in fibrous tissue and size *(myocardial hypertrophy)*. Atrophy of the cells of the conduction system results in the increased incidence of cardiac dysrhythmias. In particular, the normal reflexes in the heart that respond to hypotension diminish with age, resulting in the inability of elderly patients to increase their heart rate appropriately. Maximal heart rate also begins to decrease starting at age 40 years, calculated by the formula 220 minus the age in years. Patients with a permanent pacemaker have a fixed heart rate and cardiac output that cannot meet the demands of increased myocardial oxygen consumption accompanying the stress of trauma.

In the elderly trauma patient, this reduced circulation contributes to cellular hypoxia. The result is cardiac dysrhythmias, acute heart failure, and even sudden death. The body's ability to compensate for blood loss or other causes of shock is significantly lowered in the elderly person because of a diminished inotropic (cardiac contraction) response to catecholamines. In addition, total circulating blood volume decreases, creating less physiologic reserve for the blood loss of trauma. Diastolic dysfunction makes the patient more dependent on atrial filling to augment cardiac output, which is diminished in hypovolemic states.

The reduced circulation and circulatory defense responses, coupled with increasing cardiac failure, produce a significant problem in managing shock in the elderly trauma patient. Fluid resuscitation needs to be carefully monitored because of the reduced compliance of the cardiovascular system and the often "stiff" right ventricle. Care must be taken while treating hypotension and shock so as not to cause volume overloading with aggressive fluid resuscitation.[10]

Nervous System

As individuals age, brain weight and the number of neurons (nerve cells) decrease. The weight of the brain reaches its peak (1.4 kg, or 3 lb) at approximately 20 years of age. By 80 years of age, the brain loses about 10% of weight, with progressive cerebral atrophy.[11] The body compensates for the loss of space with increased cerebrospinal fluid. Although this additional space around the brain can protect it from contusion, it also allows for more brain movement in response to acceleration/deceleration injuries. The increased space in the cranial vault also explains why the elderly patient may have significant volumes of blood accumulate around the brain with minimal symptomatology.

The speed with which nerve impulses are conducted along certain nerves also decreases. These decreases result in only small effects on behavior and thinking. Reflexes are slower, but not to a significant degree. Compensatory functions can be impaired, particularly in patients with diseases such as Parkinson's disease, resulting in an increased incidence of falls. The peripheral nervous system is also affected by the slowing of nerve impulses, resulting in tremors and an unsteady gait.

General information and vocabulary abilities increase or are maintained, whereas skills requiring mental and muscular activity (psychomotor ability) may decline. The intellectual functions that involve verbal comprehension, arithmetic ability, fluency of ideas, experiential evaluation, and general knowledge tend to increase after 60 years of age in those who continue learning activities. Exceptions are those who develop senile dementia and other disorders such as Alzheimer's disease.

The normal biologic aging of the brain is not a predictor for diseases of the brain. However, decreases in the cortical structure of the brain may be involved in mental impairment. As changes occur in the brain, memory can be affected, and personality changes and other reductions in brain function can occur. These changes may involve the need for some form of mental health service. About 10% to 15% of elderly persons require professional mental health services. However, when assessing an elderly trauma patient, any impairment in mentation should be assumed to be the result of an acute traumatic insult, such as shock, hypoxia, or brain injury.

Sensory Changes
Vision and Hearing

Overall, approximately 28% of elderly persons have hearing impairment, and approximately 13% have visual impairment. Men tend to be more likely to have hearing difficulties, whereas both genders have a similar incidence of eye-related impairment.

Loss of vision is challenging at any age, and it may be even more problematic for the elderly person. The inability to read directions (e.g., on a prescription label) can lead to a disastrous effect. In addition, elderly persons experience decreases in visual acuity, ability to differentiate colors, and night vision.

The cells of the lens of the eye are incapable of restoration to their original molecular structure. One of the destructive agents over years of exposure is ultraviolet radiation. Eventually, the lens loses its capability to increase in thickness and curvature. The result is almost universal farsightedness *(presbyopia)* in persons over 40 years of age, requiring glasses for reading.

As a result of changes to the various structures of the eye, elderly persons have more difficulty seeing in dimly lit environments. Decreased tear production leads to dry eyes and itching, burning, and the inability to keep the eyes open for long periods.

With age, the lens of the eye begins to become cloudy and impenetrable to light. This gradual process results in what is termed a *cataract,* or a milky lens that blocks and distorts light that enters the eye and blurs vision. Some degree of cataract formation is present in 95% of elderly persons. This deterioration of vision increases the risk of an MVC, particularly while driving at night.[12]

A gradual decline in hearing *(presbycusis)* is also characteristic of aging. Presbycusis is usually caused by loss of conduction of sound into the inner ear; the use of hearing aids can compensate for this loss to some degree. This hearing loss is most pronounced when the person attempts to discriminate complex sounds, such as when many people are speaking at once or with loud ambient noise present, such as the wailing of sirens.

Pain Perception

Because of the aging process and the presence of diseases such as diabetes, elderly persons may not perceive pain normally, placing them at increased risk of injury from excesses in heat and cold exposure. Many elderly persons have conditions such as arthritis that result in chronic pain. Living with daily pain can cause an increased tolerance to pain, which may result in a patient's failure to identify areas of injury. In evaluating patients, especially those who usually "hurt all over" or who appear to have a high tolerance to pain, areas where the pain has increased or where the painful area has enlarged should be located. The provider also notes whether the pain's characteristics or exacerbating factors have changed since the trauma occurred.

Renal System

Changes common with aging include reduced levels of filtration by the kidneys and a reduced excretory capacity. These changes should be considered when administering drugs normally cleared by the kidneys. Chronic renal inhibition typically affects elderly persons and contributes to a reduction in a patient's overall health status and ability to withstand trauma. For example, renal dysfunction may be one cause of chronic anemia, which would lower a patient's physiologic reserve.

Musculoskeletal System

Bone loses mineral as it ages. The loss of bone *(osteoporosis)* is unequal among the genders. During young adulthood, bone mass is greater in women than in men. However, bone loss is more rapid in women and accelerates after menopause. With this higher incidence of osteoporosis, older women have a greater probability of fractures, particularly of the neck of the femur (hip). Causes of osteoporosis include loss of estrogen levels, increased periods of inactivity, and inadequate intake and inefficient use of calcium.

Osteoporosis contributes significantly to hip fractures and spontaneous compression fractures of the vertebral bodies. The incidence approaches 1% per year for men and 2% for women over age 85 years.[13]

Older persons are sometimes shorter than they were in young adulthood because of dehydration of the vertebral discs. As the discs flatten, a loss of approximately 2 inches (5 cm) in height occurs between 20 and 70 years of age. *Kyphosis* (curvature of the spine) in the thoracic region can also contribute to height loss and is often caused by

FIGURE 15-3 Kyphosis, typically caused by osteoporosis.

FIGURE 15-4 Because of the elderly person's tendency to flex the legs, the arms appear longer.

osteoporosis (Figure 15-3). As the bones become more porous and fragile, erosion occurs anteriorly, and compression fractures of the vertebrae may develop. As the thoracic spine becomes more curved, the head and shoulders appear to be pushed forward (Figure 15-4). If chronic obstructive pulmonary disease (COPD), particularly emphysema, is present, the kyphosis may be more pronounced because of the increased development of the accessory muscles of breathing.

Absolute levels of growth hormones decrease with aging, in conjunction with a decline in responsiveness to anabolic hormones. The combined effect is a reduction in muscle mass after age 25 years of about 4% per decade until age 50, when the process accelerates to between 10% and 35% per decade. Muscle loss is measured microscopically by both absolute number of muscle cells and reduction in cell size.

Deficits that relate to the musculoskeletal system (e.g., inability to flex the hip or knee adequately with changes in terrain) predispose the elderly person to falls. Muscle fatigue can cause many problems that affect movement, especially falls. Changes in the body's normal posture are common, and changes in the spine make the curvature become more acute with aging. Some degree of osteoporosis is universal with aging. Because of this progressive bone resorption, the bones become less pliant, more brittle, and more easily broken. The decrease in bone strength, coupled with reduced muscle strength caused by less active exercise, can result in multiple fractures with only mild or moderate

force. The most common sites of long-bone fracture in elderly persons include the proximal femur, hip, humerus, and wrist. The increased incidence of falls as a mechanism of injury results in Colles' fractures of the distal radius, as the dorsiflexed hand is outstretched.

The entire vertebral column changes with age, primarily because of the effects of both osteoporosis and calcification *(osteophysis)* of the supporting ligaments. This calcification results in decreased range of motion and narrowing of the spinal canal. The narrowed canal and progressive osteophytic disease put these patients at high risk for spinal cord injury with even minor trauma. The narrowing of the spinal canal is called *spinal stenosis* and increases the likelihood of cord compression without any actual break in the bony cervical spine. The thoracic and lumbar spine degenerate progressively as well, and the combined forces of osteoporosis and posture changes lead to increased falls. A high level of suspicion for spinal injury is needed during patient assessment because more than 50% of vertebral compression fractures are asymptomatic.[14]

Skin

Significant changes in the skin and connective tissues are associated with aging and result in difficulties with response to trauma as well as direct wound healing. Cell numbers decrease, tissue strength is lost, and the skin has impaired functional status. As the skin ages, sweat and sebaceous glands are lost. Loss of sweat glands reduces the body's ability to regulate temperature. Loss of sebaceous glands, which produce oil, makes the skin dry and flaky. Production of melanin, the pigment that gives color to skin and hair, declines, causing an aging pallor. The skin thins and appears translucent, primarily because of changes in connective tissue. The thinning and drying of the skin also reduce its resistance to microorganisms, resulting in an increased infection rate with minor trauma. As elasticity is lost, the skin stretches and falls into wrinkles and folds, especially in areas of heavy use, such as those overlying the facial muscles of expression.

Loss of fatty tissue can predispose the elderly person to *hypothermia*. The loss of up to 20% of dermal thickness with advanced aged and an associated loss in vascularity are also responsible for impaired thermoregulatory dysfunction. However, hypothermia should also suggest the possibility of occult sepsis, hypothyroidism, or phenothiazine overdose in the elderly population. This loss of fatty tissue also leads to less padding over bony prominences, such as the head, shoulders, spine, buttocks, hips, and heels. Prolonged immobilization without additional padding can result in tissue necrosis and ulceration as well as increased pain and discomfort during treatment and transport. Thinning of the skin also results in the potential for significant tissue loss and injury in response to relatively low energy transfers.

Nutrition and the Immune System

With aging, reductions in lean body mass and decreases in metabolic rate cause a reduction in caloric needs. However, because of inefficient utilization mechanisms, protein needs may actually increase. These competing changes often result in preexisting malnutrition in the elderly trauma patient. The financial status of retired individuals may also affect their choices of and access to quality nutrition.

As the immune system ages, its ability to function decreases. Grossly, organs associated with the immune response (thymus, liver, and spleen) all decrease in size. A decrease in cell-mediated and humoral responses also results. Coupled with any preexisting nutritional problems common in the elderly population, this leads to an increased susceptibility to infection. *Sepsis* is a common cause of late death after severe or even insignificant trauma in the elderly patient.

Assessment

Prehospital assessment of the elderly patient is based on the same method used for all trauma patients. Although the methodology is unchanged, the process may be altered in elderly patients. As with all trauma patients, however, the mechanism of injury should be considered first. This

section discusses some special considerations in assessing an elderly trauma patient.

Mechanism of Injury
Falls

Falls are the leading cause of trauma death and disability in those over 75 years of age. Approximately one third of community-dwelling people over 65 years of age fall each year, increasing to 50% by 80 years of age. Men and women fall with equal frequency, but women are more than twice as likely to sustain a serious injury because of more pronounced osteoporosis.

Most falls result from the inherent nature of aging, with the changes in posture and gait.[15] Declining visual acuity from cataracts, glaucoma, and loss of night vision contributes to the loss of visual clues used by elderly persons to navigate safely. Diseases of the central and peripheral nervous systems and the vascular instability of cardiovascular disease further precipitate falls. However, the most important variables contributing to falls in elderly persons are physical barriers in their environment, such as slippery floors, stairs, poorly fitting shoes, and poor lighting.

Long-bone fractures account for the majority of injuries, with fractures of the hip resulting in the greatest mortality and morbidity rates. The mortality rate from hip fractures is 20% at 1 year after the injury and rises to 33% at 2 years. Mortality is most often secondary to pulmonary embolus and the effects of decreased mobility.

Vehicular Trauma
MVCs are the leading cause of trauma death in the geriatric population between 65 and 74 years of age. An elderly patient is five times more likely to be fatally injured in an MVC than a younger driver, even though excessive speed is rarely a causative factor in the older age group.[16] For many reasons, elderly persons are often involved in collisions during daylight hours, during good weather, and close to their domicile.

These high fatality rates have been attributed to certain physiologic changes. In particular, subtle changes in memory and judgment together with impaired visual and auditory acuity can result in delayed reaction time. A common finding at crash investigations is that the elderly driver failed to yield to traffic. The National Highway Traffic Safety Administration has produced a CD-ROM program to assist physicians in assessing and counseling older drivers.

Alcohol is rarely involved, unlike with MVCs in younger persons. Only 6% of fatally injured elderly persons are intoxicated, compared with 23% for all other age categories.[16]

Elderly pedestrians represent more than 20% of all pedestrian fatalities. Because of slower walking speeds, the time allowed by traffic signals may be too short for the elderly person to traverse the crosswalk safely. This may explain the observation that more than 45% of all elderly pedestrian fatalities occur near a crosswalk.

Assault and Domestic Abuse

Abuse is defined as willful infliction of injury, unreasonable confinement, intimidation, or cruel punishment resulting in physical or psychological harm or pain, or the withholding of services that would prevent these. The elderly are highly vulnerable to crime. Violent assaults have been estimated to account for more than 10% of trauma admissions in elderly patients. The need for chronic care because of debilitation may predispose an elderly person to abuse or neglect from his or her caregivers. It is estimated that only about 15% of cases are reported to the proper authorities[17,18] (see later discussion).

Burns

Elderly patients represent 20% of burn unit admissions, with an estimated 1500 fire-related deaths per year. Burn fatalities in elderly patients occur from burns of smaller size and severity compared with other age groups. Fatality rates are seven times those of younger burn victims.

Because of impairments in visual and auditory acuity, elderly persons may have delayed recognition of house fires. Decreased pain perception can result in more significant burns. Thinning of dermal elements may result in a deeper thickness of burns.

The presence of preexisting medical conditions, such as cardiovascular disease and diabetes, results in poor tolerance to the resuscitative care of burns. Vascular collapse and infection are the most common causes of death from burns in elderly patients.

Traumatic Brain Injury

The brain has undergone a 10% reduction in mass by 70 years of age. The dura mater adheres more closely to the skull, resulting in a loss of some brain volume. The dural bridging veins become more stretched and thus susceptible to tearing. This results in a lower frequency of epidural hemorrhage and a higher frequency of subdural hemorrhage. Because of brain atrophy, a fairly large subdural hemorrhage can exist with minimal clinical findings. The combination of head trauma and hypovolemic shock yields a greater fatality rate. Preexisting medical conditions or their treatment may be a cause of altered mentation in elderly patients. When in doubt as to whether confusion represents an acute or chronic process, the injured patient should be preferentially transported to a trauma center for evaluation when possible.

Airway

Evaluation of the elderly patient begins with assessment of the airway. Changes in mentation may be associated with the tongue blocking the airway. The oral cavity should be examined for foreign bodies, such as dentures, that have become dislodged.

Breathing

Elderly patients who breathe at a rate of less than 10 or greater than 30 breaths/min, similar to any other adult, will not have adequate minute volume and will require positive-pressure assisted ventilations. In most adults a ventilatory rate between 12 and 20 breaths/min is normal and confirms that an adequate minute volume is present. However, in an elderly patient, reduced tidal volume capacity and pulmonary function may result in an inadequate minute volume even at rates of 12 to 20 breaths/min. Breath sounds should be immediately assessed if the ventilatory rate is abnormal.

Circulation

Delayed capillary refilling time is common in the elderly because of less efficient circulation; therefore it is a poor indicator of acute circulatory changes in these patients. Some degree of decreased distal motor, sensory, and circulatory ability in the extremities represents a common normal finding in elderly patients.

Some findings can only be interpreted properly by knowing the individual patient's preevent, or "baseline," status. Expected ranges of normal vital signs and other findings usually accepted as standard (normal) are not "normal" in every individual, and deviation is much more common in the elderly patient. Although the typical ranges are broad enough to include most individual adult differences, an individual of any age may vary beyond these norms; therefore, such variation in elderly patients should be expected. Medication may contribute to these changes. For example, in the average adult, a systolic blood pressure (SBP) of 120 mm Hg is considered normal and generally unimpressive. However, in the chronically hypertensive patient who normally has SBP of 150 mm Hg, a pressure of 120 mm Hg would be a concern, suggestive of hidden bleeding (or some other mechanism) of such a degree that decompensation has occurred. Likewise, heart rate is a poor indicator of trauma in elderly patients because of the effects of medications and the heart's poor response to circulating catecholamines (epinephrine). Quantitative information or signs should not be used in isolation from other findings. However, failing to recognize that such a change occurred, or that it is a serious pathologic finding in a particular patient, can produce a poor outcome for the patient.

Disability

All findings should be viewed as a group to maintain an increased level of suspicion in the elderly patient. Wide differences in mentation, memory, and orientation (to the past and present) can exist in elderly persons. Significant neurologic trauma should be identified in light of the individual's preinjury, normal status. Unless someone on the scene can describe this status, it should be assumed that the patient has a neurologic injury, hypoxia, or both. The ability to distinguish between a patient's chronic status and acute changes is an essential factor to prevent underreaction or overreaction to the patient's present neurologic status as a key index in evaluating his or her overall condition. However, unconsciousness remains a serious sign in all cases.

The elderly patient's orientation to time and place should be assessed by careful and complete questioning. People who work 5 days a week with weekends off usually know the day of the week. If they do not, it can be assumed that they have some level of disorientation. For those who no longer work a traditional job and who are often surrounded by others who do not, a lack of distinction between days of the week or even months of the year may not indicate disorientation but only of a lack of "calendar" importance in the structure of their lives. Similarly, people who no longer drive pay less attention to roads, town borders, locations, and maps. Although normally oriented, they may not be able to identify their present location. Confusion or the inability to recall events and details long past may be more indicative of how long ago the events occurred rather than how forgetful the individual is. Similarly, the repeated retelling of events long past and more attention paid to the far past than the immediate past often simply represent a nostalgic lingering on years and events. Such social and psychological compensations should not be considered as signs of senility or a diminished mental capacity.

Expose/Environment

Elderly persons are more susceptible to ambient environmental changes. They have a decreased ability to respond to changes, decreased heat production, and a decreased ability to rid the body of excessive heat. Thermoregulatory problems are related to an imbalance of electrolytes (e.g., potassium depletion, hypothyroidism, diabetes mellitus). Other factors include a decreased basal metabolic rate, decreased ability to shiver, arteriosclerosis, and effects of drugs and alcohol. Hyperthermia is affected by cerebrovascular accidents (strokes) and administration of diuretics, antihistamines, and antiparkinsonian drugs. Hypothermia is affected by decreased metabolism, fat, less efficient peripheral vasoconstriction, and poor nutrition.

Secondary Survey (Detailed History and Physical Examination)

In the assessment of acute illness, the following factors are important to consider after management of urgent life-threatening conditions. The prehospital care provider may take more than the average time in gathering information and taking a history with elderly patients.

- *The body may not respond the same as in younger patients.* Typical findings of serious illness, such as fever, pain, or tenderness, may take longer to develop and make it more difficult to evaluate the elderly patient. In addition, many medications will alter the body's response. Often a prehospital care provider will have to depend on history alone.

- *Additional patience may be needed because of the elderly patient's hearing or visual deficits.* Empathy and compassion are essential. A patient's intelligence should not be underestimated merely because communication may be difficult or absent. If the patient has close associates or relatives, they may participate in giving information or may stay nearby to help validate information. However, not all elderly patients have significant deficits. Speaking in a louder tone or slower cadence to the elderly patient may be unnecessary and insulting.

- *Assessment of the elderly patient requires different questioning tactics.* The patient should be asked for specific versus general information because elderly persons tend to respond "yes" to all questions during the assessment process. Asking open-ended questions is a useful tool in evaluating most patients. When dealing with a problem, however, providing specific details from which to choose can be helpful. For example, instead of saying, "Describe the pain in your hip," ask, "Is the pain in your hip sharp, stabbing, or dull?" or "On a scale of 1 to 10, with 10 being the most intense pain, how would you rate the pain?"

- *A significant other may need to be involved.* With the patient's permission, involving the caregiver or spouse may be necessary to gather valid information. It is important, however, to not approach elderly patients as if they were small children. A common mistake by health care professionals in both prehospital and emergency department settings is to treat the elderly in this way. Often, well-meaning relatives are so aggressive in reporting the events for an elderly loved one that they take over as the respondent to all inquiries. In such a situation, the provider can easily overlook that the clinical impression and history are from someone other than the patient and may not be correct. Not only does this increase the danger of obtaining incomplete or inaccurate information through a third party's impressions and translation, but it also discounts the patient as a mature adult. Some elderly patients may be reluctant to give information without the assistance of a relative or support person. However, the elderly patient may not want any other person present for many reasons, including abuse problems. The elderly patient may fear punishment for telling someone, in the presence of the abuser, why he or she has multiple bruise marks. Also, some problems may embarrass the elderly patient, and the person may not want any family members to know about them.

■ *Altered comprehension or neurologic disorders are a significant problem for many elderly patients.* These impairments can range from confusion to senile dementia of the type associated with Alzheimer's disease. Not only may these patients have difficulty in communicating, but they may also be unable to comprehend or help in the assessment. They may be restless and sometimes combative.

■ *Firmness, reassurance, and clear, simple (and repeated) questioning may be helpful.* Often a family member or friend can be of assistance.

■ *Pay attention to impaired hearing, sight, comprehension, and mobility capabilities.* Eye contact should be made with the patient. The patient may be hearing impaired and depend on watching your lips and other facial movements. Noise, distractions, and interruptions should be minimized. Fluency in speech, an involuntary movement, cranial nerve dysfunction, or difficulty breathing should be noted. Is the patient's movement easy, unsteady, or unbalanced?

■ *Shake the patient's hand to feel for grip strength, skin turgor, and body temperature.* The patient should be addressed by his or her last name, unless otherwise told by the patient. Phrases such as, "Now, now, you'll be fine," should be avoided. Open-ended questions such as, "Describe the pain in your abdomen, is it . . . ?" should be used, and such questions as, "Where does it hurt?" should be avoided.

■ *Look for behavioral problems or manifestations that do not fit the scene.* Look at grooming. Are the patient's attire and grooming appropriate for where and how the patient was found? The ease of rising or sitting should be observed. Is there the potential for elder abuse or neglect?

■ *Look at the patient's state of nourishment.* Does the patient appear to be well, thin, or emaciated? Elderly patients have a decreased thirst response. The kidneys have a problem in meeting the challenge of injury. The kidney's ability to concentrate urine is decreased, leading to dehydration even before injury. Urine output is a poor measure of perfusion in elderly persons. They also have a decreased amount of body fat (15%-30%) and total body water.

■ *Elderly patients have a decrease in skeletal muscle weight, widening and weakening of bones, degeneration of joints, and osteoporosis.* They have an increased probability of fractures with minor injuries and a greatly increased risk of fractures to the vertebrae, hip, and ribs.

■ *Elderly patients have degeneration of heart muscle cells and fewer pacemaker cells.* Elderly persons are prone to dysrhythmias as a result of a loss of elasticity of the heart and major arteries. Widespread use of beta and calcium channel blockers and diuretics further complicates this problem. Often after injury, elderly patients present with low cardiac output with hypoxia and have no lung injury. Cardiac stroke volume and rate decrease, as does cardiac reserve, all leading to morbidity and mortality in the elderly trauma patient. An elderly patient with SBP of 120 mm Hg should be considered to be in hypovolemic shock until proved otherwise.

■ *An elderly patient's vital capacity is diminished by 50%.* Kyphotic changes in the spine (anteroposterior) result in a ventilation-perfusion mismatch at rest. Hypoxia is much more likely to be a consequence of shock than in younger patients. Elderly patients also have a decreased ability for chest excursions. Lower tidal volumes and lower minute volumes are typical. Reductions in capillary oxygen and carbon dioxide exchange are significant. Hypoxemia tends to be progressive.

Medications

Knowledge of a patient's medications can provide key information in determining prehospital care. Preexisting disease in the elderly trauma patient is a significant finding. The following classes of drugs are of particular interest because of their frequent use by elderly persons and their potential to affect care of the trauma patient:

■ Beta blockers (e.g., propranolol, metoprolol) may account for a patient's absolute or relative bradycardia. In this situation, an increasing tachycardia as a sign of developing shock may not occur. The drug's inhibition of the body's normal sympathetic defense mechanisms can mask the true level of the patient's circulatory deterioration. Such patients can rapidly decompensate, seemingly without warning.

■ Calcium channel blockers (e.g., verapamil) may prevent peripheral vasoconstriction and accelerate hypovolemic shock.

■ Nonsteroidal antiinflammatory agents (e.g., ibuprofen) may contribute to platelet dysfunction and increase bleeding.

■ Anticoagulants (e.g., clopidogrel, aspirin, warfarin) may increase blood loss. Data suggest that use of warfarin increases the risk of isolated head injury and adverse outcome. Any bleeding from trauma will be more brisk and difficult to control when a patient is taking an anticoagulant. More importantly, internal bleeding can progress rapidly, leading to shock and death.

■ Hypoglycemic agents (e.g., insulin, metformin, rosiglitazone) may be causally related to the events that caused injury and may make blood glucose therapy difficult if their use is unrecognized.

FIGURE 15-5 Vial of Life program sticker to alert EMS providers that medical history and medication list is attached to the refrigerator door.

■ Herbal preparations are frequently used by elderly persons. Their inclusion in the list of medications is often omitted by patients, who should be specifically questioned about their use. These preparations are unregulated and thus have unpredictable dose effects and possible drug-drug interactions. Complications of these agents include bleeding (garlic) and myocardial infarction (ephedrine/Ma-Huang).

The difficulty in assessing the elderly trauma patient's medication list may include loss of consciousness and an extensive list of medications with difficult names. In some communities, emergency medical services (EMS) has promoted programs such as the Vial of Life Project (www.vialoflife.com).[19] In this program, the patient's detailed medical history is placed in a common location in any house, the refrigerator door. A sticker is applied to the front door of the home, alerting the prehospital team to the Vial of Life (Figure 15-5).

Management

Airway

The presence of dentures, common in the elderly population, may affect airway management. Ordinarily, dentures should be left in place to maintain a better seal around the mouth with a mask. However, partial dentures (plates) may become dislodged during an emergency and may occlude or partially block the airway; these should be removed.

Friable nasopharyngeal mucosal tissues and the possible use of anticoagulants put the elderly trauma patient at increased risk of bleeding from placement of a nasal trumpet. This hemorrhage may further compromise the patient's airway and result in aspiration. Arthritis may affect the temporomandibular joints and cervical spine. The

decreased flexibility of these areas may make endotracheal intubation more difficult.

The objective of airway management is primarily to ensure a patent airway for the delivery of adequate tissue oxygenation. Early mechanical ventilation by either bag-valve-mask (BVM) or endotracheal intubation should be considered early in elderly trauma patients because of their greatly limited physiologic reserve.[20]

Breathing

In all trauma patients, supplemental oxygen should be administered as soon as possible. The elderly population has a high prevalence of COPD. In the presence of COPD, the ventilatory drive of some patients is not dependent on the level of carbon dioxide (CO_2) in the blood but on diminished blood oxygen levels. However, oxygen should never be withheld from a seriously injured patient based on these concerns. If elevated CO_2 results in somnolence, assisted ventilation by BVM or even intubation is appropriate. Oxygen saturation (Spo_2) should generally be kept at greater than 95%.

Elderly persons experience increased stiffness of the chest wall. In addition, reduced chest wall muscle power and stiffening of the cartilage makes the chest cage less flexible. These and other changes are responsible for reductions in lung volumes. The elderly patient may need ventilatory support by assisted ventilations with a BVM device earlier than younger trauma patients. The mechanical force applied to the resuscitation bag may need to be increased by the prehospital provider to overcome the increased chest wall resistance.

Circulation

Hemorrhage in the elderly patient is controlled somewhat differently than in other patients. Elderly persons have poor cardiovascular reserve. Vital signs are a poor indicator of shock in the elderly patient because the patient who is normally hypertensive may be in shock with SBP of 110 mm Hg. Reduced circulating blood volume, possible chronic anemia, and preexisting myocardial and coronary disease leave the patient with very little tolerance for even modest amounts of blood loss. Early control of hemorrhage through direct pressure on open wounds, stabilization or immobilization of fractures, and rapid transport to a trauma center are essential. Fluid resuscitation should be guided by the index of suspicion for serious bleeding based on the mechanism of injury and an overall appearance of shock.

Immobilization

Protection of the cervical spine, particularly in trauma patients who have sustained multisystem injury, is an expected standard of care. In the elderly population, this standard of care must apply not only in trauma situations but also during acute medical problems in which attempts to maintain airway patency is a priority. Degenerative arthritis of the cervical spine may subject the elderly patient to spinal cord injury from maneuvering the neck, even if the patient has no injury to the bony spine. Another consideration with improper movement of the cervical spine is the possibility of occlusion of the arteries to the brain, which can result in unconsciousness and even stroke.

A cervical collar applied to an elderly patient with severe kyphosis should not compress the airway or carotid arteries. Less traditional means of immobilization, such as a rolled towel and head block, can be considered if standard collars are inappropriate.

Padding may need to be placed under the patient's head and between the shoulders when immobilizing the supine elderly patient. Because of the lack of adipose tissue in the frail elderly patient, additional padding will be required when the patient is immobilized to a long backboard. The prehospital care provider will check for pressure points where the patient is resting on the board and pad appropriately. When applying the straps to secure the patient, the elderly patient may not be able to straighten the legs fully because of decreased range of motion of the hips and knees. This may require the placement of padding under the legs for comfort and security of the patient during transport.[21]

Temperature Control

The elderly patient should be monitored closely for hypothermia and hyperthermia during treatment and transportation. Although it is appropriate to expose the patient to facilitate a thorough examination, elderly persons are especially prone to heat loss. The effects of various medications may mean that a patient is more prone to overheating; therefore, some means of cooling the patient should be considered if the patient is unable to be moved quickly to a controlled environment. Prolonged extrication in the extremes of heat and cold may also place the elderly patient at risk and should be rapidly addressed. External methods of heating or cooling the elderly trauma patient should be balanced by the possibility of direct thermal injury to the site of application with the patient's attenuated skin structure.

Legal Considerations

Several legal distinctions can become issues when giving care to the elderly trauma patient. Recent evidence demonstrates that although mortality increases with age, 80% of discharged geriatric trauma patients return to a high functional level. Under certain circumstances, the patient or family member may forego potentially lifesaving interventions and provide comfort measures only (e.g., elderly patient with extensive burns). The patient's most appropriate care plan can be assisted by identifying a living will, advance directives, or other legal documents, if provided to them at the scene.

In most of the United States, spouses, siblings, children, spouses of children, and parents have no legal standing in making medical decisions for an adult. Persons with power of attorney or court-appointed conservators may have authority over an individual's financial affairs, but they do not necessarily have control over that individual's personal medical decisions. Court-appointed custodians or guardians may or may not have the power to make medical decisions, depending on the local laws and the specific charge of their appointment. Such powers are considered to exist only when a guardianship of person or a durable power of attorney for health care is specified and clear documentation of such third-party powers is present.

In the midst of a trauma scene, it may be difficult to make such a fine legal distinction. Because the ambulance was summoned and a "call for help" was made, the basis of "implied consent" to care for the patient applies in cases of patients who are unconscious or have reduced mental capacity.

Should further clarification be necessary or should anyone attempt prehospital care, the problem should be presented to the police officer in charge at the scene. The law generally provides a protocol for an officer to make a timely decision at the scene, with clarification to occur later at the hospital when time allows. Such events should be documented carefully and completely as a part of the run report.

Elder Abuse and Neglect

Elder abuse is defined as any action by an elderly person's family member (any relative), associated persons who have daily household contact (housekeeper, roommate), anyone on whom the elderly person is reliant for daily needs of food, clothing, and shelter, or a professional caregiver who takes advantage of the elderly person's property or emotional state.

Reports and complaints of abuse, neglect, and other related problems among the elderly population are increasing. The exact extent of elder abuse is not known for the following reasons:

1. Elder abuse has been largely hidden from society.
2. Abuse and neglect of elderly persons have varying definitions.
3. Elders are uneasy or fearful of reporting the problem to law enforcement agencies or human and social welfare personnel. A typical victim of elder abuse may be a

parent who feels ashamed or guilty because he or she raised the abuser. The abused may also feel traumatized by the situation or fear continued reprisal by the abuser.
4. Some jurisdictions lack formal reporting mechanisms. Some areas do not even have a statutory provision requiring the reporting of elder abuse.

The physical and emotional signs of abuse, such as rape, beating, or nutritional deprivation, are often overlooked or perhaps are not accurately identified. Older women in particular are not likely to report incidents of sexual assault to law enforcement agencies. Sensory deficits, senility, and other forms of altered mental status (e.g., drug-induced depression) may make it impossible or extremely difficult for the elderly patient to report the maltreatment.

Profile of the Abused

The elderly adult most likely to be abused falls into the following profile:

- Over 65 years of age, especially women over 75 years of age
- Frail
- Multiple chronic medical conditions
- Demented
- Impaired sleep cycle, sleepwalking, or loud shouting at night
- Incontinent of feces, urine, or both
- Dependent on others for activities of daily living or incapable of independent living

Profile of the Abuser

Because many elderly people live in a family environment and are typically women older than 75 years of age, that environment may provide clues. The abuser is frequently the spouse of the patient or the middle-age daughter-in-law of the patient who is caring for dependent children and dependent parents while perhaps holding full-time or part-time employment. Most of these abusers are untrained in the particular care required by the elderly and have little relief time from the constant care demands of their family.

Abuse is not restricted to the home. Other environments such as nursing, convalescent, and continuing care centers are sites where the elderly may sustain physical, chemical, or pharmacologic harm. Care providers in these environments may consider elderly persons to represent management problems or categorize them as obstinate or undesirable patients. The usual profile of the abuser includes the following signs:

- Existence of household conflict
- Marked fatigue
- Unemployment

- Financial difficulties
- Substance abuse
- Previous history of being abused

Categories of Abuse

Abuse can be categorized in the following three ways:

1. *Physical abuse* includes assault, neglect, malnutrition, poor maintenance of the living environment, and poor personal care. The signs of physical abuse or neglect may be obvious, such as the imprint left by an item (e.g., fireplace poker), or may be subtle (e.g., malnutrition). The signs of elder abuse are similar to those of child abuse (Figure 15-6) (see Chapter 14).
2. *Psychological abuse* can take on the forms of neglect, verbal abuse, infantilization, or deprivation of sensory stimulation.
3. *Financial abuse* can include theft of valuables or embezzlement.

Important Points

Many abused patients are terrorized into making false statements for fear of retribution. In the case of elder abuse by family members, fear of removal from the home environment can cause the elderly patient to lie about the origin of the abuse. In other cases of elder abuse, sensory deprivation or dementia may deter adequate explanation. The prehospital care provider should identify abuse and uncover any pathology reported by the patient.

Further trauma may be reduced to a patient by identifying an abusive situation. Reporting a high index of suspicion for abuse can allow for referral and protective services from human, social, and public safety agencies (Box 15-1).

Disposition

One of the greatest challenges with prehospital care of the injured patient is defining which patients are most likely to benefit from the surgeons and advanced treatment options available at a trauma center. For many of the reasons mentioned previously, triage criteria may be less reliable in the elderly patient because of physiologic or pharmacologic effects. A major recommendation in the *Guidelines for Geriatric Trauma* of the Eastern Association for the Surgery of Trauma is that trauma patients of advanced age should have a lower threshold to be triaged directly to a trauma center.[22] Data from several states demonstrate that a disproportionate number of elderly trauma patients are receiving care at trauma centers. Furthermore, potentially preventable mortality in the geriatric trauma population is lower at trauma centers.

FIGURE 15-6   Signs of physical abuse of elderly persons. **A,** Bruising caused by a punch. This woman agreed to go the hospital only because she was advised to by the police. When about to leave, she mentioned discomfort in her neck. X-ray examination showed a fracture of the body of C6. **B,** Wound of the scalp. The scalp is a common site of elder abuse that often causes hemorrhagic shock.
(From London PS: *A colour atlas of diagnosis after recent injury,* London, 1990, Wolfe.)

BOX 15-1   **Reporting Elder Abuse and Neglect**
In many states, EMS personnel are legally considered to be mandated reporters of suspected elder (or *adult*) abuse, neglect, and exploitation. *Abuse* is considered the deliberate infliction of pain, injury, mental anguish, unreasonable confinement, or nonconsensual sexual contact. *Neglect* involves living in conditions in which the adult or responsible caretaker is not providing care required to maintain the elderly person's physical and mental health and well-being. *Exploitation* is the illegal use of an adult's resources for another's gain or advantage. In recent years, elder abuse has been increasingly recognized. However, younger adults who have incapacitating conditions such as mental illness, mental retardation, and physical disability are also at risk for abuse and neglect.
Signs of abuse and neglect include unexplained or unusual injuries; conflicting accounts of how an injury occurred; a caregiver who prevents the adult from speaking with others; dehydration or malnutrition; depression; lack of access to medications, eyeglasses, dentures, or other aids; lack of personal hygiene; unkempt environment; and lack of adequate heating and cooling.
Mandated reporters must report directly to the social services agency responsible for investigating adult abuse, rather than relying on intermediaries such as hospital personnel. If the individual is in immediate danger or has been sexually assaulted, law enforcement must be notified as well. In the event that a death appears to have been caused by abuse or neglect, mandatory reporters generally must notify the office of the medical examiner or coroner and law enforcement. Mandatory reporters are liable for failing to report suspected abuse, neglect, and exploitation. However, they are protected against civil and criminal liability associated with reporting, may be able to keep their identity confidential, and are allowed to share medical information that is related to the case, although this information would be protected under the Health Insurance Portability and Accountability Act (HIPAA) in normal circumstances. Laws governing the mandatory reporting of elder abuse are enacted at the state level. All EMS providers must be aware of the laws in the state in which they work.

Prolonged Transport

The majority of care of the elderly trauma patient follows general guidelines for prehospital care of the injured patient. However, several special circumstances exist in prolonged transport scenarios. These concerns are particularly important for the recommendations to triage patients with less significant anatomic injuries directly to trauma centers.

Treatment of shock in the prehospital environment over an extended period requires careful reassessment of vital signs during transport. After control of hemorrhage with local measures, fluid resuscitation should be titrated to physiologic response to optimize resuscitation of intravascular volume status while avoiding potential volume overload in a patient with impaired cardiac function. A pneumatic antishock garment (PASG) is used less often than in the past but may be used in transport from remote areas to stabilize pelvic and lower extremity fractures. However, the PASG may precipitate congestive heart failure in patients with preexisting disease. It may also impair ventilation by increasing pressure on the diaphragm that elderly persons rely on for ventilation to a great extent because of decreased chest wall compliance. The decision to place the PASG on an elderly trauma patient requires increased vigilance in observing for associated complications.

Immobilization on a long backboard places these patients at increased risk for pressure-related skin breakdown over extended transports. Weakened skin structure and impaired vascular supply may lead to earlier complications than expected. Over long transports, consideration should be given to appropriate padding to protect the patient. Agencies in remote regions should consider purchasing a specially designed, low-pressure backboard that immobilizes the patient while limiting the potential for skin breakdown.

Environmental control is essential in geriatric patients with a lengthy transport. Limiting body exposure and controlling ambient temperature of the vehicle may limit hypothermia. The hypothermic patient may shiver, producing anaerobic metabolism, leading to lactic acidosis, and accelerating shock.

Finally, transport of the geriatric trauma patient from remote regions may be a valid use of aeromedical transport. Transport via helicopter may limit the duration of environmental exposure, reduce the duration of shock, and ensure earlier access to hospital-based care, including early surgery and blood transfusion.

SUMMARY

Elderly persons are living healthier, more active, and longer lives than ever before. As a result, trauma has become a significant cause of morbidity and mortality among older adults. The elderly represent a unique population of trauma patients. Although general guidelines for care of the injured patient remain the same, several specific approaches are unique to care of the injured geriatric patient. Anatomic and physiologic changes associated with aging, chronic disease, and medications can make certain types of trauma more likely, complicate traumatic injuries, and cause a decreased ability to compensate for shock. Older patients have less physiologic reserve and tolerate physical insult poorly.

Knowledge of the elderly trauma patient's medical history and medications is an essential component of care. Many factors in elderly trauma patients can mask early signs of deterioration, increasing the possibility of sudden, rapid decompensation without apparent warning. Even simple isolated trauma can progress to an acute systemic condition and produce potentially life-threatening conditions in elderly patients. Awareness of the unique patterns of injury in elderly patients, including elder abuse is needed. Proactive, timely care is particularly important in the treatment of the elderly trauma patient. A lower threshold for direct triage of these patients to trauma centers is important.

With an elderly trauma patient, more serious injury may have occurred than indicated by the initial presentation. The injuries and conditions found will have a more profound effect than in a younger patient. By including these considerations, the prehospital care provider will be forewarned, will manage the patient in a more anticipatory manner, and will provide better, safer care to the older trauma patient.

SCENARIO SOLUTION

When dealing with trauma in the elderly patient, you cannot always determine immediately whether the trauma was the primary event or whether it was secondary to a medical event, such as a stroke, myocardial infarction, or syncopal episode. However, you always need to consider the possibility that a significant medical event preceded the trauma. This patient could also have sustained significant blunt force trauma before the collapse (e.g., abuse, violent crime). Because this patient is receiving anticoagulant therapy and has evidence of impaired blood clotting, you are alerted that any bleeding from traumatic brain injury or internal injury will be increased as a result.

Trauma in the elderly patient may be exacerbated by the effects of aging, disease, and medications. These factors may also distort the normal findings associated with shock. Similarly, preexisting illness and physiologic changes caused by aging may be aggravated by otherwise less serious trauma, creating a more serious situation in the older trauma patient than the same injury in a younger patient.

You approach the elderly trauma patient with an index of suspicion for injuries in which the signs and symptoms may be masked by the effects of aging, disease, or medications. You are also alert to the possibility of injuries sustained with less significant mechanisms than in younger patients. Of particular concern is modification of cervical spine immobilization because of increased curvature of the spine. Airway management may be more challenging because changes in facial structure may make it difficult to achieve a seal with a mask. In addition, for a variety of reasons, elderly patients are more prone to aspiration. This scenario involves an elderly patient with injuries serious enough to warrant direct transport to a trauma center. However, elderly patients with even less apparent physiologic compromise should be considered for immediate triage to a trauma center. ∎

References

1. Scommegna P: US growing bigger, older, and more diverse, Population Reference Bureau, 2005, http://www.prb.org/.
2. Champion H et al: The Major Trauma Outcome Study: establishing national norms for trauma care, *J Trauma* 30(11):1356, 1990.
3. Weigelt J: Trauma. Advanced trauma life support for doctors. In *Advanced trauma life support,* ed 6, Chicago, 1997, ACS.
4. Jacobs D: Special considerations in geriatric injury, *Curr Opin Crit Care* 9(6):535, 2003.
5. US Department of Health and Human Services, Centers for Disease Control and Prevention, National Center for Health Statistics: *Access to health care.* Part 3. Older adults, 2005, http://www.cdc.gov/nchs/.
6. Milzman DP, Boulanger BR, Rodriguez A, et al: Pre-existing disease in trauma patients: a predictor of fate independent of age and injury severity score, *J Trauma* 32:236, 1992.
7. Smith T: Respiratory system: aging, adversity, and anesthesia. In McCleskey CH, editor: *Geriatric anesthesiology,* Baltimore, 1997, Williams & Wilkins.
8. US Department of Health and Human Services, Centers for Disease Control and Prevention, National Center for Health Statistics: *Stroke and cerebrovascular diseases,* 2005, http://www.cdc.gov/nchs/.
9. US Department of Health and Human Services, Centers for Disease Control and Prevention, National Center for Health Statistics: *Hypertension,* 2005, http://www.cdc.gov/nchs/.
10. Abrams K et al: Management of trauma in the geriatric patient, *Curr Opin Anaesthesiol* 17(2):165, 2004.
11. Carey J: *Brain facts: a primer on the brain and nervous system,* Washington, DC, 2002, Society for Neuroscience, www.sfn.org.
12. US Department of Health and Human Services, National Institutes of Health, National Eye Institute: *Cataract: what you should know,* 2005, http://www.nei.nih.gov/health/cataract/cataract_facts.asp.
13. Alexander J, Shneiderman A: *Vertebral fracture,* 2004, http://www.emedicine.com/med/topic2895.htm.
14. Blackmore C: Cervical spine injury in patients 65 years old and older: epidemiologic analysis regarding the effects of age and injury mechanism on distribution, type, and stability of injuries, *Am J Roentgenol* 178:573, 2002.
15. Tinetti M: Preventing falls in elderly persons, *N Engl J Med* 348:42, 2003.
16. US Department of Health and Human Services, Centers for Disease Control and Prevention, National Center for Health Statistics: *Older adult drivers: fact sheet,* 2005, http://www.cdc.gov/nchs/.
17. US Department of Health and Human Services, US Administration on Aging, National Center on Elder Abuse, 2005, http://www.elderabusecenter.org/.
18. US Department of Health and Human Services, US Administration on Aging: *Elder rights and resources,* 2005, http://www.aoa.gov/eldfam/Elder_Rights/Elder_Rights.asp.
19. Vial of Life, 2005, http://www.vialoflife.com/index_old.html.
20. Heffner J, Reynolds S: Airway management of the critically ill patient, *Chest* 127:1397, 2005.
21. American Geriatric Society: *Geriatric education for emergency medical services (GEMS),* Sudbury, Mass, 2003, Jones & Bartlett.
22. Eastern Association for the Surgery of Trauma: Guidelines for geriatric trauma. In *Practice management guidelines,* www.east.org/tpg/geriatric.pdf.

Suggested Reading

American College of Surgeons Committee on Trauma: Extremes of age: geriatric trauma. In *Advanced trauma life support for doctors, student course manual*, ed 7, Chicago, 2004, ACS.

Lavoie A, Ratte S, Clas D, et al: Preinjury warfarin use among elderly patients with closed head injuries in a trauma center, *J Trauma* 56:802, 2004.

Tepas JJ 3rd, Veldenz HC, Lottenberg L, et al: Elderly trauma: a profile of trauma experience in the sunshine (retirement) state, *J Trauma* 48:581, 2000.

Victorino GP, Chong TJ, Pal JD: Trauma in the elderly patient, *Arch Surg* 138:1093-1097.

Chapter Objectives

*At the completion of this chapter, the reader
will be able to do the following:*

✓ Give the reason why heat stroke is considered a life-threatening condition.

✓ Differentiate between heat stroke and hyponatremia.

✓ List two effective cooling procedures for heat exhaustion and heat stroke.

✓ List the five factors that place prehospital care providers at risk for heat illness.

✓ Explain the fluid hydration guidelines and how they should be used to prevent dehydration in hot or cold environments.

✓ Differentiate the management of mild hypothermia from that of severe hypothermia.

✓ List the signs of mild frostbite, and discuss how to prevent its progression.

✓ Discuss the rationale for the statement, "patients are not dead until they are warm and dead."

CHAPTER 16

Environmental Trauma I: Heat and Cold

SCENARIO

On a sunny, hot, and humid summer afternoon (98° F [36.6° C], 65% relative humidity), a medic unit responds to a dispatch for an unconscious patient. On arrival, two paramedics find a lethargic, overweight, 60-year-old male lying prone on a neighborhood hiker-biker trail, appearing flushed, with hot and moist face and forearms. The lead paramedic conducts the initial assessment and finds rapid and shallow respirations and a rapid pulse while the second paramedic asks the bystanders about the patient and any events preceding this incident. A fellow hiker states that the patient was acting confused and did not understand what was being said just before he passed out, and that he takes prescription medications for allergies and depression.

What is your general impression of this patient? Is this an emergency situation? What factors make this patient susceptible to this condition? How would you assess the patient, and what are the initial treatment interventions? What is the heat index when the paramedics arrived at the scene, and how does this impact the patient's condition? Do you have any concern about the prehospital care providers working in this hot environment? ■

This chapter focuses on recognizing and treating exposure to heat and cold temperatures because the most significant morbidity and mortality in the United States from all environmental trauma are caused by thermal trauma.[1-3]

Thermal Trauma

Environmental extremes of heat and cold have a common outcome of injuries and potential death that can affect many individuals during the peak summer and winter months. Individuals who are susceptible to both highs and lows of temperature are very young persons, the elderly population, urban poor people, individuals who take specific medications, chronically ill patients, and alcoholic persons.[3-6] The majority of emergency medical services (EMS) responses in the United States for heat and cold injuries are for the *hyperthermic* and *hypothermic* patient in an urban setting. However, emerging interest in recreational and high-risk adventure activities in the wilderness backcountry during periods of environmental extremes places more individuals at risk for heat-related and cold-related injuries and fatalities.[7-10]

Epidemiology

Heat-Related Illness

During a 20-year period (1979-1999) in the United States, 8015 heat-related deaths from all causes were recorded.[2] More deaths were caused by heat stress than by hurricanes, lightning, tornadoes, floods, and earthquakes combined. Of these, 3829 (48%) deaths were related to high ambient temperatures. This averages to about 182 heat-related deaths per year during the four warmest months (May through August). The greatest percentage of deaths (1891, or 45%) occurred in those 65 years of age and older. Furthermore, morbidity and mortality can be extremely high when periodic seasonal heat waves occur (≥3 consecutive days of air temperatures ≥90° F [≥32.2° C]).

In 1995, a record heat wave occurred during a 17-day period in Chicago, Illinois.[11,12] The Chicago Medical Examiner's office reported 1177 heat-related deaths during this short period. These cases included deaths where heat was determined to be the underlying cause (primary) of death and where cardiovascular disease was listed as the cause of death and heat as a contributing factor (secondary). Compared with the same period in 1994, this was an 84% increase in heat-related deaths. Of these 1177 cases, heat was the primary cause of death in 465 (39.5%).[12]

Cold-Related Illness

Mild to severe cold weather conditions caused 13,970 unintentional hypothermia-related deaths in the United States between 1978 and 1998 (an average of 699 deaths per year), and 6857 of these deaths occurred in persons 65 years of age and older.[3] When adjusted for age, death from hypothermia occurred approximately 2.5 times more often in men than women. The incidence of hypothermia related-deaths progressively increases with age and is three times higher in males than females after age 15 years. In 2003, 599 deaths were reported from exposure to cold weather in the United States, and 67% were males and 51% were older than 65 years of age.[6] Major contributing factors for accidental hypothermia are urban poverty, socioeconomic conditions, alcohol intake, malnutrition, and age (very young, senior citizens).[3,6]

FIGURE 16-1 The skin is composed of three tissue layers—epidermis, dermis, and subcutaneous layer—and associated muscle. Some layers contain structures such as glands, hair follicles, blood vessels, and nerves. All these structures are interrelated to the maintenance, loss, and gain of body temperature.

Labels in figure: Oil gland, Hair follicle, Sweat gland, Blood vessel, Epidermis, Dermis, Subcutaneous, Muscle

Anatomy

The skin, the largest organ of the body, interfaces with the external environment and serves as a layer of protection. It controls the invasion of microorganisms, maintains fluid balance, and regulates temperature. Skin is composed of three tissue layers—the epidermis, dermis, and subcutaneous tissue (Figure 16-1). The outermost layer, called the *epidermis,* or the stratum corneum, is made up entirely of epithelial cells, with no blood vessels. Underlying the epidermis is the thicker dermis. The *dermis,* or deeper layer of skin, is 20 to 30 times thicker than the epidermis. The dermis is made up of a framework of connective tissues that contain blood vessels, blood products, nerves, sebaceous glands, and sweat glands. The innermost layer, the *subcutaneous* layer, is a combination of elastic and fibrous tissue as well as fatty deposits, and below this layer is skeletal muscle. The skin, nerves, blood vessels, and other underlying anatomic structures have major roles in regulating body temperature.

Physiology
Thermoregulation and Temperature Balance

Humans are considered *homeotherms,* or warm-blooded animals. A key feature of homeotherms is that they are able to regulate their own internal body temperature independent of varying environmental temperatures. The body is essentially distributed in a warmer inner *core* layer (including the brain and the thoracic and abdominal organs) and the skin and subcutaneous outer *shell* layer. *Core temperature* is regulated through a balance of heat production and heat dissipation mechanisms. The temperatures on the skin surface and the thickness of the shell depend on the *environmental temperature,* so the shell becomes thicker in the colder temperatures and thinner in the warmer temperatures based on shunting blood away or to the skin, respectively. This shell or tissue insulation, as induced by vasoconstriction, has been estimated to be about the same outer protection as wearing a light business suit, compared with six to eight times the insulation created when wearing heavy, insulated clothing in cold temperatures.

Metabolic heat production will vary based on activity levels. Independent of the variation of external temperature, the body normally functions within a narrow temperature range, known as *steady-state metabolism,* of about 1° on either side of 98.6° F (37° C ±0.6° C). Normal body temperature is maintained in a narrow range by homeostatic mechanisms regulated in the *hypothalamus,* which is located in the brain. The hypothalamus is known as the *thermoregulatory center* and functions as the body's thermostat to control neurologic and hormonal regulation of body temperature. As noted in preceding chapters, trauma to the brain can disrupt the hypothalamus, which in turn causes an imbalance in the regulation of the body temperature.

Humans have two systems to regulate body temperature: *behavioral regulation* and *physiologic thermoregulation.* Behavioral regulation is governed by the individual thermal sensation and comfort, and the distinguishing feature is the conscious effort to reduce thermal discomfort (e.g., adding additional clothing, seeking shelter in cold environments). The processing of sensory feedback to the brain of thermal information in behavioral thermoregulation is not well understood, but the feedback of thermal sensation and comfort responds more quickly than physiologic responses to changes in environmental temperature.[13]

Heat Production and Dissipation

Basal metabolic rate is the heat produced primarily as a byproduct of metabolism, principally from the large organs of the core and from skeletal muscle contraction. The heat generated is transferred throughout the body by blood in the circulatory system. Heat transfer and dissipation by the cardiopulmonary system from the body are important in the assessment and management of heat illness, as discussed later. At rest, an average size male will generate approximately 80 to 90 calories per hour. Individuals performing steady-state, moderate to heavy work will increase heat production four to five times greater than resting levels. Maximum metabolic heat production is generated at approximately 10 times the resting level (≈1000 calories per hour) when performing short-term, intense aerobic exercise. By comparison, metabolic heat production generated by shivering will increase metabolic rate up to six times the resting level.

Shivering increases the metabolic rate by increasing muscle tension, which leads to repeated bouts of muscular contraction and relaxation. There is a wide range of individual differences in the point at which shivering starts and stops, but typically, shivering starts when the core temperature is 94° to 97° F (34.4°-36° C) and continues until the core temperature is 84° to 88° F [29°-31° C].[14] With maximal shivering, heat production is increased by five to six times the resting level.[14,15] When there is a slight core temperature reduction, shivering effectively increases the metabolic rate, but the heat generated can be lost quickly to the environment. The increased muscular activity from shivering causes an increase in extremity blood flow, which in turn decreases the insulating effect of the "shell" caused by vasoconstriction, and heat loss is increased by convection, conduction, radiation, and evaporation. Maximal shivering can also interfere with any coordinated muscular activity.

Thermal Balance

The physiologic thermoregulation systems that control heat production and heat-loss responses are well documented.[13,15,16] Two principles in thermoregulation are key to understanding how the body regulates core temperature: thermal gradient and thermal equilibrium. A *thermal gradient* is the difference in temperature (high vs. low temperature) between two objects. A *thermal equilibrium* is the transfer of heat from a warmer object to a colder object in an effort to create the same temperature between them.

When body temperature rises, the normal physiologic response is to increase skin blood flow and to begin sweating. The majority of body heat is exchanged to the environment at the skin surface by conduction, convection, radiation, and evaporation, as defined next. Because heat is transferred from greater temperature to lower temperature, the human body can gain heat by radiation and conduction during hot weather conditions. Methods to maintain and dissipate body heat are important concepts for prehospital care providers. They must understand how both heat and cold are transferred to and from the body so that they can effectively manage a patient who has hyperthermia or hypothermia (Figure 16-2).

- *Radiation* is the loss or gain of heat in the form of electromagnetic energy; it is the transfer of energy from a warm object to a cooler one. Radiation does not use an intermediary source such as air or water. The sun warms the earth through space by this method of energy transfer. A patient with heat illness can acquire additional body heat from the hot ground or directly from the sun. These sources of heat will increase body heat and impede inventions to cool the patient until the prehospital care provider eliminates these sources of radiant heat when assessing and treating the patient.

- *Conduction* is the transfer of heat between two objects in direct contact with each other, as with a patient lying on a frozen lawn after a fall. A patient will generally lose heat faster when lying on the cold ground than when exposed to cold air. Therefore, prehospital care providers need to lift the patient off the ground in cold temperatures rather than merely cover the patient with a blanket.

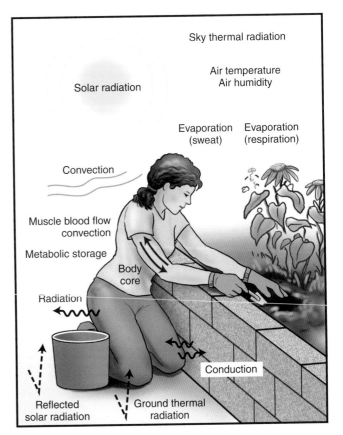

FIGURE 16-2 How humans exchange thermal energy with the environment.

- *Convection* is the transfer of heat from a solid object to a source that moves across that solid object. Air or water currents are the two sources generally considered in convective heat loss because they come into contact with the human body. The movement of cool air or water across the warmer skin provides for the continuous elimination of heat from the warmer skin. Furthermore, a patient will lose body heat 25 times faster in water than in air of the same temperature, so it is important to keep the patient dry and to remove wet clothing in mild to cold temperatures. A scuba diver's wetsuit helps to minimize the loss of body heat from convection heat loss while diving in water colder than skin temperature. When prehospital care providers are effectively managing a heat illness patient, they use the principle of convective heat loss by moistening and fanning their patient to dissipate body heat quickly.

- *Evaporation* of sweat from a liquid to a vapor is an extremely effective method of heat loss from the body, depending on the relative humidity or moisture in the air. A basal level of both water and accompanying heat loss from exhaled air, skin, and mucous membranes is called *insensible loss* and is caused by evaporation. This insensible loss is normally about 10% of basal heat production, but when the body temperature rises, this process becomes more active (sensible), and sweat is produced. Evaporative heat loss increases in cool, dry, and windy conditions (e.g., southwestern U.S. deserts). Collectively, convection and evaporation are more important than other methods of heat transfer because they are regulated by the body to control core temperature.[4]

Increases (*hyperthermia)* and decreases (*hypothermia)* in body temperature beyond the steady-state range [98.6°F ± 1.0° F (37° C ± 0.6° C)] can result from different internal and external causes and return to steady-state temperature without complications.[16] Hyperthermia occurs primarily in one of three ways: (1) as a normal response to sustained exercise, in which the heat produced elevates core temperature and is the stimulus for heat-dissipating responses (e.g., sweating, increased blood flow in skin); (2) when the sum of heat production and heat gained from the environment is greater than the body's heat dissipation; and (3) from a fever. Unlike the first two ways, fever usually occurs in response to inflammation because of a change in the thermoregulatory set point, and the body responds by elevating body temperature to a higher value (100°-106° F [38°-41° C]). Heat production increases only temporarily to achieve a new set point temperature in an attempt to make the environment less hospitable for the invading infection.[16]

Homeostasis

All these anatomic structures and physiologic systems are interacting so that the body functions properly when exposed to temperature changes. The body is in a constant state of neurologic feedback from peripheral and internal regions to the thermoregulatory center and other regions in the brain, all in an effort to maintain constant, stable internal conditions, or *homeostasis,* in the body, but at times this does not occur. For example, when an imbalance occurs in the cardiovascular and thermoregulatory adjustments to eliminate excessive body heat, one outcome is the loss of excessive body fluid through sweating, which causes acute dehydration and may lead to signs and symptoms of heat illness.

Injuries Produced by Heat

Risk Factors in Heat Illness

Many studies on humans have demonstrated large individual differences in their tolerance to hot environments.[17] These differences can be partially explained by both physical characteristics and medical conditions that are associated with an increased risk for heat illness (Box 16-1). Transient conditions include those affecting individuals who travel from cooler climates and are not heat-acclimatized to warmer climates on arrival. Factors during flight that contribute to the onset of heat illness during the first few days are

travel fatigue, jet lag, alcohol consumption, dehydration, inadequate diet, and sleep loss. Other transient factors that place individuals at risk for heat illness are common illnesses, including colds and other conditions that cause fever, vomiting, and diarrhea, along with poor dietary and fluid intake.[18,19]

Factors considered to be *chronic* conditions that place individuals at greater risk for heat illness are fitness, body size, age, medical condition, and medications.

Fitness and Body Mass Index

Low levels of physical fitness caused by genetic factors or a sedentary lifestyle with inadequate daily physical activity will reduce tolerance to heat exposure. Being physically fit provides a cardiovascular reserve to maintain cardiac output as needed to sustain thermoregulation. Overweight individuals have a normal response to vasodilate skin blood vessels and a sweat response to heat exposure, but the combination of low fitness, lack of heat acclimatization, and excessive body weight (higher body mass index) increases the energy cost of movement, placing them at greater risk for heat illness.

Age

Thermoregulatory capacity and tolerance to heat diminish with age. However, this state can be improved by maintaining a low body weight and a high level of physical fitness.

Gender

A long-held belief was that women were less tolerant to heat compared with men. Although wide variation was reported previously, these differences resulted from women who were less physically fit and had less exposure to heat compared with men in conditions that would induce full *heat acclimatization.* More recent studies have controlled for differences in physical fitness and heat acclimatization between men and women and indicate that women demonstrate equal work tolerance in heat and, in some studies, are more tolerant to heat than men.

Medical Conditions

A mild form of heat illness seen in individuals is "prickly heat rash" and has been shown to cause reduced heat tolerance. Other medical conditions that can increase the risk for heat intolerance and heat illness are diabetes mellitus, thyroid disorders, and renal disease. Cardiovascular disease and circulatory problems that increase cutaneous blood flow and circulatory demand are aggravated by heat exposure.

Medications

The use of specific prescription or over-the-counter medications can place individuals at a greater risk for heat illness (see Box 16-1). Certain medications can increase metabolic heat production, suppress body cooling, reduce cardiac reserve, and alter renal electrolyte and fluid balance. Sedative and narcotic drugs will affect mental status and can

---

BOX 16-1 Heat Illness Risk Factors

CONDITIONS
Cardiovascular disease
Dehydration
Autonomic neuropathies
Parkinsonism
Dystonias
Skin disorders: psoriasis, sunburn, burns
Endocrine disorders
Fever
Delirium tremens
Psychosis
Neonates, elderly persons
History of heat stroke
Obesity
Low fitness

TOXINS/DRUGS
Increase Heat Production
Thyroid hormone
Cyclic antidepressants
Hallucinogens (e.g., LSD)
Cocaine
Amphetamines

Decrease Thirst
Haloperidol
Angiotensin-converting enzyme (ACE) inhibitors

Decrease Sweating
Antihistamines
Anticholinergics
Phenothiazines
Glutethimide
Beta blockers

Increase Water Loss
Diuretics
Ethanol
Nicotine

BEHAVIOR
Injudicious exertion
Inappropriate clothing
Poor acclimatization
Poor fluid intake
Poor supervision
High motivation
Athletic profile
Military recruit profile

Modified from Tek D, Olshaker JS: Heat illness, *Emerg Med Clin North Am* 10(2):299, 1992.

affect logical reasoning and judgment, suppressing decision-making ability, when the individual is exposed to heat.

Dehydration

Body water is the largest component of the human body, representing 45% to 70% of body weight; for example, a 165-lb (75-kg) man contains 45 liters of water, representing 60% of body weight. Excessive changes in the normal body water balance *(euhydration)* resulting from either over-consumption of water *(hyperhydration;* see section on hyponatremia) or fluid loss (causing acute dehydration) alter homeostasis, producing specific signs and symptoms. Acute dehydration *(hypohydration,* a chronic form of dehydration) can be a serious outcome of both heat and cold exposure, but it is also seen as a dangerous side effect of diarrhea, vomiting, and fever.

Dehydration is a common finding in many cases of heat illness occurring over many days, as seen in senior citizens, or during physical activity, as seen with profuse sweating in athletes. Generally, these individuals consume no fluid or low volumes of fluid during daily activities, not replacing the depleted body water. Children and persons over age 60 are particularly susceptible to dehydration. We lose body water daily through sweat, tears, urine, and stool. Normally, drinking fluids and eating foods that contain water replace body water. When a person becomes sick with fever, diarrhea, or vomiting, or an individual is exposed to heat, dehydration occurs. Occasionally, drugs that deplete body fluids and electrolytes, such as diuretics, can cause dehydration.

During heat exposure, body water is primarily lost as sweat. Individuals can sweat 0.8 to 1.4 liters per hour (L/hr), and it has been reported that some elite athletes who are heat-acclimatized can sweat up to 3.7 L/hr during competition in hot environments.[20] The keys to avoiding the onset of heat illness are to maintain a body fluid balance and to minimize dehydration during daily activities, particularly during any physical activity in moderate to high heat exposure. Individuals normally do not perceive thirst until a deficit of approximately 2% body weight loss has resulted from sweating.[21] Thus, thirst provides a poor indicator of body water needs during rest or physical activity.

With mild to moderate levels of acute dehydration (2%-6% body weight), individuals experience fatigue, decreased heat tolerance, and cognitive deterioration, along with reductions in strength and aerobic physical capacity.[22,23] Without some form of fluid hydration guidelines (see Prevention of Heat-Related Illness) to assist individuals with the amount of fluids to consume per hour when exposed to mild or high heat exposure, people will consistently underconsume fluids and remain dehydrated at approximately 1% to 2% of body weight. The underconsumption of fluid to restore normal water balance is currently known as "voluntary" dehydration.[21]

When individuals are encouraged to drink fluids frequently during heat exposure, the rate at which fluids can be replaced by mouth is limited by the rate of gastric emptying and the rate of fluid absorption in the small intestine.[24] Fluids empty from the stomach at a maximal rate of approximately 1 to 1.2 L/hr to the small intestine, where absorption occurs into the bloodstream.[24] Furthermore, gastric emptying rates are decreased approximately 20% to 25% when sweat-induced weight loss causes dehydration of 5% of total body weight (e.g., 5% of 200-lb male = 10-lb weight loss).[25] The important message is that once dehydration occurs, it becomes more challenging to rehydrate the individual adequately with oral fluids. The keys to minimizing the amount of dehydration during heat exposure is to begin consuming oral fluids before heat exposure and to maintain fluid intake frequently during and after heat exposure.

The following are the most common signs and symptoms of dehydration in infants, children, and adults, although each individual may experience symptoms differently:

- Less frequent urination
- Thirst
- Dry skin
- Fatigue
- Lightheadedness
- Dizziness
- Confusion
- Dry mouth and mucous membranes
- Increased heart rate and breathing

In infants and children, additional symptoms may include the following:

- Dry mouth and tongue
- No tears when crying
- No wet diapers for more than 3 hours
- Sunken abdomen, eyes, or cheeks
- High fever
- Listlessness
- Irritability
- Skin that does not flatten when pinched and released

Heat-Related Disorders

Heat-related disorders can range from minor to severe in patients with heat illness.[8,26,27] It is important to note that prehospital care providers may or may not see a progression of signs and symptoms, starting with minor syndromes (e.g., heat cramps) and then advancing to major heat-related illness (e.g., classic heat stroke). In the majority of these heat exposures, the patient is able to dissipate core body heat adequately and maintain core temperature within the normal range. However, when heat-related conditions do result in a call for EMS assistance, the minor heat-related conditions may be apparent to the prehospital care provider

during patient assessment, along with signs and symptoms of a major heat illness (Table 16-1).

Minor Heat-Related Disorders
The minor heat-related disorders include heat rash, heat edema, heat tetany, muscle (heat) cramps, and heat syncope.

Heat Rash
Heat rash, also known as "prickly heat" and *miliaria rubra,* is a red, pruritic, papular rash normally seen on the skin in areas of restrictive clothing and heavy sweating. This condition is caused by inflammation of the sweat gland that blocks the sweat duct. Affected areas cannot sweat, putting individuals at an increased risk of heat illness depending on the amount of skin surface involved.

Management. Treatment is by cooling and drying the affected area and by preventing further conditions that cause sweat in these areas.

Heat Edema
Heat edema is a mild, dependent edema in the hands, feet, and ankles seen during early stages of heat acclimatization while plasma volume is expanding to compensate for the increased need for thermoregulatory blood flow. This form of edema does not indicate excessive fluid intake or cardiac, renal, or hepatic disease. In the absence of other diseases, this condition is of no clinical significance and is self-limiting. Heat edema is observed more often in females.

Management. Treatment consists of loosening clothes and elevating the legs. Diuretics are not indicated and may increase risk of heat illness.

Heat Tetany
Heat tetany is a rare and self-limiting condition that may occur in patients acutely exposed to short, intense heat conditions. The hyperventilation that results from these conditions is considered to be the principal cause. Respiratory alkalosis, paresthesias, carpopedal spasm, and tetany may develop.

Management. Treatment consists of removal from the source of heat and controlling hyperventilation. Dehydration is not a common occurrence with these short heat exposures. Heat tetany may be seen along with signs and symptoms of heat exhaustion and heat stroke.

Muscle (Heat) Cramps
Muscle (heat) cramps are short-term, painful muscle contractions frequently seen in the calf (gastrocnemius) muscles but also in the voluntary muscles of the abdomen and extremities. This occurs in individuals during exercise that produces profuse sweating or during the exercise recovery period. Smooth muscle, cardiac, diaphragm, and

TABLE 16-1 **Common Heat-Related Disorders**

Disorder	Cause/problem	Signs/symptoms	Treatment
Muscle (heat) cramps	Failure to replace NaCl lost through sweating; electrolyte and muscle problems	Painful muscle cramps, usually in legs or abdomen	Move to cool place; massage/stretch muscle; drink athletic drinks or drinks with NaCl (e.g., tomato juice); transport those with signs or symptoms listed below.
Dehydration	Failure to replace sweat loss with fluids	Thirst, nausea, excessive fatigue, hypovolemia, decreased thermoregulation; reduces physical and mental capacity	Replace sweat loss with lightly salted fluids; rest in cool place until body weight and water losses are restored.
Heat exhaustion	Excessive heat strain with inadequate water intake; cardiovascular problems with venous pooling, decreased cardiac filling time, reduced cardiac output	Low urine output, tachycardia, weakness, unstable gait, extreme fatigue, wet clammy skin, headache, dizziness, nausea, collapse; untreated, may lead to heat stroke	Remove from heat source and place in cooler location; cool body with water and fanning; drink lightly salty fluids (e.g., athletic drinks); IV 0.9 % NaCl or lactated Ringer's solution.
Heat stroke	High core temperatures >105° F (40.6° C); cellular disruption; dysfunction of multiple organ systems common; neurologic disorder with thermoregulatory center failure	Mental status changes; irrational behavior or delirium; possible shivering; tachycardia initially, then bradycardia late; hypotension; rapid and shallow breathing; dry or wet, hot skin; loss of consciousness; seizures and coma	*Emergency:* Rapid, immediate cooling by water immersion, or wet patient or wrap in cool wet sheets and fan vigorously. Continue until core temperature is <102° F (39° C). Treat for shock if necessary once core temperature is lowered. Immediately transport to emergency department.
Exertional (dilutional) hyponatremia	Low plasma sodium concentration; typically seen in individuals during prolonged activity in hot environments; drinking water (>1 L/hr) that exceeds sweat rate; failure to replace sodium loss in sweat.	Nausea, vomiting, malaise, dizziness, ataxia, headache, altered mental status, polyuria, signs of intracranial pressure, seizures, and coma; core temperature <102° F; mimics signs of heat illness	Restrict water intake; eat salty foods; unresponsive patients receive "ABC" standard care, 15 L/min O$_2$ NRM; IV 0.9 % NaCl at TKO rate; immediate transport alert; patient in situp position or left lateral position if unresponsive.

bulbar muscles are not involved. Muscle (heat) cramps can occur alone or in heat exhaustion patients. The cause is unknown, but it is believed that body sodium and other electrolyte depletion is associated with this condition. Salt supplementation in the diet has been shown to reduce the incidence of heat cramps.

Management. Treatment consists of rest in a cool environment, stretching the affected muscle, and consuming oral fluids. Sport drinks that contain sodium or other fluids (e.g., tomato juice containing sodium) should be consumed. Intravenous (IV) fluids are rarely needed, but prolonged and severe muscle cramps can be resolved rapidly with IV normal saline. Avoid the use of salt tablets because these can cause gastrointestinal (GI) distress.

Heat Syncope

Heat syncope is seen with prolonged standing in warm environments and is caused by low blood pressure that results in fainting or feeling faint or lightheaded. Heat causes vasodilation, and venous blood pools in the legs, causing low blood pressure.

Management. After removal to a cool environment, patients rest in a recumbent position and are provided oral or IV rehydration. If a fall occurred, patients should be thoroughly evaluated for any injury. Patients with a significant history of cardiac or neurologic disorders need further evaluation for the cause of their syncopal episode. Monitoring of vital signs and the electrocardiogram (ECG) during transport is essential.

Major Heat-Related Disorders

The major heat-related disorders include exertion-associated collapse, heat exhaustion, and heat stroke (classic and exertional forms).

Exertion-Associated Collapse

This disorder occurs when an individual collapses after strenuous exercise.[28,29] During exercise, muscular contraction of the lower extremities assist in venous blood return to the heart. When exercise stops, such as at the end of a jog, the muscle contraction assisting blood return to the heart slows significantly. This in turn causes venous blood return to the heart to decrease, resulting in a decreased cardiac output to the brain.

Assessment. Signs and symptoms include nausea, lightheadedness, collapse, or syncope. Patients may feel better while lying down but become lightheaded when they attempt to stand or sit *(orthostatic hypotension)*. Profuse sweating is not unusual. Ventilations and pulse rates may be rapid. The patient's core body temperature may be normal or slightly elevated. It is difficult to rule out dehydration, but this type of postexercise collapse is not from hypovolemia. In contrast, the type of collapse that occurs during exercise needs immediate evaluation for other causes (e.g., cardiovascular).

Management. The patient is removed to a cool environment and rests in a recumbent position. Oral or IV rehydration is provided as needed. Because many of these patients experienced collapse because of the decreased venous return at the end of exercise and not from dehydration, it is recommended to withhold IV therapy until further assessment is completed following recumbent rest and "cool down." As with any form of collapse, further evaluation is necessary to rule out other disorders (e.g., cardiac or neurologic causes). Monitoring of vital signs and ECG during transport is essential to detect cardiac arrhythmias.

Heat Exhaustion

Heat exhaustion is the most common heat-related disorder seen by prehospital care providers. This condition can develop over days of exposure, as in elderly persons living in poorly ventilated spaces, or acutely, as in athletes. This condition results from cardiac output insufficient to support the increased circulatory load caused by competing demands of thermoregulatory heat dissipation, with increased skin blood flow, reduced plasma volume, reduced venous return to the heart from vasodilation, and sweat-induced depletion of salt and water.[19] Patients with heat exhaustion normally present with a rectal temperature less than 104° F (<40° C), but this is a guide and not always a reliable finding.[29]

Distinguishing severe heat exhaustion from *heat stroke* often may be difficult, but a quick mental status assessment will determine the level of neurologic involvement. If heat exhaustion is not effectively treated, it can lead to heat stroke, a life-threatening form of heat illness. Heat exhaustion is a *diagnosis of exclusion* when there is no evidence of heat stroke. These patients will need further physical and laboratory evaluation in the emergency department (ED).

Assessment. Signs and symptoms include low fluid intake, decreased urine output, frontal headache, drowsiness, euphoria, nausea, lightheadedness, anxiety, fatigue, and apathy. Patients may feel better while lying down but may become lightheaded when they attempt to stand or sit (orthostatic hypotension). Profuse sweating is not unusual. Ventilation and pulse rates may be rapid, and the radial pulse may feel thready. Systolic blood pressure (SBP) may be normal or slightly decreased. The patient's core body temperature may be either normal or slightly elevated, but generally below 104° F (40° C). It is important to obtain a good history of prior heat illness and the current heat exposure incident because these patients may display signs and symptoms of other conditions of fluid and sodium loss (e.g., hyponatremia; see later discussion).

Management. Immediately remove the patient from the hot environment to a cooler location. Place the patient in a supine resting position. Remove anything restricting heat dissipation, such as a hat or clothing. Oral rehydration should be considered for any patient who can take fluids by mouth and who is not at risk of aspirating vomit, using sport electrolyte fluids diluted to half-strength. Large amounts of oral fluids may increase bloating, nausea, and vomiting. If IV fluids are needed, lactated Ringer's (LR) solution or normal saline (NS) should be used. IV solutions produce more rapid fluid recovery than fluids by mouth due to delays in gastric emptying and absorption in the small intestine caused by dehydration.

Because heat exhaustion may be difficult to distinguish from heat stroke, and because heat stroke patients should be cooled, the best course of action is to provide active cooling procedures to all heat exhaustion patients. Active cooling can be done quickly by wetting the head and upper torso with water and fanning the patient to increase *convective* body heat dissipation. Transport all patients who are unconscious, who do not recover rapidly, or who have a significant medical history. Proper environmental temperature control and monitoring of vital signs and mental status are essential during transport.

Heat Stroke

Heat stroke is considered the most emergent and life-threatening form of heat illness. Heat stroke is defined as an abnormal form of hyperthermia resulting in a total failure of the thermoregulatory system—a failure of the body's physiologic systems to dissipate heat and cool down. Heat stroke is characterized by an elevated core temperature of 104° F or greater (≥40° C) and central nervous system (CNS) dysfunction, resulting in delirium, convulsions, or coma.[27,30]

The most significant difference in heat stroke compared with heat exhaustion is *neurologic disability*, which presents to the prehospital care provider as mental status changes. The degree of complications in patients with heat stroke is not entirely related to the magnitude of core temperature elevation, because pathophysiologic changes can result in multiorgan dysfunction syndrome.[27,31] Consequently, heat stroke is distinguished clinically from heat exhaustion in most patients only after further evaluation at the hospital. Morbidity and mortality are directly associated with the duration of elevated core temperature. Even with aggressive prehospital intervention and in-hospital management, heat stroke can be fatal, and many patients who survive have permanent neurologic disability.

Heat stroke has two different clinical presentations: classic heat stroke and exertional heat stroke (Table 16-2).

Classic heat stroke is a disorder of infants, febrile children, poor people, the elderly population, alcoholic persons, and sick patients that may be compounded by the risk factors listed in Box 16-1 (e.g., medications). A classic presentation is a patient who is exposed to elevated humidity and high room temperatures over several days without air conditioning, leading to dehydration and high core temperature. Often their sweating mechanism has stopped, known as *anhidrosis*. This is especially common in large cities during summer heat waves, when effective home ventilation is either not possible or not used.[11] Scene assessment will provide information helpful in the identification of classic heat stroke.

Exertional heat stroke is a preventable disorder often seen in poorly acclimatized young individuals involved in short-term, strenuous physical activity (e.g., industrial workers, athletes, military recruits) during a combination of high environmental temperature and high humidity. These conditions can rapidly elevate internal heat production and limit the body's ability to dissipate heat. Compared with the classic heat stroke patient, these patients usually present with profuse sweating and thus may be mistaken for having only heat exhaustion.[4]

Assessment. Heat stroke patients typically present with hot, flushed skin. They may or may not be sweating, depending on where they are found and whether they have classic or exertional heat stroke. Blood pressure may be elevated or diminished, and the pulse is usually tachycardic and thready; 25% of these patients are hypotensive. The patient's level of consciousness (LOC) can range from confused to unconscious, and seizure activity may also be present, particularly during cooling.[30] As confirmed in hospitals, rectal temperature may range from 104° to 116° F (40°-47° C).[27,30]

The keys to distinguishing heat stroke from one of the other heat-related conditions are the elevation in body temperature and altered mental status. Any patient who is warm to the touch with an altered mental status (confused, disoriented, combative, or unconscious) should be suspected of having heat stroke and managed immediately and aggressively.

Management. Heat stroke is a true emergency. Cooling the patient should begin as the prehospital care provider assesses and stabilizes airway, breathing, and circulation (ABCs). The provider immediately begins cooling the patient with whatever means is available (e.g., garden hose, fire hose, bottled water), even before removing clothing. Ideally, ice-water immersion is the fastest method of cooling, but this is generally limited to an in-hospital setting.[32-34] If ice is not

TABLE 16-2 Classic versus Exertional Heat Stroke

	Classic	Exertional
Age group	Elderly	Men (15-45 yr)
Health status	Chronically ill	Healthy
Concurrent activity	Sedentary	Strenuous exercise
Drug use	Diuretics, antidepressants, antihypertensives, anticholinergics, antipsychotics	Usually none
Sweating	May be absent	Usually present
Lactic acidosis	Usually absent; poor prognosis if present	Common
Hyperkalemia	Usually absent	Often present
Hypocalcemia	Uncommon	Frequent
Hypoglycemia	Uncommon	Common
Creatine	Mildly elevated	Greatly elevated
Rhabdomyolysis	Mild	Frequently severe

Modified from Knochel JP, Reed G: Disorders of heat regulation. In Kleeman CR, Maxwell MH, Narin RG, editors: *Clinical disorders of fluid and electrolyte metabolism,* New York, 1987, McGraw-Hill.

immediately available, cool-water spraying of the patient with fanning is the next most effective technique and will provide evaporation and convective heat loss.[32] Since the late 1950s it has been thought that cold- or ice-water immersion will cause vasoconstriction sufficient to decrease heat loss from the body and cause the onset of shivering so that internal heat is produced. However, recent research has shown that this does not interfere with the critical lowering of the elevated core temperature.[32,34] *The most important intervention prehospital care providers can deliver to a heat stroke patient (along with ABCs) is immediate and rapid whole-body cooling to reduce core temperature.*

Rapid cooling should begin before transport. During transport, the patient should be placed in a prepared air-conditioned ambulance. Remove any additional clothing, cover the patient with a sheet, and wet down the sheet with irrigation fluids along with continuous fanning. Ice packs should be placed in the groin area, in the axillae, and around the anterior lateral neck because blood vessels are closest to the skin surface in these areas. However, ice packs alone are insufficient to lower core body temperature rapidly and should be considered only as extra cooling.[4,32] Rectal temperature should be measured every 5 to 10 minutes during transport to ensure effective cooling and prevent hypothermia. Active cooling should stop when rectal temperature reaches 102.2° F (39° C).[4,34] Provide high-flow oxygen, support ventilations with a bag-valve-mask (BVM) device as needed, and monitor cardiac rhythm.

Heat stroke patients generally do not require extensive fluid resuscitation and typically are initially given IV fluids consisting of 1.0 to 1.5 L of NS. Provide a 500-mL fluid challenge and assess vital signs. Fluid volume should not exceed 1 to 2 L in the first hour, or follow local medical protocol. Monitor blood glucose because these patients are frequently hypoglycemic and may require a bolus of dextrose. Seizures can be managed with 5 to 10 mg of diazepam. Transport patient in a right or left lateral recumbent position to maintain an open airway and to avoid aspiration.

Exertional Hyponatremia

Exertional hyponatremia, formerly called *water intoxication*, is a life-threatening condition that has increasingly been described in recreational hikers, marathoners, ultra-marathoners, triathletes, adventure racers, and military infantry personnel.[35-37] Low plasma sodium concentration disturbs the osmotic balance across the blood-brain barrier, resulting in rapid influx of water into the brain, which in turn causes cerebral edema.[38] As with similar signs and symptoms of intracranial pressure (ICP) in head trauma (see Chapter 8), a progression of neurologic symptoms with hyponatremia will occur, from headache, malaise, confusion, and seizures to coma, permanent brain damage, brainstem herniation, and death.[38] Symptomatic patients generally have a serum sodium concentration below 125 mEq/L (normal range, 135-145 mEq/L) with rapidly

developing (<48 hours) hyponatremia, as seen frequently in prolonged endurance events.[35]

Studies have reported that 18% to 23% of ultra-marathoners and 29% of the Hawaiian Ironman Triathletes finishers had exertional hyponatremia.[39-41] In 2003, 32 cases of exertional hyponatremia were reported in hikers in the Grand Canyon National Park, requiring an extensive rescue efforts by park rangers and paramedics in many cases.[42]

Exertional hyponatremia can occur in the following situations:

1. Excessive sodium and water loss in sweat throughout an endurance event, resulting in dehydration and sodium depletion.
2. Athletes overhydrate solely with water while maintaining plasma sodium, creating a dilution of sodium concentration.
3. Combination of excessive sodium and fluid loss in sweat and an excessive overhydration only with water.

The evidence indicates that exertion-induced hyponatremia is a result of fluid retention in the extracellular space (dilutional) rather than fluid remaining unabsorbed in the intestine.[35] Typically these patients have not consumed sport electrolyte drinks or have consumed energy food supplements containing no salt or in quantities insufficient to balance the loss of sodium in sweat or the dilution from excessive water intake.

A few plausible risk factors for the development of exertional hyponatremia have been identified. Slower runners are at a greater risk for hyponatremia than faster racers, possibly because of the greater opportunity to consume water and a greater volume consumed, but a lower fluid requirement, by the slower racers. Another factor that may place endurance athletes at greater risk is the use of nonsteroidal antiinflammatory drugs (NSAIDs; e.g., ibuprofen) during these activities. NSAIDs decrease renal prostaglandin production, leading to a decrease in kidney glomerular filtration rate.[43] However, based solely on observations, the most common risk factor is gender: the female population of endurance athletes.[44]

Exertional hyponatremia has been described as the "other heat-related illness" because the symptoms are nonspecific and are similar to those seen in minor and major heat-related disorders.[42] Many endurance events and multi-day adventure activities are conducted in warm to hot environments; therefore, it is assumed that the signs and symptoms of exertional hyponatremia are some form of heat illness and patients are managed with standard protocols that address the presumed hypovolemia and excessive body heat. Standard protocols that provide body cooling and IV fluid challenge to correct hyperthermia, sweat-induced dehydration, and mental status changes can complicate the dilutional hyponatremia and place the patient at further risk for seizure and coma. Treating a hyponatremic patient with fluids and rest will worsen their condition, unlike the heat exhaustion patient.

This "other heat-related disorder" is becoming more widely recognized and correctly treated today by EMS and ED personnel, largely because of an increased effort to educate medical personnel and the public in its prevention, early recognition, and management. Prehospital care providers directly supporting or responding to dispatches at these athletic endurance events need to be aware that exertional hyponatremia is common and potentially serious.

Assessment

A wide range of signs and symptoms may be found in the endurance athlete population with hyponatremia (see Table 16-1). Core temperature is usually normal but can be low or slightly elevated, depending on the ambient temperature, body heat dissipation, and recent exercise intensity at assessment. Heart rate and blood pressure can be low, normal, or elevated, depending on core temperature, exercise intensity, hypovolemia, or shock. Respiratory rate ranges from within normal limits to slightly elevated. Hyperventilation observed with exertional hyponatremia can account for vision disturbances, dizziness, tingling in hands, and paresthesia in the extremities. The hallmark assessment and findings are mental status changes, fatigue, malaise, headache, and nausea. Other forms of neurologic changes include slowed speech, ataxia, and cognitive changes, including irrational behavior, combativeness, and fear. These patients also often report that they have a sense of "impending doom."

Management

The first step in treatment is recognizing the disorder and determining the severity. Management is based on the severity of exertional hyponatremia. Figure 16-3 provides an algorithm for assessing patients to determine whether hyponatremia or a heat illness is present. Mild symptoms should be managed conservatively by observing the patient and waiting for normal diuresis of excessive fluid. Symptomatic patients should be placed in an upright position to maintain airway and to minimize any positional effect on ICP. These patients are known to have projectile vomiting when transported. Place unconscious patients in left lateral recumbent position and anticipate vomit. Monitor for seizures and administer anticonvulsant therapy (e.g., diazepam, 2-5 mg intravenously or intramuscularly [IV/IM]), per medical protocol. After gaining IV access at the keep vein open (KVO) rate, check with your medical control for volume of NS fluid, if any, depending on patient severity and transport time to hospital. Because these patients are already fluid-overloaded, a rapid infusion or infusion of a large volume of fluid is contraindicated. Patients with extensive signs and symptoms of cerebral edema need to have their plasma sodium concentration increased, which generally takes administration of a hypertonic (3%) saline solution in the ED or intensive care unit (ICU). Keep the patient calm while en route to the ED, and continue to monitor for mental status changes or seizures.

Prevention of Heat-Related Illness

Because heat stress is a significant public health factor in the United States, methods for preventing heat illness are vital to any community, particularly for those who must work in high-heat occupational settings. Prehospital care providers and their EMS agencies are a good source as partners of community education on heat stress prevention strategies in many different formats, including educational handouts, agency website or newsletter, community presentations, and local newspaper.

As with the general public, it may not be possible to prevent all forms of heat-related illness in prehospital care providers; therefore, EMS and other public safety personnel need to use prevention strategies and prepare for exposure to high ambient temperature and high occupational exposures. These strategies, which include administrative policies, procedures, engineering controls, use of equipment, and medical surveillance programs, are designed to help minimize the overall impact from acute or chronic heat exposure. The implementation of simple preventive procedures can have a dramatic impact on lowering the incidence of heat illness, but individuals in an organization often do not consider these strategies. Box 16-2 provides an overview of heat stress prevention strategies for EMS providers, firefighters, and other public safety personnel.[45]

A complex interaction of factors that combine to exceed the tolerance limits for individual heat exposure can eventually lead to the onset of signs and symptoms of heat illness. The capacity of humans to work in moderate to hot environments can be maximized through advanced preparation of physical fitness, heat acclimatization, living and working conditions, personal hygiene, and use of food and beverages to maintain and replace electrolytes and water in the body. Environment, fluid hydration, physical fitness, and heat acclimatization are essential factors to understand.

Environment

Prehospital care providers and other public safety personnel are subjected to high-heat environments as part of their occupational requirements. During training or an emergency response, many personnel will encounter high levels of heat stress while working in *personal protection equipment* (PPE) (impermeable clothing), such as turnout gear, hazardous material (hazmat) suit, or chemical/biologic protective garment. This heat stress is further compounded by the need to enter poorly ventilated or confined spaces or to work on a multivehicle crash in the sun on a hot, humid day. PPE compromises the body's ability to dissipate body heat and prevents the evaporation of sweat during a heavy workload.

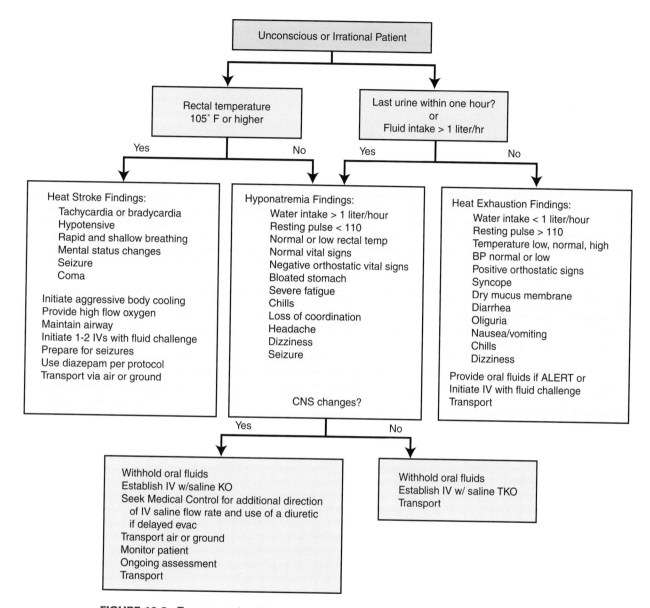

FIGURE 16-3   Treatment algorithm for heat exhaustion, heat stroke, and hyponatremia.

With high sweat rates from internal heat production during physically demanding tasks and the external heat exposure, personnel are at a high risk of dehydration and heat illness. Thus the use of PPE diminishes the physiologic advantage gained through heat acclimatization and physical fitness.

These risks can be minimized by measuring the environmental heat conditions and, where applicable, following the recommended work/rest and hydration guidelines for work in highly thermal environments.[17,46]

One traditional method for measuring the thermal load is by use of the *heat stress index* (Figure 16-4). This index uses the combination of ambient temperature (read on a thermometer) and relative humidity. This is a better method of predicting potential systemic heat injury than the ambient temperature alone. If working in direct sunlight,

near surfaces that radiate large amounts of heat, or in heavy protective clothing, 10° F should be added to the value in the table.

A more widely used method for measurement of environmental heat strain used in many industrial and military settings is the *wet-bulb globe temperature* (WBGT) *index*[4,17,47] (Table 16-3). This index uses the combination of a dry bulb for ambient temperature, wet bulb for humidity measurement, black globe for radiant heat, and air movement to provide a more accurate impact of the environmental conditions. Integrated in the five-level WBGT index range of temperatures are hourly work/rest (minutes) and hydration (quarts) guidelines. A color flag (no flag, green, yellow, red, black) represent each of the five WBGT ranges of temperatures. The WBGT can be monitored hourly and the

BOX 16-2   Prevention of Heat-Related Disorders in Prehospital Care Providers

You can prevent the serious consequences of heat disorders by improving your level of fitness and becoming acclimated to the heat.

Maintaining a high level of aerobic fitness is one of the best ways to protect you against heat stress. The fit worker has a well-developed circulatory system and increased blood volume. Both are important to regulate body temperature. Fit workers start to sweat sooner, so they work with a lower heart rate and body temperature. They adjust to the heat twice as fast as the unfit worker. They lose acclimatization more slowly and regain it quickly.

Heat acclimatization occurs in 5 to 10 days of heat exposure as the body:

- Increases sweat production
- Improves blood distribution
- Decreases the heart rate, and lowers the skin and body temperatures

You can acclimatize by gradually increasing work time in the heat, taking care to replace fluids, and resting as needed. You maintain acclimatization with periodic work or exercise in a hot environment.

ON THE JOB
The heat stress index (Figure 16-4) illustrates how temperature and humidity combine to create moderate-heat or high-heat stress conditions.

Be alert for heat stress when radiant heat from the sun or nearby flames is high, the air is still, or when you are working hard, creating large amounts of metabolic heat.

Some organizations use the WBGT heat stress index (Table 16-3). The index uses dry bulb, wet bulb, and black globe temperatures. The temperatures are weighted to indicate the impact of each measure on the worker:

- *Wet bulb* (humidity) accounts for 70%
- *Black globe* (radiant heat and air movement) accounts for 20%
- *Dry bulb* (air temperature) accounts for 10%

Heat stress indexes do not take into account the effects of long hours of hard work, dehydration, or the impact of personal protective clothing and equipment.

When heat stress conditions exist, you must modify the way you work or exercise. Pace yourself. There are individual differences in fitness, acclimatization, and heat tolerance. Push too hard and you will be a candidate for a heat disorder. When possible:

- Avoid working close to heat sources

- Do harder work during cooler morning and evening hours
- Change tools or tasks to minimize fatigue
- Take frequent rest breaks

Most important, maintain hydration by replacing lost fluids.

HYDRATION
Maintaining body fluids is essential for sweating and the removal of internal heat generated during work. To minimize dehydration and the risk of heat illness, you must hydrate before, during, and after work.

Before work, you should take extra fluids to prepare for the heat. Drink 1 to 2 cups of water, juice, or a sport drink before work. Avoid excess caffeine. It hastens fluid loss in the urine.

While working, take several fluid breaks every hour, drinking at least 1 quart of fluid. Water is your greatest need during work in the heat. Studies show that workers drink more when lightly flavored beverages are available. Providing a portion of fluid replacement with a carbohydrate/electrolyte sport beverage will help you retain fluids and maintain energy and electrolyte levels.

After work, you need to continue drinking to replace fluid losses. *Thirst always underestimates fluid needs,* so you should drink more than you think you need. Rehydration is enhanced when fluids contain sodium and potassium, or when foods with these electrolytes are consumed along with the fluid.

Sodium lost in sweat is easily replaced at meals with liberal use of the salt shaker. Unacclimatized workers lose more salt in the heat, so they need to pay particular attention to salt replacement. Do not overdo salt intake; too much salt impairs temperature regulation. Excessive salt can cause stomach distress, fatigue, and other problems.

Make potassium-rich foods like bananas and citrus fruits a regular part of your diet, and drink lots of lemonade, orange juice, or tomato juice. Limit the amount of caffeine drinks such as coffee and colas because caffeine increases fluid loss in the urine. Avoid alcoholic drinks. They also cause dehydration. Avoid sharing water bottles except in emergencies.

You can assess your hydration by observing the volume, color, and concentration of your urine; low volumes of dark, concentrated urine and painful urination indicate a serious need for rehydration. Other signs of dehydration include a rapid heart rate, weakness, excessive fatigue, and dizziness. Rapid loss of several pounds of body weight is a certain sign of dehydration. Rehydrate before returning to work. Continuing to work in a dehydrated state can lead to serious

BOX 16-2 Prevention of Heat-Related Disorders in Prehospital Care Providers—Cont'd

consequences, including heat stroke, muscle breakdown, and kidney failure.

CLOTHING

Personal protective clothing strikes a balance between protection and worker comfort. Australian researchers have concluded that *the task for personnel wearing personal protection equipment is not to keep heat out, but to let it out.* About 70% of the heat load comes from within, from metabolic heat generated during hard work. Only 30% comes from the environment and the fire. Wear loose-fitting garments to enhance air movement. Wear cotton T-shirts and underwear to help sweat evaporate. Avoid extra layers of clothing that insulate, restrict air movement, and contribute to heat stress.

INDIVIDUAL DIFFERENCES

Individuals differ in their response to heat. Some workers are at greater risk for heat disorders. The reasons include inherited differences in heat tolerance and sweat rate. Excess body weight raises metabolic heat production. Illness, drugs, and medications can also influence your body's response to work in a hot environment. Check with your physician or pharmacist if you are using prescription or over-the-counter medications, or if you have a medical condition.

You should always train and work with a partner who can help in the event of a problem. Remind each other to drink lots of fluids, and watch each other. If your partner develops a heat disorder, start treatment immediately.

SUMMARY
Prevention
- Improve or maintain aerobic fitness
- Acclimate to the heat

On the Job
- Be aware of conditions (temperature, humidity, air movement)
- Take frequent rest breaks
- Avoid extra layers of clothing
- Pace yourself

Hydrate
- Before work, drink several cups of water, juice, or a sport drink
- During work, take frequent fluid breaks
- After work, keep drinking to ensure rehydration
- Remember, only you can prevent dehydration

Partners
- Always work or train with a partner

Drinks
- Sport drinks with carbohydrates and electrolytes encourage fluid intake, provide energy, and diminish urinary water loss. The carbohydrates also help maintain immune function and mental performance during prolonged arduous work. Drinks with caffeine and alcohol interfere with rehydration by increasing urine production.

Modified from US Department of Agriculture, US Forest Service: Heat stress brochure, http://www.fs.usda.gov/fire/safety/fitness/heat_stress/hs_pg1.html.

Temperature (°F) versus Relative Humidity (%)

°F	90%	80%	70%	60%	50%	40%
80	85	84	82	81	80	79
85	101	96	92	90	86	84
90	121	113	105	99	94	90
95		133	122	113	105	98
100			142	129	118	109
105				148	133	121
110						135

High	Possible Heat Disorder
80°F - 90°F	Fatigue possible with prolonged exposure and physical activity.
90°F - 105°F	Sunstroke, heat cramps, and heat exhaustion possible.
105°F - 130°F	Sunstroke, heat cramps, and heat exhaustion likely, and heat stroke possible.
130°F or greater	Heat stroke highly likely with continued exposure.

Due to the nature of the heat index calculation, the values in the tables have an error +/− 1.3° F

FIGURE 16-4 Heat stress index.
(Courtesy National Weather Service, Pueblo, Colo, www.crh.noaa.gov/pub/heat.htm.)

TABLE 16-3   Fluid Replacement Guidelines for Warm Weather Training

Heat category	WBGT Index (°F)	Easy work		Moderate work		Hard work	
		Work/rest (min)	Water intake (qt/hr)	Work/rest (min)	Water intake (qt/hr)	Work/rest (min)	Water intake (qt/hr)
1	78-81.9	NL	$1/2$	NL	$3/4$	40/20	$3/4$
2	82-84.9	NL	$1/2$	50/10	$3/4$	30/30	1
3	85-87.9	NL	$3/4$	40/20	$3/4$	30/30	1
4	88-89.9	NL	$3/4$	30/30	$3/4$	20/40	1
5	>90	50/10	1	20/40	1	10/50	1

The work/rest times and fluid replacement volumes will sustain performance and hydration for at least 4 hours of work in the specified heat category. Individual water needs will vary ±qt/hr.

NL, No limit to work time per hour.

Rest means minimal physical activity (sitting or standing), accomplished in shade if possible.

Caution: Hourly fluid intake should not exceed 1.5 quarts. Daily fluid intake should not exceed 12 quarts.

Wearing body armor add 5° F to WBGT index in humid climates.

Wearing personal protective equipment (PPE) over garment add 10° F to WBGT index for easy work and 20° F for moderate and hard work.

Easy work	Moderate work	Hard work
Walking on hard surface at 2.5 mph, <31-lb load.	Walking on hard surface at 3.5 mph, <41-lb load. Walking in loose sand at 2.5 mph, no load. Calisthenics.	Walking on hard surface at 3.5 mph, >40-lb load. Walking in loose sand at 2.5 mph with load.

Current version of WBGT, hydration, and work/rest guidelines as updated by US Army Research Institute for Environmental Medicine (USARIEM) and published by Montain SJ, Latzka WA, Sawka MN: *Mil Med* 164:502, 1999.

corresponding colored flag placed on a flagpole outdoors for all personnel to see throughout the day. Where applicable, the appropriate adjustments of clothing, physical activity, work/rest cycles, and fluid intake can then be made based on these WBGT conditions. This integrated WBGT system and related policies can easily be developed at various public safety locations and training sites to ensure that effective heat illness prevention programs are in use to reduce fatigue, injuries, and heat illness.

Hydration

If the WBGT flag system is not used to provide guidelines for hydration, another excellent resource is published by the American College of Sports Medicine (ACSM), based on years of research.[48] These guidelines are easily applied to any individual engaged in physical activity. These guidelines should be established within an agency in an effort to minimize dehydration by creating easy access to water and sport electrolyte drinks, particularly during activity in warm environments (Box 16-3). Studies show that individuals do not drink sufficient quantities of fluids before, during, and after work or exercise to recover body fluids lost from sweating, even though they believe they are consuming enough fluids.[48]

Fitness

To increase heat tolerance effectively in high-heat conditions, individuals should increase their aerobic fitness (e.g., walk, jog, bike, swim, stair stepping, elliptical exercise machines) through individualized programs.[17] These programs will provide the cardiac reserve to sustain the cardiac output required in meeting the competing demands of physical (muscular) work and heat dissipation mechanisms (thermoregulation) in a high-temperature environment.[49] The ACSM and the Centers for Disease Control and Prevention (CDC) have collaborated to establish a nationwide recommendation of 30 minutes a day of physical activity to maintain health and well-being.[50] Boxes 16-4 and 16-5 summarize the consensus reports by the ACSM and the U.S. Surgeon General, respectively, for recommendations for the general adult population.

Heat Acclimatization

A policy and protocol for heat acclimatization should be provided within a public safety organization.[51] Heat acclimatization can be achieved with 60 to 90 minutes of exercise a day in hot conditions for approximately 7 to 14 days.[8,52] The outcomes of heat acclimatization are increased work performance, heat tolerance, and reduced physiologic

BOX 16-3   Hydration Guidelines to Minimize Dehydration

1. Start exercise well hydrated.
Drink 2 to 3 cups (16-24 oz) of fluid 2 to 3 hours before physical activity to allow excess fluid to be lost as urine. About one-half hour before physical activity, drink 5 to 10 oz. There is no benefit to overconsumption of fluids (hyperhydration), so do not drink excessively.

2. Weigh yourself.
The best way to determine if you have replaced sweat loss during heavy work or exercise is to check to see how much weight you have lost. Determine your body weight before and after physical activity. Minimal weight loss means that you have done a good job staying hydrated. Remember that weight loss during exercise or work is water loss, not fat loss, and must be replaced.

3. Drink during physical activity.
Drink 5 to 10 oz of water or sport electrolyte drink every 10 to 20 minutes during a workout. Heavy sweaters can benefit from drinking more often (e.g., every 10 minutes) and light sweaters should drink less often (every 20+ minutes).

4. Ingest sodium during physical activity.
The best time to begin replacing the sodium lost in sweat is during exercise. That is one reason why a good sports electrolyte drink is better than plain water.

5. Follow your own plan.
Everybody sweats differently, so everybody needs a drinking plan tailored to his or her individual needs.

6. Drink plenty during meals.
If you were not able to drink enough during heavy work or exercise to keep from losing weight, be sure to drink enough before the next practice or returning to work. Mealtime is the best time to do that because of the ease of drinking and the sodium that comes along with food.

7. Do not rely solely on water.
Drinking only water keeps you from replacing the electrolytes lost in sweat and from ingesting carbohydrates that help you work or exercise longer and stronger. Excessive water drinking can lead to dangerous electrolyte disturbances (hyponatremia).

8. Do not overdrink.
Water is definitely a good thing, but you can get too much of a good thing. Drinking large amounts of fluid not only is unnecessary, but can be dangerous (hyponatremia). Bloated stomach, puffy fingers and ankles, a bad headache, and confusion are warning signs of hyponatremia.

9. Do not gain weight during exercise.
A sure sign of drinking too much is weight gain during heavy work or exercise. If you weigh more after work or exercise than you did before, that means that you drank more than you needed. Be sure to cut back the next time so that you do not gain weight.

10. Do not restrict salt in your diet.
Ample salt (sodium chloride) in the diet is essential to replace the salt lost in sweat. Because athletes sweat a lot, their need for salt is much greater than for nonathletes. (This principle holds true for those who work and sweat heavily each day in occupations conducted in moderate to hot environments.)

11. Do not use dehydration to lose weight.
Restricting fluid intake during work or exercise impairs physical performance and increases the risk of heat-related problems. Dehydration should be kept to a minimum by following a wise fluid replacement plan.

12. Do not delay drinking during exercise or work.
Stick to a drinking schedule so that you avoid dehydration early in exercise or work. Once dehydrated, it is almost impossible to catch up to what your body needs, because dehydration actually slows the speed at which fluid exits the stomach.

Modified from Murray B, Eichner ER, Stofan J: Hyponatremia in athletes, *Sports Sci Exchange* 16(1):88, 2003, http://www.gssiweb.com/.

strain. These adjustments include increased blood volume, increased stroke volume, decreased heart rate at a given activity level, reduced sodium concentration in sweat, sodium conserved in the body, earlier onset of sweating, and *increased* sweat volume rate (Box 16-6). These changes improve the transfer of body heat from the core to the skin in effort to increase the heat transfer from the skin to the environment. Although heat tolerance is improved in these individuals and considered desirable (e.g., endurance athletes, military infantry personnel), the greater sweat volume production (1-2 L/hr) results in large fluid losses, leading to dehydration. Consequently, the greater volume of sweat loss in heat-acclimatized individuals increases the hydration requirements during heat exposure, particularly

BOX 16-4 American College of Sports Medicine (ACSM) Fitness Recommendations for General Adult Population

CARDIORESPIRATORY FITNESS

1. *Frequency of training:* 3 to 5 days per week.
2. *Intensity of training:* 55%/65% to 90% of maximum heart rate. The lower-intensity values, 55% to 64% of maximum heart rate, are most applicable to individuals who are unfit and starting a fitness program.
3. *Duration of training:* 20 to 60 minutes of continuous or intermittent (minimum of 10-minute bouts accumulated throughout the day) aerobic activity. Duration is dependent on the intensity of the activity; thus, lower-intensity activity should be conducted over a longer period (≥30 minutes), and, conversely, individuals training at higher levels of intensity should train at least 20 minutes or longer. Because of the importance of "total fitness" and that it is more readily attained with exercise sessions of longer duration, and because of the potential hazards and adherence problems associated with high-intensity activity, moderate-intensity activity of longer duration is recommended for adults not training for athletic competition.
4. *Mode of activity:* Any activity that uses large muscle groups, can be maintained continuously, and is rhythmical and aerobic in nature, including walking-hiking, running-jogging, cycling-bicycling, cross-country skiing, aerobic dance/group exercise, rope skipping, rowing, stair climbing, swimming, skating, and various endurance game activities.

MUSCULAR STRENGTH AND ENDURANCE, BODY COMPOSITION, AND FLEXIBILITY

1. *Resistance training:* Resistance exercises should be an integral part of an adult fitness program and of a sufficient intensity to enhance strength, muscular endurance, and maintain fat-free mass (FFM). Resistance training should be progressive and individualized and provide a stimulus to all the major muscle groups. One set of 8 to 10 exercises that conditions the major muscle groups 2 or 3 days per week is recommended. Multiple-set regimens (e.g., 2-3 sets) may provide greater benefits if time allows. Most persons should complete 8 to 12 repetitions of each exercise; however, for older and more frail persons (≥age 50-60), 10 to 15 repetitions may be more appropriate.
2. *Flexibility training:* Flexibility exercises should be incorporated into the overall fitness program sufficient to develop and maintain range of motion. These exercises should stretch the major muscle groups and be performed a minimum of 2 or 3 days per week. Stretching should include appropriate static and/or dynamic techniques.

From American College of Sports Medicine: *Med Sci. Sports Exerc* 30(6):975, 1998.

BOX 16-5 U.S. Surgeon General's Fitness Recommendations for General Adult Population

This is the first Surgeon General's report to address physical activity and health. The main message of this report is that Americans can substantially improve their health and quality of life by including moderate amounts of physical activity in their daily lives. Health benefits from physical activity are thus achievable for most Americans, including those who may dislike vigorous exercise and those who may have been previously discouraged by the difficulty of adhering to a program of vigorous exercise. For those who are already achieving regular moderate amounts of activity, additional benefits can be gained by further increases in activity level.

This report grew out of an emerging consensus among epidemiologists, experts in exercise science, and health professionals that physical activity need not be of vigorous intensity for it to improve health. Moreover, health benefits appear to be proportional to amount of activity; thus, every increase in activity adds some benefit. Emphasizing the amount rather than the intensity of physical activity offers more options for people to select from in incorporating physical activity into their daily lives. Thus, a moderate amount of activity can be obtained in a 30-minute brisk walk, 30 minutes of lawn mowing or raking leaves, a 15-minute run, or 45 minutes of playing volleyball, and these activities can be varied from day to day. It is hoped that this different emphasis on moderate amounts of activity, and the flexibility to vary activities according to personal preference and life circumstances, will encourage more people to make physical activity a regular and sustainable part of their lives.

The information in this report summarizes diverse literature from the fields of epidemiology, exercise physiology, medicine, and the behavioral sciences. The report highlights what is known about physical activity and health, as well as what is being learned about promoting physical activity among adults and young people.

BOX 16-5   U.S. Surgeon General's Fitness Recommendations for General Adult Population—cont'd

Finally, physical activity is only one of many everyday behaviors that affect health. In particular, nutritional habits are linked to some of the same aspects of health as physical activity, and the two may be related lifestyle characteristics. This report deals solely with physical activity; a Surgeon General's Report on Nutrition and Health was published in 1988.

MAJOR CONCLUSIONS

1. People of all ages, both male and female, benefit from regular physical activity.
2. Significant health benefits can be obtained by including a moderate amount of physical activity (e.g., 30 minutes of brisk walking or raking leaves, 15 minutes of running, or 45 minutes of playing volleyball) on most, if not all, days of the week. Through a modest increase in daily activity, most Americans can improve their health and quality of life.
3. Additional health benefits can be gained through greater amounts of physical activity. People who can maintain a regular regimen of activity that is of longer duration

or of more vigorous intensity are likely to derive greater benefit.

4. Physical activity reduces the risk of premature mortality in general, and of coronary heart disease, hypertension, colon cancer, and diabetes mellitus in particular. Physical activity also improves mental health and is important for the health of muscles, bones, and joints.
5. More than 60% of American adults are not regularly physically active. In fact, 25% of all adults are not active at all.
6. Nearly half of American youths 12 to 21 years of age are not vigorously active on a regular basis. Moreover, physical activity declines dramatically during adolescence.
7. Daily enrollment in physical education classes declined among high school students from 42% in 1991 to 25% percent in 1995.
8. Research on understanding and promoting physical activity is at an early stage, but some interventions to promote physical activity through schools, worksites, and health care settings have been evaluated and found to be successful.

Pate RR, Pratt M, Blair SN, et al: Physical activity and public health. A recommendation from the Centers for Disease Control and Prevention and the American College of Sports Medicine. *JAMA* 273(5):402, 1995.

BOX 16-6   Benefits of Heat Acclimatization

1. Thermal comfort: improved
2. Core temperature: reduced
3. Skin blood flow: earlier
4. Heart rate: lowered
5. Salt losses (sweat and urine): reduced
6. Exercise performance: improved
7. Sweating: earlier and greater
8. Body heat production: lower
9. Thirst: improved
10. Organ protection: improved

From the Heat Acclimatization Guide, Ranger and Airborne School Students, 2003, www.usariem.army.mil/download/heatacclimatizationguide.pdf.

when the person does not adhere to a rigorous oral hydration schedule. Box 16-7 provides an overview of heat acclimatization guidelines.

Emergency Incident Rehabilitation

The United States Fire Administration (USFA) created a standardized approach for evaluating and rehabilitating

firefighters and emergency personnel during environmental extremes (Box 16-8). In 1992 the USFA stated the following:

The physical and mental demands of EMS, firefighting and emergency operations that are associated with extreme heat and humidity create conditions that can have an adverse impact upon the safety and health of the individual emergency responder. Members who are not provided adequate rest and rehydration during emergency operations and training exercises are at increased risk for illness, and may jeopardize the safety of others on the incident scene. When emergency responders become fatigued, their ability to operate safely is impaired. As a result, their reaction time is reduced, and their ability to make critical decisions diminishes. Rehabilitation is an essential element on the incident scene to prevent more serious conditions such as heat exhaustion or heat stroke from occurring.[53]

EMS Drug Storage in Thermal Extremes

Prehospital care providers work in regions within the United States where annual extremes range from below freezing to high heat and humidity. Their vehicles, including mobile intensive care units, paramedic units, and medical helicopters, and the medications stored in those vehicles are also subjected to the environmental extremes unless a temperature-controlled storage device is on board. Medications used by prehospital care providers are intended

BOX 16-7 Heat Acclimatization Guidelines

The following is a modified version of the heat acclimatization guidelines designed for healthy and physically fit infantry personnel in preparation for physical activity in hot environments.

Should You Be Concerned About Hot Weather?
If you are used to working in cool or temperate climates, exposure to hot weather will make it much more difficult to complete your advanced training course. Hot weather will make you feel fatigued, make it more difficult to recover, and increase your risk of being a heat casualty. Individuals with the same abilities but who are used to training in hot weather will have a greater heat tolerance and physical ability during heat exposure.

What Is Heat Acclimatization?
Heat acclimatization refers to biologic adaptations that reduce physiologic strain (e.g., heart rate, body temperature), improve physical work capabilities, improve comfort and protect vital organs (brain, liver, kidneys, muscles) from heat injury. The most important biologic adaptation from heat acclimatization is an earlier and greater sweating response, and for this response to improve, it needs to be invoked.

Heat acclimatization is specific to the climate (desert) and physical activity level. However, acclimatization to desert climates greatly improves the ability to work in other climates. Individuals who only perform light or brief physical work will achieve the level of heat acclimatization needed to perform that task. If they attempt a more strenuous or prolonged task, additional acclimatization and improved physical fitness will be needed to perform that task successfully in the heat.

How Do You Become Heat Acclimatized?
Heat acclimatization occurs when repeated heat exposures are sufficiently stressful to elevate body temperature and provoke perfuse sweating. Resting in the heat, with limited physical activity to that required for existence, results in only partial acclimatization. Physical exercise in the heat is required to achieve optimal heat acclimatization for that exercise intensity in a given hot environment.

Generally, about 2 weeks of daily heat exposure is needed to induce heat acclimatization. Heat acclimatization requires a minimum daily heat exposure of about 2 hours (can be broken into two 1-hour exposures) combined with physical exercise that requires cardiovascular endurance (e.g., jogging) rather than strength training. Gradually increase the exercise intensity or duration each day. Work up

to an appropriate physical training schedule adapted to the required physical activity.

The benefits of heat acclimatization will be retained for about 1 week and then decay, with about 75% lost by about 3 weeks, once heat exposure ends. One or 2 days of intervening cool weather will not interfere with acclimatization to hot weather.

How Fast Can You Become Heat Acclimatized?
For the average individual, heat acclimatization requires about 2 weeks of heat exposure and progressive increases in physical work. By the second day of acclimatization, significant reductions in physiologic strain are observed. By the end of the first week and second week, >60% and >80% of the physiologic adaptations are complete, respectively. Less fit individuals or those unusually susceptible to heat exposure may require several days or weeks more to fully acclimatize.

Physically fit individuals should be able to achieve heat acclimatization in about 1 week. However, several weeks of living and working in the heat (seasoning) may be required to maximize tolerance to high body temperatures.

What Are the Best Heat Acclimatization Strategies?
1. Maximize physical fitness and heat acclimatization before hot weather exposure. Maintain physical fitness with maintenance programs tailored to the environment, such as physical training in the cooler morning or evening hours.
2. Integrate training and heat acclimatization. Train in the coolest part of the day and acclimatize in the heat of the day. Start slowly by reducing training intensity and duration (compared to what you could achieve in temperate climates). Increase training and heat exposure volume as your heat tolerance permits. Use interval training to modify your activity level.
3. If the new climate is much hotter than what you are accustomed to, recreational activities may be appropriate for the first 2 days with periods of run/walk. By the third day, you should be able to integrate training runs (20-40 minutes) at a reduced pace.
4. Consume sufficient water to replace sweat losses. Sweat rates of more than 1 quart per hour are common. Heat acclimatization increases the sweating rate, and therefore increases water requirements. As a result, heat-acclimatized individuals will dehydrate faster if they do not consume fluids. Dehydration negates many of the thermoregulatory advantages conferred by heat acclimatization and high physical fitness.

For the complete report, see: http://www.usariem.army.mil/download/heatacclimatizationguide.pdf.

BOX 16-8   **U.S. Fire Administration (USFA) Standard Operating Procedure (SOP) on Emergency Incident Rehabilitation**

PURPOSE

To ensure that the physical and mental conditions of members operating at the scene of an emergency or a training exercise do not deteriorate to a point that affects the safety of each member or that jeopardizes the safety and integrity of the operation.

SCOPE

This procedure will apply to all emergency operations and training exercises where strenuous physical activity or exposure to heat or cold exists.

RESPONSIBILITIES

The Incident Commander will consider the circumstances of each incident and make adequate provisions early in the incident for the rest and rehabilitation for all members operating at the scene. These provisions will include medical evaluation, treatment, and monitoring; food and fluid replenishment; mental rest; and relief from extreme climatic conditions and the other environmental parameters of the incident. The rehabilitation will include the provision of emergency medical services (EMS) at the basic life support (BLS) level or higher. The Incident Commander will establish a rehabilitation sector or group when conditions indicate rest and rehabilitation is needed for persons operating at the incident scene or training evaluation.

GUIDELINES

Climatic or environmental conditions of the emergency scene should not be the sole justification for establishing a rehabilitation area. Any activity or incident that is large in size, long in duration, or labor intensive will rapidly deplete the energy and strength of personnel and therefore merits consideration for rehabilitation. Climatic or environmental conditions that indicate the need to establish a rehabilitation area are a heat stress index above 90° F (32° C) (see Figure 16-4) or windchill index below 10° F (−12° C) (see Figure 16-10).

Hydration

During heat stress, the member should consume at least 1 quart per hour. The rehydration should be a 50/50 mixture of water and a commercially prepared activity beverage (sport electrolyte beverage) and administered at about 40° F (4.4° C). Alcohol and caffeine beverages should be avoided before and during heat stress because both interfere with the body's water conservation mechanisms. Carbonated beverages should also be avoided.

Nourishment

The department will provide food at the scene of an extended incident when units are engaged for 3 or more hours. A cup of soup, broth, or stew is highly recommended because it is digested much faster than sandwiches and fast-food products.

Rest

The "two-bottle rule," or 45 minutes of work time, is recommended as an acceptable level before mandatory rehabilitation. Members will rehydrate (at least 8 ounces) while SCBA cylinders are being charged. Firefighters having worked for two full 30-minute–rated bottles, or 45 minutes, will be immediately placed in the rehabilitation area for rest and evaluation. Rest will not be less than 10 minutes and may exceed an hour, as determined by the Rehab Officer.

Recovery

Members in the rehabilitation area should maintain a high level of hydration. Certain drugs impair the body's ability to sweat, and extreme caution must be exercised if the member has taken antihistamines, such as Actifed or Benadryl, or has taken diuretics or stimulants.

Medical Evaluation

EMS should be provided and staffed by the most highly trained and qualified prehospital care providers on the scene (at a minimum of BLS level). They will evaluate vital signs, examine members, and make proper disposition (return to duty, continued rehabilitation, or medical treatment and transport to medical facility). Continued rehabilitation should consist of additional monitoring of vital signs, providing rest, and providing fluids for rehydration. Prehospital care providers will be assertive in an effort to find potential medical problems early. If a member's heart rate exceeds 110 beats/min, an oral temperature should be taken. If the member's temperature exceeds 100.6° F (38° C), he or she should not be permitted to wear protective equipment. If it is below 100.6° F and heart rate remains above 110 beats/min, rehabilitation time should be increased. If the heart rate is less than 110 beats/min, the chance of heat stress is negligible. Document all medical evaluations.

Modified from SOP for USFA Emergency Incident Rehabilitation, www.smemsc.org/Emergency Incident Rehabilitation.pdf.

for storage at controlled room temperature according to recommendations of the drug manufacturers. The *United States Pharmacopeia (USP)* has oversight responsibilities in the United States for establishing drug standards intended to ensure the quality of medications, and *USP* defines controlled room temperature as follows:

A temperature maintained thermostatically that encompasses the usual and customary working environment of 68° to 77° F (20° to 25° C); that results in a mean kinetic temperature calculated to be not more than 77° F (25° C); and allows for excursions between 59° to 86° F (15° to 30° C) that are experienced in pharmacies, hospitals and warehouses. Provided the mean kinetic temperature remains in the allowed range, transient spikes up to 104° F (40° C) may be permitted if the manufacturer so instructs.[54]

Manufacturers will guarantee a medication's stability, quality, and potency only when the drugs are stored within the recommended temperature range. In many cases across the country, EMS vehicles have been shown periodically to have stored medications at temperatures outside the *USP*-recommended range.[55-58] These studies have examined thermal exposure of drugs in both field and laboratory settings for short (1-4 weeks) and long (12-26 weeks) durations.[55] What remains unclear is the effect of these thermal excursions on the bioavailability of many common prehospital drugs. However, laboratory assessment shows that the majority of these drugs remain stable, except for epinephrine, which significantly degrades in extreme cold and heat.[55,59,60]

To improve compliance with the *USP* standards and manufacturers' recommendations, the New Jersey Office of Emergency Medical Services (Department of Health and Senior Services) passed regulations requiring the following:

Each vehicle and cabinet or other storage place for medications shall be sufficiently climate controlled so that the medications and solutions are kept within temperature range recommended by the manufacturer. Each vehicle shall have a temperature recording device which shall, at least, record the highest and lowest temperature during a specified time period.[61]

EMS agencies will need to consider how they will respond to this concern for the efficacy of the medications used in their vehicles. Will these drugs always work as intended when used by the EMS personnel? Specifically, will epinephrine work as indicated to provide the rapid bronchial dilation for the asthmatic teenager? The cost for implementing environmentally controlled storage for all advanced life support (ALS) units, as recommended by each drug manufacturer and the *USP*, may be beyond the financial capability of many EMS agencies, but to take no action based on these studies may be ethically unacceptable as well. It is suggested that each EMS agency develop a policy to investigate the thermal conditions in the vehicle

medication storage area and consider a medication rotation system during periods of extreme cold and heat, or some other system to minimize the exposure of medications to thermal extremes in their region.[55]

Injuries Produced by Cold

Dehydration
Dehydration occurs very easily in the cold, particularly with increased physical activity. This occurs for three primary reasons: (1) evaporation of sweat, (2) increased respiratory heat and fluid losses caused by the dryness of cold air, and (3) cold-induced diuresis.

Cold-induced diuresis is a normal physiologic outcome of prolonged cold exposure resulting from skin vasoconstriction. This is the body's response to reduce body heat loss by shunting blood from the periphery to deeper veins of the body, which causes a central blood volume expansion.[62] This results in a rise in the mean arterial pressure (MAP), stroke volume, and cardiac output. The expanded blood volume can produce a cold-induced diuresis, as experienced by frequent urination. Cold-induced diuresis can reduce plasma volume by 7% to 15%, resulting in hemoconcentration and acute dehydration from almost a twofold fluid loss.

Prehospital care providers can experience cold-induced diuresis in the winter months while working for many hours in the cold. Consider, for example, the scene of a motor vehicle crash (MVC) on an interstate highway on a cold, windy day (42° F [6° C] and 25-mph NE winds). The provider is exposed suddenly to cold air after exiting the heated ambulance and is wearing only a windbreaker jacket. This sudden cold exposure can result in an acute response, with skin vessel vasoconstriction leading to transient muscle shivering. As work continues at the scene, skin temperature adjusts to the colder ambient temperature, the physiologic responses to the cold air moderate, and shivering stops. Skin temperature will soon accommodate to the colder air temperature over time, and the sensation of cold will become more tolerable.

As with exposure to heat, adherence to fluid hydration guidelines (see Box 16-3) while working in cold environments is necessary to minimize dehydration and the associated fatigue and physical and cognitive changes.

Cold-Related Disorders
Minor Cold-Related Disorders
Contact Freeze Injury
When cold material comes into contact with unprotected skin, it can produce local frostbite immediately. Do not touch any metal surface, alcohol, gasoline, antifreeze, ice, or snow

with the hands. (See the frostbite section for assessment and management.)

Frostnip

Frostnip is a precursor to *frostbite* and produces reversible signs of skin blanching and numbness in localized tissue. It is typically seen on areas of the face, nose, and ears.[9] Frostnip is a self-limiting tissue change as long as cold exposure does not continue; it does not require prehospital care provider intervention and transport.

Cold Urticaria

Cold urticaria ("hives") is a disorder characterized by the rapid onset (within minutes) of itchiness, redness, and swelling of the skin after exposure to cold. The sensation of burning may be a prominent feature. This condition, caused by a local release of histamine, is sometimes observed when ice is applied directly to the skin during cold therapy for sprains and strains. Individuals with a history of cold urticaria are recommended to avoid cold-water immersion, which could potentially cause death from systemic anaphylaxis. Treatment includes avoiding the cold and possibly taking antihistamines.

Chilblains (Pernio)

Chilblains are small skin lesions that are itchy and tender, red or purple bumps that occur on the extensor skin surface of the finger or any skin surface (e.g., ears, face) from chronic cold exposure. Chilblains occur several hours after exposure to the cold in temperate humid climates. They are sometimes aggravated by sun exposure. Cold causes constriction of the small arteries and veins in the skin, and rewarming results in leakage of blood into the tissues and swelling of the skin.

Chilblains are more likely to develop in those with poor peripheral circulation. Some contributing factors are a familial tendency, peripheral vascular disease caused by diabetes, smoking, hyperlipidemia, poor nutrition (e.g., anorexia nervosa), connective tissue disease, and bone marrow disorders. Each chilblain comes up over a few hours as an itchy, red swelling and subsides over the next 7 to 14 days. In severe cases, blistering, pustules, scabs, and ulceration can occur. Occasionally the lesions may be ring shaped. They may become thickened and persist for months.

Symptoms will subside with the elimination of cold. Management involves protection from cold with appropriate gloves and clothing.

Solar Keratitis (Snow Blindness)

Without protection from dry air and from exposure to bright reflections on snow, the risk of ultraviolet burns to skin and eyes increases. This risk is greatly enhanced at higher altitudes. Solar keratitis is insidious during the exposure phase, with corneal burns occurring within 1 hour, but not becoming apparent until 6 to 12 hours after exposure.

Management of snow blindness is based on symptoms, which include excessive tearing, pain, redness, swollen eyelids, pain when looking at light, headache, a gritty sensation in the eyes, and decreased (hazy) vision. Prehospital care providers need to consider patching affected eyes if there is no other method to prevent further ultraviolet exposure (e.g., sunglasses), then transport the patient. Medical attention is required to determine the level of severity and the need for antibiotics and analgesics.

Major Cold-Related Disorders

Localized Cutaneous Cold Injury

Cold injuries occur at peripheral sites on the body and are classified as either freezing (e.g., frostbite) or nonfreezing (e.g., immersion foot) injuries. Localized cold injuries are preventable with proper preparation for cold exposure, early recognition of cold injury, and effective medical care. However, frostbite, potentially the most serious form of freezing injury because of the risk of limb loss, is the primary injury of interest in this section.

It is imperative to recognize, manage, and prevent further tissue freezing in mild to severe forms of freezing injury. Nicotine, alcohol intoxication, homelessness, and major psychiatric disorders remain important predisposing factors.[63] When comparing cold weather injuries by ethnicity, African Americans are reported to be at greater risk for cold weather injuries, including frostbite. This relationship is related to the greater susceptibility of pigmented cells to freeze compared with nonpigmented cells.[64,65] Tight or constricting clothes, too many socks, and tight-fitting footwear are predicable factors in the onset of frostbite. With an increase in adventure sports and other recreational activities conducted in the winter season, localized cold injuries are now seen more often. Prehospital care providers need to prevent body heat loss and protect exposed skin from frostbite in patients during prolonged exposure to cold conditions. For example, in patients needing vehicular extrication, in scenarios resulting in the inability to move the patient, and in patients in cold environments with soft tissue swelling, impaired circulation can lead to an increased incidence of localized cold injury.

Nonfreezing Cold Injury

Nonfreezing cold injury (NFCI), a syndrome also called immersion foot and trench foot, results from damage to peripheral tissues caused by prolonged (hours to days) wet/cold exposure.[66-68] NFCI does not involve freezing of tissue but may coexist with freezing injury such as frostbite. This syndrome involves primarily the feet and is reflected in two types of NFCI. *Trench foot* occurs primarily in military personnel during infantry operations and is related to the combined effects of prolonged cold exposure and restricted circulation in the feet.[66] *Immersion foot* is caused by prolonged immersion of extremities to wet and cool to cold temperatures. Prehospital care providers may see immersion foot in homeless, alcoholic, or elderly persons; hikers and hunters; multiday adventure sport athletes; and ocean survivors.[66,69,70] Frequently this syndrome goes unrecognized during assessment of individuals who have been exposed to cold or wet conditions because of the lack of formal medical training in NFCI.[66]

Clinical Manifestations. This syndrome occurs as a result of many hours of cooling of the lower extremities in temperatures ranging from 32° to 65° F (0°-18° C). Soft tissue injury occurs to the skin of the feet, known as *maceration.* The breakdown of the skin will predispose individuals to infection as well. The greatest injury is seen to the peripheral nerves and blood vessels, caused by secondary ischemic injury. Mild NFCI is self-limiting initially, but with continued prolonged cold exposure, it becomes irreversible. When the feet are wet and cold, this increases the risk and accelerates the injury because wet socks insulate poorly, and water cools more effectively than air at the same temperature. Any factors that reduce circulation to the extremities also contribute to the injury, such as constrictive clothing, boots, prolonged immobility, hypothermia, and crouched posture.

NFCI is classified in four degrees of severity, as follows[66]:

- *Minimal.* Hyperemia or engorgement caused by an increase in blood flow to the feet and slight sensory change will remain 2 to 3 days after injury. Condition is self-limiting, and no signs of injury remain after 7 days. Occasionally, cold sensitivity will remain.
- *Mild.* Edema, hyperemia, and slight sensory change remain 2 to 3 days after injury. Seven days after injury, anesthesia is found on the plantar surface of the foot and tips of the toes and lasts 4 to 9 weeks. Blisters and skin loss are not observed. Ambulation is possible when walking does not cause pain.
- *Moderate.* Edema, hyperemia, blisters, and mottling are present 2 to 3 days after injury. At 7 days, anesthesia to touch is present to both dorsal and plantar surface and toes. Edema persists 2 to 3 weeks, and pain and hyperemia last up to 14 weeks. Some blister sloughing occurs, but no loss of deep tissue. Some patients will have permanent injury.
- *Severe.* Severe edema, blood forced into surrounding tissues *(extravasation),* and gangrene are present 2 to 3 days after injury. Complete anesthesia of entire foot remains at 7 days, with paralysis and muscle wasting in the affected extremities. The injury goes beyond the foot into the lower leg. This severe injury produces significant tissue loss, resulting in autoamputation. Gangrene is a constant risk until tissue loss is complete. The patient is expected to have prolonged convalescence and a permanent disability.

Assessment. Because the patient has experienced mild or moderate cold exposure, it is essential to rule out hypothermia and assess for dehydration. Even though this is not a freezing injury, NCFI still is an insidious injury; the common finding with these two localized cold injuries is that the extremity is cooled to the point of anesthesia or numbness while the injury is occurring.

The key to management of NFCI is detection during assessment. During the initial assessment, injured tissue appears macerated, edematous, pale, anesthetized, pulseless, and immobile, but not frozen. Patients complain of clumsiness and stumbling when attempting to walk. After removal from cold and during or after rewarming, peripheral blood flow increases as reperfusion of ischemic tissue begins. Extremities change color from white to mottled pale blue while remaining cold and numb. The diagnosis of trench foot or immersion foot is generally made when these signs have not changed after passive rewarming of the feet. From 24 to 36 hours after rewarming, a marked hyperemia develops, along with severe burning pain and reappearance of sensation proximally, but not distally. This is caused by venous vasodilation. Edema and blisters develop in the injured areas as perfusion increases. Skin will remain poorly perfused after hyperemia appears, and the skin is likely to slough as the injury evolves. Any pulselessness after 48 hours in the injured extremity suggests severe, deep injury and a greater chance of substantial tissue loss.

Management. Once a possible NFCI is detected, the priorities are to eliminate any further cooling, prevent further trauma to the extremity, and transport the patient. Do not allow the patient to walk on an injured extremity. Carefully remove the footwear and socks. Cover the injured part or extremity with loose, dry, sterile dressing, protect from cold, and begin passive rewarming of injured tissue during transport. The affected area may be aggravated by the weight of a blanket. No active rewarming is necessary. Do not massage the affected area because this may cause further damage. As needed, treat for dehydration with a bolus of IV fluids, and reassess. Depending on length of transport during passive rewarming, severe pain may develop as tissues begin to reperfuse, and before rewarming it may be necessary to manage with adequate opiate analgesia (e.g., begin initially with 5 mg morphine IV as needed).

Freezing Cold Injury

Clinical Manifestations. On the continuum of further peripheral cold tissue exposure from frostnip, *frostbite* ranges from mild to severe tissue destruction and possibly the loss of tissue.[5,9] The most susceptible body parts for frostbite are those tissues with large surface-to-mass ratios, such as the ears and nose or areas farthest from the body's core, such as the hands, fingers, feet, toes, and male genitalia. These structures are most susceptible to cold injury because they obtain many arteriovenous capillary *anastomoses* that easily shunt blood away during vasoconstriction. The body's normal response to lower-than-desirable temperatures is to reduce blood flow to the skin surface to reduce heat exchange with the environment. The body accomplishes this by vasoconstriction of peripheral blood vessels in an attempt to shunt warm blood to the body's core to maintain a normal body temperature. Reduction of this blood flow greatly reduces the amount of heat delivered to the distal extremities.

The longer the period of exposure, the more the blood flow is reduced to the periphery. The body conserves core temperature at the expense of extremity and skin temperature. The heat loss from the tissue becomes greater than the heat supplied to that area.

When an extremity is cooled to 59° F (15° C), maximal vasoconstriction and minimal blood flow occur. If cooling continues to 50° F (10° C), vasoconstriction is interrupted by periods of *cold-induced vasodilation* (CIVD), known as the "hunting response," and an associated increase in tissue temperature caused by an increase in blood flow. CIVD recurs in 5- to 10-minute cycles to provide some protection from the cold. Individuals show differences in susceptibility to frostbite when exposed to the same cold conditions, which may be explained by the amount of CIVD.[9]

Tissue does not freeze at 32° F (0° C) because cells contain electrolytes and other solutes that prevent tissue from freezing until skin temperature reaches approximately 28° F (−2° C). In cases of below-freezing temperatures when the extremities are left unprotected, the intracellular and extracellular fluids can freeze. This results in the formation of ice crystals. As the ice crystals form, they expand and cause damage to local tissues. Blood clots may also form, further impairing circulation to the injured area.

The type and duration of cold contact are the two most important factors in determining the extent of freezing injury. Frostbite is classified by depth of injury and clinical presentation.[9] The degree of injury in many cases will not be known for at least 24 to 72 hours, except in very minor or severe exposures. Cold exposure to skin that is short in duration but very intense will create a superficial injury, whereas severe frostbite to a whole extremity can occur during prolonged exposures. Direct cold injury is usually reversible, but permanent tissue damage occurs during rewarming. In more severe cases, even with appropriate rewarming of tissue, microvascular thrombosis can develop, leading to early signs of gangrene and necrosis. When the injured site freezes, thaws, and then refreezes, the second freezing causes a greater amount of severe thrombosis and vascular damage and tissue loss. For this reason, prehospital care providers need to prevent any frozen tissue that thaws during initial field treatment from being subjected to refreezing.

Traditional methods of frostbite classification present four degrees of injury based on initial physical findings

FIGURE 16-5 Edema and blister formation 24 hours after frostbite injury.
(From McCauley RL, Smith DJ, Robson MC, Heggers JP: Frostbite. In Auerbach PS: *Wilderness medicine: management of wilderness and environmental emergencies,* ed 4, St Louis, 2001, Mosby. Photograph courtesy Cameron Bangs, MD.)

FIGURE 16-6 Deep second-degree and third-degree frostbite with hemorrhagic blebs, 1 day after thawing.
(From McCauley RL, Smith DJ, Robson MC, Heggers JP: Frostbite. In Auerbach PS: *Wilderness medicine: management of wilderness and environmental emergencies,* ed 4, St Louis, 2001, Mosby. Photograph courtesy Murray P. Hamlet, DVM.)

after freezing and rewarming[9] (Figures 16-5 and 16-6), as follows:

- *First-degree frostbite.* An epidermal injury; limited to skin that has brief contact with cold air or metal; skin appears white or as yellowish plaque at site of injury; no blister or tissue loss; skin thaws quickly, feels numb, and appears red with surrounding edema; healing occurs in 7 to 10 days.
- *Second-degree frostbite.* Involves all the epidermis and superficial dermis; initially appears similar to first-degree injury, and frozen tissues are deeper; thawing is rapid; results in superficial skin blister or vesiculation that has clear or milky fluid after several hours; surrounded by erythema and edema; no permanent loss of tissue; healing occurs in 3 to 4 weeks.
- *Third-degree frostbite.* Involves the epidermis and dermis layers; frozen skin is stiff with restricted mobility; after tissue thaws, skin swells along with blood-filled blister (hemorrhagic bullae), indicating vascular trauma to deep tissues; swelling restricts

mobility; skin loss occurs slowly, leading to mummification and sloughing; healing is slow.

■ *Fourth-degree frostbite.* Frozen tissue involves full thickness completely through the dermis, with muscle and bone involvement; no mobility when frozen, and passive movement when thawed, with no intrinsic muscle function; poor skin perfusion; blisters and edema do not develop; early signs of necrotic tissue; slow mummification process will occur along with sloughing of tissue and autoamputation of nonviable tissue.

Although traditional classification of frostbite is by the four degrees of injury, it is easiest for EMS providers in the prehospital setting to classify as either superficial or deep.[71-73] *Superficial frostbite* (first and second degree) affects the skin and subcutaneous tissues, resulting in clear blisters when rewarmed. *Deep frostbite* (third and fourth degree) affects skin, muscle, and bone, and the skin has hemorrhagic blisters when rewarmed.

In special situations, frostbite may occur rapidly, and prehospital care providers may respond to the following:

■ Hydrocarbon fluid spills on skin; for example, gasoline will cause rapid evaporation and conduction in below-freezing temperatures
■ Touching extremely cold metal with warm skin
■ Intense windchill on exposed skin caused by rotary wind from a medical helicopter

Assessment. On arrival, assess scene safety and then the patient for ABCs. Remove the patient from the cold, and place in an area protected from moisture, cold, and wind. Many frostbite victims may have other medical conditions, such as dehydration, hypovolemia, hypothermia, hypoglycemia, and traumatic injury. Remove any wet clothing to minimize further body heat loss. When in doubt, treat hypothermia first. Superficial frostbite is usually assessed through a combination of recognizing the environmental conditions, locating the patient's chief complaint of pain or numbness, and observing discolored skin in the same area. The environmental conditions during exposure must be below freezing.

Frostbite injuries are insidious because the patient may have no pain at the injury site when skin is frozen and covered by a glove or footwear. Detection of the affected area requires direct visual inspection of highly suspect body regions, as previously listed. Gentle palpation of the area can determine if the underlying tissue is compliant or hard. Ensure that the patient or prehospital care provider does not rub or massage the affected skin, because this will cause further cellular damage to frozen tissues. The patient with superficial freezing will usually complain of discomfort during the manipulation of the frostbitten area. In patients with deep frostbite the frozen tissue will be hard

and usually is not painful when touched. After inspection of the affected area, a decision is necessary about the method of rewarming.

Management. Patients with superficial frostnip or frostbite should be placed with the affected area against a warm body surface, such as covering the patient's ears with warm hands or placing affected fingers into armpits, axillae, or groin regions. Superficial frostbite only needs to be warmed at normal body temperatures. Management in the prehospital care of deep frostbite includes the following:

1. Provide supportive care and appropriate shelter for the patient and the affected part to minimize heat loss
2. Cover with loose, dry, sterile dressing that is noncompressive and nonadherent
3. Do not allow patient to walk on affected feet
4. Fingers and toes should be separated and protected with sterile cotton gauze
5. Do not drain blisters
6. Hands and feet should be splinted and elevated to reduce edema
7. Intravenous opiate analgesics are usually required for pain relief and should be initiated before tissues have thawed
8. Initiate normal saline IV with a 250-mL bolus to treat dehydration and reduce blood viscosity and capillary sludging
9. Protect fragile tissues from further trauma during patient movement
10. Do not use a direct heat source greater than 102° F (>39° C) on the affected area
11. Do not allow the thawed part to thaw and refreeze
12. Ensure early transport to an appropriate facility

The patient can drink something warm (and nonalcoholic) if it is available, depending on the patient's LOC and other injuries. Tobacco use (smoking, chewing, using nicotine patches) should be discouraged because nicotine causes further vasoconstriction.

Attempts to begin rewarming of deep frostbite patients in the field can be hazardous to the patient's eventual recovery and are not recommended unless delayed transport times are involved.

Accidental Hypothermia

Hypothermia is defined as the condition in which the core body temperature is below 95° F (35° C), as measured by a rectal thermometer placed at least 6 inches (15 cm) into the rectum.[10] Hypothermia can be viewed as a decrease in core temperature that renders a victim unable to generate sufficient heat production to return to homeostasis or normal bodily functions. Hypothermia can occur in many different situations, resulting from cold ambient air, cold-water immersion, or cold-water submersion (cold-water near-drowning), and can be intentionally induced during surgery.[10,74,75] Immersion ("head out") hypothermia typically occurs when an individual is accidentally placed into a cold environment without preparation or planning. For example, a person who has fallen into ice water is immediately in danger of becoming a submersion casualty, resulting from "cold shock" gasp reflex, loss of motor skills, hypothermia, and drowning. These unique aspects of submersion incidents can lead to hypoxia and hypothermia (see later discussion and Chapter 17).

The progression of hypothermia in cold air or cold water can be delayed as long as the metabolic heat production can match heat loss. Surviving an overwhelming cold exposure is possible, with many reported cases of survival at sea and in other extreme situations.[62,76] Many factors are known to increase survival after cold exposure, including age, gender, body composition (e.g., body surface area–to–body mass ratio), onset and intensity of shivering, level of physical fitness, nutritional state, and alcohol consumption.

Unlike frostbite, hypothermia can occur in environments with temperatures well above freezing. *Primary hypothermia* generally occurs when healthy individuals are in adverse weather conditions unprepared for overwhelming acute or chronic cold exposure. Deaths by primary hypothermia are a direct result of cold exposure and are documented by the medical examiner as accidental, homicidal, or suicidal.[10]

Secondary hypothermia is considered a normal consequence of a patient's systemic disorders, including hypothyroidism, hypoadrenalism, trauma, carcinoma, and sepsis. If unrecognized or improperly treated, hypothermia can be fatal, in some cases within 2 hours. Mortality is greater than 50% in cases of secondary hypothermia caused by complications of other injuries and in severe cases in which the core body temperature is below 90° F (32° C).[10]

Hypothermia is a common finding in severely injured patients arriving at a trauma center.[77,78] The combination of multisystem trauma and hypothermia has a significant impact on patient survival. The development of hypothermia is related to the effect of trauma on thermoregulation and the inhibition of shivering as a primary mechanism for heat production.[79] One cause of higher mortality in hypothermic trauma patients is related to the lethal combination of *hypothermia, acidosis,* and *coagulopathy* (inability of blood to clot normally). This is known as the "lethal triad" in trauma patients.[80] Consequently, it is essential to assess and treat patients equally for trauma and hypothermia because the coagulopathy is reversible with patient rewarming.[78] A detailed discussion of hypothermia pathophysiology in trauma patients is beyond the scope of this chapter; see further discussions on trauma and hypothermia in Chapters 5 and 7, respectively.

Immersion Hypothermia

During immersion, if there is no heat gain or heat loss by the body, water temperature is considered *thermoneutral.*

Thermoneutral water temperature is 91° to 95° F (33°-35° C), at which temperatures a nude individual passively standing in neck-level water can maintain a nearly constant core temperature for at least 1 hour.[81,82] Individuals in thermoneutral water are at almost no risk for the initial immersion "cold shock" and hypothermia experienced in sudden cold-water exposure.[83]

When immersion occurs in water temperature colder than the lower thermoneutral limit, the immediate physiologic changes are a rapid decline in skin temperature, peripheral vasoconstriction resulting in shivering and increased metabolism, ventilation, heart rate, cardiac output, and MAP. To offset any heat loss in water, heat production must occur by increasing physical activity, shivering, or both. If not, core temperature continues to fall and shivering ceases, and these physiologic responses decrease proportionally with the fall in core temperature.[75]

The greatest risk of immersion hypothermia usually begins in water temperature less than 77° F (25° C).[84] Because the heat dissipation capacity of water is 24 times greater than that of air, individuals are at more rapid risk for hypothermia in water. However, continued physical activity in cold water will eventually become a detriment by increasing convective heat loss to the colder water surrounding the body, resulting in a faster onset of hypothermia. This understanding has lead to the recommendation for individuals to minimize heat loss during cold-water immersion by using the *heat escape lessening posture* (HELP) or the *huddle position* when multiple immersion victims are together[85] (Figure 16-7).

A **B**

FIGURE 16-7 Techniques for decreasing cooling rates of survivors in cold water. **A,** Heat escape lessening posture (HELP). **B,** Huddle technique.

The lowest recorded core temperature for an infant with an intact neurologic recovery from accidental hypothermia is 59° F (15° C).[86] In an adult, 56.8° F (13.7° C) is the lowest recorded core temperature for a survivor of accidental hypothermia. This occurred in a 29-year-old female who struggled to self-rescue for more than 40 minutes before symptoms of severe hypothermia affected muscular contraction.[76] She was immersed for more than 80 minutes before a rescue team arrived and cardiopulmonary resuscitation (CPR) was initiated during transport to a local hospital. During the first 5 minutes of rewarming, her core temperature further decreased to 57° F (13.7° C). After 3 hours of continuous rewarming, her core temperature returned to normal, and she survived with normal physiologic function.

This case of accidental hypothermia illustrates why all prehospital care providers managing hypothermic patients should not stop treatment interventions and declare the patient deceased until they have been rewarmed to over 95° F (>35° C) and still have no evidence of cardiorespiratory and neurologic function. This is one of many hypothermic survivor scenarios where patients are discharged from the hospital with full neurologic function after prolonged CPR in the field. The lessons from this case and others with a similar outcome are that the initial impression of these patients is not sufficient justification to withhold basic or advanced life support until core temperature has returned to normal; advanced lifesaving procedures are initiated as well. This is the reason the following phrase was created:

"Patients are not dead until they are warm and dead."

Whether intentional or unintentional, cold-water immersion (head out) occurs throughout the year in the United States as a result of recreational and industrial activities, as well as from accidents. If the individual survives the initial submersion incident without drowning, he or she is at risk for hypothermia depending on the water temperature. The body's responses to cold-water immersion can be divided into the following three phases[84]:

- *First phase.* This phase begins with a cardiovascular reflex known as "cold shock" response that occurs quickly (within 2-4 minutes) after immersion and begins with rapid skin cooling, peripheral vasoconstriction, a gasp reflex and the inability to breath-hold, hyperventilation, and tachycardia.[75,87] The gasp response may lead to aspiration and drowning, depending on the individual's head location above or below water. These responses can lead to immediate sudden death or death within minutes following immersion because of several conditions in this setting, including syncope or convulsions resulting in drowning, vagal arrest, and ventricular fibrillation.[75,87-89]
- *Second phase.* If a victim survives the cold shock phase, significant cooling of peripheral tissues occurs over the first 30 minutes of immersion. This cooling has a deleterious effect on gross and fine motor skills of the extremities, causing finger stiffness, poor coordination, and loss of power, making it nearly impossible to swim, grasp a rescue line, or perform other survival motor skills.[75,84]
- *Third phase.* Surviving the first two phases without drowning places an individual at risk of hypothermia from continuous heat loss and core temperature reduction from immersion longer than 30 minutes. If the victim is not able to remain above the water surface because of fatigue and hypothermia, the individual is at risk to become a submersion casualty, leading to aspiration and drowning.[75,90] How long an individual can survive in cold water depends on many factors. It has been estimated that a submersion victim cannot survive for more than 1 hour at a water temperature of 32° F (0° C), and at a water temperature of 59° F (15° C), survival is uncommon after 6 hours.[91]

The U.S. Coast Guard and other search and rescue organizations use guidelines to assist in estimating how long individuals can survive in the cold water. Theses guidelines are mathematical models that estimate core temperature cooling rate based on the influence of the following variables: (1) water temperature and sea state, (2) clothing insulation, (3) body composition (amount of fat, muscle, and bone), (4) amount of the body immersed in water, (5) behavior (e.g., excessive movement) and posture (e.g., HELP, huddle) of the body in the water, and (6) shivering thermogenesis.[92-94]

Clinical Manifestations. The influence hypothermia has on the body affects all major organ systems, particularly the cardiac, renal, and central nervous systems. As the body's core temperature decreases to 95° F (35° C), maximal rate of vasoconstriction, shivering, and metabolic rate occurs, with increases in heart rate, respiration, and blood pressure. Cerebral metabolism oxygen demand decreases by 6% to 10% per 1° C drop in core temperature, and cerebral metabolism is preserved. When core temperature falls between 86° F (30° C) and 95° F (35° C), cognitive function, cardiac function, metabolic rate, respiratory rate, and shivering rate are all significantly decreased or completely inhibited. At this point, the limited physiologic defensive mechanisms prevent heat loss from the body, and core temperature falls rapidly. At a core temperature of 85° F (29.5° C), cardiac output and metabolic rate are reduced approximately 50%. Ventilation and perfusion are inadequate and do not keep up with the metabolic demand, causing cellular hypoxia, increased lactic acid, and an eventual metabolic and respiratory acidosis. Oxygenation and blood flow are maintained in the core and brain.

Bradycardia occurs in a large percentage of patients as a direct effect of cold on the depolarization of pacemaker cells and their slower propagation through the conduction system. It is important to note that the use of atropine is often ineffective to increase the heart rate when the myocardium is cold.[5] When core temperature falls below 86° F (30° C), the myocardium becomes irritable. The PR, QRS, and QTC intervals are prolonged. ST-segment and T-wave changes and J (or Osborne) waves may be present and may mimic other ECG abnormalities, such as an acute myocardial infarction (AMI). The J waves are a striking ECG feature in hypothermic patients and are seen in approximately one third of moderately to severely hypothermic patients (<90° F [<32° C]). The J wave is described as a "humplike" deflection between the QRS complex and the early part of the ST segment.[95] The J wave is best viewed in the aVL, aVF, and left lateral leads (Figure 16-8).

Atrial fibrillation and extreme bradycardias develop and may continue between 83° and 90° F (28° and 32° C). When the core temperature reaches 80° to 82° F (26.7°-28° C), any physical stimulation of the heart can cause ventricular fibrillation (VF). CPR or rough handling (patient assessment and movement) of the patient could be sufficient to cause VF. At these extremely low core temperatures, pulse and blood pressure are not detectable, and the joints are stiff. The pupils become fixed and dilated at extremely low core temperatures. Again, a patient should not be assumed to be dead until he or she is rewarmed and still has no signs of life (ECG, pulse, ventilation, and CNS function).

With acute cold exposure, renal blood flow increases because of the shunting of blood during vasoconstriction. At 81° to 86° F (27°-30° C), renal blood flow is depressed by 50%. At this moderate to severe hypothermic level, the decrease in cardiac output causes a fall in renal blood flow and glomerular filtration rate, which in turn results in acute renal failure (ARF).

Assessment. It is imperative to assess scene safety on arrival. All responders need to ensure their safety and protection from cold exposure while working in this environment. There should be a high suspicion for hypothermia even when the environmental conditions are not highly suggestive (e.g., wind, moisture, temperature). Some patients may present with vague complaints of fatigue, nausea, vomiting, and dizziness. With trauma and critically ill patients, it is important to begin assessment and assume hypothermia by protecting the patient from the cold environment; assessment starts with the ABCs. Neurologic function is assessed and monitored frequently. Severely hypothermic patients generally present with tachypnea, stupor, and coma. Rectal temperatures are not usually assessed in the field or widely used as a vital sign in most prehospital systems. Ambulances usually carry a standard-range oral or rectal (for infants) thermometer with a lower limit of 96° F (35.5° C). Electronic thermometers are not useful in hypothermic situations for accurate readings. To obtain hypothermic temperatures, a low-range rectal thermometer is necessary. Table 16-4 provides the anticipated physiologic responses with decreasing core temperature.

FIGURE 16-8 J wave, or Osborne wave, of hypothermia.
(From Danzl DF: Accidental hypothermia. In Auerbach PS: *Wilderness medicine: management of wilderness and environmental emergencies,* ed 4, St Louis, 2001, Mosby.)

TABLE 16-4   Physiologic Characteristics of Hypothermia

°C	°F	Characteristics
37.6	99.6 ±1	Normal rectal temperature
37.0	98.6 ±1	Normal oral temperature
36.0	96.8	Increase in metabolic rate and blood pressure and preshivering muscle tone
35.0	95.0	Urine temperature 34.8° C; maximum shivering thermogenesis
34.0	93.2	Amnesia, dysarthria, and poor judgment develop; maladaptive behavior; normal blood pressure; maximum respiratory stimulation; tachycardia, then progressive bradycardia
33.3	91.4	Ataxia and apathy develop; linear depression of cerebral metabolism; tachypnea, then progressive decrease in respiratory minute volume; cold diuresis
32.0	89.6	Stupor; 25% decrease in oxygen consumption
31.0	87.8	Extinguished shivering thermogenesis
30.0	86.0	Atrial fibrillation and other arrhythmias develop; poikilothermia; pupils and cardiac output two thirds of normal; insulin ineffective
29.0	84.2	Progressive decrease in level of consciousness, pulse, and respiration; pupils dilated; paradoxical undressing
28.0	82.4	Decreased ventricular fibrillation threshold; 50% decrease in oxygen consumption and pulse; hypoventilation
27.0	80.6	Loss of reflexes and voluntary motion
26.0	78.8	Major acid-base disturbances; no reflexes or response to pain
25.0	77.0	Cerebral blood flow one third of normal; loss of cerebrovascular autoregulation; cardiac output 45% of normal; pulmonary edema may develop
24.0	75.2	Significant hypotension and bradycardia
23.0	73.4	No corneal or oculocephalic reflexes; areflexia
22.0	71.6	Maximum risk of ventricular fibrillation; 75% decrease in oxygen consumption
20.0	68.0	Lowest resumption of cardiac electromechanical activity; pulse 20% of normal
19.0	66.2	Electroencephalographic silencing
18.0	64.4	Asystole
15.0	59.0	Lowest infant accidental hypothermia survival
13.7	56.8	Lowest adult accidental hypothermia survival
10.0	50.0	92% decrease in oxygen consumption
9.0	48.2	Lowest therapeutic hypothermia survival

Modified from Danzl DF: Accidental hypothermia. In Auerbach PS: *Wilderness medicine: management of wilderness and environmental emergencies*, ed 4, St Louis, 2001, Mosby.

Signs of shivering and mental status change are important in the assessment of suspected hypothermia. Mildly hypothermic patients (core temperature >90° F, or 32° C) will be shivering and usually show signs of altered LOC (e.g., confusion, slurred speech, altered gait, clumsiness). They will be slow in their actions and are usually found in a nonambulatory state, sitting or lying. Law enforcement personnel and prehospital care providers may misinterpret this condition as drug or alcohol intoxication or as cerebrovascular accident (CVA, stroke) in elderly patients. However, a patient's LOC is not a reliable indicator of the degree of hypothermia; some patients have remained conscious at core temperature below 80° F (27° C).

When the patient's core temperature falls below 90° F (32° C), moderate hypothermia is present, and the patient will probably not complain of feeling cold. Shivering will be absent, and the patient's LOC will be greatly decreased, possibly to the point of unconsciousness and coma. The patient's pupils will react slowly or may be dilated and fixed. The patient's palpable pulses may be diminished or absent, and SBP may be low or indeterminate. The patient's ventilations may have slowed to as few as 2 breaths/min.

An ECG may show atrial fibrillation, the most common dysrhythmia. As the myocardium becomes progressively colder and more irritable at about 82° F (28° C), VF is more often observed. Because of the changes in cerebral metabolism, evidence of "paradoxical undressing" may be observed before the patient loses consciousness. This is an attempt by the patient to remove the clothing while in the cold environment, and it is thought to represent a response to an impending thermoregulatory failure.

The clinical management of hypothermia is based on the following three ranges of rectal body temperature[96]:

- *Mild hypothermia* is >93° to <97° F (>34° to <36° C)
- *Moderate hypothermia* is 86° to 93° F (30° to 34° C)
- *Severe hypothermia* is <86° F (<30° C)

Management. Prehospital care of the hypothermic patient consists of preventing further heat loss, gentle handling, initiating rapid transport, and rewarming. This includes moving the patient away from any cold source to a warm ambulance or to a warm shelter if transportation is not immediately available (see Prolonged Transport section). Wet clothing should be removed by cutting with trauma shears to avoid unnecessary movement and agitation of the patient. Concern for initiating ventricular arrhythmias based on the handling of the patient should not delay any critical interventions. This concern becomes more realistic in severe hypothermic patients (<86° F, or 30° C). The patient's head and body should be covered with warm blankets or sleeping bags, followed by an outer windproof layer to prevent convective and evaporative heat loss.

If the patient is conscious and alert, anticipate hypoglycemia and provide warm, high-caloric or glucose fluids. The patient should avoid alcohol and caffeine drinks. Hypothermic patients need high-flow oxygen because they have a decreased oxygen delivery to the tissues; the oxyhemoglobin dissociation curve shifts to the left with a decrease in core temperature. High-flow oxygen should be delivered using a nonrebreather mask or BVM. Ideally, the patient may benefit more if the oxygen can be warmed and humidified (108°-115° F [42°-46° C]). If possible, warmed oxygen administered before movement may prevent VF during transport.

In unresponsive hypothermic patients, passive rewarming will be insufficient to increase core temperature. These patients will need an airway adjunct to protect the airway, and this should be initiated depending on jaw rigidity. If endotracheal intubation cannot be successfully achieved without rough handling, continue ventilation with a BVM and consider another advanced airway adjunct (e.g., Combitube, laryngeal mask airway, nasal intubation). At a minimum, use an oral or nasal pharyngeal airway with bag-mask ventilation.

Intravenous NS, ideally with 5% dextrose, should be warmed to 109° F (43° C) and administered without agitating the patient. *The hypothermic patient should not be given cold (room-temperature) fluids* because this could make the patient colder or could delay rewarming. When NS and dextrose solutions are unavailable, any warm crystalloid solution is satisfactory. Provide a fluid challenge of 500 to 1000 mL, and prevent the solution from freezing or becoming colder by placing the IV bag under the patient to infuse warm fluids under pressure. These two forms of therapy are minimal at best for rewarming, and the prehospital care provider should use good judgment to decide whether fluids (orally or IV) are worth the risks of aspiration, coughing, and painful stimuli to the patient. Hot packs or massaging of the patient's extremities are not recommended. Typically, active external rewarming occurs only to the thoracic region, with no active rewarming of the extremities. This will prevent increased peripheral circulation, causing an increase amount of colder blood to the thorax before central core rewarming. Increased return of peripheral blood can increase acidosis and hyperkalemia and can actually decrease the core temperature ("afterdrop"). This complicates resuscitation and may precipitate VF.

National Guidelines for Treatment of Cold-Related Disorders

Emergency Cardiovascular Care: Basic and Advanced Lifesaving Guidelines for Management of Hypothermia

Guidelines for resuscitation of the hypothermic patient have evolved over many decades. The most recent revision of the Emergency Cardiovascular Care (ECC) guidelines by the American Heart Association in collaboration with the International Liaison Committee on Resuscitation represents the latest findings in cardiovascular care research. The current ECC guidelines were published by the American Heart Association in the journal *Circulation* in December 2005.[97]

The hypothermic victim can present many challenges to the EMS provider, particularly the unconscious, moderately to severely hypothermic patient. Because severe hypothermia is a core temperature less than 86° F (<30° C), the patient can present with no detectable pulse or respiration because of the reduced cardiac output and decreased arterial pressure. Historically, the challenge has been to determine whether to initiate basic (BLS) or advanced (ALS) life support interventions on these patients based on the viability of the patient. Furthermore, it may be difficult to determine from any bystanders whether these patients had a primary hypothermic exposure or, for example, a cardiac arrest or stroke, that preceded the hypothermia. Other concerns for a prehospital care provider are protecting the hypothermic patient with a potential irritable myocardium from any rough handling and initiating chest compression for the patient with nondetectable pulse, in whom both these interventions may initiate VF.[96]

However, it is now recommended that independent of any scenario that created the primary or secondary hypothermia, *do not* withhold lifesaving procedures on the basis of clinical presentation, whether in an urban setting with short transport distances or in the backcountry environment with potentially significant delays in transport, where extended patient care may be necessary (see later discussion).

Updates to Basic Life Support Guidelines for Treatment of Mild to Severe Hypothermia

Hypothermic patients should be kept in a horizontal position at all times to avoid aggravating hypotension because these patients are often volume-depleted from cold diuresis. It may be difficult to feel or detect respiration and a pulse in the hypothermic patient. Therefore it is recommended initially to assess for breathing and then a pulse for 30 to 45 seconds to confirm one of the following:

- Respiratory arrest
- Pulseless cardiac arrest (asystole, ventricular tachycardia, VF)
- Bradycardia (requiring CPR)

If the patient is not breathing, start rescue breathing immediately. Start chest compressions immediately in any hypothermic patient who is pulseless and has no detectable signs of circulation.[96] If there is a doubt about detecting a pulse, begin compressions. Never withhold BLS interventions until the patient is rewarmed. If the patient is determined to be in cardiac arrest, use the current BLS guidelines, as outlined elsewhere.[97]

An automated external defibrillator (AED) should be used if pulseless ventricular tachycardia or VF is present. The current ECC guidelines recommend that these patients should be treated by providing up to 5 cycles (2 minutes) of CPR (one cycle is 30 compressions to 2 breaths) before checking the ECG rhythm and attempting to shock when an AED arrives.[98] If a shockable rhythm is determined, give one shock, then reassess the pulse. If the hypothermic patient does not respond to one shock with a detectable pulse, further attempts to defibrillate the patient should be deferred and efforts directed toward effective CPR with an emphasis on rewarming the patient. When performing chest compression in a hypothermic patient, a greater force is required because chest wall elasticity is decreased when cold.[98] If core temperature is below 86° F (30° C), the conversion to normal sinus rhythm does not normally occur until rewarming above this core temperature is accomplished.[99]

The importance of not declaring patients dead until they have been rewarmed and remain unresponsive is even greater today, with new evidence from studies of hypothermic victims indicating that cold exerts a protective effect on the vital organs.[99,100] (See further discussion on cardiac arrest and the protective effect of mild hypothermia in the section on prolonged transport.)

Updates to ACLS Guidelines for Treatment of Hypothermia

The treatment of severe hypothermia in the field remains controversial.[96] However, the guidelines for administering advanced cardiac life support (ACLS) procedures are different than with a normothermic patient. Unconscious hypothermic patients need a protected airway and should be intubated. Do not delay intubation based on concern for initiating VF. As noted earlier, if a shockable rhythm is detected, defibrillate once at 360 joules, resume CPR, and then defer cardiac drugs and subsequent defibrillation attempts until core temperature is above 86° F (30° C). If possible, initiate active rewarming procedures with warm, humid oxygen and warm IV solutions, and package the patient for transport by preventing further heat loss.

The challenge with ACLS procedures in a hypothermic patient is that the heart may be unresponsive to ACLS drugs, pacing, and defibrillation.[101] Furthermore, ACLS drugs, (e.g., epinephrine, amiodarone, lidocaine, procainamide) can accumulate to toxic levels in the circulation with repeated administration in the severely hypothermic patient, particularly when the patient rewarms.[96] Consequently, it is recommended to withhold IV medications in patients with a core temperature below 86° F (30° C). If a hypothermic patient initially presents with a core temperature above 86° F, or if a severely hypothermic patient has been rewarmed above this temperature, IV medications may be administered. However, longer intervals between drug administration are recommended than with standard drug intervals in ACLS.[96] The use of repeated defibrillation is indicated if the core temperature continues to rise above 86° F (30° C), consistent with the current ACLS guidelines.[97]

Finally, BLS/ACLS procedures performed in the field should be withheld only in patients with injuries incompatible with life or if the body is frozen such that chest compressions are impossible, or if the mouth and nose are blocked with ice.[10,96] Figure 16-9 provides an algorithm of mild, moderate, and severe hypothermia guidelines for both pulse and pulseless patients.[96]

Prevention of Cold-Related Injuries

The prevention of cold injuries in patients, yourself, and other prehospital care providers is vital when on the scene. Recommendations to prevent cold-related injuries include the following[102]:

1. Note the risk factors generally accepted for cold injury:
   - Fatigue
   - Dehydration
   - Undernutrition
   - Lack of cold weather experience
   - Black race
   - Tobacco use
   - Wind chill

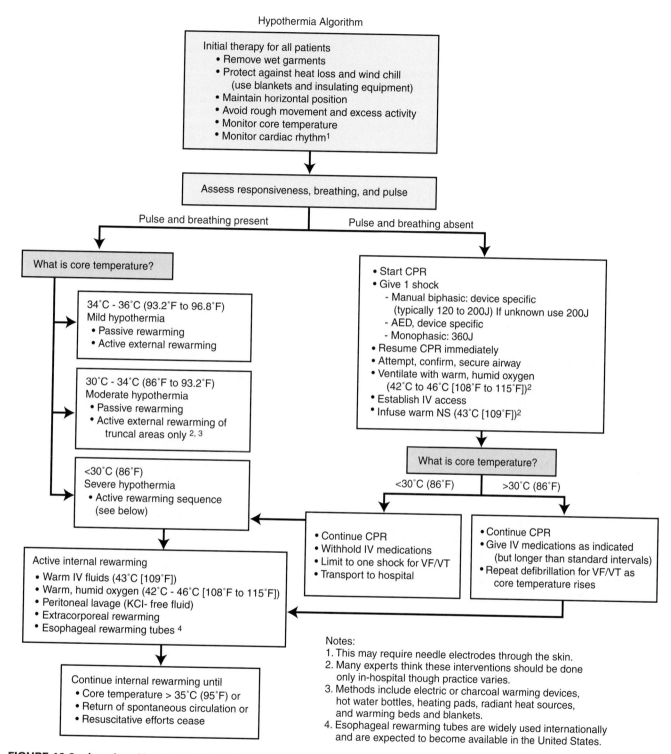

Hypothermia Algorithm

Initial therapy for all patients
- Remove wet garments
- Protect against heat loss and wind chill
  (use blankets and insulating equipment)
- Maintain horizontal position
- Avoid rough movement and excess activity
- Monitor core temperature
- Monitor cardiac rhythm[1]

Assess responsiveness, breathing, and pulse

Pulse and breathing present   Pulse and breathing absent

What is core temperature?

34°C - 36°C (93.2°F to 96.8°F)
Mild hypothermia
- Passive rewarming
- Active external rewarming

30°C - 34°C (86°F to 93.2°F)
Moderate hypothermia
- Passive rewarming
- Active external rewarming of
  truncal areas only [2, 3]

<30°C (86°F)
Severe hypothermia
- Active rewarming sequence
  (see below)

- Start CPR
- Give 1 shock
  - Manual biphasic: device specific
    (typically 120 to 200J) If unknown use 200J
  - AED, device specific
  - Monophasic: 360J
- Resume CPR immediately
- Attempt, confirm, secure airway
- Ventilate with warm, humid oxygen
  (42°C to 46°C [108°F to 115°F])[2]
- Establish IV access
- Infuse warm NS (43°C [109°F])[2]

What is core temperature?

<30°C (86°F)   >30°C (86°F)

- Continue CPR
- Withhold IV medications
- Limit to one shock for VF/VT
- Transport to hospital

- Continue CPR
- Give IV medications as indicated
  (but longer than standard intervals)
- Repeat defibrillation for VF/VT as
  core temperature rises

Active internal rewarming
- Warm IV fluids (43°C [109°F])
- Warm, humid oxygen (42°C - 46°C [108°F to 115°F])
- Peritoneal lavage (KCl- free fluid)
- Extracorporeal rewarming
- Esophageal rewarming tubes [4]

Continue internal rewarming until
- Core temperature > 35°C (95°F) or
- Return of spontaneous circulation or
- Resuscitative efforts cease

Notes:
1. This may require needle electrodes through the skin.
2. Many experts think these interventions should be done
   only in-hospital though practice varies.
3. Methods include electric or charcoal warming devices,
   hot water bottles, heating pads, radiant heat sources,
   and warming beds and blankets.
4. Esophageal rewarming tubes are widely used internationally
   and are expected to become available in the United States.

FIGURE 16-9 American Heart Association (AHA) hypothermia algorithm from the 2005 Cardiopulmonary Resuscitation and Emergency Cardiovascular Care guidelines.
(American Heart Association: *Handbook of emergency cardiovascular care for healthcare providers,* Chicago, 2006, AHA.)

2. When you cannot stay dry under conditions of cold, wet, and wind, end your session outdoors and seek shelter as soon as possible.

3. Remember that individuals with a history of cold injury are at a greater risk of a subsequent cold injury.

4. Avoid dehydration.

5. Avoid alcohol in cold environments.

6. Use the huddle technique with others if accidental water immersion in cold water occurs. You are more likely to survive if you remain still in cold water less

Wind Chill Chart

Wind (MPH) \ Temperature (°F)	40	35	30	25	20	15	10	5	0	-5	-10	-15	-20	-25	-30	-35	-40	-45
5	36	31	25	19	13	7	1	-5	-11	-16	-22	-28	-34	-40	-46	-52	-57	-63
10	34	27	21	15	9	3	-4	-10	-16	-22	28	-35	-41	-47	-53	-59	-66	-72
15	32	25	19	13	6	0	-7	-13	-19	-26	-32	-39	-45	-51	-58	-64	-71	-77
20	30	24	17	11	4	-2	-9	-15	-22	-29	-35	-42	-48	-55	-61	-68	-74	-81
25	29	23	16	9	3	-4	-11	-17	-24	-31	-37	-44	-51	-58	-64	-71	-78	-84
30	28	22	15	8	1	-5	-12	-19	-26	-33	-39	-46	-53	-60	-67	-73	-80	-87
35	28	21	14	7	0	-7	-14	-21	-27	34	-41	-48	-55	-62	-69	-76	-82	-89
40	27	20	13	6	-1	-8	-15	-22	-29	-36	-43	-50	-57	-64	-71	-78	-84	-91
45	26	19	12	5	-2	-9	-16	-23	-30	-37	-44	-51	-58	-65	-72	-79	-86	-93
50	26	19	12	4	-3	-10	-17	-24	-31	-38	-45	-52	-60	-67	-74	-81	-88	-95
55	25	18	11	4	-3	-11	-18	-25	-32	-39	-46	-54	-61	-68	-75	-82	-89	-97
60	25	17	10	3	-4	-11	-19	-26	-33	-40	-48	-55	-62	-69	-76	-84	-91	-98

Frostbite Times: ☐ 30 minutes ☐ 10 minutes ☐ 5 minutes

$$\text{Wind Chill (°F)} = 35.74 + 0.6215T - 35.75(V^{0.16}) + 0.4275T(V^{0.16})$$
Where, T = Air temperature (°F) V = Wind speed (mph)

FIGURE 16-10 Wind chill index.
(Courtesy National Weather Service.)

than 68° F (20° C), and do not attempt to swim to shore unless it is nearby.

7. Increase your likelihood of survival in cold environments by:
   - Maintaining a will to survive
   - Adaptability and improvisation
   - Optimism and belief that event is only a temporary situation
   - Maintaining a calm rationality to bizarre experiences and a sense of humor

8. Cold or nearly frozen extremities may be warmed with body heat by placing fingers in the armpits or groin area. Toes and feet can be placed on another person's stomach.

9. Keep protective cold weather clothing (e.g., boots, socks, gloves, winter hat, insulated pants and jacket, windproof outer shell) in your car for unexpected car emergencies during cold weather months.

10. Frostbite can occur rapidly when touching metal objects in the cold with your bare hands; always wear gloves.

11. Understand that the wind chill index (Figure 16-10) is composed of wind speed and air temperature, and be able to dress for extreme cold with insulated clothing and a windproof garment.

12. Keep feet dry with socks that transfer moisture from your feet to the footwear.

13. Do not walk through snow with low-cut shoes; if you lack appropriate shoes and protective clothes, attempt to stay in a protected area; do not lie or rest directly on snow. Lie on tree boughs, a sleeping pad, or a poncho.

14. Use a sleeping bag outdoors, and do not wear clothing; any sweat will be retained in your clothes and will increase heat loss and cause shivering.

15. Water-based lotions on face, hands, and ears will increase the risk for frostnip and frostbite. Use an oil-based lotion (e.g., Chapstick, Vaseline).

16. Mittens are more effective at trapping warm air around all fingers than a five-finger glove.

17. When protecting the lower extremities from cold weather, it is common not to consider protecting the genital region. Use of sweat pants, long underwear, Lycra tights, Gore-Tex pants, and any combination of these garments work well.

18. To prevent frostbite:
   - Do not wear tight clothing, gloves, or boots that restrict circulation
   - Exercise fingers, toes, and face periodically to keep them warm and to detect numb areas
   - Work or exercise with a partner, who watches for warning signs of cold injury and hypothermia

- Wear properly insulated clothing, and keep it dry; carry extra undergarments, socks, and shoes at all times
- Watch for numbness and tingling

Prolonged Transport

At times, the location of a patient will result in a delay in transport or a prolonged transport to an appropriate facility, necessitating extended prehospital care. Consequently, EMS providers may need to consider management options beyond what would be used with a rapid transport. How the patient is managed will depend on the time to definitive care, approved medical protocols, equipment and supplies on hand, additional personnel and resources, and location of the patient and severity of the injuries.

Some extended-care considerations for moderately to severely injured patients from each of the environments discussed in this chapter are provided here. As with all patient care, it is understood that the first priorities are scene safety, ABCDEs, and the use of standard assessment and management procedures appropriate to these environments. If medical control is available, always obtain a consult early, and communicate routinely throughout the extended-care period. Any of the procedures listed that fall outside the scope of practice are to be used by other, credentialed medical providers.

Also, it is important to know that all agencies have established guidelines for discontinuation of CPR. (See a discussion by the American Heart Association on the ethical issues arising from withholding or withdrawing BLS or ALS resuscitation efforts.[97]) The Wilderness Medical Society recommends that once CPR is initiated, it should be continued until resuscitation is successful, rescuers are exhausted, rescuers are placed in danger, the patient is turned over to more definitive care, or the patient does not respond to prolonged (≈30 minutes) resuscitative efforts.[103] The National Association of EMS Physicians also provides guidelines for the termination of CPR in the prehospital environment.[104] If medical control is available, begin patient consult early, if possible, for consideration of CPR termination after a total time of 20 minutes, depending on special patient circumstances (see Chapter 17 for further situations [e.g., cold-water submersion, lightning strike] in which CPR may be extended longer than 20 to 30 minutes).[103]

Heat-Related Illness

Heat Stroke
- Provide whole-body cooling as quickly as possible. Think about using any available access to water. Immerse the body to neck level in cool water (maintain body control and protect the airway), or spray the whole body with water (e.g., IV fluids, saline, water bottles, water from hydration backpacks), and provide a source of continuous wind current (e.g., natural wind current, fanning with towel, fire ventilation fans).
- When possible, keep medical control informed of patient status and to receive further medical directions.
- Stop body cooling when rectal temperature reaches 102° F (39° C). Then, protect the patient from shivering and hypothermia.
- As you are cooling, intubate unresponsive patients and initiate good ventilation with BVM with high-flow oxygen. Insert an IV line, provide a 500-mL NS fluid challenge, and assess vital signs. Patient should have vital signs assessed after every 500 mL. Total fluid volume should not exceed 1 to 2 L in the first hour. An additional liter can be considered during the second hour if prehospital care is extended.[8]
- The next priorities are to manage any seizure activity and hypoglycemia per medical protocol with diazepam and dextrose, respectively.
- Place the patient in recovery position, and continue assessment to include AVPU, vital signs, rectal temperature, and blood glucose. Provide supportive care and basic bodily needs throughout the remaining extended-care period.

Hyponatremia
- Correct the presumed low blood sodium concentration. If the patient can take food by mouth, and if available, provide potato chips, pretzels, or other salty food, a sport electrolyte or other sodium-containing beverage, or give 2 teaspoons of salt mixed in 16 ounces of water. Establish an IV line. Start NS with a flow rate of TKO. Check with medical control to consider a flow rate of 250 to 500 mL/hr based on the estimated delay in transporting the patient to the hospital. Do not use hypotonic IV fluids because this will exacerbate cerebral edema.
- In a patient with severe signs or symptoms (seizure or coma), consider administration of furosemide (a diuretic) to reduce extracellular body water content while providing some sodium by infusing NS, 250 to 500 mL/hr IV.
- Assess cerebral edema and increased ICP. Establish a baseline Glasgow Coma Scale (GCS) score, and reassess every 10 minutes as an indicator of progressive cerebral edema and increased ICP (manage per recommendation for cerebral edema; see Chapter 8).
- Be prepared to manage nausea and projectile vomiting. Take one side of a large trash bag and make a hole for the patient's head about 12 inches (30 cm) below the rim of the bag. Place the patient's head through the hole so that the patient can look down into the center of the bag.
- Be prepared to manage urine when diuresis begins. Use a large trash bag as a diaper or use a bucket or other container.

- Give supplemental oxygen to lethargic or obtunded patients. Intubate unresponsive patients, and initiate good ventilation with BVM (no hyperventilation; see Chapter 8), with oxygen at 10 breaths/min.
- Measure blood sugar, and provide IV dextrose per protocol to hypoglycemic patients.
- Monitor for seizures, and administer an anticonvulsant (e.g., diazepam, initially 2-5 mg IV/IM, and titrate per medical protocol).
- Place unconscious patients in left lateral recumbent position. Continue ongoing assessment of patient.

Cold-Related Illness

Frostbite

- Start IV fluids (KVO) before initiation of rewarming procedures.
- In a situation of significant transport delay, active rewarming should be considered. Rapid, active rewarming can reverse the direct injury of ice crystals in tissues, but it may not change the injury severity.[9] It is critical to keep the thawed tissue from refreezing because this significantly worsens the outcome compared with passive thawing. Thus, when and where to begin active rewarming becomes critical in the decision making, if it is to be done at all.
- A standard rewarming procedure is to immerse the affected extremity in circulating water warmed between 104° and 108° F (40° and 42° C).[9] If available, an oral or rectal thermometer should be used to measure water temperature. A temperature below that recommended will thaw tissue but is less beneficial for rapid thawing and for tissue survival. Any greater temperature may cause a burn injury.[9] Avoid active rewarming with intense sources of heat (e.g., placing near campfire). Continue immersion until tissue is soft and pliable, which may take up to 30 minutes. Active motion of the extremity during immersion is beneficial, without directed rubbing or massaging of the affected part.
- Extreme pain is experienced during rapid thawing. Treat with morphine, 5 to 10 mg IV, and titrate as needed. Provide ibuprofen, 400 mg orally every 12 hours, alone or in combination with morphine. Use of aspirin is no longer recommended for frostbite injury.
- The return of normal skin color, warmth, and sensation in the affected part are all favorable signs. Dry all affected parts, and ideally, rub topical aloe vera on skin, place sterile gauze between toes or fingers, bandage, splint, and elevate extremity. Cover any extremity with insulating material, and wrap a windproof and waterproof material (e.g., trash bag) as the outer layer, particularly if continuing patient extraction outdoors to a transport location.

Hypothermia

- Start active rewarming procedures.
- Shivering is the single best way for rewarming mildly hypothermic patients in the prehospital setting compared with external methods for rewarming. Hypothermic patients who are able to shiver maximally can increase core temperature by up to 6° to 8° F (≈3°-4° C) per hour.
- However, external heat sources are often used but may provide only minimal benefit.[75] For the moderately to severely hypothermic patient, these remain important considerations in the extended-care situation when used in combination with the hypothermia insulation wrap.
- Some external heat sources are as follows:
  1. Warmed, humidified oxygen by mask can prevent heat loss during respiration and provide some heat transfer to the chest from the respiratory tract.
  2. Body-to-body contact has merit for heat transfer, but many studies fail to show any advantage except in mildly hypothermic patients.
  3. Electric and portable heating pads provide no additional advantage.
  4. Forced-air warming has some benefit in minimizing postcooling core temperature ("afterdrop"); it provides effective warming rate comparable to shivering for mildly hypothermic patients.
- Insulate all hypothermic patients in the remote setting to minimize heat loss. Prepare a multilayer hypothermia wrap. Place a large, waterproof plastic sheet on the floor or ground. Add an insulation layer of blankets or a sleeping bag on top of the waterproof layer. Lay the patient on top of the insulation layer along with any external heat sources. Add a second insulating layer on top of the patient. The left side of the hypothermia wrap is folded over the patient first, then the right side. The patient's head is covered to prevent heat loss, keeping an opening at the face to allow patient assessment.
- Assess for hypoglycemia. Providing dextrose will ensure that adequate fuel (sugar) is available for muscular metabolism during shivering and will prevent further hypoglycemia. Alert patients can consume warm sugar fluids by mouth.

SUMMARY

Prehospital care providers will inevitably be faced with unpredictable environmental encounters, such as those described in this chapter. Basic knowledge of common environmental emergencies is necessary to provide rapid assessment and treatment in the prehospital setting. It is not easy to remember this type of information because these problems are infrequently encountered. Therefore, remember the general principles involved.

For heat-related illness, treat heat stroke patients with effective, rapid, whole-body cooling to reduce core temperature quickly.

For cold-related illness, manage all moderately to severely hypothermic patients gently, taking the time to remove them from the cold environment and begin passive rewarming while monitoring core temperature. Remember, drugs and defibrillation are generally ineffective when core temperature is less than 86° F (<30° C), and "patients are not dead until they are warm and dead."

In every case, remember that you must maintain your own safety. There are too many cases in which prehospital care providers have lost their lives as a result of attempting a rescue.

SCENARIO SOLUTION

This 60-year-old male patient is experiencing a heat stroke, a life-threatening condition. Several factors can be identified that may have contributed to the development of this emergency. First, the heat index is 128° F (54° C). These environmental conditions result in elevated core temperatures when exercising outdoors and increased sweat loss, leading to moderate to severe dehydration. Next, the patient is overweight, has a low fitness level, and has been expending significant energy while hiking. Additionally, he is taking antidepressants and antihistamines, two types of medications known to interfere with the body's ability to regulate core temperature effectively.

Because this patient is unconscious, initial care would include management of the airway and support of his ventilatory status. Oxygen would be administered to maintain a pulse oximetry reading of 95% or higher. A check of the patient's temperature reveals a rectal temperature of 105.6° F (40.5° C). This patient's temperature will continue to rise, so priority should be given to immediate procedures to lower the patient's temperature rapidly. For example, the prehospital care provider could wet all skin surfaces with water and fan the whole body.

Rapid transport in an air-conditioned unit to an appropriate medical facility should begin as soon as possible. Efforts to cool the patient should continue en route. If conditions delay immediate transport, the patient should be moved to a shady area, removed from any hot surface, and have his clothing removed. After this, he should be misted with water and rigorously fanned. An IV line should be initiated with LR solution and a 250-mL bolus given. Additional fluid boluses should be titrated to a normal blood pressure. Rectal temperature should be monitored frequently. Because of possible seizures, diazepam should be available. As the patient's temperature decreases, his vital signs will slowly return to normal, and his LOC should improve. ∎

References

1. National Center for Health Statistics: Compressed mortality file, Hyattsville, Md, 2002, US Department of Health and Human Services, Centers for Disease Control and Prevention.
2. Center for Disease Control and Prevention: Heat-related deaths—Chicago, Illinois, 1996-2001, and United States, 1979-1999, *MMWR* 52(26):610, 2003.
3. Center for Disease Control and Prevention: Hypothermia-related deaths—Utah, 2000, and United States, 1979-1998, *MMWR* 51(4):76, 2002.
4. Lugo-Amador NM, Rothenhaus T, Moyer P: Heat-related illness, *Emerg Med Clin North Am* 22:315, 2004.
5. Ulrich AS, Rathlev NK: Hypothermia and localized injuries, *Emerg Med Clin North Am* 22:281, 2004.
6. Center for Disease Control and Prevention: Hypothermia-related deaths—United States, 2003, *MMWR* 53(8):172, 2004.
7. Speedy DB, Noakes TD: Exercise-associated hyponatremia: a review, *Emerg Med* 13:17, 2001.
8. Moran DS, Gaffen SL: Clinical management of heat-related illnesses. In Auerbach PS: *Wilderness medicine: management of wilderness and environmental emergencies*, ed 3, St Louis, 1995, Mosby.
9. McCauley RL, Smith DJ, Robson MC, Heggers JP: Frostbite. In Auerbach PS: *Wilderness medicine: management of wilderness and environmental emergencies*, ed 4, St Louis, 2001, Mosby.
10. Danzl, DF: Accidental hypothermia. In Auerbach PS: *Wilderness medicine: management of wilderness and environmental emergencies*, ed 4, St Louis, 2001, Mosby.
11. Semenza JC, Rubin CH, Flater KH, et al: Heat-related deaths during the July 1995 heat wave in Chicago, *N Engl J Med* 335(2):84, 1996.
12. Center for Disease Control and Prevention: Heat related mortality—Chicago, July 1995, *MMWR* 44 (21):577, 1995.
13. Hardy JD: Thermal comfort: skin temperature and physiological thermoregulation. In Hardy JD, Gagge AP, Stolwijk JAJ, editors: *Physiological and Behavioral Temperature Regulation*, Springfield, Ill, 1970, Charles C Thomas.
14. Pozos RS, Danzl DF: Human physiological responses to cold stress and hypothermia. In: Pandolf KB, Burr RE, editors: *Medical aspects of harsh environments,* Vol 1, Washington, DC, 2001, Office of The Surgeon General, Borden Institute/TMM Publications.
15. Stocks JM, Taylor NAS, Tipton MJ, Greenleaf JE: Human physiological responses to cold exposure, *Aviat Space Environ Med* 75:444, 2004.
16. Wenger CB: The regulation of body temperature. In Rhoades RA, Tanner GA, editors. *Medical physiology*, Boston, 1995, Little, Brown.
17. Nunnelely SA, Reardon MJ: Prevention of heat illness. In Pandolf KB, Burr RE, editors: *Medical aspects of harsh environments,* Vol 1, Washington, DC, 2001, Office of The Surgeon General, Borden Institute/TMM Publications.
18. Sonna LA: Practical medical aspects of military operations in the heat. In Pandolf KB, Burr RE, editors: *Medical aspects of harsh environments,* Vol 1, Washington, DC, 2001, Office of The Surgeon General, Borden Institute/TMM Publications
19. Tek D, Olshaker JS: Heat illness, *Emerg Med Clin North Am* 10(2):299, 1992.
20. Armstrong LE, Hubbard RW, Jones BH, Daniels JT: Preparing Alberto Salazar for the heat of the 1984 Olympic marathon, *Phys Sportsmed* 14:73, 1986.

21. Hubbard RW, Sandick BL, Matthew WT: Voluntary dehydration and alliesthesia for water, *J Appl Physiol* 57:868, 1984.

22. Johnson RF, Kobrick JL: Psychological aspects of military performance in hot environments. In Pandolf KB, Burr RE, editors: *Medical aspects of harsh environments*, Vol 1, Washington, DC, 2001, Office of The Surgeon General, Borden Institute/TMM Publications.

23. Sawka MN, Pandolf KB: Physical exercise in hot climates: physiology, performance, and biomedical issues. In: Pandolf KB, Burr RE, editors: *Medical aspects of harsh environments*, Vol 1, Washington, DC, 2001, Office of The Surgeon General, Borden Institute/TMM Publications.

24. Dutchman SM, Ryan AJ, Schedl HP, et al: Upper limits of intestinal absorption of dilute glucose solution in men at rest, *Med Sci Sport Exerc* 29:482, 1997.

25. Neufer PD, Young AJ, Sawka MN: Gastric emptying during exercise: effects of heat stress and hypohydration, *Eur J Appl Physiol* 58:433, 1989.

26. Wenger CB: Section I: Hot environments. In Pandolf KB, Burr RE, editors: *Medical aspects of harsh environments*, Vol 1, Washington, DC, 2001, Office of The Surgeon General, Borden Institute/TMM Publications.

27. Bouchama A, Knochel JP: Medical progress: heat stroke, *N Engl J Med* 346(25):1978, 2002.

28. Holtzhausen LM, Noakes TD: Collapsed ultraendurance athlete: proposed mechanisms and an approach to management, *Clin J Sport Med* 7(4):292, 1997.

29. Gardner JW, Kark, JA: Clinical diagnosis, management and surveillance of exertional heat illness. In: Pandolf KB, Burr RE, editors: *Medical aspects of harsh environments*, Vol 1, Washington, DC, 2001, Office of The Surgeon General, Borden Institute/TMM Publications.

30. Knochel JP, Reed G: Disorders of heat regulation. In Narins RE, editor: *Maxwell & Kleenman's clinical disorders of fluid and electrolyte metabolism*, ed 5, New York, 1994, McGraw-Hill.

31. Gaffin SL, Hubbard RW: Pathophysiology of heatstroke. In Pandolf KB, Burr RE, editors: *Medical aspects of harsh environments*, Vol 1, Washington, DC, 2001, Office of The Surgeon General, Borden Institute/TMM Publications.

32. Armstrong LE, Crago AE, Adams R, et al: Whole-body cooling of hyperthermic runners: Comparison of two field therapies, *Am J Emerg Med* 14:335, 1996.

33. Costrini A: Emergency treatment of exertional heatstroke and comparison of whole body cooling techniques, *Med Sci Sports Exerc* 22:15, 1984.

34. Gaffin SL, Gardner J, Flinn S: Current cooling method for exertional heatstroke, *Ann Intern Med* 132:678, 2000.

35. Speedy DB, Noakes TD: Exercise-associated hyponatremia: a review, *Emerg Med* 13:17, 2001.

36. Backer HD, Shopes E, Collins SL, Barkan H: Exertional heat illness and hyponatremia in hikers, *Am J Emerg Med* 17(6):532, 1999.

37. Gardner JW: Death by water intoxication, *Mil Med* 164(3):432, 2002.

38. Adrogue HJ, Madias NE: Hyponatremia, *N Engl J Med* 342(21):1581, 2000.

39. Hiller WDB: Dehydration and hyponatremia during triathlons, *Med Sci Sports Exerc* 21:S219, 1989.

40. Speedy DB, Noakes TD, Rodgers IR: Hyponatremia in ultra-distance triathletes, *Med Sci Sports Exerc* 31:809, 1999.

41. Laird RH: Medical care at ultraendurance triathlons, *Med Sci Sports Exerc* 21:S222, 1989.

42. Collins S, Reynolds, B: The other heat-related emergency, *JEMS*, July 2004.

43. Irving RA, Noakes TD, Buck R: Evaluation of renal function and fluid homeostasis during recovery from exercise-induced hyponatremia, *J Appl Physiol* 70:342, 1991.

44. Eichner ER: Exertional hyponatremia: why so many women? *Sports Med Digest* 24:54, 2002.

45. US Department of Agriculture, US Forest Service: Heat stress brochure, http://www.fs.fed.us/fire/safety/fitness/heat_stress/hs_pg1.html.

46. Montain SJ, Latzka WA, Sawka MN: Fluid replacement recommendations for training in hot weather, *Mil Med* 164(7):502, 1999.

47. Parson KC: International standards for the assessment of the risk of thermal strain on clothed workers in hot environments, *Ann Occup Hyg* 43(5):297, 1999.

48. American College of Sports Medicine: Position stand on exercise and fluid replacement, *Med Sci Sports Exerc* 28(1):i, 1996.

49. American College of Sports Medicine: Position stand on the recommended quantity and quality of exercise for developing and maintaining cardiorespiratory and muscular fitness, and flexibility in adults, *Med Sci Sports Exerc* 30(6):975, 1998.

50. Pate RR, Pratt M, Blair SB, et al: Physical activity and public health: a recommendation from the Centers for Disease Control and Prevention and the American College of Sports Medicine, *JAMA* 273(5):402, 1995.

51. Heat acclimatization guide, Ranger and Airborne school students, 2003, www.usariem.army.mil/download/heatacclimatizationguide.pdf.

52. Eichna LW, Park CR, Nelson N, et al: Thermal regulation during acclimatization in a hot, dry (desert type) environment, *J Appl Physiol* 163:585, 1950.

53. Federal Emergency Management System, United States Fire Administration: Emergency incident rehabilitation, Report #FA-114, July 1992, www.smemsc.org/Emergency Incident Rehabilitation.pdf.

54. US Pharmacopeia, National Formulary, USP-25/NF-20, Rockville, Md, US Pharmacopeia Convention, 2000.

55. Brown LH, Krumperman K, Fullagar CJ: Out of hospital medical storage temperature, *Prehosp Emerg Care* 8:200, 2004.

56. Mehta SH, Doran JV, Lavery RF, Allegra JR: Improvements in prehospital medication storage practices in response to research, *Prehosp Emerg Care* 6:319, 2002.

57. Allegra JR, Brennan J, Lanier V: Storage temperatures of out-of-hospital medications, *Acad Emerg Med* 6:1098, 1999.

58. Palmer RG, Zimmerman J, Clawson JJ: Altered states: the influence of temperature on prehospital drugs, *J Emerg Med Serv* 10(12):29, 1985.

59. Johansen RB, Schafer NC, Brown PI: Effects of extreme temperature on drugs for prehospital ACLS, *Am J Emerg Med* 11:450, 1993.

60. Church WH, Hu SS, Henry AJ: Thermal degradation of injectable drugs, *Am J Emerg Med* 12:306, 1994.

61. New Jersey Department of Health and Senior Services, Suppl Section 8:41-3.12, paragraph (f); Aug 17, 1998.

62. Stocks JM, Taylor NAS, Tipton MJ, Greenleaf JE: Human physiological responses to cold exposure, *Aviat Space Environ Med* 75:444, 2004.

63. Ulrich AS, Rathlev NK: Hypothermia and localized injuries, *Emerg Med Clin North Am* 22:281, 2004.

64. Chandler W, Ivey H: Cold weather injuries among US soldiers in Alaska: a five-year review, *Mil Med* 162:788, 1997.

65. DeGroot DW, Castellani JW, Williams JO, Amoroso PJ: Epidemiology of US Army cold weather injuries, 1980-1999, *Mil Med* 74:564, 2003.

66. Thomas JR, Oakley EHN: Nonfreezing cold injury. In Pandolf KB, Burr RE, editors: *Medical aspects of harsh environments*, Vol 1, Washington, DC, 2001, Office of The Surgeon General, Borden Institute/TMM Publications.

67. Montgomery H: Experimental immersion foot: review of the physiopathology, *Physiol Rev* 34:127, 1954.

68. Francis TJR: Non-freezing cold injury: a historical review, *J R Nav Med Serv* 70:134, 1984.

69. Wrenn K: Immersion foot: a problem of the homeless in the 1990s, *Arch Intern Med* 151:785, 1991.

70. Ramstead KD, Hughes RB, Webb AJ: Recent cases of trench foot, *Postgrad Med J* 56:879, 1980.

71. Biem J, Koehncke N, Classen D, Dosman J: Out of cold: management of hypothermia and frostbite. *Can Med Assoc J* 168(3):305, 2003.

72. Vogel JE, Dellon AL: Frostbite injuries of the hand, *Clin Plast Surg* 16:565, 1989.

73. Mills WJ: Clinical aspects of freezing injury. In Pandolf KB, Burr RE, editors: *Medical aspects of harsh environments*, Vol 1, Washington, DC, 2001, Office of The Surgeon General, Borden Institute/TMM Publications.

74. Sessler DI: Mild preoperative hypothermia, *N Engl J Med* 336:1730, 1997.

75. Giesbrecht GG: Cold stress, near drowning and accidental hypothermia: a review, *Aviat Space Environ Med* 71:733, 2000.

76. Gilbert M, Busund R, Skagseth A, et al: Resuscitation from accidental hypothermia of 13.7° C with circulatory arrest, *Lancet* 355:375, 2000.

77. Danzl DF, Pozos RS, Auerbach PS: Multicenter hypothermia survey, *Ann Emerg Med* 16:1042, 1987.

78. Tsuei BJ, Kearney PA: Hypothermia in the trauma patient, *Injury Int J Care Injured* 35:7, 2004.

79. Stoner HB: Effects of injury on the responses to thermal stimulation of the hypothalamus, *J Appl Physiol* 33:665, 1972.

80. Ferrara A, MacArthur J, Wright H: Hypothermia and acidosis worsen coagulopathy in the patient requiring massive transfusion, *Am J Surg* 160:515, 1990.

81. Epstein M: Renal effects of head-out immersion in man: implications for understanding volume homeostasis, *Physiol Rev* 58:529, 1978.

82. Carlson LD: Immersion in cold water and body tissue insulation, *Aerospace Med* 29:145, 1958.

83. Wittmers LE, Savage M: Cold water immersion. In Pandolf KB, Burr RE, editors: *Medical aspects of harsh environments*, Vol 1, Washington, DC, 2001, Office of The Surgeon General, Borden Institute/TMM Publications.

84. Steinman AM, Giesbrecht GG: Immersion into cold water. In Auerbach PS: *Wilderness medicine: management of wilderness and environmental emergencies*, ed 4, St Louis, 2001, Mosby.

85. Hayward JS, Eckerson JD, Collis ML: Effect of behavioral variables on cooling rate of man in cold water, *J Appl Physiol* 38:1073, 1975.

86. Nozaki R, Ishibashi K, Adachi N, et al: Accidental profound hypothermia, *N Eng J Med* 315:1680, 1986 (letter).

87. Tipton MJ: The initial responses to cold water immersion in man, *Clin Sci* 77:581, 1989.

88. Keatinge WR, McIlroy MB, Goldfien A: Cardiovascular responses to ice-cold showers, *J Appl Physiol* 19:1145, 1964.

89. Mekjavic IB et al: Respiratory drive during sudden cold water immersion, *Respir Physiol* 70:21, 1987.

90. Golden FSC, Tipton MJ, Scott RC: Immersion, near-drowning and drowning, *Br J Anaesth* 79:214, 1997.

91. Newman AB: Submersion incidents. In Auerbach PS: *Wilderness medicine: management of wilderness and environmental emergencies*, ed 4, St Louis, 2001, Mosby.

92. Wissler EH: Probability of surviving during accidental immersion in cold water, *Aviat Space Environ Med* 74:47, 2003.

93. Tikuisis P: Predicting survival time at sea based on observed body cooling rates, *Aviat Space Environ Med* 68:441, 1997.

94. Hayward JS, Errickson JD, Collis ML: Thermal balance and survival time prediction of man in cold water, *Can J Physiol Pharmacol* 53:21, 1975.

95. Van Mieghem C, Sabbe M, Knockaert D: The clinical vales of the ECG in noncardiac conditions, *Chest* 125:1561, 2004.

96. American Heart Association, International Liaison Committee on Resuscitation: Guidelines 2000 for cardiopulmonary resuscitation and emergency cardiovascular care, *Circulation* 102(suppl 8):I-229, 2000.

97. International Liaison Committee on Resuscitation: 2005 International consensus on cardiopulmonary resuscitation and emergency cardiovascular care science with treatment recommendations, *Circulation* 112(suppl 1):IV-1, 2005.

98. Danzl DF, Lloyd EL: Treatment of accidental hypothermia. In Pandolf KB, Burr RE, editors: *Medical aspects of harsh environments*, Vol 1, Washington, DC, 2001, Office of The Surgeon General, Borden Institute/TMM Publications.

99. Southwick FS, Dalglish PH: Recovery after prolonged asystolic cardiac arrest in profound hypothermia: a case report and literature review, *JAMA* 243:1250, 1980.

100. Bernard MB, Gray TW, Buist MD, et al: Treatment of comatose survivors of out-of-hospital cardiac arrest with induced hypothermia, *N Engl J Med* 346(8):557, 2002.

101. Reuler JB: Hypothermia: pathophysiology, clinical setting, and management, *Ann Intern Med* 89:519, 1978.

102. Armstrong LE: Cold, windchill, and water immersion. In *Performing in extremes environments*, Champaign, 2000, Human Kinetics.

103. Wilderness Medical Society: Cardiopulmonary resuscitation. In Forgey WW, editor: *Practice guidelines for wilderness emergency care*, Guilford, 2001, Globe Pequot Press.

104. Bailey DE, Wydro GC, Cone DC: Position paper of the National Association of EMS Physicians: Termination of resuscitation in the prehospital setting for adult patients suffering nontraumatic cardiac arrest, *Prehosp Emerg Care* 4:190, 2000.

Suggested Readings

Auerbach PS: *Wilderness medicine: management of wilderness and environmental emergencies,* ed 4, St Louis, 2001, Mosby.

Fregly MJ, Blatteis CM: *Environmental physiology,* Vols I & II, American Physiological Society, New York, 1996, Oxford University Press.

Pandolf KB, Burr RE, editors: *Medical aspects of harsh environments,* Vol 1, Washington, DC, 2001, Office of the Surgeon General, Borden Institute/TMM Publications.

Chapter Objectives

*At the completion of this chapter, the reader
will be able to do the following:*

✓ List five risk factors for a near-drowning incident.

✓ List three signs or symptoms that can occur in a patient after a near-drowning incident.

✓ List five methods for preventing a drowning incident.

✓ Explain the "30-30" rule in lightning injury prevention.

✓ Differentiate the use of "reverse" triage for multiple lightning casualties from its use for other multiple-casualty scenarios.

✓ Differentiate signs and symptoms of Type I and Type II decompression sickness.

✓ Explain two primary treatment interventions for Type II decompression sickness and arterial gas embolism.

✓ List two key risk factors for high-altitude illness.

✓ Discuss the similarities and differences between acute mountain sickness and high-altitude cerebral edema.

CHAPTER 17

Environmental Trauma II: Drowning, Lightning, Diving, and Altitude

SCENARIO

You and your partner are returning to the summit of Pike's Peak (4299 m [14,110 ft]) after transporting a patient to the hospital down in the city when you receive a dispatch at 1035 hours for trouble breathing in a 48-year-old female near the summit. This is the day of the annual Pike's Peak marathon (26.2 miles). The runners start at 0700 hours and run to Pike's Peak summit, an elevation gain of 2382 m (7815 ft), turn around at the 13.2-mile marker, and run back down the trail to the finish line.

You arrive on scene and notice a downed female runner on the trail who is being assisted by race volunteers. As your partner approaches the patient, you ask the bystanders if anyone observed her before she stopped. A race official stated he first observed her 10 miles into the race, appearing unsteady and swaying while walking. He continued to observe her over the next 2 miles. Your partner finds out that she flew in yesterday from San Francisco. She currently presents with a dry cough, dsypnea, and facial sunburn and is irritable. She complains of a severe headache and nausea and had vomited earlier. She expresses her desire to rest and then continue in the marathon, knowing that it is downhill to the finish line. She refuses transport to the hospital, but you explain that her running is unsteady and she might fall and injure herself. She reluctantly agrees to be transported by ambulance to the hospital.

Are these signs and symptoms indicative of anything more than fatigue and nausea from running continuously uphill from an altitude of 1918 m (6295 ft)? Should the runner be allowed to rest a little longer and continue toward the turnaround point? What medical condition might she be experiencing? How would you manage this patient? ■

Each year in the United States, significant morbidity and mortality are caused by a variety of environmental conditions, including drowning or near-drowning, lightning, recreational scuba diving, and high altitude (see Chapter 16 for heat and cold conditions). Thus, it is important for prehospital care providers to know minor and major disorders associated with each type of environment; understand the anatomy, physiology, and pathophysiology involved; and perform patient assessment and management, as well as prevent injury to themselves and other public safety personnel.

Drowning or Near-Drowning

Submersion incidents in water that lead to injury are all too common in the United States. Drowning remains a leading cause of death across all age groups[1] but is an epidemic in children.[2] Submersion injuries have a substantial cost to society; an estimated $450 to $650 million or more is spent on these patients each year.[3] The terminology describing these patients continues to evolve. Thirty-five years ago, "drowning" was defined as the process by which air-breathing animals succumb on submersion in a liquid, and "near-drowning" was defined as submersion with at least temporary survival.[4] The term "secondary drowning" was

used to describe patients who recovered initially from a submersion injury, but then died from respiratory failure secondary to submersion.[5,6] However, this latter term has come under question lately, and some suggest that it should not be used.[5]

The more accepted definitions for drowning and near-drowning are as follows:

- **Drowning:** death within 24 hours of the submersion incident.
- **Near-drowning:** surviving for at least 24 hours after the submersion.

Because the role of prehospital care providers for all water-related casualties is to initiate resuscitative care at the scene, it may be more practical to avoid any confusion of these two terms and use the term *submersion incident*, which encompasses drowning *and* near-drowning. Furthermore, the term submersion incident implies no particular outcome of the patient at the scene, en route to the hospital, or later at the hospital. This should help prevent prehospital care providers from making any judgment on withholding resuscitative efforts based on the mechanism of injury, length of submersion, water temperature, or the patient who presents without vital signs.[7] This last point is critical because there are numerous reports of those who have survived prolonged periods (>30 minutes) of cold-water submersion.[8-10] Immediate and effective delivery of cardiopulmonary resuscitation (CPR) and the activation of emergency medical services (EMS) from bystanders are two important factors that influence the survival of a submersion patient.[11]

Prevention strategies are vital in the effort to lower the rates of submersion incidents in the United States. Many education programs are emphasizing the reduction of *unintentional* water entry of infants and children by encouraging the installation of various types of barriers around pools (e.g., isolation fences, pool covers, alarms). Furthermore, CPR initiated by a bystander before the arrival of prehospital care personnel is associated with improved patient prognosis.[12]

Epidemiology

Death by unintentional drowning is the seventh leading cause of death for all ages, the second leading cause of death for ages 1 to 14 years, and the fifth leading cause of death of infants (<1 year of age).[1] Infants are at risk from drowning in bathtubs, buckets, and toilets.[13] The incidence of near-drowning may be 500 to 600 times the rate of drowning.[14] In 2000, there were 3281 cases of unintentional drowning in the United States, and for every child who drowned, three others survived and required emergency care for the near-drowning incident. Each week, approximately 40 children die from drowning, 115 are hospitalized, and 12 have irreversible brain injury.[2]

The Centers for Disease Control and Prevention (CDC) reported a total of 7546 submersion casualties (fatal and nonfatal) in 2001 and 2002[1] (Table 17-1). Of these, 3372 persons experienced unintentional drowning in various recreational settings, such as pools, oceans, and rivers. In comparison, 4174 unintentional nonfatal near-drowning incidents were treated in emergency departments (EDs) in the United States. The nonfatal and fatal injury rates were the highest for children age 4 years or younger and for males of all ages. The nonfatal rate for males was almost twice that of females, whereas the fatal rate for males was almost five times that of females. Nonfatal submersion injuries in pools accounted for 75%, whereas 70% of the fatal submersions occurred in natural settings, such as oceans, lakes, and rivers.

Submersion Factors

Specific factors place individuals at an increased risk for submersion incidents.[4,5,11,15] Recognizing these factors will increase awareness and assist in the creation of preventive strategies and policies to minimize these occurrences. For infants and young children, the major risk factor is inadequate supervision, and for adolescents and adults, it is risky behavior and use of drugs or alcohol.[11]

Ability to Swim

Swimming ability is not consistently related to drowning. White males have a higher incidence of drowning than

TABLE 17-1 Unintentional Drowning/Near-Drowning—United States, 2001-2002

Characteristic	Nonfatal*	Fatal*
AGE (YR)		
0-4	2168	442
5-14	1058	333
≥15	948	2563
Unknown	—	34
GENDER		
Male	2721	2789
Female	1452	583
LOCATION		
Pool	2571	596
Natural water (ocean, lakes, rivers)	909	1467
Other	513	1309
DISPOSITION		
Treated/released	1925	—
Hospitalized	2233	—
Other	16	—
TOTAL	4174	3372

Data from Centers for Disease Control and Prevention: Nonfatal and fatal drownings in recreational water settings—United States, 2001-2002, *MMWR* 53(21):447, 2004.
*Estimated number.

white females, even though they are reported to have better swimming ability.[4] Although black females have poor swimming skills, they have a very low drowning rate.[16] One study reported that nonswimmers or beginners accounted for 73% of drownings in home swimming pools and 82% of incidents in canals, lakes, and ponds.[17]

Shallow-Water Blackout

Some swimmers desire to increase their swim distance so they will intentionally hyperventilate immediately before underwater swimming in effort to lower the partial pressure of arterial carbon dioxide ($Paco_2$).[18] This will decrease the feedback to the respiratory center in the hypothalamus to increase ventilation during breath holding. These individuals are at risk of a submersion incident because the partial pressure of arterial oxygen (Pao_2) does not change significantly with hyperventilation. As the individual continues to swim underwater, Pao_2 will decrease significantly and cause a possible loss of consciousness and cerebral hypoxia.

Accidental Cold-Water Immersion

Another situation that places individuals at greater risk of drowning or near-drowning is cold-water immersion ("head out"). The physiologic changes that occur with cold-water immersion can have either a disastrous outcome or a protective effect of cold on the body, depending on many circumstances. Adverse outcomes are more common, resulting from both cardiovascular collapse and sudden death within minutes of cold-water immersion.

Age

Drowning is recognized as a young person's accident, with the largest group being toddlers, based on their inquisitive nature and a lack of parental supervision. Children under 1 year of age have the highest drowning rate.[1,19]

Gender

Males account for more than half of submersion victims. One peak incidence for drowning occurs in males at age 2 years, decreases until age 10 years, and then rises rapidly to peak again at age 18 years. Older males may be more at risk for drowning because of higher exposure rates to aquatic activities, higher alcohol consumption while at the waterfront, and more risk-taking behavior.[4,20]

Race

Black children experience more submersion incidents than white children. Black children tend to drown in ponds, lakes, and other natural sources of water.[1] The drowning rate of black male children has been estimated to be as high as three times that of white males.[21] It is suggested the higher incidence of submersion casualties for black children is related to inadequate swimming skills, risk-taking behavior, alcohol and drug abuse, and socioeconomic conditions.

Location

Submersion incidents typically occur in backyard swimming pools and in the ocean, but also occur in buckets.[5] Houses in rural areas with open wells increase the risk of a young child drowning by sevenfold.[4] Other hazardous locations are water barrels, fountains, and underground cisterns.

Alcohol and Drugs

Alcohol is the primary drug associated with submersion incidents,[22] most likely because it causes a loss of judgment.[23] Up to 30% of adult drownings occur because of boating accidents in which occupants used poor judgment, were speeding, failed to wear life jackets, or handled the craft recklessly.[4]

Underlying Disease or Trauma

The onset of illness from underlying disease can account for submersion victims. Hypoglycemia, myocardial infarction, cardiac arrhythmias, depression and suicidal thoughts, and syncope predispose to drowning incidents.[11] Cervical spine injuries and head trauma should be suspected in all unwitnessed incidents and injuries involving body surfers, board surfers, and victims diving in shallow water or water with submerged objects such as rocks or trees.

Child Abuse

A high incidence of child abuse is reported in children from submersion incidents, particularly bathtub near-drownings. A study of children sustaining bathtub near-drownings between 1982 and 1992 found that 67% had historical or physical findings compatible with a diagnosis of abuse or neglect.[24] Consequently, it is highly recommended that any suspicious child near-drowning or drowning bathtub incident be reported to local social services for appropriate investigation.

Hypothermia

Drowning may result directly from prolonged immersion leading to hypothermia. (See Cold-Related Disorders in Chapter 16 for further discussion of accidental hypothermia.)

Mechanism of Injury

A common scenario of head-out immersion in water or a whole-body submersion incident begins with a situation that creates a panic response, leading to breath holding, air hunger, and increased physical activity in effort to stay or get above the water surface. According to most bystander reports, submersion victims are rarely seen screaming and waving for assistance while struggling to stay above the surface of the water. Rather, they are seen either floating on the surface or in a motionless position, or they dive underwater and fail to come up. As the submersion incident continues, a reflex inspiratory effort draws water into the pharynx and larynx, causing a choking response and laryngospasm. The onset of laryngospasm represents the first step in suffocation, which in turn causes the victim to lose consciousness and submerge underwater even further.

Over the years, controversies have surrounded the pathophysiology of drowning and near-drowning, mostly about the differences between drowning in freshwater versus salt water and whether water entered or did not enter the lungs.[5,7,11] Approximately 15% of drownings are termed "dry drowning" because the severe laryngospasm prevents the aspiration of fluid into the lungs. The remaining 85% of submersion incidents are considered "wet drownings," in which the laryngospasm relaxes, the glottis opens, and the victim aspirates water into the lungs.[25] Theoretically, there are different effects on the pulmonary system when freshwater (hypotonic) versus salt water (hypertonic) enters in the lung. In freshwater drowning, the hypotonic fluid enters the lung and then moves across the alveolus into the intravascular space, causing a volume overload and dilutional effect on serum electrolytes and other serum components. Conversely, in saltwater aspiration, the hypertonic fluid enters the lung, which in turn causes additional fluid from the intravascular space to enter the lung across the alveolus, causing pulmonary edema and hypertonicity of serum electrolytes.

It has since been shown that no real differences exist between wet versus dry drownings and freshwater versus saltwater aspiration.[11,26,27] For prehospital care providers, the common denominator in any of these four submersion scenarios is hypoxia caused by either laryngospasm or water aspiration. Management at the scene should be aimed at reversing any hypoxia in these patients, thereby preventing cardiac arrest.

Surviving Cold-Water Submersion

In numerous cases of prolonged submersion, in one case for as long as 66 minutes, patients have presented to the hospital with severe hypothermia and recovered with either partial or full neurologic function.[28] In these submersion incidents, the lowest recorded core temperature of a survivor is 58° F (14.4° C) in an adult female.[29] In another case, a child survived fully intact after being submerged in ice water for 40 minutes, with a core temperature of 75° F (24°C). After 1 hour of resuscitation, spontaneous circulation returned.[30]

No explanation exists for such cases, but hypothermia is thought to be protective. Immersion in cold water may lead quickly to hypothermia because of surface heat loss and core cooling. In addition, swallowing or aspiration of cold water may contribute to rapid cooling. Rapid onset of hypothermia during freshwater drowning may result from core cooling caused by pulmonary aspiration and rapid absorption of cold water and subsequent brain cooling.

Another factor that may explain why some young children survive is the mammalian diving reflex. The *mammalian diving reflex* slows heart rate, shunts blood to the brain, and closes the airway. However, recent evidence suggests that the diving reflex present in various mammals is active in only 15% to 30% of human subjects, although this still may explain in part why some children survive.[4]

Every submersion patient should have full resuscitation efforts made, regardless of the presence or absence of any of these factors. The factors described next appear to influence the outcome of a cold-water submersion patient.

Age. Many successful infant and child resuscitations have been well documented in the United States and Europe. The smaller mass of a child's body cools faster than an adult's body, thus permitting fewer harmful by-products of anaerobic metabolism to form and causing less irreversible damage.

Submersion Time. The shorter the duration of submersion, the lower is the risk for cellular damage caused by hypoxia. Accurate information concerning submersion time needs to be obtained. Immersion longer than 66 minutes is prob-

ably fatal. However, rescue and resuscitation efforts should be initiated regardless of the duration of submersion.

Water Temperature. Water temperatures of 70° F (21° C) and below are capable of inducing hypothermia. The colder the water, the better is the chance of survival, probably because of the rapid decrease in brain temperature and metabolism when the body is quickly chilled.

Struggle. Submersion victims who struggle less have a better chance of being resuscitated (unless their struggling efforts are successful enough to avoid drowning). Less struggle means less hormonal release (e.g., epinephrine) and less muscle activity, which translates to less heat (energy) production and less vasodilation. These in turn cause decreased muscular oxygen deficits (decreased deficits mean less CO_2 and lactic acid production), and thus the rate of cooling is increased.

Cleanliness of Water. Patients generally do better after resuscitation if they were submerged in clean water rather than muddy or contaminated water.

Quality of CPR and Resuscitative Efforts. Patients who receive adequate and effective CPR, combined with proper rewarming and advanced life support (ALS) measures, generally do better than patients receiving one or more substandard measures. Immediate initiation of CPR is a key factor for submersion hypothermia patients. Past and current studies reveal that poor CPR technique is directly related to poor resuscitation outcome.[31,32] See the current basic life support (BLS) guidelines as outlined elsewhere.[33]

Associated Injuries or Illness. Patients with an existing injury or illness, or who become ill or injured in combination with the submersion, do not fare as well as otherwise healthy individuals.

Assessment

The initial priorities for any submersion patient include the following:

1. Prevent injuries to the patient and emergency responders
2. Initiate plans early for water extraction and rapid transport to ED
3. Conduct a safe water rescue
4. Assess for ABCs (airway, breathing, circulation)
5. Reverse hypoxia and acidosis
6. Restore or maintain cardiovascular stability
7. Prevent further loss of body heat

Initially, it is safest to presume the submersion patient is hypoxic and hypothermic until proved otherwise. Consequently, all efforts should be made to establish effective respirations during water rescue and to remove the patient from water and other sources of cold to minimize further body heat loss. Quickly assess the torso and extremities for any life threats, and assess for head trauma and cervical spine injuries, particularly if there is suspicion of trauma associated with the submersion incident (e.g., falls, boat accidents, diving into water with underwater hazards). However, it has been shown that the typical submersion casualty has a low chance of traumatic injury. Acquire vital signs, and assess all lung fields of submersion patients because they present with a wide range of pulmonary distress, including shortness of breath, rales, rhonchi, and wheezing. These patients can present without symptoms initially and then deteriorate rapidly with signs of pulmonary edema.

Assess oxygen saturation with pulse oximetry. Assess for cardiac rhythm disturbances; submersion patients often have arrhythmias secondary to hypoxia and hypothermia. Assess for altered mental status and neurologic function of all extremities because many submersion victims develop sustained neurologic damage. Acquire a baseline Glasgow Coma Scale (GCS) score and continue to assess for trends. Remove all wet clothing and assess rectal temperature to determine the level of hypothermia, and initiate steps to minimize further heat loss (see Chapter 16 for management of hypothermia).

The following variables are predictive of a more favorable outcome in near-drowning patients:

- Children age 3 years and older
- Female
- Water temperature less than 50° F (10° C)
- Duration of submersion less than 10 minutes
- No aspiration
- Time to effective BLS less than 10 minutes
- Rapid return of spontaneous cardiac output
- Spontaneous cardiac output on arrival in ED
- Core temperature less than 95° F (35° C)
- No coma on arrival and GCS score greater than 6
- Pupillary responses present

Management

A patient who has experienced some form of submersion incident, but who is not presenting with any signs or symptoms at assessment, still needs follow-up care in a hospital after being assessed at the scene. In general, all symptomatic patients are admitted to the hospital for at least 24 hours for support care and observation because the initial clinical assessment can be misleading. Many asymptomatic patients are released in 6 to 8 hours, depending on clinical findings in the hospital. It is critical to obtain a good history of the incident detailing the estimate of submersion time and any past medical history.

All suspected submersion patients should receive high-flow oxygen (12-15 L/min) independent of their initial breathing status, based on the concern for delayed pulmo-nary distress, particularly if the patient develops shortness of breath. Monitor electrocardiogram (ECG) for arrhythmias. Obtain intravenous (IV) access and provide normal saline (NS) or lactated Ringer's (LR) solution at keep vein open (KVO) rate. Transport to the ED for evaluation because many near-drowning patients are asymptomatic for 4 to 6 hours. Asymptomatic patients may refuse transport because they have no immediate chief complaint. If so, take time to provide good patient education about the delayed signs and symptoms in a near-drowning incident, and that many victims develop secondary complications from pulmonary injury. Firm and persistent persuasion is needed for them to agree to be transported or for them to report to the closest ED for further evaluation and observation.

A symptomatic patient with a history of submersion who presents with signs of distress (e.g., anxiety, rapid respirations, trouble breathing, coughing) is considered to have a submersion pulmonary injury until hospital evaluation has proved otherwise. Emphasis should be placed on correcting hypoxia, acidosis, and hypothermia. Provide cervical spine immobilization in all patients with suspicion of trauma. In unresponsive patients, use suction to clear the airway and keep the airway open with an airway adjunct. Hypoxia and acidosis can be corrected with effective ventilation support. Apneic patients should be supported with bag-mask ventilation. Intubation should be considered early to protect the airway in patients who are apneic or cyanotic or who have a decreased mental status, since submersion victims swallow large amounts of water and are at risk of vomiting and aspirating stomach contents. The Sellick maneuver (cricoid pressure) should be applied during intubation to prevent regurgitation and aspiration. Monitor the ECG for rate and rhythm disturbances. and investigate for evidence of a cardiac event that might have preceded or followed the submersion incident. Provide 100% oxygen (12-15 L/min) with a nonrebreather mask. Obtain IV access and provide NS or LR solution at KVO rate. Provide transport to local ED.

Patient Resuscitation

Rapid initiation of effective CPR and standard ALS procedures for submersion patients in cardiopulmonary arrest is associated with the best chance of survival.[5] Victims may present in asystole, pulseless electrical activity, or pulseless ventricular tachycardia/ventricular fibrillation. Follow the current version of the American Heart Association (AHA) guidelines for pediatric ALS and advanced cardiac life support (ACLS) for managing these rhythms.[33]

The use of CPR during in-water rescue is not recommended because the depth of chest compressions is ineffective in water. Besides delaying effective CPR out of water, attempting to provide CPR in water puts rescuers at risk from fatigue, cold-water, wave, surge, and current dangers. Place a greater emphasis on establishing an open airway and providing rescue breathing for apneic patients, depending on the patient's in-water position, number of rescuers, and rescue equipment (e.g., in-water backboard).

When a beach rescue (or any location) involves sloping terrain, it is no longer recommended to place a patient in a head-down (or head-up) position in an effort to drain the airway. Resuscitation efforts are shown to be more successful when the patient is placed level on the ground in parallel position to the water, with effective ventilation and chest compressions. Maintaining a level position on the ground will prevent a decrease in forward blood flow during chest compressions in the head-up position or an increase in intracranial pressure in the head-down position. Furthermore, no evidence suggests that lung drainage is effective with any particular maneuver.

The Heimlich maneuver has been previously suggested for use in drowning victims. However, the Heimlich maneuver is designed for airway obstruction and does not remove water from the airway or lungs. Rather, it induces vomiting in drowning victims and places them at greater risk for aspiration. Currently, AHA and the Institute of Medicine advise against the Heimlich maneuver except when the airway is blocked with foreign material.[34] If the patient recovers with spontaneous breathing, the patient should be placed in the right lateral recumbent position with head slightly lower than the trunk to reduce the risk of aspiration if the patient vomits.

See Chapter 16 for ALS procedures in the resuscitation of a hypothermic patient. See Figure 16-9 for hypothermia algorithm. These guidelines are the same for all hypothermic patients regardless of the source of cold exposure.

Use the regional EMS medical protocol for established guidelines that determine the criteria for an obviously dead individual. Acceptable guidelines for an obviously dead victim are a normal rectal temperature in a patient who presents with asystole, apnea, postmortem lividity, rigor mortis, or other injuries incompatible with life. A patient who has been recovered from warm water without vital signs or resuscitative efforts lasting 30 minutes may be considered dead on the scene.[4] Consult local medical control early for any individual recovered from cold-water submersion. As stated previously, many individuals have fully recovered from more than 30 minutes of cold-water submersion. These patients should be managed as a hypothermic patient based on the rectal temperature.

Table 17-2 summarizes assessment and management of a submersion patient.

TABLE 17-2 Submersion Patient: Summary of Assessment and Management

History	Examination	Intervention
ASYSMPTOMATIC PATIENT		
Time submerged	Appearance	Administer oxygen by facemask at 8-10 L/min
Description of incident	Vital signs	Initiate IV line at KVO rate
Complaints	Head and neck trauma Chest examination: lung fields	Reexamine patient as needed
Past medical history	ECG monitor	Transport patient to ED
SYMPTOMATIC PATIENT		
Description of incident	General appearance	Administer oxygen by nonrebreather mask at 12-15 L/min
Time submerged, water temperature, water contamination, vomiting, type of rescue	Level of consciousness (AVPU)	Initiate IV line at KVO rate; intubate early as needed
Symptoms	Vital signs; monitor ECG	Transport patient to ED
On-scene field resuscitation	Assess ABCDEs; vital signs; AED or ECG monitor	Initiate CPR early; intubate; 100% oxygen at 12-15 L/min via bag-valve-mask; consider NG tube for gastric distention; use ACLS procedures for VF and asystole; use ACLS hypothermia algorithm

Modified from Newman AB: Submersion incidents. In Auerbach PS: *Wilderness medicine: management of wilderness and environmental emergencies*, ed 4, St Louis, 2001, Mosby.
IV, Intravenous; *KVO*, keep vein open; *ECG*, electrocardiogram; *ED*, emergency department; *AED*, automatic external defibrillator; *CPR*, cardiopulmonary resuscitation; *ACLS*, advanced cardiac life support; *NG*, nasogastric; *VF*, ventricular fibrillation.
AVPU, **A**lert; responds to **v**erbal stimulus; responds to **p**ainful stimulus; **u**nresponsive.
ABCDEs, Airway, breathing, circulation, disability, expose/environment.

Prevention

Prehospital care providers have great opportunities to be advocates of water safety and education in their respective communities, with an emphasis on communication of the risk factor areas previously identified. Furthermore, prevention should be emphasized to EMS providers and other public safety personnel who arrive on the scene so that they do not become additional submersion victims. A panicked and struggling near-drowning victim can be a danger to an unprepared in-water rescuer, potentially resulting in a double drowning. EMS providers need to assess the problem quickly, control the scene to prevent bystanders from entering the water, and ensure their own safety.

Many water safety organizations recommend the use of highly skilled professionals who regularly train for water rescue, retrieval, and resuscitation. If no professional water rescue teams are available, however, first responders must consider their own safety and the safety of all responders before attempting an in-water rescue. First, attempt to perform the water rescue by reaching out with a pole or throwing something to a victim, such as a life preserver or rope, before any attempt to enter the water. If a water entry is necessary, it is preferable to use a boat or paddleboard to reach the victim. Too many well-intentioned first responders have become additional victims because their own safety was not the priority.

Community education regarding submersion incidents should include the following recommendations[7]:

Beaches

- Always swim near a lifeguard
- Ask a lifeguard about a safe place to swim
- Do not overestimate your swimming capability
- Always look out for your children
- Swim away from piers, rocks, and stakes
- Avoid drinking alcohol and having a heavy meal before swimming
- Take lost children to the nearest lifeguard tower
- Be aware that more than 80% of ocean drownings occur in rip currents
- Never try to rescue someone without knowing what you are doing; many people have died in such attempts
- If you are fishing on rocks, be cautious with waves that may sweep you into the ocean
- Do not dive in shallow water; cervical injury could result
- Keep away from marine animals
- Read and heed signs posted on the beach

Residential Pools

- Adult supervision is necessary, closely observing for all children

- Never leave a child alone near a pool or a source of water
- Install a four-side (4-foot) fence around the pool with a self-closing and self-latching gate
- Do not allow children to use arm buoys or other air-filled swim aids
- Avoid toys that will attract children around pools
- Turn off pump filters when using pools
- Use cordless or cell phones near pool to prevent leaving the poolside to answer the phone elsewhere
- Keep rescue equipment (e.g., shepherd's hook, life preserver) and a telephone by the pool
- Do not try or allow hyperventilation to increase underwater swim time
- Do not dive in shallow water
- Provide swimming lessons for all children by age 2 years
- After the children have finished swimming, secure the pool so they cannot return
- All family members and others watching children should learn CPR

Lightning

Lightning is the most widespread threat to people and property during the thunderstorm season and has been second only to floods in causing storm-related death in the United States since 1959.[35] The National Weather Service estimates that 100,000 thunderstorms occur each year in the United States and that lightning is present in all storms. Lightning is reported to start approximately 75,000 forest fires annually and starts 40% of all fires.[36] The most destructive form of lightning is the cloud-to-ground strike (Figure 17-1). Based

FIGURE 17-1 A cloud-to-ground lightning strike, with streak lightning pattern.
(From Cooper MA, Andrews CJ, Holle RL, Lopez RE: Lightning injuries. In Auerbach P: *Wilderness medicine: management of wilderness and environmental emergencies*, ed 4, St Louis, 2001, Mosby.)

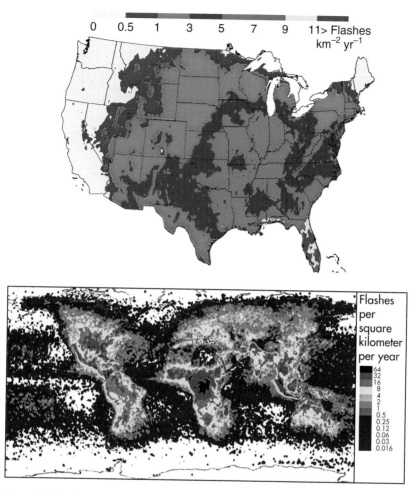

FIGURE 17-2   Distribution of lightning ground strikes in the United States, with the heaviest concentration in the southeast region.
(From Huffines GR, Orville RE: Lightning ground flash density and thunderstorm duration in the continental United States, 1989-1996, *J Appl Meteorol* 38:1013, 1999.)

on real-time lightning detection systems, it is estimated that cloud-to-ground lightning strikes occur approximately 20 million times per year, with as many as 50,000 flashes per hour during a summer afternoon.[37,38] Central Florida is the region with the highest number of lightning ground strikes each year (see Figure 17-2 for distribution of lightning flashes in the United States). Lightning occurs most frequently from June through August, but occurs in Florida and along the southeastern coast of the Gulf of Mexico throughout the year.[39]

Since the 1950s, the number of deaths from lightning have been decreasing, possibly because of fewer people working outdoors in rural areas, improved warning systems for approaching storms, increased public education on lightning safety, and improved medical care.[40] It is now reported that lightning kills 50 to 300 individuals each year and injures about 1000.[36,41] The greatest life threats from lightning strikes are neurologic and cardiopulmonary injuries.

Epidemiology

Based on the National Oceanic Atmospheric Administration (NOAA) publication called *Storm Data,* 3529 deaths (average 98 deaths per year), 9818 injuries, and 19,814 property-damage reports occurred during the 36-year period from 1959 to 1994.[35] This report showed that the top four states for casualties (death and injuries) from lightning are Florida (523), Michigan (732), Pennsylvania (644), and North Carolina (629). The highest number of deaths occurred in Florida (345), North Carolina (165), Texas (164), and New York (128). Figure 17-3 shows the ranking of lightning injuries and deaths by state from 1959 to 1994.

There were 1318 lightning deaths between 1980 and 1995 in the United States, on review of medical examiners' death certificates listing lightning as the cause of death.[42] Of those who died during this 16-year period, 1125 (85%) were male and 896 (68%) were age 15 to 44 years. The highest death rate from lightning occurred among those age 15 to 19 years (6 deaths per 10,000,000). Analysis shows that

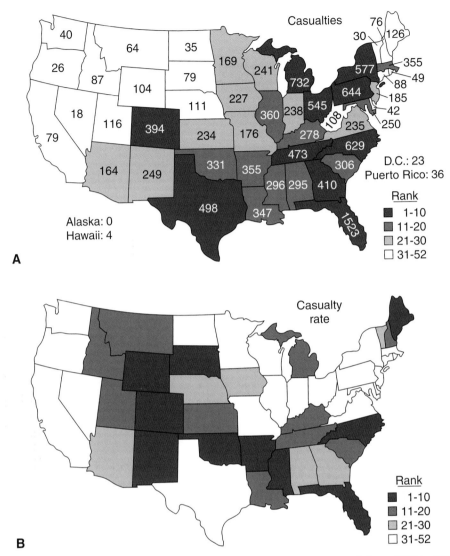

A

Casualties

Alaska: 0
Hawaii: 4

D.C.: 23
Puerto Rico: 36

Rank
■ 1-10
■ 11-20
□ 21-30
□ 31-52

B

Casualty
rate

Rank
■ 1-10
■ 11-20
□ 21-30
□ 31-52

FIGURE 17-3 Rank of each state in lightning casualties (deaths and injuries combined) from 1959 to 1994. **A,** Casualties per state. **B,** Casualties weighted by state population.
(Data from Curran EB, Holle RL, Lopez RE: Lightning fatalities, injuries, and damage reports in the United States from 1959-1994, *NOAA Tech Memo NWS SW-193*, 1997.)

about 30% die and 74% of the survivors have permanent disabilities. Furthermore, victims with cranial or leg burns are at a greater risk for death.[43] In the individuals who died from a lightning strike, 52% were outside (25% of whom were at work). Death occurred within 1 hour in 63% of the lightning victims.[40]

Mechanism of Injury

Injury from lightning can result from the following five mechanisms[36,44,45]:

- *Direct strike* occurs when a person is in the open environment unable to find shelter.
- *Side flash* or *splash contact* occurs when lightning hits an object (e.g., ground, building, tree) and splashes onto

a victim or multiple victims. The current will jump from the primary strike object and can splash over to a person. Splashes occur from person to person, tree to person, and even indoors from telephone wire to a person talking on the phone;

- *Contact* occurs when a person is in direct contact with an object that is struck directly or by a splash.
- *Step voltage,* also known as *stride voltage* or *ground current,* occurs when lightning hits the ground or a nearby object. The current will spread outward radially. Human tissue provides less resistance than the ground, and the current will travel, for example, up one leg and down the other in the path of least resistance.
- *Indirectly.* Blunt trauma can occur from a shock wave produced by lightning, which can move a person up to

10 yards. Injuries can result from lightning that causes forest fires, building fires, and explosions.

There are six known factors that determine the injury severity from electrical and lightning current: type of circuit, duration of exposure, voltage, amperage, resistance of tissue, and the pathway of current. Once contacted by lightning or other high-voltage electrical source, the heat generated within the body is directly proportional to the amount of current, tissue resistance, and the duration of contact. As resistance of various tissues increases (e.g., from nerve to muscle and bone), so does the heat generated by the passage of current.

It is easy to assume that lightning injuries are similar to high-voltage electrical injuries. However, significant differences exist between the two mechanisms of injury.

A lightning strike produces millions of volts of current, and the duration of exposure to the body is instantaneous ($1/10$ to $1/1000$ of a second). The temperature of lightning varies with the diameter, but the average temperature is approximately 14,430° F (8000° C).[41] In comparison, high-voltage electrical exposure tends to be a much lower voltage than lightning. However, the key factor that distinguishes lightning from high-voltage electrical injury and the different patterns of injury is the duration of current exposure within the body.[44] Table 17-3 lists differences between lightning and generator-produced high-voltage electrical injuries.

At times, lightning can show injury patterns similar to those seen with high-voltage electricity because of a rare lightning pattern that produces a prolonged strike lasting up to 0.5 second. This type of lightning, called "hot lightning," is capable of causing deep burns, exploding trees, and setting fires. Lightning can show entry and exit wounds on the body, but a more common pathway of lightning, once it strikes a victim, is to pass over the body. This is referred to as a "flashover" current. A flashover current can also enter the eyes, ears, nose, and mouth. It is theorized that the flashover current flow is the reason why many survive lightning strikes. It is also known that a flashover current may vaporize moisture on skin or blast a part of clothing or shoes off a victim.

Injuries from Lightning

Lightning injuries range from minor superficial wounds to major multisystem trauma and death. Table 17-4 lists common signs and symptoms of lightning injury. As a tool to determine the likely recovery or prognosis from lightning strikes, victims can be placed in one of three injury categories: minor, moderate, and severe.[46]

Minor Injury

Patients with minor injury are awake and report an unpleasant and abnormal sensation (dysesthesias) in the affected extremity. In a more serious lightning strike, victims report they have been hit in the head or state that an explosion hit them, because they are unsure of the source. A patient may present at the scene with the following:

- Confusion (short term or hours to days)
- Amnesia (short term or hours to days)
- Tympanic membrane rupture
- Temporary deafness
- Blindness
- Temporary unconsciousness
- Temporary paresthesias
- Muscular pain
- Cutaneous burns (rare)
- Transient paralysis

Victims present with normal vital signs or with mild, transient hypertension, and recovery is usually gradual and complete.[41]

TABLE 17-3 Comparison of Lightning and High-Voltage Electrical Injuries

Factor	Lightning	High voltage
Energy level	30 million volts; 50,000 amperes	Usually much lower
Time of exposure	Brief, instantaneous	Prolonged
Pathway	Flashover, orifice	Deep, internal
Burns	Superficial, minor	Deep, internal
Cardiac	Primary and secondary arrest, asystole	Fibrillation
Renal	Rare myoglobinuria or hemoglobinuria	Myoglobinuric renal failure common
Fasciotomy	Rarely if ever necessary	Common, early, and extensive
Blunt injury	Explosive thunder effect	Falls, being thrown

Modified table from Cooper MA, Andrews CJ, Holle RL, Lopez RE: Lightning injuries. In Auerbach P: *Wilderness medicine: management of wilderness and environmental emergencies*, ed 4, St Louis, 2001, Mosby.

TABLE 17-4   **Lightning Injury: Common Signs, Symptoms, and Treatment**

Injuries	Signs/symptoms	Treatment
Minor	Feeling of strange sensation in extremity; confusion; amnesia; temporary unconsciousness, deafness, or blindness; tympanic membrane rupture	Scene safety; ABCDEs; medical history and secondary exam; monitor ECG; give oxygen and transport all patients with mild injuries.
Moderate	Disoriented, combative, paralysis, fractures, blunt trauma, absent pulses in lower extremities, spinal shock, seizures, temporary cardiorespiratory arrest, comatose	Scene safety; ABCDEs; medical history and secondary exam; monitor ECG; CPR early when needed; give oxygen and transport all patients.
Severe	Any from above, otorrhea in ear canal, cardiac fibrillation or cardiac asystole	CPR and advanced lifesaving procedures; use "reverse" triage with multiple patients.

Data from O'Keefe GM, Zane RD: Lightning injuries, *Emerg Med Clin North Am* 22:369, 2004; and Cooper MA, Andrews CJ, Holle RL, Lopez RE: Lightning injuries. In Auerbach P: *Wilderness medicine: management of wilderness and environmental emergencies,* ed 4, St Louis, 2001, Mosby.

Moderate Injury

Victims with moderate injury have progressive, single or multisystem injuries, some of which are life threatening. Some patients in this category also have a permanent disability. Patients may present at the scene with the following:

- Disorientation
- Combativeness
- Comatose
- Lower extremity paralysis
- Mottling of skin
- Absent pulses
- Nonpalpable peripheral pulses
- Hypotension
- Blunt trauma (e.g., fractures)
- Spinal shock (e.g., cervical fractures)
- First- and second-degree burns, not always observed early (late finding)
- Third-degree burns (rare)
- Tympanic membrane rupture (common)

Long-term sequelae are:

- Sleep disorders
- Irritability
- Fine psychomotor dysfunction
- Paresthesias
- Generalized weakness
- Nervous system dysfunction
- Posttraumatic stress syndrome
- Spinal paralysis (rare)

Depending on the location of the lightning strike, a strike affecting the respiratory center of the brain can result in prolonged respiratory arrest that may lead to secondary cardiac arrest as a result of hypoxia.[41] Victims in this category may experience immediate cardiopulmonary arrest, although the inherent automaticity of the heart may produce a spontaneous return to normal sinus rhythm.[43] Because immediate cardiopulmonary arrest is the greatest threat, prehospital care providers need to assess the ABCs quickly in all lightning-strike victims and continuously monitor the ECG for secondary cardiac events.

Severe Injury

Victims with severe injury from a direct lightning strike (cardiovascular or neurologic injuries) or delays in CPR have a poor prognosis. On arrival at the scene, the prehospital care provider may find the patient in immediate cardiac arrest with asystole or ventricular fibrillation (VF). If prolonged cardiac and neurologic ischemia has occurred, it may be very difficult to resuscitate these patients.[41] Other common findings are tympanic membrane rupture with cerebrospinal fluid (CSF) and blood in the ear canal, ocular injuries, and various forms of blunt trauma from falls, including soft tissue contusions and fractures of the skull, ribs, extremities, and spine. Many patients in this category have no evidence of burns.

Assessment

On arrival at the scene, as with any other call, the priority is the safety of the prehospital care providers and other public safety personnel. Know whether or not there is still the chance of lightning in the area. As a storm approaches or has passed, there still is a source of danger that is not always apparent, since lightning remains a very real threat as far as 10 miles away.[47] The mechanism of injury may be unclear without a witness because lightning can strike during a perceived sunny day. When in doubt about the mechanism of injury, immediately assess for ABCDEs and any life-threatening conditions, as in any emergency. These patients do not carry an electrical charge, and touching them poses no risk in providing patient care. Assess heart rhythm with the ECG. It is common to see nonspecific

ST-segment and T-wave changes, but more specific evidence of myocardial infarction with Q-wave or ST-segment elevation is rarely seen.[48]

Once the patient is stable, a detailed head-to-toe assessment is necessary to identify the wide range of injuries that can occur with this type of trauma. Assess patient situational awareness and neurologic function of all extremities because upper and lower extremities may experience transient paralysis. Lightning victims are known to have an autonomic dysfunction causing dilated pupils, which will mimic head trauma.[49] Assess eyes because 55% of victims have some form of ocular injury. Look for blood and otorrhea in ear canals; 50% of these victims will have one or two ruptured tympanic membranes. All victims of lightning injury have a high probability of blunt trauma from being thrown against a solid object or from objects falling on the patient. Cervical spine precautions are needed during assessment to minimize further injury. Assess skin for signs of any burns, ranging from first degree to full thickness. It is common to see a feathering appearance in the skin, known as "Lichtenberg's flowers," but these patterns are not burns and resolve in 24 hours. It is more common to see burns secondary to igniting of clothes and heating of jewelry or other objects.

Management

The priorities for managing a lightning victim are to stabilize airway, breathing, and circulation. If spontaneous respiration or circulation is absent, initiate effective CPR up to 5 cycles (2 minutes), and evaluate heart rhythm with an automatic external defibrillator (AED) based on current guidelines.[33] Use ALS measures to manage lightning-induced cardiopulmonary arrest based on current AHA guidelines for ACLS and PALS, as discussed elsewhere.[33] Apply high-flow oxygen for moderately and severely injured patients. IV fluids should be started KVO, since lightning-injured patients, unlike conventional high-voltage electrical-injured patients, do not have massive tissue destruction and burns requiring a larger amount of fluids. Stabilize any fractures, and package blunt trauma patient for cervical spine immobilization. Lightning-strike victims with minor to severe injuries need to be transported to an ED for further evaluation and observation. Transport the patient by either ground or air based on availability, distance, and time to the hospital, and overall to risk to flight crew and benefit to patient.

As mentioned previously, lightning victims have a higher probability of a positive outcome from early and effective resuscitation. However, there is little evidence to suggest that these patients can regain a pulse from prolonged BLS or ALS procedures lasting longer than 20 to 30 minutes.[36] Before terminating resuscitation, all efforts should be made to stabilize the patient by establishing an airway, along with high-flow oxygen and supported ventilation, and to correct any hypovolemia, hypothermia, and acidosis.

If the incident involves multiple victims, principles of triage should be implemented immediately. The normal rules of triage are to focus limited personnel and resources on patients with moderate and severe injuries and quickly bypass those patients without respiration and circulation. However, with multiple lightning-strike patients, the rule becomes to use "reverse" triage and "resuscitate the dead," because these patients are either in respiratory arrest or cardiac arrest and have a high probability of recovery.[43,50]

Prevention

With numerous thunderstorms throughout the year, lightning ground strikes are common. The public and prehospital care providers must be educated about prevention and the many lightning myths and misconceptions (Box 17-1). Numerous lightning prevention resources are provided by such agencies as the National Weather Service/NOAA, National Lightning Safety Institute, American Red Cross, and Federal Emergency Management Agency (FEMA).[51]

Prehospital care providers and other public safety personnel should establish procedures for a severe weather watch that provides storm warnings updated through the day as one method of safety prevention.

One public education motto used for children and adults is, "If you see it, flee it; if you hear it, clear it." Another useful rule is the "30-30 rule." When the time between seeing lightning and hearing thunder is 30 seconds or less, individuals are in danger and need to seek appropriate shelter. Furthermore, it is recommended to resume outdoor activity only after 30 minutes following the last lightning or thunder, because a passing thunderstorm still is a threat and lightning can strike up to 10 miles after the storm passes. Another measure of lightning proximity is the "flash-to-bang" rule, 5 seconds = 1 mile, following lightning for every 5 seconds until the sound of thunder equals 1 mile.

The following are safety guidelines for lightning prevention as a storm develops:[36,41]

Indoors

1. Seek a building and stay away from windows, open doors, fireplaces, bath and shower, and metal objects such as sinks and appliances.
2. Turn off the radio and computer and avoid hard-wired telephones; use a telephone only in emergency.
3. Turn off all faucets, electrical appliances, and devices *before* a storm arrives.

Outdoors

1. Avoid metal objects such as bikes, tractors, and fences.
2. Avoid tall objects, and make yourself small.
3. Avoid areas near pipelines, power lines, and ski lifts.
4. Avoid open fields.

BOX 17-1 Myths and Misconceptions about Lightning

GENERAL MYTHS

■ Lightning strikes are invariably fatal
■ Major cause of death is from burns
■ A victim struck by lightning bursts into flames or is reduced to ashes
■ Victims remain charged or electrified after being struck
■ Individuals are only at risk for being struck when there are storm clouds overhead
■ Occupying a building during the storm affords 100% protection from lightning
■ The belief that lightning never strikes the same place twice is false
■ Wearing rubber-soled shoes and raincoat will protect a person
■ Rubber tires in a vehicle are what protect a person from injury
■ Wearing metal jewelry increases the risk of attracting lightning
■ Lightning always hits the highest object
■ There is no danger from lightning unless it is raining
■ Lightning can occur without thunder

MISCONCEPTIONS

Some myths and misconceptions held by prehospital care providers can adversely affect the care and outcome of their patients.

■ If you are not killed by lightning, you will be OK
■ If the victim has no outward signs of injury, the damage cannot be that serious
■ Lightning injuries should be treated similar to other high-voltage electrical injuries
■ Lightning victims who have resuscitation for several hours might still recover successfully

Modified from O'Keefe GM, Zane RD: Lightning injuries, *Emerg Med Clin North Am* 22:369, 2004; and Cooper MA, Andrews CJ, Holle RL, Lopez RE: Lightning injuries. In Auerbach P: *Wilderness Medicine: management of wilderness and environmental emergencies,* ed 4, St Louis, 2001, Mosby.

5. Avoid open shelters (e.g., carport, bus shelter), depending on overall size, because side flashes or ground strikes can occur.
6. Drop ski poles and golf clubs.
7. In large public outdoors events, seek out nearby buses or minivans.
8. Seek the inside of a hardtop vehicle, and avoid convertibles; keep windows up and avoid metal items in the vehicle.

9. Tents offer little if any protection, and avoid metal tent poles and wet objects.
10. When no immediate shelter is available, all persons should spread out 30 to 50 feet apart to avoid splash contact and ground current.
11. Seek to make smallest contact with ground, if possible, to minimize ground contact.
12. Lightning position requires squatting, feet together, ears covered with hands; squat on a ground pad, backpack, or some insulation material. An alternative position of comfort is to kneel or sit cross-legged.
13. Do not stand, hug, squat, or huddle near tall trees; seek out a low area of lower trees or saplings.
14. Seek out large caves, and stay away from the opening and side walls.
15. If on high ground or side of a mountain, seek out lower terrain in area.
16. Seek out ditches unless there is contact with water.
17. If on water, seek shore immediately; avoid swimming, boating, or tallest object on water.

Recreational Scuba-Related Injuries

Recreational diving using *self-contained underwater breathing apparatus* (scuba) is a common activity enjoyed by many age groups. The popularity of this activity continues to grow, with more than 400,000 new certified divers each year, totaling over 5 million scuba divers in the United States.[52,53] Relative to the increasing number of new divers each year, the injury rate is low, but the concern for medical fitness to dive has increased because of the diversity of divers, increasing age, low physical fitness, and underlying medical conditions. Diving is an unforgiving environment when problems occur. Currently, there are medical guidelines that indicate relative and temporary health risks and absolute contraindications for scuba diving.[53]

Injuries to divers occur from many underwater hazards (e.g., shipwrecks, coral reefs) or from handling hazardous marine life. More often, however, prehospital care providers respond to scuba-related injuries and fatalities caused by *dysbarism,* or altered environmental pressure, which accounts for the majority of the serious diving medical disorders. The mechanism of injury is based on the principles of gas laws when breathing compressed gases (e.g., oxygen, carbon dioxide, nitrogen) at varying underwater depths and pressures.

Most scuba-related injuries caused by dysbarism present with immediate signs and symptoms or within 60 minutes after surfacing, but some symptoms are delayed up to 48 hours after individuals depart the dive site and return home. Consequently, with the increasing number of scuba divers today flying to and from popular dive sites in the United States, Caribbean, and other, remote locations, there is a greater possibility of responding to diving-related injuries throughout the United States. Prehospital care providers need to recognize these scuba-related disorders, provide initial treatment, and initiate plans early for transportation to the local ED or for treatment at the closest recompression chamber.[54]

Epidemiology

Divers Alert Network (DAN) compiles an extensive morbidity and mortality database based on casualty data provided from participating recompression chambers in North America. In 2000, they published a report summarizing 11 years (1987 to 1997) of data.[55] The majority of the scuba-related diving injuries occur in the Northwest (38%) and Southeast (32%) regions of the United States during the months of May to September, with August being the peak month. Eighty-seven percent of the injuries occur in the ocean and 9% in freshwater areas (lake and quarry). Three to four times more male divers are injured than female divers. The primary cause of a diving-related injury is decompression sickness. From 1970 to 1998, the number of diving-related deaths ranged from 66 to 147 per year.[55] Eighty percent of the fatalities occurred in males with a mean age between 38 and 42 years. The causes of death were drowning (50%-70%), cardiovascular factors (6%-14%), arterial gas embolism (5%-14%), and decompression sickness (0%-2%). Even though drowning was the leading cause of fatalities, it is unclear what led to the drowning, such as equipment issues, panic, disorientation, hypothermia, heart attack, or arterial gas embolism. Many drowning deaths during scuba diving are actually arterial gas embolism leading to secondary drowning.[53] Table 17-5 summarizes the 2000 DAN report on scuba injuries and fatalities.

Mechanical Effects of Pressure

Scuba-related diving injuries incurred by the changing atmospheric pressure, or dysbarism, can be separated into two types: (1) the conditions when a change in pressure from the underwater environment results in tissue trauma or *barotrauma* in closed air spaces in the body (e.g., ears, sinuses, intestines, lungs), and (2) the problems that occur from breathing compressed gases at elevated partial pressure, such as decompression sickness.

Barotraumas associated with scuba diving are directly related to the pressure effects of air and water on the diver. When standing at sea level, the atmospheric pressure is 760 millimeters of mercury (mm Hg) or 14.7 pounds per square inch (PSI) on the body. This is also known as one atmosphere (1 atm). As a diver descends deeper in water, the absolute pressure increases 1 atm for every 33 feet of seawater.

TABLE 17-5   Eleven-Year (1987-1997) Profile of Scuba Diving Injuries

Injuries	1987-1997
Age (range of average age each year)	33-37
Percentage divers >50 yr	7% (1997)
Male/female ratio	3-4:1
DIVE PROFILES	
Mean number of days diving	1
Median number of days diving	2-4
Number of dives	1-7
Mean maximum depth	75-95 feet saltwater
SYMPTOMS	
Pain and numbness	50%-65%
Paralysis	3%-10%
Unconsciousness	4%-7%
Bladder dysfunction	0.5%-2%
DECOMPRESSION SICKNESS	
Type II	65%-70%
Type I	20%-30%
Arterial gas embolism	10%-20%
Fatalities (Range = 66-147)	**1970-1998**
Average age	38-42
Male gender	80%
CAUSES OF DEATH	
Drowning	50%-70%
Cardiovascular	6%-14%
Arterial gas emboli	5%-14%
Decompression sickness	0%-2%

Divers Alert Network: Eleven-year trends (1987-1997) in diving activity: the DAN annual review of recreational SCUBA diving injuries and fatalities based on 2000 data. In *Report on decompression illness, diving fatalities and Project Dive exploration,* Durham, NC, 2000, Divers Alert Network.

Consequently, a depth of 33 feet of seawater is equivalent to 2 atm (air [1 atm] and 33 ft water [1 atm]) of pressure on the body. Table 17-6 lists common units of pressure in the underwater environment.

When a diver descends under a column of air and increasing pressure of seawater, the forces exerted on the body are different depending on the tissue compartments. Except

TABLE 17-6 **Common Units of Pressure in Underwater Environment**

Depth (FSW)	PSIA	ATA	mm Hg (absolute)
Sea level	14.7	1	760
33	29.4	2	1520
66	44.1	3	2280
99	58.8	4	3040
132	73.5	5	3800
165	88.2	6	4560
198	102.9	7	5320

FSW, Feet seawater; *PSIA,* pounds per square inch absolute; *ATA,* atmosphere absolute; *mm Hg,* millimeters of mercury.

for air-containing spaces, the force on solid tissue acts as a fluid medium, and the diver is unaware of these forces. The air-containing spaces of the body are reduced as the diver descends and in turn expand as the diver ascends toward the surface. Boyle's law and Henry's law explain the effects of pressure on the body when underwater.

Boyle's Law

Boyle's law states that the volume of a given mass of gas is inversely proportional to the absolute pressure found in that environment. Stated another way, as a diver descends in water to a lower depth, pressure increases and the volume (e.g., volume in the lung) decreases, and the volume increases in size when the diver returns toward the surface. This is the principle behind the effects of barotrauma and arterial gas embolism in the body. Figure 17-4 shows the effects of pressure on the volume and diameter of a gas bubble.

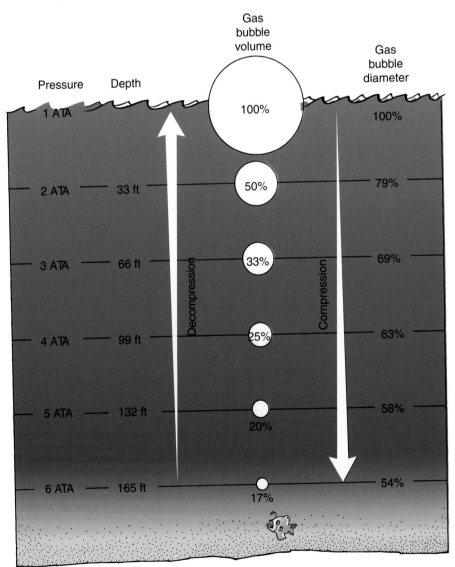

FIGURE 17-4 Boyle's law. The volume of a given quantity of gas at constant temperature varies inversely with pressure. (From Kizer KW: Diving medicine. In Auerbach PS: *Wilderness medicine: management of wilderness and environmental emergencies*, ed 4, St Louis, 2001, Mosby.)

Henry's Law

At a constant temperature, the amount of gas that will dissolve in a liquid is directly proportional to the partial pressure of gas in liquid. Henry's law is fundamental in the understanding of how gas in a compressed air cylinder (scuba tank) behaves in the body as the diver descends. For example, the partial pressure of nitrogen will dissolve in tissue fluid as the pressure increases during descent, and on return toward the surface, nitrogen will bubble out of solution in the tissues. This law describes the principles that explain why decompression sickness occurs.

Diving-Related Injuries

Barotrauma

Barotrauma, also known as "squeeze," is the most common form of scuba-related diving injury.[56] Although many forms of barotraumas cause pain, many forms resolve spontaneously and do not require EMS involvement or recompression chamber therapy. However, some pulmonary overpressurization injuries are very serious. During scuba diving, barotrauma occurs within noncompressible, gas-filled body cavities (e.g., sinuses). If the pressure in these spaces cannot equalize during a dive as ambient pressure increases, vascular engorgement, hemorrhage, and mucosal edema result from decreasing air volume when the diver descends, and tissue disruption results from increasing air volume when the diver ascends. Table 17-7 summarizes signs and symptoms of barotrauma and its treatment. The various forms of barotraumas are described next.

Barotrauma of Descent

Mask Squeeze. This generally occurs in inexperienced or inattentive divers who fail to maintain a balance of pressure equal in their facemask with increasing external water pressure during descent.

Assessment. Examine the soft tissue around the eyes and conjunctival tissues for capillary rupture. Signs and symptoms include skin ecchymoses and conjunctival hemorrhage.

Management. Mask barotrauma is self-limiting; no diving until tissue damage clears. Provide cold compresses over eyes; rest and pain medication as needed.

Tooth Squeeze. A very infrequent finding, this form of barotrauma occurs to divers when gas is trapped in the interior portion of the tooth after dental fillings, recent extractions, or a root canal or with defective restorations. During descent, the tooth can fill with blood or can implode with increasing external pressure. During ascent, any air forced into the tooth will expand, causing pain or the tooth to explode. To prevent tooth squeeze, it is recommended not to dive for 24 hours after any dental treatment.

Assessment. Examine the affected tooth to see if it is intact. Signs and symptoms include pain and fractured tooth.

Management. Refer for dental evaluation; give pain medication as needed.

Middle Ear Squeeze. This squeeze occurs in 40% of scuba divers and is considered the most common diving injury.[57] An ear squeeze occurs near surface, where the greatest changes in pressure occur as the diver descends. Divers need to begin equalizing their middle ear early as they start to descend so a pressure differential across the tympanic membrane (TM) does not occur, leading to rupture. Divers need to equalize the pressure by forcing air into the middle ear through the eustachian tube by either a Valsalva or Frenzel maneuver.[53] The diver will experience pain and vertigo if the TM ruptures, allowing water to enter the middle ear. Divers with upper respiratory infection or allergies may have difficulty equalizing their middle ear during a dive and should determine if they can perform a Valsava maneuver on the surface before the dive.

Assessment. Examine the ear canal for blood caused by ruptured TM. Signs and symptoms include pain, vertigo, conductive hearing losses with TM rupture, and vomiting.

Management. No pressure changes are permitted (diving or flying). Patient may need decongestants with no TM rupture; antibiotics may be needed with ruptured TM. Refer for audiometric evaluation. Transport in upright position or position of comfort.

Sinus Squeeze. Normally, pressure in the sinuses equalizes easily as the diver is descending and ascending. Pressure develops by the same mechanism as middle ear squeeze, but sinus squeeze is not as common. As a diver descends, there is an inability to maintain pressure in the sinuses, and a vacuum develops in the sinus cavity, causing intense pain, mucosal wall trauma, and bleeding in the sinus cavity. This squeeze may be caused by congestion, sinusitis, mucosal hypertrophy, rhinitis, or nasal poyps.[56] A reverse sinus squeeze during ascent can occur as well (see later discussion).

Assessment. Examine the nose for discharge; signs and symptoms include severe pain over the affected sinus or bloody discharge, usually from frontal sinuses.

Management. No specific management is needed at scene unless extensive bleeding is observed, in which case treat for epistaxis by pinching firmly on the fleshy part of the patient's nostrils. Transport in position of comfort.

Internal Ear Barotrauma. Although much less common than middle ear squeeze, this is the most serious form of ear

TABLE 17-7 Barotrauma: Common Signs, Symptoms, and Treatment

Type	Signs/symptoms	Treatment*
Mask squeeze	Corneal injections, conjunctival hemorrhage	Self-limiting; rest, cold compression, pain medication
Sinus squeeze	Pain, bloody nasal discharge	Pain medication, decongestants, antihistamines
Middle ear squeeze	Pain, vertigo, tympanic membrane rupture, hearing loss, vomiting	Decongestants, antihistamines, pain medication; may need antibiotics; avoid diving and flying
Internal ear barotrauma	Tinnitus, vertigo, ataxia, hearing loss	Bed rest; elevate head; avoid loud noises; stool softeners; avoid strenuous activity; no diving or flying for months
External ear barotrauma	Difficulty with Valsalva maneuver, earache, bloody discharge, possible tympanic membrane rupture	Maintain dry ear canal; antibiotics may be needed for infection
Tooth squeeze	Tooth pain while diving	Self-limiting; pain medication
Alternobaric vertigo	Pressure, pain in affected ear, vertigo, tinnitus	Usually short lived; decongestants; prohibit diving until resolution with normal hearing
Pulmonary barotrauma	Substernal pain; voice change; dyspnea; subcutaneous emphysema	Assess ABCs, neurologic functions; 100% oxygen 12-15 L/min nonrebreather mask; transport patient lying supine; need to rule out AGE
Subcutaneous emphysema	Substernal pain and crepitus, brassy voice, neck swelling, dyspnea, bloody sputum	Rest; avoid diving and flying; oxygen and recompression therapy only in severe cases
Pneumothorax	Sharp chest pain, dyspnea, diminished breath sounds	100% oxygen 12-15 L/min nonrebreather mask; monitor pulse oximetry; transport in position of comfort; assess for tension pneumothorax
Tension pneumothorax	Cyanosis, distended neck veins, tracheal deviation	14-gauge needle thoracentesis; 100% oxygen 12-15 L/min nonrebreather mask; monitor pulse oximetry
Arterial gas embolism (AGE)	Unresponsive, confusion, headache, visual disturbances, seizure	Assess ABCs, neurologic functions; initiate BLS/ALS; control seizures; 100% oxygen 12-15 L/min nonrebreather mask; transport patient lying supine; glucose-free IV fluid therapy (1-2 mL/kg /hr); monitor ECG; Consult *DAN* (919-684-8111) for closest recompression chamber (primary treatment)

From Clenney TL, Lassen LF: Recreational scuba diving injuries, *Am Fam Physician* 53(5):1761, 1996; and Kizer KW: Diving medicine. In Auerbach PS: *Wilderness medicine: management of wilderness and environmental emergencies*, ed 4, St Louis, 2001, Mosby.
*Good patient education on scene for minor barotrauma injuries because some of these injuries are self-limiting and others need physician evaluation; others need patient referral to family physician or emergency department and will not necessitate EMS transport.

barotrauma because it may lead to permanent deafness.[58] Internal ear barotrauma occurs when a diver descends and has failed attempts to equalize the middle ear. Further forceful attempts can result in a large rise in middle ear pressure and can rupture the round window structure.

Assessment. Examine the ear canal for any discharge. Signs and symptoms include roaring tinnitus, vertigo, hearing loss, feeling of fullness or "blockage" in affected ear, nausea, vomiting, pallor, diaphoresis, disorientation, and ataxia.

Management. The patient should avoid strenuous activities and loud noises, with no pressure changes (diving or flying). Transport in upright position. Early medical consult with DAN or ED is recommended because it may be difficult to determine if this is inner ear decompression sickness and if there is an immediate need for recompression chamber therapy.

Barotrauma of Ascent
Alternobaric Vertigo. This is an unusual form of barotrauma in that it occurs as expanding gas moves through the eustachian

tube and unequal pressure develops in the middle ear, which can cause vertigo. Although the symptoms are brief, vertigo can trigger panic in divers, leading to other forms of injury caused by a rapid ascent to the surface (e.g., air embolism, near-drowning, drowning).

Assessment. Examine the ear canal for any discharge; assess any hearing loss. Signs and symptoms are short in duration, resulting in transient vertigo, pressure in affected ear, tinnitus, and hearing loss.

Management. No specific intervention is required; diving is not recommended until any hearing loss returns. Provide decongestants as needed. No transport is needed if symptoms resolve quickly; arrange physician referral as needed.

Sinus Barotrauma. This form of sinus squeeze can occur on ascent when some form of blockage in the sinus openings prevents expanding gas from escaping. The expanding gas puts pressure on the mucosal lining of the sinus, causing pain with hemorrhage. Sinus barotrauma occurs in divers with upper respiratory infections or allergies. It is common for divers to take a decongestant before a dive as a preventive measure to help equalize the middle ear when diving. However, the vasoconstrictive benefits can wear off at depth, causing mucosal tissue expansion and forming a sinus blockage of expanding gas during the return to the surface.

Assessment. Examine nose for discharge. Signs and symptoms include severe pain over the affected sinus and bloody discharge, usually from frontal sinuses.

Management. No specific management is needed at the scene unless extensive bleeding is observed, in which case treat for epistaxis by pinching firmly on the fleshy part of the patient's nostrils. Transport in a position of comfort.

Gastrointestinal Squeeze. This occurs when expanding gas in the gut becomes trapped as the diver surfaces. Gastrointestinal (GI) barotrauma occurs in novice divers who frequently perform Valsalva maneuvers in the head-down position, which forces air into the stomach. It can also occur in divers who chew gum while diving or who have consumed carbonated beverages or other gas-producing foods before diving.

Assessment. Examine abdominal quadrants. Signs and symptoms include abdominal fullness, belching, and flatulence.

Management. GI squeeze normally resolves on its own and rarely needs medical attention; arrange physician referral if pain and fullness does not resolve. Only in severe cases is recompression chamber therapy needed.

Pulmonary Overinflation Barotrauma

Pulmonary overinflation is a serious form of barotrauma resulting from the expansion of gas in the lungs during ascent. Normally the diver eliminates expanding gas with normal exhalations when returning to the surface. If the expanding gas does not escape, there is a rupture of the alveoli, which in turn causes one of many forms of injury, depending on the amount of air that escapes outside the lung and its final location. A common scenario is a diver who has a rapid and uncontrollable ascent to the surface caused by running out of air, panic, or a dropped weight belt. These types of injuries are collectively called *pulmonary overpressurization syndrome* (POPS), or "burst lung."

The five forms of POPS are: (1) overdistention with local injury, (2) mediastinal emphysema, (3) subcutaneous emphysema, (4) pneumothorax, and (5) arterial gas embolism.

Overdistention with Local Injury. This is the mildest form of POPS, with only a small, isolated lung barotrauma.

Assessment. Examine lung fields for diminished breath sounds. Chest pain may or may not be present. Blood is often seen in the sputum, or *hemoptysis*.

Management. Ensure rest, and treat symptoms as needed. Monitor vital signs and oxygen saturation with pulse oximetry; provide oxygen at 2 to 4 L/min with nasal cannula. Transport patient in position of comfort. Patient needs further medical evaluation to rule out more severe form of POPS and should avoid further pressure exposure (diving or commercial flying).

Mediastinal Emphysema. This is the most common form of POPS, caused by escaping gas from ruptured alveoli entering the interstitial space to the mediastinum.

Assessment. Condition is usually benign; examine lung fields for diminished breath sounds. Signs and symptoms include hoarseness, neck fullness, and minor substernal chest pain; often a dull ache or tightness worsens with breathing and coughing. Examine chest and neck for subcutaneous emphysema. In severe cases, diver presents with chest pain, dyspnea, and difficulty swallowing.

Management. Ensure rest. Monitor vital signs and oxygen saturation with pulse oximetry; provide oxygen at 2 to 4 L/min with nasal cannula. Usually, mediastinal emphysema requires no specific treatment or recompression therapy. Rare cases of a more severe form need to be medically evaluated to rule out other causes of chest pain and severe forms of POPS. Transport the patient in a supine position; avoid further pressure exposure (diving or commercial flying).

Subcutaneous Emphysema. Air escaping from ruptured alveoli continues to move superiorly into the neck and clavicle regions.

Assessment. Examine lung fields for diminished breath sounds. Signs and symptoms include swelling, crepitus, hoarseness, sore throat, and difficulty swallowing.

Management. No specific treatment is required besides rest. Monitor vital signs and oxygen saturation with pulse oximetry; provide oxygen by nasal cannula at 2 to 4 L/min. Patient needs further medical evaluation to rule out more severe forms of POPS. Transport in supine position. Patient should avoid further pressure exposure (diving or commercial flying).

Pneumothorax. Pneumothorax is seen in less than 10% of POPS cases because air must escape through the visceral pleura around the lung, which presents greater resistance than air escaping through the interstitial space between the lung and visceral pleura. If the diver is at depth when the pulmonary rupture occurs, a tension pneumothorax can result as the volume of escaping gas surrounds the lung and expands as the diver continues toward the surface.

Assessment. Examine lung fields for diminished breath sounds. Signs and symptoms will vary based on size of the pneumothorax and include sharp chest pain, diminished breath sounds, breathlessness, and dyspnea. Provide on-going assessment for conversion from simple to tension pneumothorax.

Management. Ensure rest. Monitor vital signs and oxygen saturation with pulse oximetry; provide oxygen by nasal cannula at 2 to 4 L/min. Provide standard ALS management of tension pneumothorax with 14-gauge needle thoracentesis. Transport patient in a position of comfort. Patient needs further medical evaluation to rule out more severe form of POPS and should avoid further pressure exposure (diving or commercial flying). Recompression therapy should not be necessary.

Arterial Gas Embolism (AGE). This is the most feared complication of POPS and, after drowning, is a leading cause of death in divers, accounting for about 30% of fatalities.[59] AGE can occur from any of the four POPS conditions previously presented as a result of air escaping and forming an air embolism. AGE typically occurs in divers who have an uncontrolled ascent to the surface without appropriate exhalation, causing an overinflation pulmonary injury. However, AGE can occur in divers who surface slowly without underlying lung pathology. During ascent, once the pulmonary overinflation bursts alveoli, air enters the pulmonary venous capillary circulation, and gas bubbles enter at the left atrium, then exit the heart at the aorta and are distributed to cerebral, coronary, and other systemic vasculature. Gas bubbles can enter the coronary circulation, causing an occlusion resulting in cardiac arrhythmias, cardiac arrest, or myocardial infarction.[60] If gas bubbles enter the cerebral circulation, the diver presents with signs and symptoms similar to an acute stroke.

Unlike decompression sickness, which can present with delayed symptoms hours after diving, symptoms of AGE appear either immediately at the water surface or typically within 2 minutes. Any loss of consciousness once a diver surfaces must be presumed to be AGE until proved otherwise.[53] The primary treatment for AGE is recompression chamber therapy.

Historically, it was recommended that patients with AGE be placed in the Trendelenburg position for transport, based on the belief that this would help keep bubbles from circulating in the systemic vasculature. However, recent evidence has shown that the head-down position does not prevent systemic circulation of nitrogen bubbles, makes it more difficult to oxygenate the patient, and may worsen cerebral edema.[61] It is currently recommended that all AGE patients be placed in a supine position in the field and during transport. The supine position also provides a greater rate of nitrogen bubble washout.[62,63]

Decompression Sickness

Decompression sickness (DCS) is directly related to Henry's law. When scuba divers breathe compressed air containing oxygen (21%), carbon dioxide (0.03%), and nitrogen (79%), the amount of gas that will be dissolved in liquid is directly proportional to the partial pressure of gas in contact with liquid. Oxygen is used in the body for tissue metabolism when in solution and does not form gas bubbles during ascent from depth.

Nitrogen, an inert gas not used for metabolism, is the primary source of concern in DCS. Nitrogen is five times more soluble in fat than in water and becomes dissolved in tissue proportionately to the increasing ambient pressure. Consequently, the deeper underwater the diver goes and the longer the diver stays at depth, the greater the amount of nitrogen that dissolves into tissue. As the diver ascends toward the surface, the absorbed nitrogen must be eliminated. If there is inadequate time to eliminate nitrogen during ascent, nitrogen comes out of solution in the tissues in the form of intravascular gas bubbles, causing obstruction of the vascular and lymphatic systems and tissue distention and activating inflammatory responses.[64]

Most divers experience DCS within the first hour after surfacing, whereas other divers will present with symptoms up to 6 hours after surfacing. Only 2% of divers will have delayed symptoms between 24 to 48 hours after surfacing. Traditionally, symptoms of DCS are categorized as *Type I,* a mild form involving cutaneous, lymphatic, and musculoskeletal systems, or *Type II,* a severe form involving neurologic and cardiopulmonary systems. The term *decompression illness* (DCI) has been proposed to encompass Type I and Type II DCS and AGE.[65,66] Mild symptoms of DCS include fatigue to malaise. However, mild symptoms can be precursors to more severe signs and symptoms, such as numbness, weakness, and paralysis. Studies now suggest that it is more important clinically to describe DCS by the region of the body affected and not as Type I or Type II.[53] This suggestion is applicable for prehospital care providers to ensure that even patients with mild DCS symptoms are equally treated aggressively with 100% oxygen and an early consult for recompression therapy. Many divers with the mild form of DCS will not have a medical evaluation. Divers may delay up to 32 hours before seeking medical care for DCS because denial of DCS is a common finding in the scuba-diving population.[67]

Several factors predispose a diver to DCS.[68,69] Some risk factors are known to enhance the uptake of nitrogen in tissues during descent and slow the release of nitrogen during ascent. Certain host and environmental factors, as well as equipment failures and improper technique, increase the risk for DCS (Box 17-2).

Limb Pain (Type I DCS). This form of DCS results from bubble formation in the musculoskeletal system, typically occurring in one or more joints. The most common joints involved are the shoulder and elbow, followed by the knee, hip, wrist, hand, and ankle.[52] This pain is described as a severe tendonitis joint pain with a grating sensation on movement. The pain starts gradually, presenting as a deep, dull ache of mild to severe intensity. Although this form of DCS is not life threatening, it indicates that bubbles are present in the venous circulation. It can lead to more severe forms if left untreated.

Cutaneous and Lymphatic (Type I DCS). This form of DCS is uncommon. It represents inadequate bubble elimination forming in the skin or lymphatic systems. Cutaneous "skin bends" are uncommon and usually not serious, but signs of mottling and marbling are considered precursors of delayed neurologic problems.[53] Symptoms include an intense rash that progresses to a red patchy or bluish discoloration of the skin.[70] Lymphatic obstruction can result in swelling and an orange-peel appearance (peau d'orange).

Cardiopulmonary (Type II DCS). This severe form of DCS is referred to as the "chokes" and results when venous bubbles overwhelm the pulmonary capillary system. Hypotension can occur from a massive venous air embolism in the lung. Symptoms include nonproductive cough, substernal chest pain, cyanosis, dyspnea, shock, and cardiopulmonary arrest. This disorder resembles acute respiratory distress syndrome (ARDS).[71]

Spinal Cord (Type II DCS). The white matter of the spinal cord is vulnerable to bubble formation, and nitrogen is highly

---

BOX 17-2 Factors Related to Decompression Sickness (DCS)

HOST FACTORS
Lack of fitness
Advancing age
Female sex
Hypothermia
Alcohol or drug use
Patent foramen
Obesity
Sleep deprivation
Dehydration
Inadequate nutrition
Heavy exertion at depth or fatigue
Underlying medical illness (e.g., asthma)
Prior history of DCS

ENVIRONMENTAL FACTORS
Extremes of temperature
Rough seas
Flying after diving
Heavy exercise at depth
Nitrogen narcosis
Elevated arterial carbon dioxide tension
Low water temperature

EQUIPMENT FAILURES AND IMPROPER TECHNIQUE
Violating the decompression tables
Difficulty with buoyancy
Rapid ascent
Running out of air
Regulator malfunction
Unfamiliar or improper equipment

Barratt DM, Harch PG, Van Meter K: Decompression illness in divers: a review of the literature, *Neurologist* 8:186, 2002.

---

soluble in spinal cord tissue (myelin). The most common site for this form of DCS is the lower thoracic spine, followed by the lumbar/sacral and cervical regions.[67] Common signs and symptoms include low back pain and "heaviness" in the legs. With this form of DCS, the patient often gives a vague statement in an effort to describe "strange sensations," or *paresthesias,* which can progress to weakness, numbness, and paralysis. Bowel and bladder dysfunction leading to urinary retention also has been reported.[72]

Table 17-8 summarizes signs and symptoms of decompression sickness and its treatment.

Assessment

A standardized approach for patients with AGE and DCS is provided to ensure that consistent care is given. It is

TABLE 17-8 Decompression Sickness (DCS): Common Signs, Symptoms, and Treatment

Condition	Signs/symptoms	Treatment
DCS TYPE I		
Skin bends	Intense itching (pruritus); red rash patches over shoulders and upper chest; skin marbling may precede burning sensation and itching over shoulders and torso; localized cyanosis and pitting edema.	Self-limiting; resolves on its own; observe for delayed signs of limb-pain DCS.
Limb-pain DCS	Large joint tenderness; mild to severe joint or extremity pain; pain is usually steady but may throb and present in 75% of cases; grating sensation on joint motion; worse with movement. DCS Type I may progress to DCS Type II.	Mild pain only often resolves on its own; observe 24 hours; moderate to severe pain. Start with 100% oxygen, 12-15 L/min nonrebreather mask; transport all patients in supine position; glucose-free IV fluid therapy (1-2 mL/kg/hr); early consult *DAN* (919-684-8111) for closest recompression chamber for definitive treatment.
DCS TYPE II		
Cardiopulmonary "Chokes"	Substernal pain, mild cough, dyspnea, nonproductive cough, cyanosis, tachypnea, tachycardia, shock and cardiac arrest	ABCs; 100% oxygen, 12-15 L/min nonrebreather mask; BLS or ALS as needed; glucose-free IV fluid therapy (1-2 mL/kg/hr); transport all patients in supine position; early consult *DAN* (919-684-8111) for closest recompression chamber for definitive treatment.
Neurologic		
Brain	Many visual changes, headache, confusion, disorientation, nausea and vomiting	
Spinal cord	Back pain, heaviness or weakness, numbness, paralysis, urine retention, fecal incontinence	
Inner ear	Vertigo, ataxia	

Barratt DM, Harch PG, Van Meter K: Decompression illness in divers: a review of the literature, *Neurologist* 8:186, 2002; and Kizer KW: Diving medicine. In Auerbach PS: *Wilderness medicine: management of wilderness and environmental emergencies*, ed 4, St Louis, 2001, Mosby.

recommended that all patients with scuba-related diving injuries be examined for signs and symptoms of AGE and DCS because the primary and essential lifesaving treatment is recompression chamber therapy.

Arterial Gas Embolism

About 5% of all AGE patients present with immediate apnea, unconsciousness, and cardiac arrest. Others present with signs and symptoms similar to acute stroke, with loss of consciousness, stupor, confusion, hemiparesis, seizure, vertigo, visual changes, sensory changes, and headache.

Decompression Sickness

Type I DCS is characterized by deep pain in a joint, including minor forms of cutaneous pruritus (severe itching) and obstruction of lymph vessels (lymphedema). Type II DCS is characterized by symptoms involving the central nervous system, ranging from weakness and numbness to paralysis. Obtain a dive profile and medical history of the events that led to the diving-related injury from a fellow diver, including[73] (1) time of onset of signs and symptoms; (2) source

of breathing medium (e.g., air or mixed gases; Heliox); (3) dive profile (dive activity, depth, duration, dive frequency, surface interval, interval between dives); (4) dive location and water conditions; (5) dive risk factors; (6) underwater medical and equipment problems on ascent and descent; (7) whether a no-decompression dive or a decompression dive; (8) rate of ascent; (9) decompression stop(s); (9) post-dive activity level; (10) postdive aircraft travel, with type and duration; (11) past and present medical history (DCI); (12) medication use; and (13) current use of alcohol or illicit drugs.

Management

Provide ABCs, protect the airway, and initiate BLS or ALS procedures as required. Initiate 100% oxygen at 12 to 15L/min, and give NS or LR (no dextrose) IV fluid therapy (1-2 mL/kg/hr). Monitor vital signs, pulse oximetry, and ECG; control seizures. Protect the patient from hypothermia, and consult early with local medical control or DAN for closest recompression chamber (primary treatment) (see Box

17-3 for DAN contact information). Standard recompression therapy with 100% hyperbaric oxygen is given according to the U.S. Navy treatment tables.[74] Transport the patient in a supine position. For any scuba-related diving injury, if air evacuation is provided by helicopter or other nonpressurized aircraft, it is recommended to fly as low as possible (e.g., 500 feet), but not to exceed 1000 feet to minimize further expansion of air bubbles (Boyle's law) and further dysbarism trauma.[53,63]

Definitive treatment for specific barotraumas, including AGE and DCS, is to administer 100% oxygen by mask at two to three times the atmospheric pressure at sea level in a recompression chamber.[75] (For further discussion of recompression chamber treatment methods for scuba-related diving injuries, see the U.S. Navy Diving Manual or other sources.[53,74]) The patient immediately benefits, based on the principles of Boyle's law, by increasing the ambient pressure and decreasing the size of bubbles formation and increasing the oxygen concentration in tissues. Box 17-4 describes recompression and hyperbaric oxygen therapy (HBO).

Prevention of Scuba-Related Diving Injuries

Millions of certified scuba divers need frequent skill-refresher training to prevent and recognize scuba-related dive injuries. This includes many professional scuba dive teams in the United States, such as lifeguards, fire and law enforcement personnel, search and rescue, Coast Guard, and Department of Defense, who depend on local EMS providers to provide initial and follow-up medical care and transport to local hospitals or recompression chambers. Collaboration between dive teams and among local EMS agencies to develop medical scenarios during dive training is strongly encouraged. This should include frequent scuba training in varying underwater conditions and locations, along with in-water rescue scenarios and initial medical care, which are paramount to responding safely and effectively for in-water swimmer/diver rescues and recoveries. Scuba-training coordination among medical dive team members and local EMS providers will ensure effective communication and appropriate field care continuity. This should be included with scenario-based consults with local medical control and with DAN.

Medical Fitness to Dive

All new divers should be cleared medically before the start of scuba training. Five general medical screening recommendations for identifying individuals who are at an increased risk for a diving-related problem are listed below. These recommendations are based on consensus of medical diving specialists.[76] Also refer to Box 17-5 for the absolute, relative, and temporary contraindications for diving.

- Inability to equalize pressure in one or more of the body's air spaces increases the risk for barotrauma.
- Medical or psychiatric conditions may manifest underwater or at a remote diving site and can endanger the diver's life because of the condition itself, because it occurs in the water, or because inadequate medical help is available.
- Impaired tissue perfusion or diffusion of inert gases increases the risk of DCS.
- Poor physical condition increases the risk of DCS or exertion-related medical problems. The factors compromising physical condition may be physiologic or pharmacologic.
- In women who are pregnant, the fetus may be at increased risk of dysbaric injury.

Flying after Diving

Because diving is conducted at many popular dive locations in the United States and at remote locations outside the United States, persons may dive the day before flying. Because of Boyle's principle, flying too soon after a dive can increase the risk of decompression sickness during flight or after arriving at the destination because of the

---

BOX 17-4   Hyperbaric Oxygen (HBO) Recompression Therapy for Scuba-Related Diving Injuries

The goals of HBO therapy for scuba-related diving injuries caused by pulmonary overinflation barotrauma and decompression sickness (DCS) are to compress the bubbles and increase oxygen delivery to tissues. HBO therapy includes the following mechanisms:

- Reduces volume of the bubbles, where they are circulated to the pulmonary capillaries and filtered out
- Promotes reabsorption of bubbles in solution
- Increases oxygen delivery to the tissues
- Corrects hypoxia
- Provides an increased diffusion gradient for nitrogen
- Reduces edema
- Reduces blood vessel permeability

All divers with arterial gas embolism (AGE) and DCS must be considered early for HBO therapy because the treatment is more successful if started within 6 hours after the onset of symptoms. Divers are not always near a recompression chamber when symptoms occur, and there can be considerable delays getting to a chamber by ground or by arranging for air transport. Contact Diver's Alert Network (DAN) to consult for diving medical assistance and to determine the closest recompression chamber.

In the meantime, place the patient in a supine position. Nitrogen washout can be increased by providing 100% oxygen by mask and by starting an IV fluid line with isotonic or lactated Ringer's solution at 1 to 2 mL/kg/hr to ensure

intravascular volume and capillary perfusion. During recompression treatment, patients with AGE or DCS normally will receive HBO therapy at 2.5 to 3.0 atm for 2 to 4 hours while breathing 100% oxygen. Longer and repeated treatment will be necessary if the patient has no clinical improvement of symptoms. HBO treatment principles include the following:

- Any painful or neurologic signs or symptoms occurring within 24 hours of a dive are caused by decompression sickness (DCS) until proved otherwise.
- Any painful or neurologic signs or symptoms occurring within 48 hours of flying after diving are caused by DCS until proved otherwise.
- Contact the Diver's Alert Network 24-hour emergency hotline for consultation at 919-684-8111.
- Every diver with signs or symptoms of DCI should receive HBO therapy.
- Never fail to treat doubtful cases.
- Early treatment improves outcomes, whereas delayed treatment worsens outcomes.
- Long delays should never preclude treatment because divers respond to HBO therapy days to weeks after injury.
- Monitor patient closely for signs of relief or progression of symptoms.
- Inadequate treatment can lead to a recurrence.

Continue to treat until clinical plateau.

Modified from Tibbles PM, Edelsberg JS: Hyperbaric oxygen therapy, *N Engl J Med* 334(25):1642, 1996; and Barratt DM, Harch PG, Van Meter K: Decompression illness in divers: a review of the literature, *Neurologist* 8:186, 2002.

---

reduced atmospheric pressure in either a pressurized or a nonpressurized commercial aircraft. Box 17-6 lists the current guidelines recommended by DAN for flying safely after diving.

High Altitude

More than 40 million people each year in the United States travel above 2400 m (about 8000 ft) to participate in activities that include snow boarding, alpine skiing, hiking, camping, concerts, and festivals. Thus, many people are at risk for altitude-related illness, which can develop within hours to days after they arrive. Prehospital care providers therefore need to become familiar with the predisposing factors, signs and symptoms, medical management, and prevention techniques to reduce the morbidity and mortality of high-altitude illness. This section presents three *altitude-related* medical conditions directly caused by the high-altitude

environment and highlights specific underlying medical conditions that worsen as a result of high altitude–induced hypoxia, also known as *altitude-exacerbated* medical conditions.[77]

Epidemiology

High-altitude illness is a term that encompasses two cerebral and one pulmonary syndrome: (1) acute mountain sickness (AMS), (2) high-altitude cerebral edema (HACE), and (3) high-altitude pulmonary edema (HAPE). Even though the risks of acquiring high-altitude illness are low, once it develops, progression can be fatal.[78]

AMS is a mild form of high-altitude illness rarely experienced at altitudes below 2000 m (6540 ft), but the incidence increases to 1.4% to 25% with increasing altitudes of 2060 to 2440 m (6754-8000 ft).[79,80] AMS develops in 20% to 25% of cases above 2500 m (8200 ft) and in 40% to 50% of cases at 14,000 m (3123 ft).[77] The incidence of AMS is greater than 90% when the rate of ascent to approximately

---

BOX 17-5   Fitness to Dive: Disqualifying Conditions for Scuba Diving

ABSOLUTE*
History of epilepsy or other seizure disorder
Insulin-dependent diabetes mellitus
Symptomatic coronary artery disease
Sickle cell disease or trait
Unexplained syncope
Inability to equalize pressure in the middle ear by autoinflation
Bullous lung disease
Significant pulmonary obstructive disease
Substance abuse
Reactive airway disease (asthma)
Spontaneous pneumothorax
Perforation of the tympanic membrane

RELATIVE†
Migraine and other vascular headaches
Middle ear surgery with placement of a prosthesis in the conduction chain
History of overpressure accident in previous diving
Hypertension
Decreased visual acuity

TEMPORARY
Bronchitis
Pregnancy
Abdominal hernias
Poor physical fitness

Davis JC: Hyperbaric medicine: critical care aspects. In Shoemaker WC, editor: *Critical care: state of the art,* Aliso Viejo, Calif, 1984, The Society of Critical Care Medicine; and Kizer KW: Diving medicine. In Auerbach PS: *Wilderness medicine: management of wilderness and environmental emergencies,* ed 4, St Louis, 2001, Mosby.
*Absolute disqualifications for scuba diving based on expert panel of diving experts.
†Relative disqualification of scuba diving requires further consideration or represents subjects of ongoing debate.

BOX 17-6   Current Guidelines Recommended by Diver's Alert Network for Flying Safely after Diving

The following guidelines are the consensus of attendees at the 2002 Flying after Diving Workshop. They apply to air dives followed by flights at cabin altitudes of 610 to 2438 m (2000-8000 ft) for divers who do not have symptoms of decompression sickness (DCS). The recommended preflight surface intervals do not guarantee avoidance of DCS. Longer surface intervals will reduce DCS risk further.

- For a single no-decompression dive, a minimum preflight surface interval of 12 hours is suggested.
- For multiple dives per day or multiple days of diving, a minimum preflight surface interval of 18 hours is suggested.

For dives requiring decompression stops, there is little evidence on which to base a recommendation, and a preflight surface interval substantially longer than 18 hours appears prudent.

14,000 m (3123 ft) occurs over hours versus days.[81] Furthermore, a small number of AMS cases (5%-10%) progress from mild symptoms to become HACE, a severe form of AMS.[82] HACE is a severe neurologic form of high-altitude illness and has a low incidence rate of 0.01% in the general population at an altitude above 2500 m (8200 ft), which increases to 1% to 2% in more physically active individuals.[77]

HAPE is rare but accounts for the most deaths from high-altitude illness.[82] The incidence rate for HAPE is 0.01% to 0.1% at 2500 m (8200 ft) in the general population and increases to 2% to 6% in climbers at an altitude of 4000 m (13,120 ft). The overall mortality for HAPE is 11%

and increases to 44% when no treatment interventions are made.[83] Forty-seven cases of HAPE were reported in Vail, Colorado, from 1975 to 1982. These were young, healthy males who skied at an average altitude of 2330 m (7644 ft).[84]

Hypobaric Hypoxia

There are three defined levels of altitude. *High altitude* is defined as an elevation above 1500 m up to 3500 m (5000-11,480 ft). This is a common altitude in the western mountain ranges of the United States, where high-altitude illness is reported with greater frequency than in other U.S. regions.[85] *Very high altitude* is defined as an elevation between 3500 and 5500 m (11,480-18,045 ft) and is the more common altitude for serious forms of high-altitude illness.[86] *Extreme altitude* is defined as elevations higher than 5500 m (18,045 ft).[82] With a progressive increase in altitude, the environment becomes very hostile to an individual not acclimatized to the decreased availability of oxygen, also known as *hypobaric hypoxia.*

High altitude is a unique environment because there is a decreased availability of oxygen for respiration, which results in cellular *hypoxia.* Boyle's law states that the volume of gas is inversely proportional to external pressure applied to it, and thus air is less dense in higher altitudes (see section on scuba-related diving injuries for gas laws). Compared to sea level, or 1 atm, atmospheric pressure at 5500 m (18,045 ft) is reduced by approximately 50% (0.5 atm).[82,87] This relationship relates to Henry's law, which states that the concentration of gas in solution is proportional to the partial pressure of that gas.

Even though the concentration of oxygen remains at 21% at all altitudes, decreased atmospheric pressure at higher altitude results in a decreased partial pressure of oxygen (Po_2). For example, Po_2 is 160 mm Hg at sea level (1 atm) and 80 mm Hg at 5500 m (18,045 ft) (0.5 atm), resulting in less oxygen being available during respiration. Table 17-9 shows that as altitude increases from sea level to extreme altitude, there is a proportional decrease in barometric pressure, arterial blood gases, and arterial oxygen saturation (Sao_2). It is worth noting that Sao_2 remains, on average, above 91% in a healthy, acclimatizing adults until reaching an altitude above 2810 m (9200 ft). *Prehospital care providers are trained to provide aggressive ventilatory support with 100% oxygen for all patients who are symptomatic with a pulse oximetry reading of 91% Sao_2, because this is indicative of moderate hypoxia (86%-91%).*

This relationship between increasing altitude and progressive hypoxia forms the basis for the acute physiologic adjustments in respiratory rate and cardiac output and biochemical changes.[88] Consequently, it is the hypobaric hypoxia and hypoxemia that set up nonacclimatized individuals for high-altitude illness.[78]

High-Altitude Illness
Factors Related to High-Altitude Illness

The development of high-altitude illness depends on many factors specific to each high-altitude exposure.

Increased Altitude and Ascent Rate. The incident and severity of high-altitude illness are primarily related to the speed of ascent, altitude reached, and the length of stay because these three factors increase the hypoxic stress in the body.[78,88]

Previous History of High-Altitude Illness. A documented past history of high-altitude illness is a valuable predicator of who is susceptible for subsequent high-altitude illness when returning to the same altitude at the same ascent rate.[89] Incidence rates for HAPE increase from 10% to 60% for those with a previous history of HAPE who abruptly ascend to an altitude of 4560 m (14,960 ft).[90]

Preacclimatization. Having a permanent residence above 900 m (2950 ft) provides some preacclimatization and is associated with a lower rate and severity of high-altitude illness when ascending to higher altitudes. However, this protection is limited if the ascent rate is rapid or reaches an extreme altitude.[88,89]

Age and Gender. Age, but not gender, is a factor in developing AMS; the incidence is lower in those older than 50 years. HAPE occurs more frequently and with greater severity in children and young adults and is reported in equal proportions of males and females in these age groups.[78,91]

Physical Fitness and Exertion. The onset and severity of high-altitude illness is independent of physical fitness; fitness does not accelerate altitude acclimatization. A high level of fitness does allow individuals to exert themselves more, but vigorous exertion on arrival at high altitude further exacerbates hypoxemia and hastens the onset of high-altitude illness.[85,92]

Medications and Intoxicants. Any substance that depresses ventilation and disrupts sleep patterns at altitude should be avoided because this will further exacerbate altitude-induced hypoxemia. These substances include alcohol, barbiturates, and opiates.[82,93]

TABLE 17-9 Relationship of Altitude, Barometric Pressure (PB), Arterial Blood Gases, and Oxygen Saturation*

Altitude (meters)	Altitude (feet)	PB (mm Hg)	Pao₂ (mm Hg)	Sao₂ (%)	Paco₂ (mm Hg)
Sea level	Sea level	760	100	98.0	40.0
1646	5400	630	73.0	95.1	35.6
2810	9200	543	60.0	91.0	33.9
3660	12,020	489	47.6	84.5	29.5
4700	15,440	429	44.6	78.0	27.1
5340	17,500	401	43.1	76.2	25.7
6140	20,140	356	35.0	65.6	22.0

Modified from Hackett PH, Roach RC: High-altitude medicine. In Auerbach PS: *Wilderness medicine: management of wilderness and environmental emergencies*, ed 4, St Louis, 2001, Mosby.
*Data are mean values for subjects age 20 to 40 years.
Pao₂, Arterial oxygen partial pressure; *Sao₂*, arterial oxygen saturation; *Paco₂*, arterial carbon dioxide partial pressure.

Preexisting Medical Conditions. Box 17-7 lists underlying medical conditions that are aggravated by high altitude (low risk, caution, and contraindicated). Additionally, specific medical conditions known to increase susceptibility to high-altitude illness include the following:

- Cardiopulmonary congenital abnormalities: absent pulmonary artery, primary pulmonary hypertension, congenital heart defects
- Carotid artery surgery: irradiation or abolishing carotid bodies

---

BOX 17-7 Common Medical Conditions That Worsen at High Altitude without Supplemental Oxygen

PROBABLY NO EXTRA RISK
Young and old
Fit and unfit
Obesity
Diabetes
After coronary artery bypass grafting (without angina)
Mild chronic obstructive pulmonary disease (COPD)
Asthma
Low-risk pregnancy
Controlled hypertension
Controlled seizure disorder
Psychiatric disorders
Neoplastic diseases
Inflammatory conditions

CAUTION
Moderate COPD
Compensated congestive heart failure (CHF)
Sleep apnea syndromes
Troublesome arrhythmias
Stable angina/coronary artery disease
High-risk pregnancy
Sickle cell trait
Cerebrovascular diseases
Any cause for restricted pulmonary circulation
Seizure disorder (not receiving medication)
Radial keratotomy

CONTRAINDICATED
Sickle cell anemia (with history of crises)
Severe COPD
Pulmonary hypertension
Uncompensated CHF

From Hackett PH, Roach RC: High-altitude medicine. In Auerbach PS: *Wilderness medicine: management of wilderness and environmental emergencies*, ed 4, St Louis, 2001, Mosby.

Cold. Exposure to cold ambient temperatures increases the risk for HAPE because cold increases the pulmonary arterial pressure.[94]

Acute Mountain Sickness

AMS is a self-limiting, nonspecific syndrome that is easily mistaken for a number of other conditions because of common symptoms, including influenza, hangover, exhaustion, and dehydration. A consensus panel defined AMS as the presence of headache in an unacclimatized person who has recently arrived at an altitude above 2500 m (8202 ft) and has one or more symptoms of AMS.[95] However, AMS can occur at levels as low as 2000 m (6562 ft). AMS is now viewed as a mild form of cerebral edema, often preceding both HACE and HAPE (at the other end of the spectrum, HACE is a severe form of AMS).[96,97] The majority of AMS cases do not progress to more severe forms of high-altitude illness unless there is continued exposure to higher altitude.

The hallmark symptom of AMS is a mild to severe, protracted headache believed to be caused by the hypoxic-induced cerebral vasodilation.[98] Patients describe their headache as throbbing, as located in the occipital or temporal regions, and as worsening at night or on awakening. Other symptoms include nausea, vomiting, insomnia, dizziness, lassitude, fatigue, and difficulty sleeping. Malaise and lack of appetite may be present along with a decrease in urine output. It is important to recognize early symptoms of AMS so that continued ascent does not cause a preventable condition to progress into a severe form of HACE.

The onset of symptoms in AMS can occur as early as 1 hour after arriving at high altitude but typically develop after 6 to 10 hours of exposure. Symptoms usually peak in 24 to 72 hours and subside in 3 to 7 days. If the onset of symptoms occurs beyond 3 days after arriving at altitude and does not include headache, and if oxygen therapy provides no benefit, the condition is probably not AMS.[78]

Assessment. If patients are alert, the key is to obtain a good medical history, including the onset and severity of symptoms, rate of ascent, duration of exposure, and level of physical exertion. Obtain vital signs, including pulse oximetry. Also, assess the status of any underlying medical condition, as determined by the medical history.

Because a headache is the most common finding with AMS, assess for location and quality. Findings of a dry cough and dyspnea on exertion are common at altitude and may not always be specific for AMS. Auscultate all lung fields because crackles are common with AMS. Assess neurologic function, and assess specifically for ataxia and excessive lethargy; these symptoms are indicative of HACE.

Management. Descending 500 to 1000 m (1640-3280 ft) will provide the quickest resolution of symptoms. Mild AMS will resolve on its own, but patients should avoid further ascent and any exertion until symptoms resolve. Provide analgesics for headache and antiemetics for nausea. For moderate symptoms, descend to lower altitude and provide oxygen at 2 to 4 L/min by nasal cannula initially. Assess pulse oximetry for SaO_2 greater than 90%. If lower than 90%, titrate oxygen to 1 to 2 L/min and reassess. For patients with neurologic symptoms, see management of HACE. Patients with underlying medical problems exacerbated by altitude should be transported on oxygen for medical evaluation of their primary illness and the secondary development of high-altitude illness.

Table 17-10 summarizes the signs and symptoms, management, and prevention of AMS.

High-Altitude Cerebral Edema

HACE is a very serious neurologic syndrome that can develop in individuals with AMS or HAPE. At altitudes above 2438 m (8000 ft), cerebral blood flow increases as a result of hypoxia-induced vasodilation. The mechanism of injury appears to be related to a combination of sustained cerebral vasodilation, increased capillary permeability across the blood-brain barrier, and the inability to compensate sufficiently for the excess cerebral edema.[99]

HACE can occur within 3 to 5 days after arrival at 2750 m (9022 ft), but generally it occurs at altitudes above 3600 m (12,000 ft), with an onset of symptoms within hours. Some mild to moderate symptoms of AMS may be present, but the hallmark features of HACE are altered level of consciousness (LOC) and ataxia, along with drowsiness, stupor, and irrational behavior progressing to coma. Death results from brain herniation.[100]

Assessment. If patients are alert, as with AMS, the key in HACE patients is to obtain a good medical history, including the onset and severity of symptoms, rate of ascent, duration of exposure, and level of physical exertion. Obtain vital signs, including pulse oximetry. Also, assess the status of any underlying medical condition, as determined by the medical history. It is important to assess lung sounds because a strong association exists between HACE and HAPE.

Management. Do not delay planning for treatment and evacuation at the first signs or symptoms of HACE. The highest priority for any patient with HACE is immediate descent, along with initiation of high-flow oxygen (15 L/min) by nonrebreather mask and monitoring of SaO_2 until 90% or greater. Unconscious patients should be managed as a patient with head injury (see Chapter 8), including intubation and other ALS procedures.[86]

See Table 17-10 for a summary of the signs and symptoms, management, and prevention of HACE.

TABLE 17-10 High-Altitude Illness (AMS, HACE, HAPE): Signs, Symptoms, Treatment, and Prevention

Signs/symptoms	Treatment	Prevention
ACUTE MOUNTAIN SICKNESS (AMS)		
Mild: Headache, nausea, dizziness, and fatigue in first 12 hours *Moderate:* Moderate to severe headache, marked nausea, vomiting, decreased appetite, dizziness, insomnia, fluid retention for ≥12 hours	Oxygen 1-2 L/min by nasal cannula, and/or descend 500-1000 m (1700-3300 ft); avoid further ascent until symptoms resolve Give analgesics and antiemetics as needed	Ascend at slow rate; spend night at intermediate altitude; avoid overexertion; avoid direct transport to 2750 m (9000 ft) Consider acetazolamide (125-250 mg twice daily); begin 1 day before ascent and continue for 2 days Treat AMS early
HIGH-ALTITUDE CEREBRAL EDEMA (HACE)		
AMS for ≥24 hours, ataxia, confusion, bizarre behavior, severe lassitude	Immediately descend or evacuate ≥1000 m (3300 ft) Give oxygen 2-4 L/min; titrate to maintain SaO_2 ≥90% with pulse oximetry	As for AMS
HIGH-ALTITUDE PULMONARY EDEMA (HAPE)		
Dyspnea at rest, moist cough, rales, severe exercise limitation, cyanosis, drowsiness, tachycardia, tachypnea, desaturation	Start oxygen 4-6 L/min, then titrate to maintain SaO_2 ≥90% with pulse oximetry Minimize exertion; keep warm; descend or evacuate 500-1000 m (1700-3300 ft)	Ascend at a slow rate; avoid overexertion Consider nifedipine (20-30 mg extended-release dose every 12 hours) in person with repeated episodes of HAPE

Modified from Gallagher SA, Hackett PH: High altitude illness *Emerg Med Clin North Am* 22:329, 2004; and Hackett PH: High altitude illness, Roach RC, *N Engl J Med* 345(2):107, 2001.

High-Altitude Pulmonary Edema

The onset of HAPE follows a pattern similar to that seen with AMS and HACE, occurring in unacclimatized individuals after a rapid ascent to high altitude. This high-altitude illness has a different mechanism of injury than AMS and HACE, however, because HAPE is induced by hypobaric hypoxia. HAPE is a form of noncardiogenic pulmonary edema associated with pulmonary hypertension and elevated capillary pressure.[101] More than 50% of patients with HAPE have AMS, and 14% have HACE.[102] The signs and symptoms generally appear during the second night (1-3 days onset) and rarely occur 4 days after arriving at a given altitude.[103] The development of HAPE and the rate of progression are hastened by cold exposure, vigorous exertion, and continued ascent. Compared with the other two high-altitude illnesses, HAPE accounts for the greatest number of fatalities.

Assessment. Patient assessment, including vital signs, lung sounds, and medical history, are vital in the determination of HAPE, which is defined by at least two or more symptoms (e.g., dyspnea at rest, cough, weakness, or decreased exertion performance; chest tightness or congestion) and at least two signs (e.g., crackles or wheezing, central cyanosis, tachypnea, or tachycardia).[104] Rales are generally present in lung fields starting in the right axilla and eventually become bilateral. Assess for fever, which is a common sign with HAPE. Late findings as HAPE progresses are resting tachycardia, tachypnea, and blood-tinged sputum. If treatment interventions are not provided, symptoms will progress over hours to days to include audible gurgling, respiratory distress, and eventually death.

Management. Descending to a lower altitude by at least 500 to 1000 m (1640-3280 ft) provides the fastest recovery, but initially patients show good improvement with rest and oxygen. Keep patients warm, and prevent any exertion. These patients need to improve their arterial oxygenation; start oxygen at 4 to 6 L/min or titrate oxygen flow until Sao_2 is 90% or greater. Reassess vital signs after starting oxygen because improved arterial oxygenation decreases the tachycardia and tachypnea.

See Table 17-10 for a summary of the signs and symptoms, management, and prevention of HAPE.

Prevention

Acute high-altitude illness in unacclimatized individuals is preventable. The common factor for the onset of AMS, HACE, and HAPE is the rate of ascent to higher altitude. Altitude illness may be experienced by skiers traveling by commercial airlines who start in the early morning from cities at sea level, arrive at high altitude, and by early afternoon begin skiing at 2100 m to 4500 m (about 7000-

14,000 ft). Another scenario with risk of high altitude illness is a call for mutual aid to various public safety personnel living below 1000 m (3300 ft). They quickly assemble and then arrive at 2750 m (9000 ft) or higher to assist local volunteer search and rescue teams trekking to higher altitudes in search of a missing backcountry hiker. Therefore, prehospital care personnel, whether ground crew or flight crew, who have responsibilities at high altitude for patient transfer to another hospital or for medical evacuation from the backcountry need to possess the knowledge to minimize the risk of high-altitude illness for their own safety and the safety of co-workers.

General guidelines for prevention of high-altitude illness in those who fly to altitudes above 2500 m (8200 ft) include the following[86]:

- Perform minimal activity during the first 24 hours at altitude
- A layover at 1500 to 1800 m (4900-5900 ft) for 24 to 36 hours is more beneficial
- Conduct graded ascent with no more than 600 m (1900 ft)/day
- Take a rest day every 600 to 1200 m (1900-3950 ft)
- Avoid heavy exertion for the first 3 days
- Keep well hydrated with water
- Avoid alcohol, sleeping pills, and other sedatives
- Eat a high-carbohydrate diet
- Avoid overexertion
- Avoid smoking
- Physical training is not preventive for high-altitude illness

The "golden rules" of high-altitude illness are as follows[86]:

1. If you are ill at altitude, your symptoms are caused by the altitude until proved otherwise.
2. If you have altitude symptoms, do not go any higher.
3. If you are feeling ill or are getting worse, or if you cannot walk heel-to-toe in a straight line, descend immediately.
4. A person ill with altitude illness must always be accompanied by a responsible companion who can accomplish or arrange for descent should it become necessary.

Medications as Prophylaxis for High-Altitude Illness

For the prevention of AMS and HACE, individuals traveling from sea level to over 3000 m (9850 ft) as their sleeping altitude in 1 day or individuals who have a history of AMS should consider prophylactic treatment. The drug of choice is oral acetazolamide (Diamox), 125 to 250 mg two times a day, beginning 1 day before ascent and continuing for 2 days at maximum altitude. The alternative drug is dexamethasone (Decadron), 4 mg orally or intramuscularly (IM) every 6 hours and continuing for 2 days at maximum altitude. The combination of both drugs has been shown to be more effective than either drug alone.[105,106] Other studies have shown the benefit of *Ginkgo biloba* to prevent AMS during gradual ascent to 5000 m (16,400 ft) or reduce AMS symptoms by 50% during rapid ascent to 4100 m (13,450 ft).[107,108] Aspirin (325 mg) taken every 4 hours for three doses reduced the incidence of headache from 50% to 7%.[109] For the prevention of HAPE in individuals with a history of repeated episodes, prophylaxis with oral nifedipine, 20 to 30 mg (extended-release formulation) every 12 hours, is recommended.

PROLONGED TRANSPORT

Near Drowning

- Asymptomatic patients can become symptomatic in an extended-care situation.
- Obtain a pulse oximetry reading before and after administration of oxygen. Provide high-flow oxygen via a nonrebreather mask at 12 to 15 L/min.
- Any patient with pulse oximetry values less than 90%, altered mental status, apnea, or coma should be intubated early to protect from aspiration. Any patient who continues to be hypoxic with pulse oximetry readings less than 85% after administration of high-flow oxygen is a candidate for rapid-sequence intubation (RSI) protocol.
- Liberal use of suction through the endotracheal tube is necessary to remove pulmonary secretions and water aspirated during submersion.
- Consult with medical control, if available, to sedate and paralyze the patient to ensure successful intubation, oxygenation, and effective ventilation.
- Another effective method to ensure effective oxygenation and ventilation is the use of positive end-expiratory pressure (PEEP) in apneic submersion patients.[4,11] PEEP increases the diameter of small and large airways and improves the ventilatory/perfusion ratio and arterial oxygenation.
- Determine the GCS score and assess routinely for trends because it is predictive of patient outcome.
- Monitor for hypothermia and hypoglycemia. Any comatose patient should receive IV dextrose.
- The placement of a nasogastric tube may be needed to reduce gastric content and water swallowed during submersion.

Lightning Injury

- Initiate CPR very quickly.
- When in the extended-care situation with multiple victims, use "reverse triage" and first resuscitate those who appear dead. However, prolonged (multiple hours) CPR on these victims has a poor patient outcome, and there is little benefit from CPR or ACLS procedures lasting longer than 20 to 30 minutes. All measures to stabilize the patient to correct for hypoxia, hypovolemia, hypothermia, and acidosis should be attempted before terminating resuscitative efforts.[36]
- Assess cerebral edema and increased intracranial pressure (ICP). Establish a baseline GCS score, and reassess every 10 minutes as an indicator of progressive cerebral edema and increased ICP (manage per recommendation for cerebral edema; see Chapter 8).

Recreational Scuba-Related Diving Injuries

- The standard treatment protocol for scuba-related injuries causing pulmonary overpressurization syndrome (e.g., AGE, DCS) is to provide high-flow oxygen (12-15 L/min via nonrebreather mask) at the scene and continue oxygen therapy during transport of the patient to the closest recompression chamber for hyperbaric oxygen (HBO) therapy.
- Conduct an extensive neurologic evaluation, and reassess frequently for progression of signs and symptoms.
- Use analgesics for pain control. Also consider giving aspirin (325 or 650 mg) for its antiplatelet activity.[53] Anecdotal data suggest benefits for DCS and AGE patients with cerebral edema, shock, and other conditions after treatment with HBO and high-dose parenteral corticosteroids.[53,110] The standard regimen used has been to administer hydrocortisone hemisuccinate (1000 mg) or methylprednisolone sodium succinate (125 mg), followed by dexamethasone, 4 to 6 mg every 6 hours, with continuation of the dexamethasone for 72 hours. However, this therapeutic approach is lacking acceptance because there are no published clinical trials demonstrating the efficacy of these drugs in these patients.[53]
- Use Divers Alert Network (DAN, telephone 919-684-8111) and local medical control for the closest location of a functional recompression chamber. Before transporting a patient for HBO therapy, contact the chamber directly because the status of chamber readiness can change without notification. DAN is the primary medical source for diving consultation and for recommending recompression chamber location and availability worldwide. When transporting by

air, use aircraft that can preferably maintain sea-level atmosphere during flight. Any nonpressurized aircraft should maintain an altitude below 1000 feet en route to the chamber site.

High-Altitude Illness

- Mild to moderate acute mountain sickness (AMS) can be managed with low-volume oxygen at 2 to 4 L/min by nasal cannula, titrated to 1 to 2 L/min (>90% Sao_2), with a combination of analgesics (e.g., aspirin, 650 mg; acetaminophen, 650-1000 mg; ibuprofen, 400-600 mg) for headache and prochlorperazine (5-10 mg IM) for nausea. Other medications used for treating mild to moderate AMS include oral acetazolamide (125-250 mg twice daily) and dexamethasone (4 mg PO or IM every 6 hours) until symptoms resolve. Treat HACE with oxygen at 2 to 4 L/min by nasal cannula, to maintain greater than 90% Sao_2, and with dexamethasone (8 mg PO, IV, or IM initially, then 4 mg every 6 hours); consider using oral acetazolamide (125-250 mg twice daily) with prolonged delays to descent.
- If a severe form of HACE develops and the patient is comatose, manage according to recommendations for cerebral edema (see Chapter 8).

- Prolonged management of HAPE primarily consists of administering oxygen at 4 to 6 L/min by nasal cannula (>90% Sao_2) until improvement of symptoms, then 2 to 4 L/min for conserving oxygen. If oxygen is not available, give oral nifedipine (10 mg initially, then 30 mg extended-release dose every 12 to 24 hours). If the patient acquires HACE, add dexamethasone (8 mg PO or IM every 6 hours).
- Use of portable hyperbaric chambers, such as the Gamow bag (Altitude Technologies) or HELP system (Live High, Boulder, Colo), has been successful for treating high-altitude illness.[82] These lightweight, fabric pressure bags simulate descending to a lower altitude with or without the use of supplemental oxygen or medication (e.g., acetazolamide, dexamethasone, nifedipine). They inflate with manual pumps up to 2 psi, which is equivalent to descending 1600 m (5250 ft), depending on the initial altitude. The use of these chambers for 2 to 3 hours can effectively improve symptoms. This is an ideal use of technology while waiting for transportation to definitive care.

SUMMARY

Prehospital care providers will inevitably be faced with unpredictable environmental encounters, such as those described in this chapter. Basic knowledge of common environmental emergencies is necessary so that rapid assessment and treatment in the prehospital setting can be provided. It is not easy to remember this type of information because these problems are not frequently encountered. Therefore, remember the general principles involved, as follows:

- *Drowning or near-drowning.* Assume all near-drowning patients have pulmonary distress until proved otherwise; correct hypoxia, acidosis, and hypothermia as indicated.
- *Lightning.* Patients with severe lightning injury need rapid assessment of cardiopulmonary status. Use the "reverse triage" principle for multiple victims. Initiating CPR early is the key to survival.
- *Recreational scuba-related diving injuries.* Patients with severe decompression sickness and arterial gas embolism need high-flow oxygen and rapid treatment in a recompression chamber for the best outcome. Consult early with medical control and Divers Alert Network (919-684-8111).
- *High-altitude illness.* Key interventions for acute mountain sickness and high-altitude cerebral or pulmonary edema are to descend at least 500 to 1000 m in altitude (1640-3280 feet) and provide rest and oxygen.

In every case, remember that personal safety must be maintained. There are too many cases in which EMS and other prehospital care providers have lost their lives as a result of attempting a rescue.

SCENARIO SOLUTION

Assess this patient's ABCDEs quickly to obtain an initial impression of her cardiopulmonary status. The key is obtaining a good medical history from this 48-year-old runner as a partner assesses vital signs. Remind your partner to give specific attention to lung sounds, oxygen saturation, and neurologic status. This patient has nearly completed a half-marathon, running uphill for approximately the last 3.5 hours and starting at a high-altitude elevation of 1918 m (6295 ft), and she was approaching the summit (4300 m [14,000 ft]).

The concern is whether her signs and symptoms are based on severe fatigue, a medical condition made worse at altitude, by high-altitude illness, or by a combination of these two factors. Based on her symptoms, the feedback from the race official, and her unsteady running at altitude, this is more than fatigue from running. She should stop running in the race. Suspect that she is very fit to run

this grueling marathon, the concern is that she may not be prepared to run at high altitude because she arrived yesterday from sea level. She has two major risk factors for acute mountain sickness (AMS): rapid ascent and physical exertion. Furthermore, consider that in combination with her rapid ascent to altitude, her physical exertion, and continued ascent toward the summit, she could also be at risk for severe high-altitude illness (e.g., HACE, HAPE) if she continues.

Her condition can be managed well by providing three interventions important for any high-altitude illness: (1) immediate descent, (2) oxygen, and (3) rest. After good patient education, start her on oxygen at 4 to 6 L/min (nasal cannula), reassess oxygen saturation with pulse oximetry, and transport her down from Pike's Peak summit to the hospital in town (1918 m [6295 ft]) in a position of comfort. ■

References

1. Centers for Disease Control and Prevention: Nonfatal and fatal drowning in recreational water settings—United States, 2001-2002, *MMWR* 53(21):447, 2004.
2. Zuckerman GB, Conway EE Jr: Drowning and near drowning, *Pediatr Ann* 29:6, 2000.
3. Zamula WW: In *Social costs of drowning and near drowning from submersion accidents occurring to children under five in residential swimming pools,* Washington, DC, 1987, US Consumer Product Safety Commission.
4. Newman AB: Submersion incidents. In Auerbach PS: *Wilderness medicine: management of wilderness and environmental emergencies,* ed 4, St Louis, 2001, Mosby.
5. DeNicola LK, Falk JL, Swanson ME, Kissoon N: Submersion injuries in children and adults, *Crit Care Clin* 13(3):477, 1997.
6. Olshaker JS: Near drowning, *Emerg Med Clin North Am* 10(2):339, 1992.
7. Orlowski JP, Szppilman D: Drowning, *Pediatr Clin North Am* 48(3):627, 2001.
8. Gilbert M, Busund R, Skagseth A: Resuscitation from accidental hypothermia of 13.7° C with circulatory arrest, *Lancet* 355:375, 2000.
9. Bolte RG, Black PG, Bowers RS: The use of extracorporeal rewarming in a child submerged for 66 minutes, *JAMA* 260:377, 1988.
10. Lloyd EL: Accidental hypothermia, *Resuscitation* 32:111, 1996.
11. Olshaker JS: Submersion, *Emerg Med Clin North Am* 22:357, 2004.
12. Kyriacou DN, Arcinue EL, Peek C, Kraus JF: Effect of immediate resuscitation on children with submersion injury, *Pediatrics* 94:137, 1994.
13. Brenner RA, Trumble AC, Smith GS, et al: Where children drown, United States, 1995, *Pediatrics* 108:85, 2001.
14. Karkal MB, Rasch DK, Gilbert J: Optimizing salvage in drowning and near drowning victims, *Emerg Med Rep* 10(16), 1989.
15. Lavelle JM: Ten-year review of pediatric bathtub near-drownings: evaluation for child abuse and neglect, *Ann Emerg Med* 25:344, 1995.
16. Schuman SH et al: The iceberg phenomenon of near-drowning, *Crit Care Med* 4:127, 1976.
17. Rowe MI, Arango A, Allington G: Profile of pediatric drowning victims in a water-oriented society, *J Trauma* 17:587, 1977.
18. Craig AB Jr: Underwater swimming and loss of consciousness, *JAMA* 176:255, 1961.
19. Jensen LR et al: Submersion injuries in children younger than 5 years in urban Utah, *West J Med* 157:641, 1992.
20. Howland J, Smith GS, Mangione TW, et al: Why are most drowning victims men? Sex differences, aquatic skills and behaviors, *Am J Public Health* 86:93, 1996.
21. Schuman SH et al: The iceberg phenomenon of near-drowning, *Crit Care Med* 4:127, 1976.
22. Howland J, Smith GS, Mangione T, et al: Missing the boat on drinking and boating, *JAMA* 270:91, 1993.
23. Mackie I: Alcohol and aquatic disasters, *Med J Aust* 1:652, 1978.
24. Lavelle JM et al: Ten-year review of pediatric bathtub near-drownings: evaluation for child abuse and neglect, *Ann Emerg Med* 25:344, 1995.
25. Karch KB: Pathology of the lung in near-drowning, *Am J Emerg Med* 4(1):4, 1986.
26. Orlowski JP, Drowning, near-drowning, and ice water submersion, *Pediatr Clin North Am* 34(1):75, 1987.

27. Modell JH, Moya F: Effects of volume of aspirated fluid during chlorinated fresh-water drowning, *Anesthesiology* 27:663, 1966.
28. Bolte RG, Black PG, Bowers RS: The use of extracorporeal rewarming in a child submerged for 66 minutes, *JAMA* 260:377, 1988.
29. Gilbert M, Busund R, Skagseth A: Resuscitation from accidental hypothermia of 13.7° C with circulatory arrest, *Lancet* 355:375, 2000.
30. Siebke H, et al: Survival after 40 minutes submersion without cerebral sequelae, *Lancet* 1:1275, 1975.
31. Abella BS, Alvarado JP, Myklebust H, et al: Quality of cardiopulmonary resuscitation during in-hospital cardiac arrest, *JAMA* 293(3):305, 2005.
32. Wik L, Kramer-Johansen J, Myklebust H, et al: Quality of cardiopulmonary resuscitation during out-of-hospital cardiac arrest, *JAMA* 293(3):299, 2005.
33. International Liaison Committee on Resuscitation: 2005 International Consensus on Cardiopulmonary Resuscitation and Emergency Cardiovascular Care Science with Treatment Recommendations, *Circulation* 112(suppl 1):IV-1, 2005.
34. Rosen P, Stoto M, Harley J: The use of the Heimlich maneuver in near drowning: Institute of Medicine report, *J Emerg Med* 13:397, 1995.
35. Curran EB, Holle RL, Lopez RE: Lightning fatalities, injuries and damage reports in the United States, 1959-1994, *NOAA Tech Memo NWS SR-193*, 1997, http://www.nssl.noaa.gov/papers/techmemos/NWS-SR-193/techmemo-sr193.html.
36. Gatewood MO, Zane RD: Lightning Injuries, *Emerg Med Clin North Am* 22:369, 2004.
37. Huffins GR, Orville RE: Lightning ground flash density and thunderstorm duration in the contiguous United States, *J Appl Meteorol* 38:1013, 1999.
38. Cummins KL, Krider EP, Malone MD. A combined TOA/MDF technology upgrade of the US National Lightning Detection Network, *J Geophys Res* 103:9035, 1998.
39. MacGorman, DR, Rust WD: Lightning strike density for the contiguous United States from thunderstorm duration records, Pub No NUREG/CR03759, Washington, DC, 1984, Office of Nuclear Regulatory Research.
40. Dulcos PJ, Sanderson LM, Klontz KC: Lightning-related mortality and morbidity in Florida, *Pub Health Rep* 105:276, 1990.
41. Cooper MA, Andrews CJ, Holle RL, Lopez RE: Lightning injuries. In Auerbach P: *Wilderness medicine: management of wilderness and environmental emergencies*, ed 4, St Louis, 2001, Mosby.
42. Centers for Disease Control and Prevention: Lightning associated deaths—1980-1995, *MMWR* 47(19):391, 1998.
43. Cooper MA: Lightning injuries: prognostic signs of death, *Ann Emerg Med* 9:134, 1980.
44. Andrews CJ, Darveniza M, Mackerras D. Lightning injury: a review of the clinical aspects, pathophysiology and treatment, *Adv Trauma* 4:241, 1989.
45. Andrews CJ, Darveniza M, Mackerras D: *Lightning injuries: electrical, medical, and legal aspects*, Boca Raton, Fla, 1992, CRC Press.
46. Cooper MA: Electrical and lightning injuries, *Emerg Med Clin North Am* 2:489, 1984.
47. Holle RL, Lopez RE, Howard KW, et al: Safety in the presence of lightning, *Semin Neurol* 15:375, 1995.
48. Kleiner JP, Wilkin JH: Cardiac effects of lightning stroke, *JAMA* 240:2757, 1978.
49. Casten JA, Kytilla J: Eye symptoms caused by lightning, *Acta Ophthalmol* 41:139, 1963.
50. Taussig HB: Death from lightning and the possibility of living again, *Ann Intern Med* 68:1345, 1968.
51. Zimmerman C, Cooper MA, Holle RL: Lightning safety guidelines, *Ann Emerg Med* 39:660, 2002.
52. Melamed Y, Shupak A, Bitterman H: Medical problems associated with underwater diving, *N Engl J Med* 326:30, 1992.
53. Kizer, KW: Diving medicine. In Auerbach PS: *Wilderness medicine: management of wilderness and environmental emergencies*, ed 4, St Louis, 2001, Mosby.
54. Strauss MB, Borer RC Jr: Diving medicine: contemporary topics and their controversies, *Am J Emerg Med* 19:232, 2001.
55. Divers Alert Network: Eleven-year trends (1987-1997) in diving activity: the DAN annual review of recreational SCUBA diving injuries and fatalities based on 2000 data. In *Report on decompression illness, diving fatalities and Project Dive exploration*, Durham, NC, 2000, Divers Alert Network.
56. Hardy KR: Diving-related emergencies, *Emerg Med Clin North Am* 15(1):223, 1997.
57. Green SM: Incidence and severity of middle ear barotraumas in recreational scuba diving, *J Wilderness Med* 4:270, 1993.
58. Shupak A, Doweck I, Greenberg, E, et al: Diving-related inner ear injuries, *Laryngoscope* 101:173, 1991.
59. Kizer KW: Dysbaric cerebral air embolism in Hawaii, *Ann Emerg Med* 16:535, 1987.
60. Cales RH, Humphreys N, Pilmanis AA, Heilig RW: Cardiac arrest from gas embolism in scuba diving, *Ann Emerg Med* 10(11):589, 1981.
61. Butler BD, Laine GA, Leiman BC, et al: Effect of Trendelenburg position on the distribution of arterial air emboli in dogs, *Ann Thorac Surg* 45(2):198, 1988.
62. Moon RE: Treatment of diving emergencies, *Crit Care Clin* 15:429, 1999.
63. Van Meter K: Medical field management of the injured diver, *Respir Care Clin North Am* 5(1):137, 1997.
64. Francis TJ, Dutka AJ, Hallenbeck JM: Pathophysiology of decompression sickness. In Bove AA, Davis JC, editors: *Diving medicine*, ed 2, Philadelphia, 1990, Saunders.
65. Neuman TS: DCI/DCS: does it matter whether the emperor wears clothes? *Undersea Hyperb Med* 24:2, 1997.
66. Bove AA: Nomenclature of pressure disorders, *Undersea Hyperb Med* 24:1, 1997.
67. Spira A: Diving and marine medicine review. Part II. Diving diseases, *J Travel Med* 6:180, 1999.
68. Clenney TL, Lassen LF: Recreational scuba diving injuries, *Am Fam Physician* 53(5):1761, 1996.
69. Kizer KW: Women and diving, *Physician Sportsmed* 9(2):84, 1981.
70. Baratt DM, Harch PG, Van Meter K: Decompression illness in divers: a review of the literature, *Neurologist* 8:186, 2002.
71. Francis TJ, Dutka AJ, Hallenbeck JM: Pathophysiology of decompression sickness. In Bove AA, Davis JC, editors: *Diving medicine*, ed 2, Philadelphia, 1990, Saunders.
72. Greer HD, Massey EW: Neurologic injury from undersea diving, *Neurol Clin* 10(4):1031, 1992.
73. Kizer KW: Management of dysbaric diving casualties, *Emerg Med Clin North Am* 1:659, 1983.

74. Department of the Navy: *U.S. Navy diving manual,* Vol 1, Rev 4, Washington, DC, 1999, US Government Printing Office.

75. Tibbles PM, Edelsberg JS: Hyperbaric-oxygen therapy, *N Engl J Med* 334(25):1642, 1996.

76. Davis JC: Hyperbaric medicine: critical care aspects. In Shoemaker WC, editor: *Critical care: state of the art,* Aliso Viejo, Calif, 1984, Society of Critical Care Medicine.

77. Gallagher SA, Hackett PH: High altitude illness, *Emerg Med Clin North Am* 22:329, 2004.

78. Hackett PH, Roach RC: High altitude illness, *N Engl J Med* 345(2):107, 2001.

79. Houston CS: High altitude illness disease with protean manifestations, *JAMA* 236:2193, 1976.

80. Montgomery AB, Mills J, Luce JM: Incidence of acute mountain sickness at intermediate altitude, *JAMA* 261:732, 1989.

81. Gertsch JH, Seto TB, Mor J, Onopa J: Ginkgo biloba for the prevention of severe acute mountain sickness (AMS) starting day one before rapid ascent, *High Alt Med Biol* 3(1):29, 2002.

82. Hackett PH, Roach RC: High-altitude medicine. In Auerbach PS: *Wilderness medicine: management of wilderness and environmental emergencies,* ed 4, St Louis, 2001, Mosby.

83. Tso E: High-altitude illness, *Emerg Clin North Am* 10(2):231, 1992.

84. Sophocles AM: High-altitude pulmonary edema in Vail, Colorado, 1975-1982, *West J Med* 144:569, 1986.

85. Honigman B, Theis MK, Koziol-McLain J, et al: Acute mountain sickness in a general tourist population at moderate altitudes, *Ann Intern Med* 118(8):587, 1993.

86. Zaphren K, Honigman B: High-altitude medicine, *Emerg Clin North Am* 15(1):191, 1997.

87. Sutton JR, Reeves JT, Wagner PD, et al: Operation Everest II: oxygen transport during exercise at extreme stimulated altitude, *J Appl Physiol* 64(4):1309, 1988.

88. Hultgren HN: *High altitude medicine,* Stanford, Calif, 1997, Hultgren Publications.

89. Schneider M, Bernasch D, Weymann J, et al: Acute mountain sickness: influence of susceptibility, preexposure, and ascent rate, *Med Sci Sports Exerc* 34(12):1886, 2002.

90. Bartsch P: High altitude pulmonary edema, *Med Sci Sports Exerc* 31(suppl 1):S23, 1999.

91. Roach RC, Houston CS, Honigman B: How well do older persons tolerate moderate altitude? *West J Med* 162 (1):32, 1995.

92. Roach RC, Maes D, Sandoval D, et al: Exercise exacerbates acute mountain sickness at simulated high altitude, *J Appl Physiol* 88(2):581, 2000.

93. Roeggla G, Roeggla H, Roeggla M, et al: Effect of alcohol on acute ventilation adaptation to mild hypoxia at moderate altitude, *Ann Intern Med* 122:925, 1995.

94. Roach RC, Wagner J, Zafren K, et al. Seasonal variation in barometric pressure and temperature in Summit County: effect on altitude illness: In Sutton JR, Houston CS, Coates G, editors: *Hypoxia and molecular medicine,* Burlington, 1993, Charles S Houston.

95. Roach RC, Bartcsh P, Oelz O, Hackett PH, Lake Louise Scoring Committee: The Lake Louise Acute Mountain Sickness Scoring System: In Sutton JR, Houston CS, Coates G, editors: *Hypoxia and molecular medicine,* Burlington, 1993, Charles S Houston.

96. Muza SR, Lyons TP, Rock PB: Effect of altitude on exposure on brain volume and development of acute mountain sickness (AMS). In Roach RC, Wagner PD, Hackett PH, editors: *Hypoxia: into the next millennium.* Vol 474, Advances in experimental medicine and biology, New York, 1999, Kluwer Academic/Plenum.

97. Hacket PH: High altitude cerebral edema and acute mountain sickness: a pathological update. In Roach RC, Wagner PD, Hackett PH, editors: *Hypoxia: into the next millennium.* Vol 474, Advances in experimental medicine and biology, New York, 1999, Kluwer Academic/Plenum.

98. Sanchez del Rio M, Moskkowitz MA: High altitude headache: lessons from aches at sea level. In Roach RC, Wagner PD, Hackett PH, editors: *Hypoxia: into the next millennium.* Vol 474, Advances in experimental medicine and biology, New York, 1999, Kluwer Academic/Plenum.

99. Hackett PH: The cerebral etiology of high-altitude cerebral edema and acute mountain sickness, *Wilderness Environ Med* 10(2):97, 1999.

100. Yarnell PR, Heit J, Hackett PH: High-altitude cerebral edema (HACE): the Denver/Front Range experience, *Semin Neurol* 20(2):209, 2000.

101. Maggiorini M, Melot C, Pierre S, et al: High altitude pulmonary edema is initially caused by an increase in capillary pressure, *Circulation* 103(16):2078, 2011.

102. Hultgren HN, Honigman B, Theis K, Nicholas D: High-altitude pulmonary edema at ski resort, *West J Med* 164:222, 1996.

103. Stenmark KR, Frid M, Nemenoff R, et al: Hypoxia induces cell-specific changes in gene expression in vascular wall cells: implications for pulmonary hypertension. In Roach RC, Wagner PD, Hackett PH, editors: *Hypoxia: into the next millennium.* Vol 474, Advances in experimental medicine and biology, New York, 1999, Kluwer Academic/Plenum.

104. The Lake Louise Consensus on the Definition and Quantification of Altitude Illness. In Sutton JR, Coates G, Houston C, editors: *Hypoxia and mountain medicine,* Burlington, 1992, Queen City Press.

105. Reid LD, Carter KA, Ellsworth A: Acetazolamide and dexamethasone for the prevention of acute mountain sickness: a meta-analysis, *J Wilderness Med* 5:34, 1994.

106. Bernhard WN, Schalick LM, Delaney PA, et al: Acetazolamide plus low-dose dexamethasone is better than acetazolamide alone to ameliorate symptoms of acute mountain sickness, *Aviat Space Environ Med* 69:883, 1998.

107. Maakestad K, Leadbetter G, Olsen S, Hackett PH: *Ginkgo biloba* reduced the incidence of and severity of acute mountain sickness, *Wilderness Environ Med* 12:51, 2001.

108. Rankin JP, Schwartz F, D'Aubigne P: EGB 761 in control and acute mountain sickness and vascular reactivity to cold exposure, *Avita Space Environ Med* 67:445, 1996.

109. Burtscher M., Likar R, Nachbauer W, Philadelphy M: Aspirin for the prophylaxis against headache at high altitude: randomized, double blind, placebo controlled trial, *BMJ* 316:1057, 1998.

110. Kizer KW: Corticosteroids in the treatment of serious decompression sickness, *Ann Emerg Med* 10:485, 1981.

Suggested Reading

Bennett P, Elliott D: *The physiology and medicine of diving,* ed 4, Philadelphia, 1993, Saunders.

Bove AA: *Bove and Davis' diving medicine,* ed 5, Philadelphia, 2003, Saunders.

Sutton JR, Coates G, Remmers JE, editors: *Hypoxia: the adaptations,* Philadelphia, 1990, BC Dekker.

CHAPTER 18

Golden Principles of Prehospital Trauma Care

n the late 1960s, R. Adams Cowley, MD, conceived the idea of a crucial time period during which it was important to begin definitive patient care for a critically injured trauma patient. In an interview he said, "There is a 'golden hour' between life and death. If you are critically injured, you have less than 60 minutes to survive. You might not die right then—it may be 3 days or 2 weeks later—but something has happened in your body that is irreparable."

Is there a basis for this concept? The answer is definitely "yes." However, an important realization is that a patient does not always have the luxury of a "Golden Hour." A patient with a penetrating wound of the heart may have only a few minutes to reach definitive care before the shock caused by the injury becomes irreversible. At the other end of the spectrum is a patient with slow, ongoing internal hemorrhage from an isolated femur fracture. Such a patient may have several hours to reach definitive care and resuscitation. Because the "Golden *Hour*" is not a strict 60-minute time frame and varies from patient to patient based on the injuries, the more appropriate term is the "Golden *Period*." If a critically injured patient is able to obtain definitive care, that is, hemorrhage control and re-suscitation, within the patient's Golden Period, the chance of survival is greatly improved.[1]

No call, scene, or patient is the same. Each requires flexibility of the health care team members to act and react to situations as they develop. The management of prehospital trauma must reflect these contingencies. The goals, however, have not changed: (1) gain access to the patient, (2) identify and treat life-threatening injuries, and (3) package and transport to the closest appropriate facility in the least amount of time. The majority of the techniques and principles discussed are not new, and most are taught in an initial education program. This text is different in the following ways:

1. It provides current, evidence-based practices of management of the trauma patient.
2. It provides a systematic approach for establishing priorities of patient care for trauma patients who have sustained injury to multiple body systems.
3. It provides an organizational scheme for interventions.

The Prehospital Trauma Life Support (PHTLS) program teaches that the prehospital care provider can make correct judgments leading toward a good outcome only if the provider is supplied with a good base of knowledge. The foundation of the PHTLS program is that patient care should be *judgment* driven, not protocol driven; thus the medical detail provided in this course. This chapter addresses the key aspects of prehospital trauma care and "brings it all together."

Why Trauma Patients Die

Studies that analyze the causes of death in trauma patients have several common themes. A study from Russia of more than 700 trauma deaths found that most patients who rapidly succumbed to their injuries fall into one of three categories: massive acute blood loss (36%), severe injury to vital organs such as the brain (30%), and airway obstruction and acute ventilatory failure (25%).[2] In an analysis of 753 trauma patients who died of their injuries at a Level I trauma center, Stewart and co-workers[3] found that 51% of trauma patients died from severe trauma to the central nervous system (CNS, e.g., traumatic brain injury), 21% from irreversible shock, 25% from both severe CNS trauma and irreversible shock, and 3% from multiple organ failure.

But what is happening to these patients on a cellular level? As discussed in Chapter 7, the metabolic processes of the human body are driven by energy, similar to any other machine. As with machines, the human body generates its own energy but must have fuel to do this. Fuel for the body is oxygen and glucose. The body can store glucose as complex carbohydrates (glycogen) and fat to use at a later time. However, oxygen cannot be stored. It must be constantly supplied to the cells of the body. Atmospheric air, containing oxygen, is drawn into the lungs by the action of the diaphragm and intercostal muscles. Oxygen then diffuses across the alveolar and capillary walls, where it binds to the hemoglobin in the red blood cells (RBCs) and is transported to the body's tissues by the circulatory system. In the presence of oxygen, the cells of the tissues then "burn" glucose though a complex series of metabolic processes (glycolysis, Krebs cycle, and electron transport) to produce the energy needed for all body functions. This energy is stored as adenosine triphosphate (ATP). Without sufficient energy (ATP), essential metabolic activities cannot function normally, and organs begin to fail.

Shock is viewed as a failure of energy production in the body. The sensitivity of the cells to oxygen deprivation varies from organ to organ. The cells within an organ can be fatally damaged but can continue to function for a period of time (see Chapter 7 for complications of prolonged shock). This delayed death of cells, leading to organ failure, is what Dr. Cowley referred to in his statement quoted earlier. The condition he described, shock, resulted in death if a patient was not treated promptly. His definition included transporting the patient to the operating room for control of internal hemorrhage. The American College of Surgeons (ACS) Committee on Trauma has used this concept of a "Golden Hour" to emphasize the importance of transporting a patient to a facility where expert trauma care is immediately available.

The Golden Period represents a time interval during which shock is worsening, but this condition is almost always **reversible** if proper care is received. Failure to

When the heart is deprived of oxygen, the myocardial cells cannot produce enough energy to pump blood to the other tissues. For example, a patient has lost a significant number of red blood cells and blood volume from a gunshot wound to the aorta. The heart continues to beat for several minutes before failing. Refilling the vascular system, after the heart has been without oxygen for several minutes, will not restore the function of the injured cells of the heart. This process is called *irreversible shock*. The specific condition in the heart is known as *pulseless electrical activity* (PEA). Cellular function is still present; however, it is not sufficient to pump blood to the body's cells. The patient has an ECG rhythm but not enough contractile power to force blood out of the heart to the rest of the body.

Another example of this same process but with a less severe outcome is congestive heart failure. Many of the cells of the heart have been damaged by ischemia secondary to coronary artery disease, but some are not. The damage is not complete, so enough functioning cells are left for the pumping process to continue.

Although ischemia, as seen in severe shock, may damage virtually all tissues, the damage to the organs does not become apparent at the same time. In the lungs, acute respiratory distress syndrome (ARDS) often develops within 48 hours after an ischemic insult, whereas acute renal failure and hepatic failure typically occur several days later. Although all body tissues are affected by insufficient oxygen, some tissues are more sensitive to ischemia. For example, a patient who has sustained a traumatic brain injury may develop cerebral edema (swelling) that results in permanent brain damage. Although the brain cells cease to function and die, the rest of the body may survive for years.

initiate appropriate interventions aimed at improving oxygenation and controlling hemorrhage allows shock to progress, becoming **irreversible.** For trauma patients to have the best chance of survival, interventions should start in the field with prehospital care providers and then continue in the emergency department (ED), the operating room (OR), and the intensive care unit (ICU). Trauma is a "team sport." The patient "wins" when all members of the trauma team—from those in the field to those in the trauma center—work together to care for the individual patient.

The Golden Principles of Prehospital Trauma Care

The preceding chapters discuss the assessment and management of patients who have sustained injury to specific body systems. Although this text presents the body systems individually, most severely injured patients have injury to more than one body system, thus the name *multisystem trauma patient* (also known as *polytrauma*). A prehospital care provider needs to recognize and prioritize the treatment of patients with multiple injuries, following the "Golden Principles of Prehospital Trauma Care" described next.

1. Ensure the Safety of the Prehospital Care Providers and the Patient.

Prehospital care providers need to ensure that scene safety remains their highest priority. This includes not only the safety of the patient, but their own safety as well. Based on information provided by dispatch, potential threats can often be anticipated before arrival at the scene. For a motor vehicle crash (MVC), threats may include traffic, hazardous materials, fires, and downed power lines; for a shooting victim, providers need to be aware that the perpetrator may still be in the area. When a violent crime is involved, law enforcement personnel should first enter the scene and secure the area. A prehospital care provider who takes needless risk may also become a victim; in doing so, the provider is no longer of help to the original trauma patient. Except in the most unusual circumstances, only those with proper training should attempt rescues.

Another fundamental aspect of safety involves the use of standard precautions. Blood and other body fluids can transmit infections, such as human immunodeficiency virus (HIV) and hepatitis B virus (HBV). Protective gear should always be worn, especially when caring for trauma patients in the presence of blood.

The safety of the patient and possible hazardous situations should also be identified. Even if a patient involved in an MVC has no life-threatening conditions identified in the primary survey, rapid extrication is appropriate if threats to patient safety are noted, such as a significant potential for fire or a precarious vehicle position.

2. Assess the Scene Situation to Determine the Need for Additional Resources.

During the response to the scene and immediately on arrival, a quick assessment is performed to determine the need for additional or specialized resources. Examples include additional emergency medical services (EMS) units to accommodate the number of patients, fire suppression equipment, special rescue teams, power company personnel, medical helicopters, and physicians to aid in the triage of a large number of patients. The need for these resources should be anticipated and requested as soon as possible.

3. Recognize the Kinematics That Produced the Injuries.

Chapter 3 provides the reader with a foundation of how energy can translate into injury to the trauma patient. As the scene and the patient are approached, the kinematics of the situation can be noted. Understanding the principles of kinematics leads to better patient assessment. Knowledge of specific injury patterns aids in predicting injuries and knowing where to look. Consideration of the kinematics should not delay the initiation of patient assessment and care but can be included in the global scene assessment and in the questions directed to the patient and bystanders. The kinematics may also play a key role in determining the destination facility for a given trauma patient. The key aspects of the kinematics noted at the scene should also be relayed to the physicians at the receiving facility.

4. Use the Primary Survey Approach to Identify Life-Threatening Conditions.

The central concept in the PHTLS program is the emphasis on the primary survey adopted from the Advanced Trauma Life Support Program for Doctors, taught by the ACS Committee on Trauma. This brief survey allows vital functions to be rapidly assessed and life-threatening conditions to be identified through systematic evaluation of the ABCDEs: airway, breathing, circulation, disability, and expose/environment (Box 18-1). On initial approach to the scene and as field care is provided, the prehospital care provider receives input from several senses (sight, hearing, smell, touch) that must be sorted, placed in a priority scheme of life-threatening or limb-threatening injuries, and used to develop a plan for correct management.

The primary survey involves a "treat as you go" philosophy. As life-threatening problems are identified, care is initiated at the earliest possible time. Although taught in a stepwise fashion, many aspects of the primary survey can be performed simultaneously. During transport, the primary survey should be reassessed at reasonable intervals so that the effectiveness of the interventions can be evaluated and new concerns addressed.

In children, pregnant patients, and elderly persons, injuries should be considered (1) to be more serious than their outward appearance, (2) to have a more profound systemic influence, and (3) to have a greater potential for producing rapid decompensation. In pregnant patients, there are at least two patients to care for—the mother and the fetus—both of whom may have sustained injury. Compensatory mechanisms differ from younger adults and

BOX 18-1 Critical or Potentially Critical Trauma Patient: Scene Time of 10 Minutes or Less

Presence of any of the following life-threatening conditions:

1. Inadequate or threatened airway
2. Impaired ventilation as demonstrated by the following:
   - Abnormally fast or slow ventilatory rate
   - Hypoxia (Spo$_2$ <95% even with supplemental oxygen)
   - Dyspnea
   - Open pneumothorax or flail chest
   - Suspected pneumothorax
3. Significant external hemorrhage or suspected internal hemorrhage
4. Shock, even if compensated
5. Abnormal neurologic status
   - GCS score ≤13
   - Seizure activity
   - Sensory or motor deficit
6. Penetrating trauma to the head, neck, or torso, or proximal to the elbow and knee in the extremities
7. Amputation or near-amputation proximal to the fingers or toes
8. Any trauma in the presence of the following:
   - History of serious medical conditions (e.g., coronary artery disease, chronic obstructive pulmonary disease, bleeding disorder)
   - Age >55 years
   - Hypothermia
   - Burns
   - Pregnancy

may not reveal abnormalities until the patient is profoundly compromised.

The primary survey also provides a framework to establish management priorities when faced with numerous patients. At a multiple-casualty incident, for example, patients who have serious problems identified with their airway, ventilation, or perfusion are managed and transported before patients with only altered levels of consciousness.

5. Provide Appropriate Airway Management while Maintaining Cervical Spine Stabilization.

Management of the airway remains the highest priority in the management of critically injured patients. This should be accomplished while maintaining the head and neck in a neutral inline position. The "essential skills" of airway management should be performed with ease: manual clearing of the airway, manual maneuvers to open the airway (trauma jaw thrust and trauma chin lift), suctioning, and the use of oropharyngeal and nasopharyngeal airways.

For those properly trained, endotracheal intubation is the "gold standard" technique for controlling an airway. Endotracheal intubation should be considered for all trauma patients who are unable to protect their airway, including those who have a Glasgow Coma Scale (GCS) score of 8 or less, require high concentrations of oxygen to maintain oxygen saturation (SpO_2) greater than 95%, or require assisted ventilations because of a decreased ventilatory rate or decreased minute volume. Intubation may also be considered for those patients with potential threats to their airway, such as an expanding hematoma in the neck or findings consistent with airway or pulmonary burns. After performing endotracheal intubation, a combination of clinical assessments and adjunct devices should be used, if practical, to confirm that the tube has been properly placed. After moving an intubated patient, tube placement should always be confirmed.

When intubation is indicated but cannot be performed, there are several backup options (see Airway Management Algorithm, p. 125). Ventilation can be attempted using the essential skills alone, or ventilation can be attempted with a dual-lumen airway or a laryngeal mask airway. If adequate ventilation can be achieved, additional attempts at intubation using retrograde or digital techniques may be considered. If ventilation cannot be accomplished, percutaneous transtracheal ventilation is an acceptable option.

The decision to attempt intubation involves weighing the potential risks and benefits of intubation along with the distance to the closest appropriate facility. Although performing intubation in the field seems to make sense, there is no conclusive evidence that endotracheal intubation results in lower morbidity or mortality rates in the trauma patient. *In some circumstances, such as the close proximity of an appropriate receiving facility, the most prudent decision may be to focus on the essential skills of airway management and rapidly transport the patient to that facility.*

6. Support Ventilation and Deliver Oxygen to Maintain an SpO_2 Greater than 95%.

Assessment and management of ventilation is another key aspect in the management of the critically injured patient. The normal ventilatory rate in the adult patient is 12 to 20 ventilations per minute. A rate slower than this often significantly interferes with the body's ability to oxygenate the RBCs passing though the pulmonary capillaries and to remove the carbon dioxide (CO_2) produced by the tissues. These bradypneic patients require assisted or total ventilatory support with a bag-valve-mask (BVM) connected to supplemental oxygen (FiO_2 >0.85). When patients are tachypneic (adult rate >20 breaths/min), their minute ventilation (tidal volume multiplied by their ventilatory rate) should be estimated. For a patient who has a significant decrease in minute volume (rapid, shallow ventilations), ventilations should be assisted with a BVM connected to supplemental oxygen (FiO_2 >0.85). If available, end-tidal CO_2 monitoring ($ETCO_2$) can prove useful to ensure sufficient ventilatory support. A sudden decrease in the $ETCO_2$ may indicate dislodgment of the endotracheal tube or a sudden decrease in perfusion (profound hypotension or cardiopulmonary arrest).

Supplemental oxygen is administered to any trauma patient with obvious or suspected life-threatening conditions. If available, pulse oximetry can be used to titrate the oxygen administration to keep the SpO_2 greater than 95%. If concern exists about the accuracy of a pulse oximetry reading or if this technology is not available, oxygen can be administered through a nonrebreathing mask to the spontaneously breathing patient or with a BVM connected to supplemental oxygen (FiO_2 >0.85) for those patients receiving assisted or total ventilatory support.

7. Control Any Significant External Hemorrhage.

In the trauma patient, significant external hemorrhage is a finding that requires immediate attention. Because blood is not amenable to administration in the prehospital setting, hemorrhage control becomes a paramount concern for prehospital care providers in order to maintain a sufficient number of circulating RBCs; *every RBC counts.* Extremity injuries and scalp wounds, such as lacerations and partial avulsions, may be associated with life-threatening blood loss.

Most external hemorrhage is readily controlled by the application of direct pressure at the bleeding site, or if resources are limited, by the use of a pressure dressing created with gauze 4 × 4 pads and an elastic bandage. If direct pressure or a pressure dressing fails to control external hemorrhage from an extremity, the prehospital care provider may consider applying a tourniquet. Although taught for many years in first-aid and basic emergency care courses, evidence shows that elevation of an extremity or applying pressure over a pressure point adds little to direct pressure or a pressure dressing.[4] Tourniquets are routinely used in surgical procedures, with an excellent safety record, and may be lifesaving in the prehospital setting. When faced with a patient who has external hemorrhage that is difficult to control and an anticipated prolonged transport time, the provider may consider application of a topical hemostatic agent.

For a patient in obvious shock from external hemorrhage, measures aimed at resuscitation (e.g., administration of IV fluids) should be avoided before adequately controlling the bleeding. *Attempted resuscitation will never be successful in the presence of ongoing external hemorrhage.*

Control of external hemorrhage and recognition of suspected internal hemorrhage, combined with prompt transport to the closest appropriate facility, represent opportunities in which prehospital care providers can make significant impact and save many lives.

8. Provide Basic Shock Therapy, Including Restoring and Maintaining Normal Body Temperature and Appropriately Splinting Musculoskeletal Injuries.

At the end of the primary survey, the patient's body is exposed so that the prehospital care provider can quickly scan for additional life-threatening injuries. Once this is completed, the patient should be covered again because hypothermia can be fatal to a critically injured trauma patient. The patient in shock is already handicapped by a marked decrease in energy production resulting from widespread inadequate tissue perfusion. If the patient's body temperature is not maintained, severe hypothermia can ensue. Hypothermia drastically impairs the ability of the body's blood clotting system to achieve hemostasis. Blood coagulates (clots) as the result of a complex series of enzymatic reactions leading to the formation of a fibrin matrix that traps RBCs and stems bleeding. These enzymes function in a very narrow temperature range. A drop in body temperature below 95° F (35° C) may significantly contribute to the development of a *coagulopathy* (decreased ability for blood clotting to occur). Therefore it is important to maintain and restore body heat through the use of blankets and a warmed environment inside the ambulance.

When fracture of a long bone occurs, surrounding muscle and connective tissue are often torn. This tissue damage, along with bleeding from the ends of the broken bones, can result in significant internal hemorrhage. This blood loss can range from about 500 mL from a humerus fracture up to 1 to 2 L from a single femur fracture. Rough handling of a fractured extremity can worsen the tissue damage and aggravate bleeding. Splinting assists in reducing the loss of additional blood into surrounding tissues, thus helping to preserve circulating RBCs for oxygen transport. For this reason, as well as for pain management, fractured extremities are splinted.

With a critically injured trauma patient, there is no time to splint each individual fracture. Instead, immobilizing the patient to a long backboard will splint virtually all fractures in an anatomic position and diminish internal hemorrhage. The one possible exception to this is a midshaft fracture of the femur. Because of the spasm of the very strong muscles in the thigh, the muscles contract, causing the bone ends to override one another, thereby damaging additional tissue. These types of fractures are best managed by use of a traction splint if time allows its application

during transport. For the vast majority of trauma calls, when no life-threatening conditions are identified in the primary survey, each suspected extremity injury can be appropriately splinted.

9. Consider Use of Pneumatic Antishock Garment for Patients with Decompensated Shock (SBP <90 mm Hg) and Suspected Pelvic, Intraperitoneal, or Retroperitoneal Hemorrhage, and in Patients with Profound Hypotension (SBP <60 mm Hg).

When a trauma patient in *decompensated* shock has suspected pelvic, intraperitoneal, or retroperitoneal hemorrhage, application and inflation of the pneumatic antishock garment (PASG) may decrease and even tamponade serious internal bleeding. Some research data indicate that trauma patients with profound hypotension (systolic blood pressure [SBP] <60 mm Hg) might also benefit from the use of the PASG. Trauma patients with a significant mechanism of injury may be logrolled into the PASG. The device is then inflated if hypotension occurs, especially if transport times are prolonged (>15-20 minutes). The PASG is probably ineffective when used solely as a splint for the lower extremity. It is contraindicated in patients with penetrating trauma to the thorax, evisceration of abdominal organs, or impaled objects in the abdomen; in pregnant patients; and in traumatic cardiopulmonary arrest.

10. Maintain Manual Spinal Stabilization until the Patient Is Immobilized on a Long Backboard.

When contact with a trauma patient is made, manual stabilization of the cervical spine should be provided and maintained until the patient is either (a) immobilized on a long backboard, or (b) deemed not to meet indications for spinal immobilization (see Indications for Spinal Immobilization Algorithm, p. 235). Satisfactory spinal immobilization involves immobilization from the head to the pelvis. Immobilization should not interfere with the patient's ability to open the mouth and should not impair ventilatory function.

For the victim of penetrating trauma, spinal immobilization is performed if the patient has a neurologic complaint or if a motor or sensory deficit is noted on physical examination. In a patient with blunt trauma, spinal immobilization is indicated if the patient has an altered level of consciousness (GCS score <15) or a neurologic complaint, or if spinal tenderness, an anatomic abnormality, or a motor or sensory deficit is identified on physical examination. If the patient has sustained a mechanism of injury that causes concern, spinal immobilization is indicated if the patient has evidence of alcohol or drug intoxication, a significant distracting injury, or an inability to communicate because of an age or language barrier.

11. For Critically Injured Trauma Patients, Initiate Transport to the Closest Appropriate Facility within 10 Minutes of Arrival on Scene.

Numerous studies have demonstrated that delays in transporting trauma patients to appropriate receiving facilities lead to increases in mortality rates. Although prehospital care providers have become proficient at endotracheal intubation, ventilatory support, and administration of intravenous (IV) fluid therapy, most critically injured trauma patients are in hemorrhagic shock and are in need of two things that cannot be provided in the prehospital setting: blood and control of internal hemorrhage. Because human blood is a perishable product, it is impractical for administration in the field under most circumstances. Crystalloid solution restores intravascular volume but does not replace the oxygen-carrying capacity of the lost RBCs. Although some blood substitutes have shown promising results in early clinical trials, none is yet nearing approval for use in the field setting. Similarly, control of internal hemorrhage almost always requires emergent surgical intervention best performed in an OR. Resuscitation can never be achieved in the patient with ongoing internal hemorrhage. Therefore the goal of the prehospital care provider is to spend as little time on scene as possible.

This concern for limiting scene time should not be construed as a "scoop and run" mentality in which no attempts are made to address key problems before initiating transport. Instead, the PHTLS program advocates a philosophy of "limited scene intervention," focusing on a rapid assessment aimed at identifying threats to life and performing interventions that are *believed* to improve outcome. Examples include airway and ventilatory management, control of external hemorrhage, and spinal immobilization. Precious time should not be wasted on procedures that can be instituted en route to the receiving facility. Patients who are critically injured (see Box 18-1) should be transported within 10 minutes of the arrival of EMS on the scene—the "Platinum 10 Minutes" of the Golden Period. Reasonable exceptions to the Platinum 10 Minutes include situations that require extensive extrication or time needed to secure an unsafe scene, such as law enforcement ensuring that a perpetrator is no longer present.

The *closest* hospital may not be the *most appropriate* receiving facility for many trauma patients. Those patients who meet certain physiologic, anatomic, or mechanism of injury criteria benefit from being taken to a trauma center—a facility that has special expertise and resources for managing trauma. Each community, through a consensus of surgeons, emergency physicians, and prehospital care providers, must decide where these types of trauma patients should be transported. These decisions should be incorporated into protocols that designate the best destination facility—the closest *appropriate* facility. In some situations, it is appropriate to bypass non–trauma centers to reach a trauma center. Even if this causes a moderate increase in the transport time, the overall time to definitive care will be shorter. Ideally, in the urban setting, a critically injured patient arrives at a trauma center within 25 to 30 minutes of being injured. The hospital also must work equally efficiently to continue resuscitation and, if necessary, transport the patient quickly to the OR (all within the Golden Period) to control hemorrhage.

12. Initiate Warmed Intravenous Fluid Replacement En Route to the Receiving Facility.

Initiation of transport of a critically injured trauma patient should never be delayed simply to insert IV catheters and administer fluid therapy. Although crystalloid solutions do restore lost blood volume and improve perfusion, they do not transport oxygen. Additionally, restoring normal blood pressure may result in additional hemorrhage from clot disruption in damaged blood vessels that initially clotted off.

While en route to the receiving facility, the prehospital care provider can insert two large-bore IV catheters and start an infusion of warmed (102° F [39° C]) crystalloid solution, preferably lactated Ringer's. Warmed solution is given to aid in the prevention of hypothermia. Volume resuscitation is individualized to the clinical situation (see Managing Volume Resuscitation Algorithm, p. 188). For adult patients with suspected uncontrolled hemorrhage in the chest, abdomen, or retroperitoneum IV fluid therapy is titrated to maintain a mean blood pressure of 60 to 65 mm Hg (SBP of 80 to 90 mm Hg). When a TBI is suspected, a target systolic blood pressure of at least 90 mm Hg is appropriate. If hemorrhage has been controlled, patients in Class II, III, or IV shock are administered a 1- to 2-L bolus of warmed crystalloid solution. Fluid resuscitation is titrated to normal vital signs, unless the patient develops evidence of recurrent Class II or IV shock, in which case fluid is titrated to a MAP of 60 to 65 mm Hg. IV lines and fluid therapy may be initiated during extrication or while awaiting the arrival of an air medical helicopter. These situations do not result in a delay in transport to initiate volume resuscitation. Basic life support (BLS) providers should consider a rendezvous with an advanced life support (ALS) service (by air or ground units) when faced with prolonged transport time.

13. Ascertain the Patient's Medical History and Perform a Secondary Survey when Life-Threatening Problems Have Been Satisfactorily Managed or Have Been Ruled Out.

If life-threatening conditions are found in the primary survey, key interventions should be performed and the patient prepared for transport within the Platinum 10 Minutes. Conversely, if life-threatening conditions are not identified, a secondary survey is performed. The secondary survey is a systematic, head-to-toe physical examination that serves to identify all injuries. At this time an AMPLE history (**a**llergies, **m**edications, **p**ast medical history, **l**ast meal, **e**vents preceding the injury) is also obtained. For critically injured trauma patients, a secondary survey is performed if time permits and once life-threatening conditions have been appropriately managed. In some situations where the patient is located close to an appropriate receiving facility, a secondary survey may never be completed. This approach ensures that the prehospital care provider's attention is focused on the most serious problems—those that may result in death if not properly managed—and not on lower-priority injuries. The patient should be reassessed frequently because patients who initially present without life-threatening injuries may subsequently develop them.

14. Above All, *Do No Further Harm.*

The medical principle that states "Above all, do no further harm" dates back to the ancient Greek physician Hippocrates. Applied to the prehospital care of the trauma patient, this principle can take many forms: developing a backup plan for airway management before initiating rapid sequence intubation, protecting a patient from flying debris during extrication from a damaged vehicle, or controlling significant external hemorrhage before initiating volume resuscitation. Recent experience has shown that prehospital care providers can safely perform many of the life-saving skills that can be delivered in a trauma center. However, the issue is not, "What *can* providers do for critically injured trauma patients?" but rather, "What *should* providers do for critically injured trauma patients?"

When caring for a critically injured patient, prehospital care providers need to ask themselves if their actions at the scene and during transport will reasonably benefit the patient. If the answer to this question is either "no" or "uncertain," those actions should be withheld and emphasis placed on transporting the trauma patient to the closest appropriate facility. Interventions should be limited to those that prevent or treat physiologic deterioration. Trauma care must follow a given set of priorities that establish an efficient and effective plan of action, based on available time frames and any dangers present at the scene, if the patient is to survive. Appropriate intervention and stabilization should be integrated and coordinated between the field, the ED, and the OR. It is essential that every provider at every level of care and at every stage of treatment be in harmony with the rest of the team.

In discussing the issue of "do no further harm," the concept of "financial" harm should be considered in addition to the common thought of "physical" harm. Specifically, on a regular basis, manufacturers introduce new medications and devices designed to replace or improve existing modalities of treatment. It is important to consider a number of issues prior to implementing new treatments including:

■ What is the medical evidence supporting the efficacy of the new treatment?
■ Is the new intervention as good as or better than existing interventions?
■ How does the cost of providing the new intervention compare to the existing intervention?

As a general principle, there should be medical evidence that demonstrates that a new intervention is at least as good

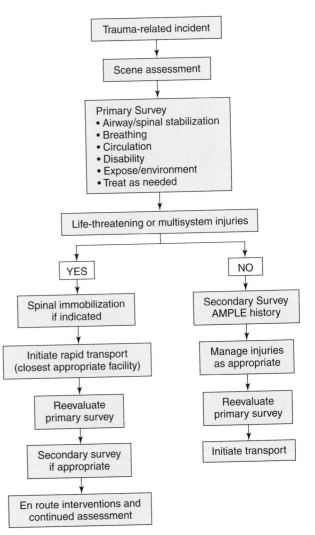

as, and preferably better, than existing treatments before it is formally accepted and implemented. As the cost of a new intervention often exceeds that of an existing intervention, the absence of evidence indicating superiority of the new intervention leads to added charges to the patient resulting in "financial" harm.

As discussed in Chapter 1, critically injured trauma patients arriving at a trauma center can have a worse outcome when transported by EMS rather than private vehicle. A significant factor that probably accounts for the increased mortality rate is the actions of well-intentioned prehospital care providers who fail to understand that trauma is a *surgical* disease; most critically injured patients require immediate surgery to save their lives. Anything that delays surgical intervention translates into more hemorrhage, more shock, and ultimately death.

Even with the best-planned and executed resuscitation, not all trauma patients can be saved. However, with attention focused on the reasons for early traumatic death, a much larger percentage of patients may survive, with a lower residual morbidity rate than would otherwise result without the benefit of correct and expedient field management. *The fundamental principles taught in PHTLS—rapid assessment, key field interventions, and rapid transport to the closest appropriate facility—have been shown to improve outcomes in critically injured trauma patients.*

SUMMARY

The following are the Golden Principles of Prehospital Trauma Care:

1. Ensure the safety of the prehospital care providers and the patient.
2. Assess the scene situation to determine the need for additional resources.
3. Recognize the kinematics that produced the injuries.
4. Use the primary survey approach to identify life-threatening conditions.
5. Provide appropriate airway management while maintaining cervical spine stabilization.
6. Support ventilation and deliver oxygen to maintain an Spo_2 greater than 95%.
7. Control any significant external hemorrhage.
8. Provide basic shock therapy, including restoring and maintaining normal body temperature and appropriately splinting musculoskeletal injuries.
9. Consider use of pneumatic antishock garment for patients with decompensated shock (SBP <90 mm Hg) and suspected pelvic, intraperitoneal, or retroperitoneal hemorrhage, and in patients with profound hypotension (SBP <60 mm Hg).
10. Maintain manual spinal stabilization until the patient is immobilized on a long backboard.
11. For critically injured trauma patients, initiate transport to the closest appropriate facility within 10 minutes of arrival on scene.
12. Initiate warmed intravenous fluid replacement en route to the receiving facility.
13. Ascertain the patient's medical history and perform a secondary survey when life-threatening conditions have been satisfactorily managed or have been ruled out.
14. Above all, **do no further harm.**

References

1. Lerner EB, Moscati RM: The Golden Hour: scientific fact of medical "urban legend"? *Acad Emerg Med* 8:758, 2001.
2. Tsybuliak GN, Pavlenko EP: Cause of death in the early post-traumatic period, *Vestn Khir Im I I Grek* 114(5):75, 1975.
3. Stewart RM, Myers JG, Dent DL, et al: 753 Consecutive deaths in a Level 1 trauma center: the argument for injury prevention, *J Trauma* 54:66, 2003.
4. 2005 International Consensus on Cardiopulmonary Resuscitation (CPR) and Emergency Cardiovascular Care (ECC) Science with Treatment Recommendations. Part 10. First aid, *Circulation* 112(suppl I):III-115, 2005.

Chapter Objectives

*At the completion of this chapter, the reader
will be able to do the following:*

✓ Describe the components of the disaster cycle

✓ Discuss common pitfalls encountered during disaster response

✓ List the components that comprise the medical response to a
disaster

✓ Recognize how disaster response may affect the psychological well-
being of prehospital care providers

CHAPTER 19

Disaster Management

SCENARIO

A group of men with a political agenda against the government purchased a fuel truck and converted it into a bomb with smuggled explosives. It contained 3000 to 5000 pounds of explosives. Late in the evening (approximately 10 PM) on the night of the attack, the individuals drove three vehicles, two cars and the bomb truck, to a parking lot adjacent to a convention center. A concert with 3000 individuals was in progress at the time. A chainlink security fence separated the parking lot from the convention center. The men parked the truck next to the fence and left the area. The bomb exploded between 3 and 4 minutes later.

The force of the explosion was enormous. It heavily damaged the convention center and left an enormous crater where the fuel truck had been. The blast was felt for miles around the area. Initial evacuation was by local security officials, and the "walking wounded" went, on their own, to the local hospital.

What safety and security concerns would first responders encounter? What triage system should be utilized? Who should be selected as incident commander? What level of personal protection should first responders utilize? What are important features of the casualty collection station? ■

Unlike system-specific injuries that have a finite period for presentation, intervention, and recovery, the response to and recovery from a disaster are all-encompassing and include not only medical and psychosocial issues, but also the rebuilding of public health, physical safety, and sociologic resources and infrastructures.

The World Health Organization (WHO) has defined a disaster as a sudden ecologic phenomenon of sufficient magnitude to require external assistance. This broad definition is in keeping with concepts devoid of specifications to the medical response but inclusive of the overall community response and sociopolitical response to any disaster of significant magnitude.

From a medical perspective, the definition can be more focused in that a disaster is defined when the number of patients presenting within a given time is such that the medical providers cannot provide care for them without external assistance.[1]

In short, the definition of a disaster identifies two key concepts: (1) a disaster is independent of a specific number of victims, and (2) the impact exceeds the available resources of the medical response.

Disasters follow no rules. No one can predict the complexity, time, or location of the next disaster. Traditionally, medical providers have held the erroneous belief that all disasters are different, especially those involving terrorism. All disasters, regardless of etiology, have similar medical and public health consequences. Disasters differ in the degree to which these consequences occur and the degree to which they disrupt the medical and public health infrastructure of the disaster scene.

The key principle of disaster medical care is to do the greatest good for the greatest number of patients, whereas the objective of conventional medical care is to do the greatest good for the individual patient.

Natural disasters, man-made disasters, and terrorism encompass the spectrum of possible disaster threats. Weapons of mass destruction, creating huge numbers of casualties and "contaminated environments," may be the greatest challenge of all (see Chapter 20).

A consistent approach to disasters, based on an understanding of their common features and the response expertise required, is becoming the accepted practice throughout the world. This strategy is called the *mass-casualty incident* (MCI) *response*. MCI response has the primary objective of reducing the morbidity (injury, disease) and mortality (death) caused by the disaster. All medical responders need to incorporate the key principles of the MCI response in their training, given the complexity of current disasters (Figure 19-1).

The Disaster Cycle

Noji[1] and others have defined a theoretic framework by which the sequence of events in a disaster can be broken down and analyzed. This provides an opportunity for learning about the process of an event and also provides for the development of the response process.[2,3] Five phases have been identified, as follows:

1. The *quiescence level*, or the interdisaster period, represents the time during which risk assessment should be undertaken and plans for response to likely events developed, tested, and implemented.

FIGURE 19-1 Mass-casualty management at Ground Zero, World Trade Center, New York, 2001.

2. The next phase is the *prodrome phase,* or warning phase. At this point, a specific event has been identified as inevitably going to occur. This could reflect a natural weather condition (e.g., impending landfall of a hurricane) or the active unfolding of a hostile and potentially violent situation. During this period, steps may be taken to mitigate the effects of the ensuing events. These defensive maneuvers may include such actions as fortifying physical structures, initiating evacuation plans, and mobilizing public health resources to mount a postevent response.

3. The third phase is the *impact phase,* or the presentation of the actual event. During this period, there is often little that can be done to alter the actual impact or outcome of what is occurring.

4. The fourth phase is the *rescue phase,* which is the time immediately after impact during which response occurs and appropriate management and intervention can save lives. The skills of the first responders, rescue teams, and medical supportive services will be brought to bear to maximize survival from the event.

5. The fifth phase is the *recovery phase,* or reconstruction phase, which addresses the community's resources to endure and emerge from the effects of the disaster through the coordinated efforts of the medical, public health, and community infrastructure (physical and political). This period is by far the longest, lasting months, and perhaps years, before a community fully recovers.

Understanding the disaster cycle allows a prehospital care provider to evaluate the postincident action report and assess the provider's individual area of responsibilities and response, as well as the response of others, to determine the efficiency and efficacy of the response process and identify areas for future improvement.

Mass-Casualty Incident Management

Mass-casualty incidents (MCIs) are events that cause casualties in numbers large enough to overwhelm the medical and public health services of the affected community. The severity and diversity of injuries, in addition to the number of victims, will be major factors in determining whether an MCI requires resources and assistance from outside the impacted community.

Today's complex disasters, especially those involving terrorism and weapons of mass destruction (chemical, biological, or nuclear), may result in an austere environment. An *austere environment* is a setting where resources, transportation, and other aspects of the physical, political, social, and economic environments impose severe constraints on the availability and adequacy of immediate care for the population in need.

Medical concerns related to MCIs include the following four elements:

- Search and rescue
- Triage and initial stabilization
- Definitive medical care
- Evacuation

Public health concerns related to MCIs include the following:

- Water
- Food
- Shelter
- Sanitation
- Security and safety
- Transportation
- Communication
- Endemic and epidemic diseases

Both medical and public health disaster response activities are coordinated through one organizational structure, the incident command system.

Incident Command System

Many different organizations participate in the response to a disaster. The incident command system (ICS) was created to allow different types of agencies and multiple jurisdictions of similar agencies (fire, police, emergency medical services [EMS]) to work together effectively using a common organizational structure and language in response to a disaster (Figure 19-2) (see Chapter 4).

FIGURE 19-2 Incident command system (ICS) allows integration of fire, police, and EMS assets at a disaster scene.

From a medical perspective, important ICS principles will help during an MCI response, as follows:

1. ICS must be started early, before an incident gets out of control.
2. Medical and public health responders, often used to working independently, need to implement the ICS management structure to better respond to an MCI.

Common Pitfalls of Disaster Response

Numerous studies performed after significant MCIs have identified several consistent shortcomings in the medical response to these events. Identification of these deficiencies has resulted from actual incidents and subsequent evaluations of the response as well as from communities performing risk, vulnerability, and needs assessments mandated by the U.S. government in order to receive funding resources to enhance the disaster response infrastructure.

Communications

Many events have demonstrated that the lack of a unified communication system significantly hinders the ability to mount a coordinated response to an MCI. Individual communication systems are effective, but relying on a single system for communication is doomed to failure. The use of cellular phones became impossible when the central communication center located in the World Trade Center was no longer in existence. Also, the failure of the police, fire, and EMS agencies to be able to communicate with each other because of different radio technologies or frequencies is a serious deficiency that significantly reduces the ability to respond to MCIs effectively. Redundancy in the system is of paramount importance, regardless of the chosen source for primary communications. Landlines, hardwired phone systems, cellular phone systems, satellite phone systems, VHF radios, and 800-MHz frequency systems all have some degree of vulnerability. The following two principles are essential:

1. A unified communication system to which all pertinent responders in the community have access.
2. System redundancy such that if one modality of communication fails or is disabled, another source can be used efficiently as an appropriate backup.

Scene Security

Scene security has become an ever-increasing problem in MCIs. Scene security is important for the following reasons:

1. To protect the response teams from a second strike resulting in further casualties.
2. To provide for the ingress and egress of rescue workers and victims unencumbered by onlookers to the disaster.
3. To protect and assist in securing the scene and physical evidence.

Scene security becomes a significant challenge during a disaster event because, by definition, all resources are being stretched to the maximum of their capabilities and limits. Coordination with local law enforcement leaders is essential for the prehospital and medical community to ensure that security will be available.

Self-Dispatched Assistance

In many MCIs, public safety and EMS agencies from adjacent and even distant communities have responded to the scene without any formal request for assistance from the impacted jurisdiction. These self-dispatched responders, although well intentioned, often serve only to further complicate and confuse an already chaotic situation. Interagency communications issues are often made more difficult by noncompatible radio systems, and coordinated rescue efforts are often impossible because of the lack of participation in the incident command structure. Ideally, public safety and EMS agencies should respond to a disaster site only if they have been specifically requested to do so by the responsible jurisdiction and incident commander.

Supply and Equipment Resources

Most municipalities have plans for the routine utilization of supplies and have purchased supplies based on this demand. Events of large magnitude will rapidly exhaust these resources. Having a seamless plan for the reconstitution of supplies is essential for the ongoing mission of treating victims. Supplies must be available in a timely fashion, and appropriate mechanisms must be in place for distribution, which cannot include the care providers in the field, who will already be utilized to their fullest availabilities. A plan for pharmaceutical replenishment must also be in place. In those communities that have been designated to receive Metropolitan Medical Response System (MMRS) funds, community stockpiles have been or are being purchased in preparation for such events (see later discussion).

Media

The media are often seen as a detriment to the physical and operational process of a disaster response. However, communities are encouraged to partner with the media because these outlets can be an asset during a disaster response. The media can provide for the dissemination of appropriate and accurate information to the population, giving them directions as to how to respond to maintain personal safety and where to report to obtain information or to reunite with family members, as well as communicating other needed information. It is inevitable that the media will broadcast information to the public, and as responders, prehospital care providers have the responsibility to partner with the media to ensure that the information provided is accurate as well as helpful to the response process.

Preparedness

As responders in a community, prehospital care providers also prepare for the devastation that can occur in a mass-casualty event and plan for such events in a variety of ways. Although one method of preparing, the tabletop drill does not truly test the ability to perform the duties as well as the ability to bring resources and assets to the site in a timely and efficient manner. Likewise, medical facilities must have realistic disaster drills during which victims are brought through the medical response process inside the hospital facility doors in a realistic fashion to test the medical, surgical, and critical care response that will be required. The ability to provide for "surge capacity" and for supplying the large number of beds and other equipment needed for victims must be appropriately addressed by the health care community.

Unfortunately, few facilities have actually tested a surge-capacity response in real time and instead have relied on tabletop drills as a measure of their ability to respond. Only through community drills that bring victims from the scene through the medical process, including admission and discharge from the hospital, can the true level of preparedness to respond to an MCI as a community be assessed. (See Disaster Education and Training.)

Medical Response to Disasters

Several actions must be initiated to respond effectively to an MCI.

Initial Response

The first step is notification and activation of the EMS response system. This is usually performed by witnesses to the event who call the local emergency dispatch center seeking response by appropriate police, fire, and emergency medical agencies.

The first medical responders to arrive have a number of important functions to fulfill; importantly, these do *not* include finding and treating the most critically injured patients. Before beginning the process of providing medical assistance, the first medical personnel should take the time to perform an overall scene assessment. The goal of this assessment is to estimate the potential number of casualties, determine what additional medical resources will be needed at the scene, and evaluate whether any specialized equipment or personnel, such as search and rescue teams, will be required.

Once this assessment is complete, the next step is to communicate the assessment to the dispatch center, where the process of acquiring and dispatching the needed resources can be performed. After this, the medical personnel should identify appropriate locations to perform triage and to stage incoming ambulances, personnel, and supplies so as not to impede rapid ingress and egress when necessary.

In addition to providing for the medical response to the disaster scene, it is essential that the responding EMS agency notify the likely receiving hospitals in the community so that they can activate their disaster plans to prepare to receive casualties.

Search and Rescue

At this point, the on-scene process of initiating patient care can begin. Generally, this will start with a search and rescue effort to identify and evacuate casualties (Figure 19-3). The local population near any disaster site is often the immediate search and rescue resource and may have already begun to search for victims. Experience has demonstrated that the local community will respond to a disaster site and begin the process of aiding victims. In addition, many countries and communities have developed specialized search and rescue teams as an integral part of their national and local disaster plans. Members of these teams receive specialized training in "confined-space environments" and are activated as needed for a particular event.

FIGURE 19-3 Search and rescue, Hurricane Katrina, 2005.

FIGURE 19-4 Triage and initial stabilization, Hurricane Katrina, Louisiana, 2005.

These search and rescue units generally include the following:

- A cadre of medical specialists
- Technical specialists knowledgeable in hazardous materials, structural engineering, heavy equipment operation, and technical search and rescue methods (e.g., listening equipment, remote cameras)
- Trained canines and their handlers

Local construction companies may provide valuable search and rescue assets by providing equipment, tools, and wooden planks that can be used at the disaster site to assist in moving heavy debris.

Triage

As patients are identified and evacuated, they are brought to the triage site, where they can be assessed and a triage category assigned (Figure 19-4). The term "triage" is a French word that means "to sort." From a medical perspective, triage means sorting casualties based on the severity of their injuries. This further serves to prioritize the patient's need for medical care and transportation to the hospital.

Triage is one of the most important missions of any disaster medical response. As noted previously, the objective of conventional triage in the nondisaster setting is to do the greatest good for the individual patient. The objective of disaster triage is to do the greatest good for the greatest number of people. Disaster triage in the field must be overseen by a trained triage officer. A *triage officer* should have a wide breadth of clinical experience in the assessment and management of field injuries; a paramedic with significant field experience usually meets this requirement. A trained physician with wide experience in the field may also function in this capacity.[4,5]

A number of different methodologies exist for evaluating and assigning the triage category. One common method is to evaluate the anatomic injuries and assign the priority for medical care and transport based on the severity of the injury and the likelihood of need for surgical intervention. Another method involves a rapid physiologic and mental status evaluation. This triage process is referred to as the "START" triage algorithm (simple triage and rapid treatment). This system evaluates the respiratory status, perfusion status, and mental status of the patient in making a prioritization for initial transfer to definitive care facilities[5,6] (see Chapter 4).

Regardless of the exact triage method used, all these systems ultimately classify patients into one of (usually) four injury severity categories. Highest-priority patients are those who are identified as having critical, but likely survivable, injuries and are usually categorized as *Class I* priority and color-coded *red*. Patients with moderate injuries are categorized as *Class II* patients and color-coded *yellow*. Patients with relatively minor injuries, often referred to as the "walking wounded," are classified as *Class III* victims and color-coded *green*. Patients who have expired on the scene or whose injuries are so severe that death is imminent or is likely are categorized as "dead" or "expectant," respectively, which is considered *Class IV* and color-coded *black*. All these color codes refer to the use of "disaster tags," which are used at disaster scenes and attached to patients once they have been triaged. The "color code" provides an immediate visual reference to their triage category.

It is important that all triage personnel keep in mind that they must avoid the temptation to stop performing triage in favor of treating a critically injured patient that they encounter. As mentioned earlier, the primary principle involved in dealing with an MCI is to do the most good for the most people. During this initial triage phase, medical interventions are limited to those actions that are performed easily and rapidly, and that are not labor intensive. Generally, this means only procedures such as manual airway opening and external hemorrhage control. Interventions such as bag-mask ventilation and closed chest compression involve the use of significant personnel and are not performed.

Once patients have been triaged, they are collected together according to their triage priority. Specifically, all the "red" category or Class I patients are grouped, as are the Class II ("yellow") and Class III ("green") patients. Casualty collection sites should be located close enough to the disaster site to offer rapid treatment but far enough away to be safe. Important features include the following:

- Proximity to the disaster site
- Safety from hazards and upwind location from contaminated environments
- Protection from climatic conditions
- Easy visibility for disaster victims
- Convenient exit routes for air and land evacuation

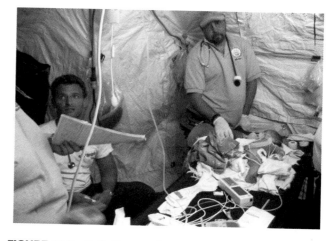

FIGURE 19-5   Definitive medical care, U.S. field hospital, Bam, Iran earthquake, 2005.

As additional medical staff and resources arrive and become available on-scene, medical care and interventions are provided according to the triage priority. Finally, as transportation resources become available, patients are then transported for definitive care according, once again, to their triage priority (Figure 19-5). A prehospital care provider never holds a critical patient for the provision of further medical care on-site if transport is available (Figure 19-6). Needed medical interventions should be conducted during transport to the definitive care facility.

Because of visible, critical patient injuries, emergency personnel often have a tendency to move patients forward for immediate treatment and transport and to bypass the triage process. This must be avoided so that the most life-threatening casualties can be treated first and the best care can be provided for the majority of victims. However, bypassing the triage process is indicated in certain situations. These conditions include (1) risk, as in bad weather; (2) potential impending darkness, without the capabilities of lighting resources; (3) the continued risk of injury as a result of natural or unnatural events; (4) no triage facility or triage officer immediately available; and (5) any tactical situation in a law enforcement scenario where the victims are rapidly moved from the impact site to the collection point for transportation.[6,7]

FIGURE 19-6   Interior of a military transport plane converted for medical evacuation with patient litters.

wounded" arriving at the hospital closest to the disaster site. In fact, approximately 70% to 80% of casualties will get to a hospital without EMS ambulance transport.

EMS systems must therefore understand that the hospital closest to a disaster scene may be overwhelmed with casualties even before the arrival of the first transporting ambulance. Before taking patient to the closest hospital, contact should be made to ascertain the status of the emergency department (ED) and the capability to accept and treat victims being transported by ambulance. If the closest hospital is overwhelmed, the EMS system should transport patients to more distant facilities, when possible. Although the transport time will be longer, the patient's care will not be complicated by the presence of numerous other casualties. Dispersal of casualties to multiple institutions will ultimately better preserve the ability of all the receiving hospitals to optimize the patient care they provide.

Transport

Another important issue in effectively responding to an MCI relates to the decision-making process for patient destination once transport is initiated. Recent events have demonstrated that casualties with non–life-threatening injuries will often depart the disaster site using any available means of transportation and make their own way to the hospital. Often this results in large numbers of "walking

FIGURE 19-7 Aerial view of devastation caused by Supertyphoon Pongsona, Guam, 2002.

FIGURE 19-8 Madrid terrorist bombing, 2004.

Medical Assistance Teams

If the disaster is of significant proportion that outside resources are needed through the state or federal government, other medical response teams are available in many municipalities (Figure 19-7). As a result of the Metropolitan Medical Response System, MMRS strike teams have been created in many cities. These strike teams comprise medical experts in emergency medicine, trauma surgery, and surgical subspecialties. These teams can respond with resources that have been purchased through state and federal funds. These teams can be used to augment and back-fill medical facilities or to staff mobile medical facilities that are established to meet surge-capacity victims.

On a larger-scale basis, the U.S. government has capabilities through the National Disaster Medical System to mobilize disaster medical assistance teams. These teams are able to provide field care as well as create mobile medical facilities with the capability to perform surgical interventions and meet the critical care needs of the victims. A request for these teams must come through the appropriate channels via the state emergency management authority and the governor's office through the federal government to the Federal Emergency Management Agency (FEMA), which houses the National Disaster Medical System's response program.

Threat of Terrorism and Weapons of Mass Destruction

Terrorism may present one of the most challenging MCIs for emergency responders. The spectrum of terrorist threats is limitless, ranging from suicide bombers, conventional explosives, and military weapons to weapons of mass destruction (nuclear, biologic, or chemical WMDs).

Terrorist events have the greatest potential of all man-made disasters to generate large numbers of casualties and fatalities.

Terrorists have demonstrated their ingenuity and capacity not to be limited by conventional technology or weaponry. During the terrorist attacks on September 11, 2001, the terrorists used fully fueled passenger jets as "flying bombs," generating massive destruction of life and property.

One of the unique features of a terrorist threat, especially involving WMDs, is that psychogenic casualties usually predominate. Terrorists do not need to kill a large number of people to achieve their goals; they only need to create a climate of fear and panic to overwhelm the medical infrastructure. In the March 1995 sarin attacks in Tokyo, 5000 casualties presented to hospitals. Of these, fewer than 1000 had physical effects of the sarin gas; the remaining presented with psychological stress. The recent anthrax incidents in the United States also dramatically increased the number of individuals presenting to EDs with nonspecific respiratory symptoms that ultimately did not result from actual anthrax infection.

Explosions and bombings continue to be the most frequent cause of mass casualties in disasters caused by terrorists. The majority of these bombings consist of relatively small explosives that produce low mortality rates. However, when strategically placed in buildings, pipelines, or moving vehicles, their impact can be much greater (Figure 19-8). The high morbidity and mortality is related not only to the intensity of the blast, but also to the subsequent structural damage that leads to collapse of the targeted buildings. A greater threat will be disasters caused by conventional explosives in combination with a chemical, biologic, or radiologic agent, such as a "dirty bomb" that combines a conventional explosive with radioactive material.

FIGURE 19-9 Decontamination of casualties in the "warm zone" by personnel in Level B personal protective equipment (PPE).

WMDs creating "contaminated environments" may prove to be the greatest disaster challenge. Emergency responders will not be able to bring victims into hospitals because of the risk of further contaminating medical facilities. Medical responders must be prepared and equipped to perform triage, not only to determine the extent of the injuries, but also to assess the potential for contamination and need for decontamination and initial stabilization. At the same time, prehospital care providers need to take appropriate steps to protect themselves from potential contamination.

Decontamination

Decontamination is an important part of all disasters involving hazardous materials (hazmat) and WMDs (Figure 19-9). Terrorist events, with their larger number of patients, unknown substances, and large numbers of "worried well," significantly increase the possibility of contaminated or potentially contaminated casualties (see Chapter 20).

Treatment Area
When responding to a disaster involving hazmat and WMDs, it is critical that the treatment area be at least 300 yards upwind and uphill of the contaminated area.

Psychological Response to Disasters

Psychological trauma and other adverse psychological sequelae are frequently the side effects of events such as natural

disasters and unintentional disasters caused by humans. With terrorism, the objective is to inflict psychological pain, trauma, and disequilibrium.

Characteristics of Disasters That Affect Mental Health

Not all disasters have the same level of psychological impact. Disaster characteristics that seem to have the most significant mental health impact are the following:

- Little or no warning
- Serious threat to personal safety
- Potential unknown health effects
- Uncertain duration of the event
- Human error or malicious intent
- Symbolism related to the terrorist target

Factors Impacting Psychological Response

Everyone who experiences a disaster, whether as a victim or as a responder, is affected by it. Fortunately, this does not mean that most will develop a mental health disorder. It does mean, however, that all individuals will have some type of psychological or emotional response to the event.

Similarly, there are both individual and collective reactions that interact as individuals and communities recover from these extraordinary events.

Factors affecting individual response to disasters include the following:

- Physical and psychological proximity to the event
- Exposure to gruesome or grotesque situations
- Diminished health status before or because of the disaster
- Magnitude of loss
- Trauma history

Factors impacting collective response to trauma are as follows:

- Degree of community disruption
- Predisaster family and community stability
- Community leadership
- Cultural sensitivity of recovery efforts

Psychological Sequelae of Disasters

Postdisaster psychological responses are wide ranging, from mild stress responses to full-blown *posttraumatic stress disorder* (PTSD), major depression, or acute stress disorder. Although many people may exhibit signs of psychological stress, relatively few (typically 15%-25%) of those most directly impacted will subsequently develop a diagnosable mental disorder.

Interventions

1. In persons with no diagnosed mental disorder, it is helpful to provide educational materials that help people understand what they and their families are experiencing.
2. Brief crisis counseling should be provided, followed by referral when treatment is indicated.
3. When a mental disorder is diagnosed, therapeutic interventions can be helpful, including cognitive-behavioral therapy and psychiatric medications.

Worker Stress

Disaster workers can also become secondary victims of stress and other psychological sequelae. This can adversely affect their functioning during and after an event. It can also adversely impact their personal well-being as well as their family and work relationships.

Signs of Stress in Workers

Some common signs of stress in workers include physiologic, emotional, cognitive, and behavioral elements.

Physiologic signs
- Fatigue, even after rest
- Nausea
- Fine motor tremors
- Tics
- Paresthesias
- Dizziness
- Gastrointestinal upset
- Heart palpitations
- Choking or smothering sensations

Emotional signs
- Anxiety
- Irritability
- Feeling overwhelmed
- Unrealistic anticipation of harm to self or others

Cognitive signs
- Memory loss
- Decision-making difficulties
- *Anomia* (inability to name common objects or familiar people)
- Concentration problems or distractibility
- Reduced attention span
- Calculation difficulties

Behavioral signs
- Insomnia
- Hypervigilance
- Crying easily
- Inappropriate humor
- Ritualistic behavior

FIGURE 19-10 Fatigue contributes greatly to worker stress.

Managing Worker Stress On-Site

The following on-site interventions can assist in reducing worker stress:

- Limited exposure to traumatic stimuli
- Reasonable hours
- Adequate rest and sleep (Figure 19-10)
- Reasonable diet
- Regular exercise program
- Private time
- Talking to somebody who understands
- Monitoring signs of stress
- Identifiable endpoint for involvement

Disaster Education and Training

The development and implementation of a formal educational and training infrastructure will improve the prehospital care provider's ability to respond efficiently to an MCI. Preparedness with regard to education and learning can be accomplished in various structured as well as unstructured learning environments. Each has its individual advantages and disadvantages, as measured by educational impact and comparative cost. For optimal learning from educational exercises, it is imperative that interdisciplinary training events be conducted often to include all the appropriate agencies and participants in a disaster response.

Independent learning is the foundation of disaster preparedness. A multitude of resources are available through printed literature as well as via the Internet. The Centers for Disease Control and Prevention (CDC), public health agencies, and the military forces all have Web-based learning opportunities that are available to individuals. Courses can be completed on an independent basis on a time-flexible schedule. The limitation of this modality of learning is that it does not allow for an interactive learning experience.

Group training is directed at specific response teams with regard to disaster response. Training programs are broadly available and include understanding command structure and WMD preparedness. Numerous professional and paraprofessional organizations have developed training programs and modules specific to their scope of professional practice, including public health, emergency medicine, critical care, and surgical and medical specialties, as well as all levels of prehospital care providers.

Simulations provide a training opportunity that brings together many individuals from varied and different backgrounds who are essential to the implementation of a disaster response. As mentioned earlier, these exercises come in two specific forms: a tabletop exercise and a fully active, field training exercise. *Tabletop exercises* are cost-effective and highly useful methods to test and evaluate a disaster response. A starting point and focused points of accomplishment and order for completion of the exercise are usually established in advance. Tabletop exercises can allow for real-time communications and interaction between multi-disciplinary agencies. These activities require direction in the form of a facilitator guiding the participants through the objective and critical evaluation of the results at the conclusion.

Field exercises are the most realistic training events, involving the actual execution and performance of the community disaster response plan. The field exercise allows for a real-time assessment of the physical capacity to meet the objectives as defined in writing. Ideally, the exercises will involve moving victims from the point of impact and injury through the EMS response system and into definitive care at medical facilities. These events, however, are labor intensive and long in duration and have significant cost.

SUMMARY

Many disasters result from natural climactic or geologic events; however they may also result from intentional or unintentional acts of man. Although disasters may be unpredictable, adequate preparation can turn an unthinkable event into a manageable situation. Appropriate disaster response involves much more than the medical component. Implementation of the Incident Command System allows multiple agencies to collaborate in the disaster response. Despite the fact that disasters occur in varying sizes and result from many different causes, common pitfalls have been identified that hinder management of such an event, including issues with communications, scene security, self-dispatched assistance, and lack of supplies. The best outcomes in response to MCIs from conventional or unconventional threats is the creation of a well-devised disaster plan that has been rehearsed, tested, and critiqued to identify and improve problem areas. Disaster response may take a heavy psychologic toll on those involved.

SCENARIO SOLUTION

After the blast event, precautionary measures are taken to evaluate the threat potential for a "dirty bomb" detonation involving a radiologic dispersion, a chemical contaminant, or a "second strike" bomb. Appropriate personal protective equipment (PPE) must be used if contamination is detected, as well as standard precautions when treating patients.

Crowd control and containment of patients are of the utmost importance after a WMD event, both for treatment purposes and for protection of evidence. The ICS should be used to manage the resources required to deal with this event. A staging area for responding units should be designated. Patients will need to be triaged using whatever triage system the EMS provider has in place. Casualty collection points will be set up and located in strategic areas to allow for rapid loading and evacuation of victims.

In addition to patient care needs, remember that rescue workers will have hydration, nutrition, and sanitary needs throughout the rescue mission. ∎

References

1. Noji EK: *The public health consequences of disasters,* New York, 1997, Oxford University Press.
2. Noji EK, Siverston KT: Injury prevention in natural disasters: a theoretical framework, *Disasters* 11:290, 1987.
3. Cuny SC: Introduction to disaster management. Lesson 5. Technologies of disaster management, *Prehosp Disaster Med* 6:372, 1993.
4. Burkle FM, editor: *Disaster medicine: application for the immediate management and triage of civilian and military disaster victims,* New Hyde Park, NY, 1984, Medication Examination Publishing.
5. Burkle FM, Hogan DE, Burstein JL: *Disaster medicine,* Philadelphia, Baltimore, 2002, Lippincott, Williams & Wilkins.
6. Super-G START: a triage training module, Newport Beach, Calif, 1984, Hoag Memorial Hospital Presbyterian.
7. Burkle FM, Newland C, Orebaugh S, et al: Emergency medicine in the Persian Gulf. Part II. Triage methodology lessons learned, *Ann Emerg Med* 23:748, 1994.

Suggested Reading

Briggs SM, Brinsfield KH: *Advanced disaster medical response: manual for providers,* Boston, 2003, Harvard Medical International.

De Boer J, Dubouloz M: *Handbook of disaster medicine, emergency medicine in mass casualty situations,* National Society of Disaster Medicine, Netherlands, 2000, Van der Wees.

De Boer J, Rutherford WH: Definition and quantification of disaster: introduction of a disaster severity scale, *J Emerg Med* 8:602, 1990.

Eachempati SR, Flomenbaum N, Barie PS: Biological warfare: current concerns for the health care provider, *J Trauma* 52:179, 2002.

Emerg Med Clin North Am 14(2), 1996 (entire issue).

Feliciano DV, et al: Management of casualties from the bombing at the centennial Olympics, *Am J Surg* 176(6):538, 1998.

Hirshberg A, Holcomb JB, Mattox KL: Hospital trauma care in multiple-casualty incidents: a critical view, *Ann Emerg Med* 37(6):647, 2001.

Rutherford WH, De Boer J: The definition and quantification of disaster, *Injury* 15:1, 1983.

Slater MS, Trunkey DD: Terrorism in America: an evolving threat, *Arch Surg* 132(10):1059, 1997.

Stein M, Hirshberg A: Medical consequences of terrorism: the conventional weapon threat, *Surg Clin North Am* 79(6):1537, 1999.

Chapter Objectives

*At the completion of this chapter, the reader
will be able to do the following:*

✓ Understand the essential considerations regarding mitigation of a
  weapon of mass destruction (WMD) event:

  Scene assessment
  Incident command
  Personal protective equipment
  Patient triage
  Principle of decontamination

✓ Understand the mechanisms of injury, evaluation and management,
  and transport considerations associated with specific categories of
  WMD agent:

  Explosive agents
  Incendiary agents
  Chemical agents
  Biologic agents
  Radiologic agents

✓ Know how to access and utilize resources for further study.

CHAPTER 20

Weapons of Mass Destruction

SCENARIO

You are dispatched to the scene of a reported explosion. The dispatcher indicates that several blasts have been witnessed by callers. The number of victims is unknown. Other public safety agencies have been dispatched to the location.

On arrival at the transit terminal, you note that you are the first EMS responder on scene. No incident command has yet been established. A burning transit train, the target of an explosive device, is sitting on the tracks. Dozens of people are running about the platform. Many are screaming for you to assist fellow passengers who are apparently trapped on the burning train. Others are lying immobile on the platform.

What will you do first? What are your priorities as you determine your course of action? How will you care for so many people? How will you save those trapped in the burning train? ■

Preparing to manage a weapon of mass destruction (WMD) event challenges emergency medical services (EMS) systems every day. Recent history has demonstrated that these events can occur at any time and in any location. The 1993 World Trade Center bombing resulted in only six deaths, but yielded 548 casualties, with more than 1000 victims being assisted by EMS. Responders sustained casualties as well, with 105 firefighters reporting injuries. The 1995 explosion at the Murrah Federal Building in Oklahoma City resulted in 168 deaths, with 700 known injuries. One third of the patients brought to one Oklahoma City hospital came by EMS, and they were the sickest, with 64% requiring admission to the hospital, compared with only 6% of those self-referring to the emergency department (ED). The 2001 World Trade Center attacks yielded over 1100 injured survivors, with almost a third of those patients arriving at the hospital by EMS. Rescue workers accounted for 29% of the injured victims.

Although conventional high explosives are the most common and most likely form of WMD event, EMS systems have also been challenged by chemical and biohazard events. The 1994 sarin gas attack in Matsumoto, Japan, killed seven, but injured more than 300. The more widely known 1995 sarin gas attack in the Tokyo subway system killed 12, but more than 5000 victims sought medical attention. The Tokyo Fire Department sent 1364 firefighters to the 16 affected subway sites; 135 responders were affected by direct or indirect exposure.

No life-threatening bioterrorism assault in the United States has yielded a large number of casualties, but this does not mean that EMS systems have not been challenged to prepare for bioterrorism threats. During 1998 and 1999, almost 6000 persons across the United States were affected by a series of anthrax-related hoaxes in more than 200 incidents. The anthrax letters delivered in the fall of 2001 resulted in only 22 cases of clinical anthrax, but generated countless calls for EMS to respond to suspicious packages and powders. Also, although not a bioterrorist event, a

naturally occurring biohazard, severe acute respiratory syndrome (SARS), seriously challenged the Toronto EMS system. During the epidemic, 526 of their paramedics had to be quarantined, the vast majority secondary to potential unprotected exposure to the virus, seriously straining that EMS system's ability to mitigate the crisis.

The threat that EMS may one day have to respond to a radiologic WMD event grows, with increasing speculation that terrorists may detonate a "dirty bomb" that will generate injuries and panic about radioactive contamination.

General Considerations

Scene Assessment and Incident Command System

The ability of the prehospital care provider to assess the scene properly will be crucial to the provider's safety and that of other responders and will ensure the best delivery of service to the patient. WMD events pose significant threats to responding emergency services. In the case of a high-explosives detonation, there may be fire, spilled hazardous materials, power line hazards, and risk of falling debris or subsidence. A rescue worker was killed by falling debris in response to the Oklahoma City bombing,[1] and many more were killed in the 2001 World Trade Center attack. Chemical attacks potentially expose the emergency responder to the offending agent not only from its primary source, the weapon, but also from contamination of victims' skin, clothing, and personal belongings. Biohazards, depending on the form of their delivery, pose a risk of injury from the offending agent (e.g., concentration of aerosolized anthrax spores) or from transmission of a communicable disease (e.g., encountering patient with smallpox). A further risk to emergency responders and patients alike is the possibility of a secondary device, for example, a second bomb placed at the scene of the incident, set to explode after arrival of emergency responders, with the intention of increasing not only injury, but also confusion and panic.

The prehospital provider will take all these factors into consideration when evaluating a scene and needs to comprehend their significance before taking action. Prehospital providers also need to communicate their observations through the chain of command so that proper steps can be taken to mount an appropriate response, increasing the safety of the responders and the delivery of care to patients. The *incident command system* (ICS) defines the chain of command through which this communication takes place. The ICS is the model tool for command, control, and coordination. It was developed to mitigate the recurring failures of response to disasters, which include the following:

1. Nonstandard terminology of responding agencies
2. Lack of capability to expand and contract as required by the situation
3. Nonstandard and nonintegrated communications
4. Lack of consolidated action plans
5. Lack of designated facilities

ICS offers a management structure that coordinates all available resources to ensure an effective response. All incidents, regardless of size or complexity, will have an *incident commander,* who may be the first responding prehospital provider, until relieved by some competent authority (see Chapter 4). It is essential that prehospital providers become familiar with and have the opportunity to practice implementation of the ICS.

Personal Protective Equipment

When responding to WMD events, proper personal protective equipment (PPE) needs to be considered. PPE requirements may range from the standard daily uniform to a fully encapsulated suit with *self-contained breathing apparatus* (SCBA). PPE is designed to protect the prehospital provider from exposure to offending agents by providing varying protection of the respiratory tract, skin, and other mucous membranes. Civilian PPE has generally been described in terms of the following levels:

- *Level A.* The respiratory tract is protected by an SCBA or *supplied air respirator* (SAR) delivering air to the prehospital provider with positive pressure. A chemical-resistant barrier that completely encapsulates the wearer protects the skin and mucous membranes. This level offers the highest respiratory and skin protection.
- *Level B.* The respiratory tract is protected in the same manner as in Level A protection, with positive-pressure–supplied air. Nonencapsulated chemical-

resistant garments, including suit, gloves, and boots, which provide splash protection only, protect the skin and mucous membranes. The highest respiratory protection is afforded, with a lower level of skin protection.
- *Level C.* The respiratory tract is protected by an *air-purifying respirator* (APR). This may be a powered air-purifying respirator (PAPR), which draws ambient air through a filter canister and delivers it under positive pressure to a facemask or hood, or a nonpowered APR, which relies on the wearer to draw ambient air through a filter canister by breathing through a properly fitted mask. The skin protection is the same as for Level B.
- *Level D.* This represents standard work clothes (i.e., uniform for prehospital care provider) and may also include a gown, gloves, and surgical mask. This level provides minimal respiratory protection and minimal skin protection.

PPE is selected based on the known hazards of the environment and proximity to the threat. Proximity to the threat has often been described in terms of the following zones:

- The *hot zone* is the area where there is immediate threat to health and life. This might include an environment contaminated with a hazardous gas, vapor, aerosol, liquid, or powder. PPE adequate to protect the prehospital care provider is determined based on potential routes of exposure to the substance. Level A protection is often used in the hot zone.
- The *warm zone* is characterized as an area where the concentration of the offending agent is limited. In the case of a hazardous materials (hazmat) scene, this is characterized as the area to which victims are brought from the hot zone and where decontamination is taking place. The prehospital care provider is still at risk for hazmat exposure in this area as it egresses from the hot zone on victims, responders, and equipment. PPE is recommended based on potential routes of exposure to the substance.
- The *cold zone* is characterized as an area that is not contaminated, where there is no risk of hazmat exposure, and thus no specific level of PPE is required.

It is important to note that it is often difficult to define these hazard zones and that they are often dynamic and not static. Factors that contribute to the dynamics of the zones include the activity of the victims and responders and ambient conditions. Unless completely incapacitated, contaminated victims might walk toward prehospital care providers in the "cold zone" or leave the scene completely, either in panic or with the intention of seeking aid at a nearby medical treatment facility or their personal physician. By design, warm zones and cold zones are designated upwind of the hot zone, but if wind direction changes, prehospital care providers would be at risk of hazmat exposure if unable to don personal PPE or to retreat. These contingencies must be anticipated when planning for or responding to a WMD event.

It might be concluded that the best protective posture for a prehospital care provider is always to respond in the highest level of protection, Level A, regardless of the threat. This is, however, not a reasonable response. Level A protection is cumbersome, often making manual tasks difficult to perform. It puts the wearer at risk for heat stress and physical exhaustion. It can make communication between responders and victims difficult. Appropriate PPE must be recommended based on the threat and the operational responsibilities of the prehospital care provider.

Patient Triage

Prehospital care providers will potentially face a large and overwhelming number of victims who will require evaluation and treatment after a WMD event. Every EMS system should identify and rehearse a mechanism for rapidly triaging victims. The objective of patient triage is to do the greatest good for the greatest number of victims. Field triage is typically based on physiologic criteria that assign patients to severity categories, identifying those who require treatment and transport to a medical treatment facility most urgently.[2] Several triage criteria are published.[3] The START (simple triage and rapid treatment) system is typically used. Patient severity is determined in an algorithmic fashion by first assessing ability to ambulate, then airway, respirations, circulation, and mental status. Patients are usually assigned to one of four severity categories. *Nonurgent/ambulatory* ("green") patients do not have life-threatening injury and will likely do well even if care is withheld several hours or days. *Urgent* ("yellow") patients have a serious injury but will likely not deteriorate with a slight delay in care. *Emergent* ("red") patients are critical and will require immediate care. *Expectant* ("black") patients are dead or have injuries not compatible with life. A fifth category ("blue") has been used on occasion for patients requiring decontamination.

Whatever patient triage system is utilized, it must be employed in routine EMS operations to promote familiarity and to ensure recognition among emergency service providers at all levels of care, including the medical treatment facility.

Principles of Decontamination

Patients and prehospital care providers alike may require decontamination after exposure to adherent solids or liquids that may pose a risk to the patient or other health care personnel. These individuals should have decontamination procedures performed in the field in a designated decontamination area. Exposure to only gases will not require decontamination to prevent secondary contamination.

Decontamination areas are typically upwind and uphill of the affected area when conditions allow.

Decontamination is a two-step process that first involves removal of all clothing, jewelry, and shoes, which are bagged and tagged for later identification. Removing clothing achieves removal of 70% to 90% of contamination. Any solid contamination should be carefully brushed away from the patient, and any liquid contamination should be blotted off. The second step involves washing the skin surfaces with water or water and a mild detergent to ensure removal of all substances from the patient's skin. Avoid using harsh detergents or bleach solutions on skin. Chemically or physically aggravating the skin may contribute to increased absorption of the offending agent. When washing, the skin folds, axillae, groin, buttocks, and feet must receive special attention because contaminants can collect in these areas and may be overlooked by patients in their cleansing efforts.

Decontamination should be performed in a systematic manner to avoid missing areas of contaminated skin. For the eyes, contact lenses should be removed and mucous membranes irrigated with copious amounts of water or saline, especially if the patient is symptomatic. Ambulatory patients should be able to assist with their own decontamination under instruction from prehospital care providers. Nonambulatory patients will require the assistance of individuals properly outfitted to decontaminate litter patients. Expeditious decontamination may be warranted in the effort to decrease exposure time to various life-threatening substances. All prehospital care providers need to be familiar with a hasty decontamination procedure that may be executed even before arrival of the formal hazmat/decon team, to minimize exposure time for both patients and responders.

Issues to consider include (1) offering privacy for males and females required to disrobe, (2) having warm water available for irrigation, (3) providing a suitable substitute for clothing at the completion of decontamination, (4) assuring victims that their personal belongings will be secure until a final disposition is made regarding their return or necessary disposal, and (5) collection of effluent, if practical.

Specific Threats

Explosive Agents

Explosions are by far the most common cause of casualties associated with terrorism. Of 93 reported terrorist attacks producing more than 30 casualties in the world from 1991 to 2000, 88% involved explosions.[4]

Categories of Explosives

Explosives are characterized as *high-order explosives* (HE) and *low-order explosives* (LE). Because they are designed to detonate and release their energy very quickly, HE are capable of producing a shock wave, or *overpressure phenomenon*, which can result in primary blast injury. Because they release their energy much more slowly, LE are not capable of producing this overpressure. Examples of HE include TNT, C-4, Semtex, nitroglycerine, dynamite, and ammonium nitrate fuel oil. Examples of LE include pipe bombs, gunpowder, and pure-petroleum–based bombs such as Molotov cocktails.[5]

Mechanisms of Injury

Traumatic injury after explosions has been divided into three categories: primary, secondary, and tertiary blast injury.[6]

Primary blast injury (PBI) is that caused by the shock wave or overpressure that is produced after detonation of HE. This is not to be confused with wind generated by a blast; a *shock wave* is significantly increased atmospheric pressure produced by the almost instantaneous combustion of HE. Overpressures from these detonations can exceed 4 million pounds per square inch (psi), compared with 14.7 psi ambient pressure. The shock wave or pressure wave then disseminates from the point of origin, gradually dissipating as the distance from the point of combustion increases. Depending on the proximity of the victim to the blast, as well as shielding or augmentation of the wave secondary to detonations in a closed space, a victim may suffer PBI.

PBI occurs in gas-filled organs such as the lung, bowel, and middle ear. Solid organs are generally not affected by this phenomenon. The injury to the tissue occurs at the gas-fluid interface, presumably from a rapid compression of the gas in the organ, causing violent collapse of that organ, followed by an equally rapid and violent expansion, resulting in tissue injury. Damage to the lung manifests as pulmonary contusions, or possibly hemopneumothoraces, resulting in hypoxemia if the patient does not immediately succumb from the injuries. Alveoli can also become disrupted, resulting in arterial gas emboli, which may cause cerebral or cardiac embolic complications. Damage to the bowel may include petechiae or hematomas of the bowel wall or even perforation of the bowel. Tympanic membrane rupture or disruption of the middle ear ossicles also may occur.

Evidence of PBI to the lung is more often found in patients who die minutes after the explosion from associated injuries; however, pulmonary PBI has been noted more frequently among surviving victims of confined-space explosions. It has also been associated with other severe injuries and is indicative of increased mortality in survivors. After an open-air explosion in Beirut, only 0.6% of survivors had evidence of PBI, and 11% of those died.[7] In a confined-space explosion in Jerusalem, 38% of survivors had evidence of PBI, with a similar mortality rate of approximately 9%.[8]

Secondary blast injury is that caused by flying debris and bomb fragments. These projectiles are components of the bomb itself, as from military weapons designed to fragment or from improvised bombs augmented with nails, screws,

and bolts. Secondary blast injury is also caused by debris that is carried by the blast wind. Blast winds associated with the force required to create enough overpressure to rupture 50% of exposed tympanic membranes (approximately 5 psi) can briefly generate winds of 145 mph. Winds associated with the force necessary to create an overpressure resulting in significant PBI may exceed 831 mph.[6] Although brief in duration, these winds can propel debris with great force and for great distances, causing both penetrating and blunt trauma.

Tertiary blast injury is that caused by the body being thrown by the blast wind, resulting in tumbling and collision with stationary objects. This can result in the whole spectrum of injuries associated with blunt trauma and even penetrating trauma, such as impalement.

Other trauma associated with a blast, such as thermal injury, inhalation injury, and injury from structural collapse, has been described as *quaternary blast injury* (see Chapter 3).[5]

Injury Patterns

The prehospital care provider will be confronted with a combination of familiar penetrating, blunt, and thermal injuries and possibly survivors with PBI. The numbers and types of injury will depend on multiple factors, including explosion magnitude, composition, environment, and location and number of potential victims at risk.

Various mortality rates have been associated with different types of bombing. One study that examined 29 terrorist bombings showed that 1 of 4 victims died immediately after structural-collapse bombings, 1 of 12 died immediately in closed-space bombings, and 1 of 25 died immediately after open-space bombings.[4] Soft tissue injuries, orthopedic trauma, and traumatic brain injury (TBI) are predominant among survivors.

For example, of 592 survivors of the Oklahoma City bombing,[9] 85% had soft tissue injuries (lacerations, puncture wounds, abrasions, contusions), 25% had sprains, 14% had head injuries, 10% had fractures/dislocations, 10% had ocular injuries (nine with ruptured globes), and 2% had burns. The most common location for soft tissue injury was extremities (74%), followed by head and neck (48%), face (45%), and chest (35%). Eighteen survivors had severe soft tissue injuries, including carotid artery and jugular vein lacerations, facial and popliteal artery lacerations, and severed nerves, tendons, and ligaments. Seventeen survivors had serious internal organ injury, including partial bowel transection, lacerated kidney, spleen, and liver, pneumothorax, and pulmonary contusion. Of patients with fractures, 37% had multiple fractures. Of those diagnosed with a head injury, 44% required admission to the hospital.[9]

Evaluation and Management

The general evaluation and management of trauma victims is applicable to the WMD patient population and are addressed in other chapters. Unique to this patient population,

Blast Lung Injury: What Prehospital Providers Need to Know

Current patterns in worldwide terrorist activity have increased the potential for casualties related to explosions, yet few civilian Emergency Medical Services (EMS) providers in the United States have experience treating patients with explosion-related injuries. Blast lung injury (BLI) presents unique triage, diagnostic, and management challenges and is a direct consequence of the blast wave from high-explosive detonations upon the body. Persons in enclosed space explosions or those in close proximity to the explosion are at a higher risk. BLI is a clinical diagnosis characterized by respiratory difficulty and hypoxia. BLI can occur, although rarely, without obvious external injury to the chest.

CLINICAL PRESENTATION
- Symptoms may include dyspnea, hemoptysis, cough, and chest pain.
- Signs may include tachypnea, hypoxia, cyanosis, apnea, wheezing, decreased breath sounds, and hemodynamic instability.
- Victims with greater than 10% BSA burns, skull fractures, and penetrating torso or head injuries may be more likely to have BLI.
- Hemothoraces or pneumothoraces may occur.
- Due to tearing of the pulmonary and vascular tree, air may enter the arterial circulation ("air emboli") and result in embolic events involving the central nervous system, retinal arteries, or coronary arteries.
- Clinical evidence of blast lung injury is typically present at the time of initial evaluation; however, it has been reported to occur over the course of 24 to 48 hours after an explosion.
- Other injuries are often present.

PREHOSPITAL MANAGEMENT CONSIDERATIONS
- Initial triage, trauma resuscitation, and transport of patients should follow standard protocols for multiple injured patients or mass casualties.
- Note the patient's location and the surrounding environment. Explosions in a confined space result in a higher incidence of primary blast injury, including lung injury.
- All patients with suspected or confirmed BLI should receive supplemental high-flow oxygen sufficient to prevent hypoxemia.
  - Impending airway compromise requires immediate intervention.
  - If ventilatory failure is imminent or occurs, patients should be intubated; however, prehospital providers must realize that mechanical ventilation and positive pressure may increase the risk of alveolar rupture, pneumothorax, and air embolism in BLI patients.
  - High-flow oxygen should be administered if air embolism is suspected, and the patient should be placed in a prone, semi-left lateral, or left lateral position.
- Clinical evidence of, or suspicion for, a hemothorax or pneumothorax warrants close observation. Chest decompression should be performed for patients clinically presenting with a tension pneumothorax. Close observation is warranted for any patient with suspicion of BLI who is transported by air.
- Fluids should be administered judiciously, as overzealous fluid administration in the patient with BLI may result in volume overload and the worsening of pulmonary status.
- Patients with BLI should be transported rapidly to the nearest, appropriate facility, in accordance with community response plans for mass casualty events.

From Centers for Disease Control and Prevention, Atlanta.

however, is the possibility of PBI. Primary blast injuries might increase the likelihood that prehospital care providers will encounter patients with hemoptysis and pulmonary contusions, pneumothorax or tension pneumothorax, or even arterial gas embolism. The likelihood of multisystem trauma is increased in bomb victims.[10] Management principles are similar to those for trauma from other mechanisms.

Transportation Considerations

Patients requiring transport must be brought to an appropriate medical treatment facility for further evaluation and management. These patients will often require the services of a designated trauma center. Prehospital providers should be aware of the epidemiology of patient transport after these events. Patient arrival at hospitals is usually bimodal, with ambulatory patients arriving first and more critically ill patients arriving later by ambulance. This was demonstrated in the Oklahoma City bombing. Patients began to arrive in the EDs 5 to 30 minutes after the bombing, with patients requiring admission taking longer to arrive. Also, the geographically closest hospitals in Oklahoma City received the majority of victims, as seen with other disasters. Nearby hospitals that are overwhelmed by the first wave of patients may experience some difficulty managing the critically ill patients that arrive in the second wave. In Oklahoma City the aggregate peak arrival rate of patients to EDs was 220 per hour at 60 to 90 minutes; 64% of patients visited EDs within a 1.5-mile radius of the event. Prehospital care providers should consider this latter fact when determining the destination of patients from the bomb scene.[1]

Incendiary Agents

Incendiary agents are typically encountered in the military and are used to burn equipment, vehicles, and structures. The three incendiaries recognized most often are magnesium, thermite, and white phosphorus. All three are highly flammable compounds that burn at extremely high temperatures.

Thermite is powdered aluminum and iron oxide that burns furiously at 3600° F and scatters molten iron.[11] Its primary mechanism of injury is partial-thickness or full-thickness burns. The primary and secondary assessment is performed with intervention directed at treating burns. Thermite wounds can be irrigated and copious amounts of water, and contaminating particles subsequently removed.

Magnesium is also a metal in powdered or solid form that burns furiously hot. In addition to its ability to cause second-degree and third-degree burns, magnesium can react with tissue fluid and cause alkali burns. The same chemical reaction produces hydrogen gas, which can cause the wound to bubble or can result in subcutaneous emphysema. Inhalation of magnesium dust can produce respiratory symptoms, including cough, tachypnea, hypoxia, wheeze, pneumonitis, and airway burns. Residual magnesium particles in a wound will react with water, so irrigation is discouraged until the wounds can be debrided and the particulate removed. If irrigation is required for other reasons, such as decontamination of another suspected material, care should be taken to ensure flushing or removal of magnesium particles from the wound.[11]

White phosphorus (WP) is a solid that spontaneously ignites when exposed to air, causing a yellow flame and white smoke. WP that comes in contact with skin can quickly result in second-degree and third-degree burns. WP can become embedded in the skin, propelled by the blast of WP munitions. The substance will continue to burn in the skin if exposed to air. Prehospital care providers can decrease the likelihood of combustion in the skin by immersing the affected areas in water or applying saline-soaked dressings to the area. Oily or greasy dressings are avoided in these patients because WP is lipid soluble, and application of these dressings may increase the likelihood of systemic toxicity. Copper sulfate has historically been used to neutralize WP and facilitate its removal because the reaction resulted in a black compound, which was easier to identify in the skin. Copper sulfate has fallen out of favor, however, because of complications from its use, specifically, intravascular hemolysis.[12]

Chemical Agents

Many scenarios could expose the prehospital care provider to chemical agents, including an industrial complex accident, a spilled tanker truck, unearthed military ordnance, or a terrorist attack. The 1984 Union Carbide industrial accident in Bhopal, India, and the sarin gas attack in Tokyo in 1995 are examples of such incidents.

Classification of Chemical Agents

Cyanides
    Hydrogen cyanide, cyanogen chloride
Nerve Agents
    Tabun (GA), sarin (GB), soman (GD), GF, VX
Lung toxicants (choking agents)
    Chlorine, phosgene, diphosgene
Vesicants (blistering agents)
    Mustard, lewisite
Incapacitating agents
    BZ
Lacrimating agents (riot control agents)
    CN, CS
Vomiting agents
    Adamsite

Physical Properties of Hazardous Materials

The physical property of a substance is affected by its chemical structure, the temperature, and ambient pressure. These factors will determine whether a substance exists as a solid, liquid, or gas. Understanding the physical state of a material is important for the prehospital care provider because it gives clues as to the likely route of exposure and the potential for transmission and contamination.

A *solid* is in a state of matter that has a fixed volume and shape; a powder is an example of a solid. When heated to a melting point, solids become *liquids*. Liquids that are heated to their boiling point become a *gas*. Solid particles and liquid particles can become suspended in the air, similar to a dust particle or a liquid mist. This is considered an *aerosol*. A *vapor* is simply a solid or liquid that is in a gaseous state, but technically would be expected to be found as a solid or liquid at standard temperature and pressure, defined as 32° F and normal atmospheric pressure (1 ATA, 14.7 psi). Some solids and liquids can therefore emit vapors at room temperature. When solids emit vapors, bypassing the liquid state, this is called *sublimation*. The likelihood that solids or liquids vaporize into a gaseous form at room temperature is defined as the *volatility* of the substance. Highly volatile substances easily convert into a gas at room temperature.

These physical properties have implications for primary and secondary contamination and possible routes of exposure. *Primary contamination* is defined as exposure to the hazardous substance at its point of release. For example, primary contamination occurs, by definition, in the "hot zone." Gases (vapors), liquids, solids, and aerosols can all play a role in primary contamination. *Secondary contamination* is defined as exposure to the hazardous substance after it has been carried away from the point of origin by a victim, a responder, or a piece of equipment. Secondary contamination occurs in the "warm zone." Solids and liquids (and sometimes aerosols) generally contribute to secondary contamination. Gases (vapors), which cause injury by inhalation of the substance, do not deposit on skin or contain substances and therefore do not typically play a role in secondary contamination, although vapors can become trapped in clothing. Volatility plays a significant role in risk of secondary contamination. More volatile substances are considered "less persistent," meaning that because they vaporize, the likelihood of long-lasting physical contamination is unlikely. Less volatile substances are considered "more persistent." These substances do not vaporize, or do so at a very slow rate, thereby remaining on exposed surfaces for a long time, increasing the risk of secondary contamination. For example, the nerve agent sarin is a nonpersistent agent, whereas the nerve agent VX is a persistent agent.[13]

Personal Protective Equipment

PPE is selected based on the threat of exposure to the hazardous substance. Level A provides respiratory and skin protection from gases (vapors), solids, liquids, and aerosols. Because it also has supplied air, Level A PPE is suitable for oxygen-deprived environments. Level B provides the same respiratory protection as Level A, but only provides skin and splash protection suitable for solids and liquids. Level C provides respiratory protection from selected vapors and aerosols and skin and splash protection from solids and liquids. Level D provides no particular respiratory or skin protection from chemical hazards.

Evaluation and Management

After ensuring the safety of the scene, and that the victim has been properly decontaminated, the prehospital care provider will often encounter patients with signs and symptoms of exposure to a hazardous substance of which the identity has not yet been determined. Victims of chemical agents can manifest signs and symptoms of exposure that affect (1) the respiratory system, affecting oxygenation and ventilation; (2) the mucous membranes, causing eye and upper airway injury; (3) the nervous system, resulting in seizures or coma; (4) the gastrointestinal (GI) tract, causing vomiting or diarrhea; and (5) the skin, causing burning and blistering.

Patients will require a primary survey to determine what lifesaving intervention may be immediately required. A secondary survey may then assist in the identification of symptom constellations that might indicate the nature of the hazardous substance and suggest a specific antidote. This constellation of signs and symptoms has been called a *toxidrome*. A toxidrome is a collection of signs and symptoms that suggest exposure to a certain class of chemical or toxin.[14]

The *irritant gas toxidrome* will include mucous membrane burning and inflammation, coughing, and difficulty breathing. Agents responsible might include chlorine, phosgene, or ammonia.

The *asphyxiant toxidrome* is caused by cellular oxygen deprivation. This can result from inadequate oxygen availability, as in an oxygen-poor atmosphere; inadequate oxygen delivery to the cells, as in carbon monoxide poisoning; or inability to utilize oxygen at the cellular level, as in cyanide poisoning. Signs and symptoms include shortness of breath, chest pain, dysrhythmias, syncope, seizures, coma, and death.

The *cholinergic toxidrome* is characterized by cough, respiratory secretions, difficulty breathing, nausea, vomiting, diarrhea, profuse sweating, pinpoint pupils and possible altered mental status, seizures, and coma. Pesticides and nerve agents can cause these cholinergic signs and symptoms.

Most often, prehospital care providers will initiate supportive therapy, without knowing the cause of the injury. If the offending agent is properly identified, or if its identity is suggested by a toxidrome, therapy specific to the agent may be delivered. Cyanide and nerve agent victims are examples of patients who can benefit from agent-specific therapy.

Transportation Considerations

Patients must be brought to an appropriate medical treatment facility for further evaluation and management. Communities may identify preferred hospitals for the management of chemical casualties. These facilities may be more capable of managing these patients by virtue of specialized training or availability of critical care services and specific antidotes. Also, considerations similar to those previously noted for HE incidents, regarding transport epidemiology, also apply to these patients. Nearby EDs may become overwhelmed by ambulatory patients. Of 640 patients presenting to one hospital in Tokyo after the sarin incident, 541 arrived without EMS assistance.[15] Hospitals closest to the event will likely receive the largest number of ambulatory patients. These factors should be considered in determining the destination of casualties via ambulance.

Selected Specific Agents[13,16,17]

Cyanides. Prehospital care providers might encounter cyanides when responding to a fire in which certain plastics are burning. Cyanide is present in large quantities in certain industrial complexes, where it is used in chemical syntheses, electroplating, mineral extraction, dyeing, printing, photography, and agriculture, and in the manufacture of paper, textiles, and plastics. Cyanide has been inventoried in military stockpiles.

Hydrogen cyanide is a highly volatile liquid and thus will most often be encountered as a vapor or gas. It therefore has greater potential for mass casualties in a confined space with poor ventilation than if released outdoors. Although a smell of bitter almonds has been associated with this agent, this is not a reliable indicator of hydrogen cyanide exposure.

Cyanide's mechanism of action is arrest of metabolism or respiration at the cellular level, quickly resulting in cell death. Patients who are ventilating will present with evidence of acyanotic hypoxia.

The organs most affected are the central nervous system (CNS) and the heart. Symptoms of mild cyanide poisoning include headache, dizziness, drowsiness, nausea, vomiting, and mucosal irritation. Severe cyanide poisoning includes alteration of consciousness, dysrhythmias, hypotension, and death. Death can occur within a few minutes after inhalation of cyanide gas.

Supportive therapy is important, including high-concentration oxygen delivery, correction of hypotension with fluids or pressors, and treatment of seizures. Cyanide antidote kits are available for patients with known or suspected cyanide poisoning. The administration of inhaled amyl nitrite, or preferably intravenous (IV) sodium nitrite, creates methemoglobin, which binds cyanide in the bloodstream, making it less available to poison the victim's cellular respiration. This is followed by IV administration of sodium thiosulfate to assist the body in the conversion of cyanide to harmless thiocyanate, which is excreted by the kidneys.

Nerve Agents. Nerve agents can be found in military stockpiles. The most recent use in a military conflict was in the Iraq-Iran war. Nerve agents have also been produced by terrorist organizations, the most notorious releases occurring in Matsumoto (1994) and Tokyo (1995), Japan. Commonly available pesticides (e.g., malathion, Sevin) and common therapeutic drugs (e.g., physostigmine, pyridostigmine) share properties with nerve agents, causing similar clinical effects.

Nerve agents are usually liquids at room temperature. *Sarin* is the most volatile of the group. *VX* is the least volatile and is found as an oily liquid. The main routes of intoxication are through inhalation of the vapor and absorption through the skin. Nerve agents can injure or kill at very low doses. A small drop of VX, the most potent nerve agent, if evenly distributed, could kill 1000 victims. Because nerve agents are liquids, they pose a risk for secondary contamination from clothes, skin, and other objects.

The mechanism of action of nerve agents is the inhibition of the enzyme acetylcholinesterase. This enzyme is necessary to inhibit the action of acetylcholine. *Acetylcholine* is a neurotransmitter that stimulates cholinergic receptors. These receptors are found in smooth muscles, skeletal muscles, the CNS, and most exocrine (secretory) glands. Some of these cholinergic receptors are termed *muscarinic* sites (because experimentally they are stimulated by muscarine), mostly found in smooth muscles and glands. Others are termed *nicotinic* sites (because experimentally they are stimulated by nicotine), mostly found in skeletal muscle. The mnemonic *DUMBELS* (**d**iarrhea, **u**rination, **m**yosis, **b**radycardia, bronchorrhea, bronchospasm, **e**mesis, **l**acrimation, **s**alivation, sweating) represents the constellation of symptoms associated with the muscarinic effects of nerve agent toxicity. The mnemonic *MTWHF* (**m**ydriasis,

tachycardia, **w**eakness, **h**ypertension, hyperglycemia, **f**asciculations) represents the constellation of symptoms associated with stimulation of nicotinic receptors. The CNS effects, a result of both muscarinic and nicotinic receptors, include confusion, convulsions, and coma.

The clinical effects depend on the dose and route of nerve agent exposure, whether inhalation or dermal. Small amounts of vapor exposure primarily cause irritation to eyes, nose, and airways. Large amounts of vapor exposure can quickly lead to loss of consciousness, seizures, apnea, and muscular flaccidity. Miosis is the most sensitive marker of exposure to vapor. Symptoms of dermal exposure also vary according to dose, as does time of onset. Small doses may not result in symptoms for several hours. Skin fasciculations and local sweating may occur, followed by GI symptoms, nausea, vomiting, and diarrhea. Large dermal doses will result in onset of symptoms in minutes, with effects similar to a large vapor exposure.

Clinical symptoms of the nerve agents include rhinorrhea, chest tightness, miosis (pupil is pinpoint, and patient complains of blurry or dim vision), shortness of breath, excessive salivation and sweating, nausea, vomiting, abdominal cramps, involuntary urination and defecation, muscle fasciculations, confusion, seizures, flaccid paralysis, coma, respiratory failure, and death.

Management of nerve agent poisoning includes decontamination, a primary survey, administration of antidotes, and supportive therapy. Ventilation and oxygenation of the patient may be difficult because of bronchoconstriction and copious secretions. The patient will likely require frequent suctioning. These symptoms improve after the antidote is administered. The three therapeutic drugs for the management of nerve agent poisoning are atropine, pralidoxime chloride, and diazepam.

Atropine is an anticholinergic drug that controls the muscarinic effects of the nerve agent, while having little effect on the nicotinic effects. Atropine is indicated for exposed victims with pulmonary complaints. Miosis alone is not an indication for atropine. Atropine will be given according to system protocols. Atropine is titrated until the patient's ability to breathe or ventilate is improved or there is a drying of pulmonary secretions. In moderate to severe exposures, it is not unusual to give 10 to 20 mg of atropine over a few hours.

Pralidoxime chloride (2-PAM chloride) is an oxime. Pralidoxime works by uncoupling the bond between the nerve agent and acetylcholinesterase, thereby reactivating the enzyme and helping to reduce the effects of the nerve agent, primarily on nicotinic receptors. The oxime therapy needs to be initiated within minutes to a few hours of the exposure to be effective; otherwise, the bond between acetylcholinesterase and the nerve agent will become permanent ("aging"), delaying recovery of the patient.

Diazepam (Valium) is a benzodiazepine and anticonvulsant. If patients develop seizures after significant exposure, benzodiazepine therapy is initiated to manage the seizures and help to reduce the brain injury and other life-threatening effects associated with status epilepticus.

The Mark-1 kit supplies two autoinjectors, one filled with atropine (2 mg) and one filled with pralidoxime chloride (600 mg). These are intended for rapid intramuscular (IM) injection in the event of a nerve agent exposure. Dosage is determined by protocol and titration of these drugs to effect. These autoinjector kits are available to the military and other government agencies.

Lung Toxicants. Lung toxicants, including chlorine, phosgene, ammonia, sulfur dioxide, and nitrogen dioxide, are present in industrial manufacturing applications. *Phosgene* has been stockpiled for military applications and was the most lethal chemical warfare agent used in World War I.

Chemical pulmonary agents may be gases (vapors) or aerosolized liquids or solids. The properties of the agent influence its ability to cause injury. For example, aerosolized particles of 2 microns (μm) or smaller readily access the alveoli of the lung, causing injury there, whereas larger particles are filtered out before reaching the alveoli. Water solubility of an agent also affects the injury pattern. Ammonia and sulfur dioxide, which are highly water soluble, cause irritation and injury to the eyes, mucous membranes, and upper airways. Phosgene and nitrogen oxides, which have low water solubility, tend to cause less immediate irritation and injury to the eyes, mucous membranes, and upper airways, thus providing little warning to the victim and allowing for prolonged exposure to these agents. Prolonged exposure makes it more likely that the alveoli will be injured, resulting in not only upper airway injury, but also alveolar collapse and noncardiogenic pulmonary edema. Moderately water-soluble agents such as chlorine can cause both upper airway and alveolar irritation.

The mechanisms of injury vary among the lung toxicants. Ammonia, for example, combines with the water in the mucous membranes to form a strong base, ammonium hydroxide. Chlorine, when combined with water, produces hydrochloric acid, causing injury to the tissues. Lung toxicants are not systemically absorbed but compromise the victim by damaging components of the pulmonary system, from the upper airway to the alveoli.

The agents with high water solubility cause burning of the eyes, nose, and mouth. Tearing, rhinorrhea, coughing, dyspnea, and respiratory distress secondary to glottic irritation or laryngospasm are possible. Bronchospasm can result in coughing, wheezing, and dyspnea. Agents with low water solubility, causing injury to the alveoli, can immediately injure the alveolar epithelium in the case of a large exposure, leading to death from acute respiratory failure, or with less massive exposure can result in a delayed onset of respiratory distress secondary to development of mild noncardiogenic pulmonary edema or fulminant acute respiratory distress syndrome (ARDS), depending on the dose.

Management of lung toxicants includes removal of the patient from the offending agent, decontamination (if solid, liquid, or aerosol), primary survey, and supportive therapy, which will likely require interventions to maximize ventilation and oxygenation. Eye irritation can be managed with copious irrigation using normal saline. Contact lenses should be removed. Expect to manage copious airway secretions, which will require suctioning. Bronchospasm may respond to inhaled β-adrenergic agonists. Hypoxia will require correction with high-flow oxygen and possibly intubation. Prehospital care providers need to be prepared to encounter a difficult endotracheal intubation secondary to copious secretions, inflammation of glottic structures, and laryngeal spasm.

Vesicant Agents. The vesicants include sulfur mustard, nitrogen mustards, and lewisite. These agents have been stockpiled for military operations. Sulfur mustard was first introduced to the battlefield in World War I. It was reportedly used by Iraq against its Kurdish population and also in its conflict with Iran (1980). It is described as easy and inexpensive to manufacture.

Sulfur mustard is an oily, clear to yellow-brown liquid that can be aerosolized by a bomb blast or a sprayer. Its volatility is low, allowing it to persist on surfaces for a week or more. This allows for easy secondary contamination. The agent is absorbed through the skin and mucous membranes, resulting in direct cellular damage, with dose-dependent clinical symptoms 1 to 12 hours after exposure. The delayed onset of symptoms can make it difficult to recognize exposure and therefore increases the likelihood of secondary contamination. Warm, moist skin increases the likelihood of skin absorption, making the groin and axillary regions particularly susceptible. The eyes, skin, and upper airways can develop a range of findings, from erythema and edema to vesicle development and necrosis. Upper airway involvement can result in cough and bronchospasm. High-dose exposures can result in nausea and vomiting, as well as bone marrow suppression.

Treatment involves decontamination, primary survey, and supportive therapy; no antidote exists for the effects of mustard agents. Eyes and skin should be decontaminated with copious amounts of water as soon as exposure is recognized, to minimize further absorption of the agent and prevent secondary contamination. Absorbed agent cannot be decontaminated and will result in cellular injury. The fluid in resulting vesicles and blisters is not a source of secondary contamination. Pulmonary bronchoconstriction may benefit from nebulized β-agonists. Skin wounds should be treated as burns, with regard to local wound care.

Lewisite has a similar constellation of symptoms, but the onset of action is much quicker than with sulfur mustard, resulting in immediate pain and irritation to the eyes, skin, and respiratory tract. Also unique to this agent is "lewisite shock," the result of intravascular volume depletion secondary to capillary leak. British anti-lewisite (BAL) is an antidote available for the treatment of lewisite-exposed patients. It is administered intravenously for patients with hypovolemic shock or pulmonary symptoms. Applied topically, BAL ointment has been reported to prevent mucous membrane and skin injury.

Biologic Agents

Biologic agents in the form of contagious disease represent a threat to prehospital care providers on a daily basis. Proper infection control procedures must be in place to prevent the contraction or transmission of tuberculosis, influenza, human immunodeficiency virus (HIV), methicillin-resistant streptococci, SARS, and a myriad of other organisms.

Preparing for bioterrorist events increases the complexity of EMS system preparation. Patients with pathogens not typically seen by EMS personnel, such as plague, anthrax, and smallpox, might be encountered, requiring appropriate PPE and precautions. Familiar infection control procedures will be effective in the safe management of these potentially contagious patients. An intentional terrorist act, however, might include delivery of a hazardous agent with the potential to cause disease or illness, such as aerosolized anthrax spores, aerosolized live organisms, or an aerosolized biologic toxin. If the prehospital care provider is responding to an overt event, appropriate precautions regarding decontamination of victims and PPE are required, similar to other hazmat events.

Classification of Biologic Agents

Bacterial agents
   Anthrax
   Brucellosis
   Glanders
   Plague
   Q fever
   Tularemia
Viral agents
   Smallpox
   Venezuelan equine encephalitis
   Viral hemorrhagic fevers
Biologic toxins
   Botulinum
   Ricin
   Staphylococcal enterotoxin B
   T-2 mycotoxins

Concentrated Biohazard Agent vs. Infected Patient

Prehospital care providers can experience bioterrorism in two forms. The first scenario is encountering an environment or a patient contaminated with a suspicious substance. The anthrax hoaxes of 1998 and 1999 and the anthrax letters of 2001 are good examples. Prehospital providers responded on countless occasions to individuals covered in "white powder" or suspected anthrax. EMS services may be summoned to suspicious activity, such as a device delivering an unknown aerosol agent. The nature of the threat at these events is usually unknown, and precautions for personal safety should always be paramount. These events must be respected as hazmat events until characterized otherwise. If the suspicious substance is in fact a concentrated aerosol of an infectious organism or toxin, PPE appropriate for the hazard and some form of decontamination will likely be required.

The second scenario is encountering a patient who has been a victim of a remote, covert bioterrorist event. Perhaps an individual inhaled anthrax spores after a covert attack at work and now, several days later, is manifesting signs of pulmonary anthrax. Perhaps a terrorist has inoculated himself with smallpox, and you are summoned to assist the unconscious victim with a suspicious rash. In these cases, personal and public safety can be assured by knowledge of proper infection control procedures and the proper donning and removal of PPE appropriate for the biohazard (Boxes 20-1 and 20-2).

BOX 20-1 Sequence for Donning Personal Protective Equipment (PPE)

The type of PPE used will vary based on the level of precautions required (e.g., Standard Precautions and contact, droplet, or airborne infection isolation).

1. GOWN
- Fully cover torso from neck to knees, arms to end of wrists, and wrap around the back
- Fasten in back of neck and waist

2. MASK OR RESPIRATOR
- Secure ties or elastic bands at middle of head and neck
- Fit flexible band to nose bridge
- Fit snug to face and below chin
- Fit-check respirator

3. GOGGLES OR FACE SHIELD
- Place over face and eyes and adjust to fit

4. GLOVES
- Extend to cover wrist of isolation gown

Use safe work practices to protect yourself and limit the spread of contamination:

- Keep hands away from face
- Limit surfaces touched
- Change gloves when torn or heavily contaminated
- Perform hand hygiene

From Centers for Disease Control and Prevention, Atlanta.

BOX 20-2 Sequence for Removing Personal Protective Equipment (PPE)

Except for the respirator, remove PPE at doorway or in an anteroom. Remove respirator after leaving patient room and closing door.

1. GLOVES
- Outside of glove is contaminated!
- Grasp outside of glove with opposite gloved hand; peel off
- Hold removed glove in gloved hand
- Slide fingers of ungloved hand under remaining glove at wrist
- Peel glove off over first glove
- Discard gloves in waste container

2. GOGGLES
- Outside of goggles or face shield is contaminated!
- To remove, handle by head band or ear pieces
- Place in designated receptacle for reprocessing or in waste container

3. GOWN
- Gown front and sleeves are contaminated!
- Unfasten gown ties
- Pull away from neck and shoulders, touching inside of gown only
- Turn gown inside out
- Fold or roll into a bundle and discard

4. MASK OR RESPIRATOR
- Front of mask/respirator is contaminated—do not touch!
- Grasp bottom, then top ties or elastics, and remove
- Discard in waste container

From Centers for Disease Control and Prevention, Atlanta.

PPE for infection control purposes should be familiar to all prehospital care providers. Different levels of PPE are recommended, depending on the potential for transmission and the likely route of transmission. Transmission-based PPE is used in addition to the Standard Precautions, which are used in the care of all patients. These include contact, droplet, and aerosol precautions.

Contact Precautions. This level of protection is recommended to reduce the likelihood of transmission of microorganisms by direct or indirect contact. Contact precautions include the use of gloves and a gown. Typically encountered organisms that require contact precautions include viral conjunctivitis, methicillin-resistant streptococci, scabies, and herpes simplex or zoster virus. Organisms that might be encountered as a result of bioterrorism include bubonic plague or the viral hemorrhagic fevers, such as Marburg or Ebola, as long as the patient does not have pulmonary symptoms or profuse vomiting and diarrhea.

Droplet Precautions. This level of protection is recommended to reduce the likelihood of transmission of microorganisms that are known to be transmitted by large droplet nuclei (>5 μm) expelled by an infected person in the course of talking, sneezing, or coughing or during routine procedures such as suctioning. These droplets infect the susceptible individual by landing on the exposed mucous membranes of the eye and mouth. Because the droplets are large, they do not remain suspended in air, and therefore contact must be in close proximity, usually defined as 3 feet or less. Droplet precautions include the gloves and gown of contact precautions, but also add eye protection and a surgical mask. Because the droplets do not remain suspended in air, no additional respiratory protection or air filtration is required. Typically encountered organisms in this category include influenza, mycoplasma pneumonia, and invasive *Haemophilus influenzae* or *Neisseria meningitidis* causing sepsis or meningitis. Pneumonic plague is an example of a possible agent encountered as a result of a bioterrorist event.

Aerosol Precautions. This level of protection is recommended to reduce the likelihood of transmission of microorganisms by the airborne route. Some organisms can become suspended in the air attached to small droplet nuclei (<5 μm) or attached to dust particles. In this case, microorganisms can become widely dispersed by air currents immediately around the source or far from the source, depending on conditions. These patients are kept in isolation rooms in which the exhaust ventilation can be filtered. Aerosol precautions include gloves, gown, eye protection, and a fit-tested high-efficiency particulate air (HEPA) filter mask, such as the N-95. Examples of illnesses typically encountered include tuberculosis, measles, chickenpox, and SARS. Smallpox or viral hemorrhagic fever with pulmonary symptoms are examples that could possibly be related to a bioterrorist event.

Note that many illnesses associated with bioterrorist events require no additional protection beyond Standard Precautions, provided there is no risk of exposure to a concentrated agent. Examples include patients with inhalational anthrax or a biologic toxin such as botulinum.

Selected Agents

Anthrax. Anthrax is a disease caused by the bacterium *Bacillus anthracis.* The disease is naturally occurring, contracted most often by persons in contact with infected animals or anthrax-contaminated animal products. The bacterium has been weaponized and is known to be inventoried in several nations' military stockpiles. The accidental release of aerosolized anthrax spores from a Soviet military facility at Sverdlovsk in 1979 resulted in approximately 79 cases of pulmonary anthrax with 68 reported deaths. Letters contaminated with anthrax spores were sent through the U.S. mail in 2001 to prominent legislators and media outlets. Although only 22 cases (11 pulmonary, 11 cutaneous) and five deaths were related to anthrax, thousands required prophylaxis with antibiotics. An efficient release of 100 kg of anthrax spores over Washington, DC, is reported to be capable of causing 130,000 to 3 million deaths.[18]

B. anthracis is a spore-forming bacterium and thus can exist as a vegetative cell or as a spore. The vegetative cell lives well in a host organism but cannot survive long outside the body, unlike the spore, which can be viable in the environment for decades.

Routes of exposure to anthrax include the respiratory tract, the GI tract, and breaks in the skin. Exposure to anthrax through the respiratory tract leads to inhalational or pulmonary anthrax. Exposure through the GI tract causes gastrointestinal anthrax, and skin exposure causes cutaneous anthrax.

Gastrointestinal anthrax is rare and would be the result of ingesting food substances contaminated with spores. Patients would have nonspecific symptoms of nausea, vomiting, malaise, bloody diarrhea, and acute abdomen; mortality is approximately 50%. Cutaneous anthrax follows deposition of spores or organisms into a break in the skin. This results in a papule, which subsequently ulcerates and causes a dry, black eschar with local edema. If not treated with antibiotics, mortality approaches 20%; with antibiotics, mortality is less than 1%.

For effectiveness, anthrax would likely be disseminated in its spore form. Anthrax spores are approximately 1 to 5 μm in size, which allows the spores to be suspended in air as an aerosol. Aerosolized spores can be inhaled into the lungs and deposited in the alveoli. They are then consumed by macrophages and brought to the mediastinal lymph nodes, where they germinate, generate toxins, and cause acute hemorrhagic mediastinitis and often death. The onset of symptoms after inhalation of spores varies, with most developing symptoms within 1 to 7 days, but there may be a latency period as long as 60 days. Symptoms are nonspecific, including fever, chills, dyspnea, cough, chest pain, headache, and vomiting. After a few days, symptoms improve, followed by a rapidly deteriorating course of fever, dyspnea, diaphoresis, shock, and death.[19] Before the 2001 anthrax attacks, mortality from inhalational anthrax was thought to be 90%, but recent experience suggests that with early antibiotic therapy and critical care services, mortality may be less than 50%.[20]

Inhalational anthrax is not contagious and does not pose a risk to the prehospital care provider. Only exposure to aerosolized spores poses a risk of infectivity. Caring for patients infected with inhalational anthrax requires only Standard Precautions. The prehospital care provider

will provide supportive therapy and transport ill patients to facilities where critical care services are available.

Often, prehospital care providers will not be caring for patients infected with the disease, but rather, victims contaminated with spores on their skin or clothing. Any person coming in direct physical contact with a substance alleged to be anthrax should remove articles of clothing and perform a thorough washing of exposed skin with soap and water.[19] Clinically significant reaerosolization of spores from victims' skin or clothing is unlikely, and the risk to the provider is negligible.[21] As a matter of routine practice, however, clothing normally removed by pulling over the face and head should instead be cut off to minimize any risk of inadvertent inhalation of contaminant.

Prophylaxis with antibiotics is only required for individuals who have been exposed to spores. Local public health officials will determine the appropriate antibiotic and length of prophylactic treatment. The latest recommendations suggest 60 days of therapy with oral doxycycline or a quinolone antibiotic.

An anthrax vaccine does exist, and an immunization program for U.S. military forces was instituted in 1998. The current regimen requires a series of six initial shots and annual boosters. It is currently recommended only for military personnel and for laboratory and industrial workers at high risk for exposure to spores.

Plague. Plague is a disease caused by the bacterium *Yersinia pestis*. It is naturally occurring, found in fleas and rodents. If an infected flea bites a human, the person can develop *bubonic plague*. If this local infection goes untreated, the patient can become systemically ill, resulting in septicemia and death. A number of patients may proceed to develop pulmonary symptoms *(pneumonic plague)*. Plague was responsible for the "Black Death" of 1346, which killed 20 to 30 million people in Europe, approximately one third of its population at that time. *Y. pestis* has been weaponized for military stockpiles with techniques developed to aerosolize the organism directly, bypassing the animal vector. The World Health Organization (WHO) reports that in a worst-case scenario, 50 kg of *Y. pestis*, released as an aerosol over a city of 5 million, would result in 150,000 cases of pneumonic plague and 36,000 deaths.[22]

Naturally occurring plague, resulting from the bite of an infected flea, will cause symptoms in 2 to 8 days, with onset of fever, chills, weakness, and acutely swollen lymph nodes (buboes) in the neck, groin, or axilla. Untreated patients can deteriorate to systemic illness and death. Twelve percent have been described as developing pneumonic plague, with complaints of chest pain, dyspnea, cough, and hemoptysis, and these patients can also succumb from systemic illness.

Plague occurring from terrorist deployment of a weapon will likely result from aerosolized organisms, and thus it will clinically present differently. Inhalation of *Y. pestis* aerosol will result in symptoms in 1 to 6 days. Patients will present with fever, cough, and dyspnea, with bloody or watery sputum. They may also develop nausea, vomiting, diarrhea, and abdominal pain. Buboes are not typically present. Without antibiotics, death occurs in 2 to 6 days after development of respiratory symptoms.[23]

Currently, no vaccine is available to protect from pneumonic plague. Treatment of the disease includes antimicrobial and supportive therapy, often requiring critical care services. Antibiotic regimens are also recommended for individuals with unprotected close exposure to patients with known pneumonic plague.

Patients with plague represent a communicable disease risk. If patients present with only cutaneous signs and symptoms (bubonic plague), contact precautions are adequate to protect the prehospital care provider. If patients present with pulmonary signs of plague (pneumonic plague), a more likely scenario after a terrorist attack, providers will be required to wear PPE suitable for respiratory droplet protection. Droplet precautions include a surgical mask, eye protection, gloves, and gown. Prehospital care providers responding to the scene of an overt *Y. pestis* aerosol delivery, which is unlikely to be a recognized event, would require PPE suitable for a hazmat environment if entering the hot zone or warm zone. Plague victims are treated with supportive therapy. Communication with the receiving facility is vital before arrival to ensure that the pneumonic plague patient can be properly isolated in the ED and that staff are prepared with the appropriate PPE. Asking the patient to wear a surgical mask, if tolerated, may also decrease the likelihood of secondary transmission.

Decontamination of the vehicle and equipment is similar to that required after transport of any patient with communicable disease. Contact surfaces should be wiped down with an Environmental Protection Agency (EPA)–approved disinfectant or 1:1000 diluted bleach solution. There is no evidence to suggest that *Y. pestis* poses a long-term environmental threat after dissolution of the primary aerosol.[23] The organism is sensitive to heat and sunlight and does not last long outside the living host. *Y. pestis* does not form spores.

Smallpox. Smallpox is also known as *variola major* and *variola minor*. This naturally occurring disease was eradicated in 1977 but still exists in at least two laboratories—Russia's Institute of Virus Preparations and the U.S. Centers for Disease Control and Prevention (CDC). It has been alleged that the Soviet government began a program in 1980 to produce large quantities of smallpox virus to be used in bombs and missiles, as well as develop more virulent strains of the virus for military purposes. There is concern that smallpox virus may have changed hands after the dissolution of the Soviet Union.[24]

The smallpox virus infects its victim by entering the mucous membranes of the oropharynx or respiratory

Day 3 of rash   Day 5 of rash   Day 7 of rash

On any part of the body, all lesions are in the same stage of development.

Most patients have lesions on the palms or soles   Umbilicated lesions   Confluent lesions

FIGURE 20-1 Smallpox.
(Courtesy Centers for Disease Control and Prevention, Atlanta.)

mucosa. After a 12- to 14-day incubation period, the patient develops fever, malaise, headache, and backache. The patient then develops a maculopapular rash that starts on the oral mucosa, but quickly progresses to a generalized skin rash with characteristic vesicles and pustules. The rash is characteristically a round, tense pustule, which tends to affect the head and extremities more densely than the trunk (centrifugal), with the stage of the lesions appearing uniform (Figure 20-1). This distinguishes smallpox from *varicella*, or chickenpox (Box 20-3), which begins and is more dense on the trunk (centripetal) and has lesions at various stages of development (new lesions appear with older, crusted lesions) (Figure 20-2). Mortality from naturally occurring smallpox was approximately 30%. Little is known about the natural course of the disease in immunocompromised patients, such as those with HIV.

Smallpox is a contagious disease that is primarily spread by droplet nuclei projected from the oropharynx of infected patients and by direct contact. Contaminated clothing and bed linens can also spread the virus. Patients are contagious beginning at the onset of the rash, although this might not always be obvious if the rash is subtle in the oropharynx. If having to manage a patient with smallpox, prehospital providers must wear PPE appropriate for contact, droplet, and aerosol precautions. This includes N-95 mask, eye protection, goggles, and gown. Ideally, persons managing patients with smallpox will have been immunized.[25]

BOX 20-3 Differentiating Chickenpox from Smallpox

Chickenpox (varicella) is the most likely condition to be confused with smallpox.

In chickenpox:

- No prodrome or mild prodrome
- Lesions are superficial vesicles: "dewdrop on a rose petal"
- Lesions appear in crops; on any one part of the body, there are lesions in different stages (papules, vesicles, crusts)
- Centripetal distribution: greatest concentration of lesions on the trunk, fewest lesions on distal extremities. Lesions may involve the face/scalp; occasionally, entire body equally affected
- First lesions appear on the face or trunk
- Patients rarely toxic or moribund
- Rapid evolution: lesions evolve from macules → papules → vesicles → crusts quickly (<24 hours)
- Palms and soles rarely involved
- Patient lacks reliable history of varicella or varicella vaccination
- From 50% to 80% of patients recall an exposure to chickenpox or shingles 10 to 21 days before rash onset

From Centers for Disease Control and Prevention, Atlanta.

Healthy child with varicella Healthy adult with varicella Bacterial super-infection of varicella lesions

Note centripetal distribution of rash Day 3 of rash Lesions are in different stages of development

Healthy adult with varicella Healthy adult with varicella Pregnant woman with varicella

FIGURE 20-2 Chickenpox.
(Courtesy Centers for Disease Control and Prevention, Atlanta.)

The smallpox vaccination program was stopped in 1972. The residual immunity provided by this vaccination program is unknown, and it is suggested that individuals whose last immunization was 40 years ago will likely not be immune from contracting smallpox.[24] Vaccination for the smallpox virus is available to certain U.S. Department of Defense and State Department members. It is also made available under a Department of Health and Human Services program to develop Smallpox Response Teams. It is currently only available to the general public for participants in clinical trials. In case of a public health emergency, the United States has stockpiles of vaccine that can be released for mass immunization of the public. Vaccination within 4 days of the exposure has been shown to offer some protection against contracting the illness and substantial protection against a fatal outcome.[24]

Prehospital care providers will provide supportive care to manage a patient with smallpox. The recommended PPE must be worn at all times, and it is imperative that there is no breach in infection control procedures. Hospitals with the appropriate isolation facilities and properly trained staff should be identified in the community. The receiving facility must be contacted to inform them of the intention

to transport the confirmed or suspected case of smallpox to their facility so that proper precautions can be taken to prevent transmission of the virus. The identification of a patient with smallpox will be considered a public health emergency of enormous significance.

Proper removal of PPE without breach in infection control procedures is important for the safety of the prehospital care provider. All contaminated disposable medical waste must be properly bagged, labeled, and disposed of as other regulated medical waste. Reusable medical equipment must be cleaned after use according to standard protocol, either autoclaved or subject to high-level disinfection. Environmental surfaces need to be cleaned only by an approved EPA-registered detergent-disinfectant. Air decontamination or fumigation of the emergency vehicle is not required.[26]

Botulinum Toxin. Botulinum toxin is produced by the bacterium *Clostridium botulinum* and is the most poisonous substance known. It is 15,000 times more toxic than VX and 100,000 times more toxic than sarin.[27] The Aum Shinrykyo cult, responsible for the Tokyo subway sarin attack, attempted to deliver an aerosol of botulinum toxin without success in 1995. Botulinum toxin has been weaponized for military use. Despite the reported difficulty of concentrating and stabilizing the toxin for dissemination, it is estimated that a terrorist point-source delivery of botulinum aerosol could incapacitate or kill 10% of persons downwind 0.5 km (0.3 mile). The toxin could also be introduced into the food supply in an attempt to poison large numbers of people.

Three forms of botulism exist naturally. *Wound botulism* occurs when toxins are absorbed from a dirty wound, often with devitalized tissue, in which *C. botulinum* is present. *Food-borne botulism* occurs when improperly canned foods allow the bacteria to grow and produce toxin, which is ingested by the victim. *Intestinal botulism* occurs when toxin is produced and absorbed within the GI tract. The fourth and man-made form of botulism is a result of aerosolized botulinum toxin, causing *inhalational botulism.*

Regardless of the route, botulinum toxin is carried to the neuromuscular junction, where it binds irreversibly, preventing binding of the neurotransmitter acetylcholine and causing a descending flaccid paralysis. Onset of symptoms is several hours to a few days. All patients will present with diplopia and multiple cranial nerve deficits, causing difficulty with sight, speech, and swallowing. The extent and rapidity of the descending paralysis depend on dose. Patients become fatigued, lose the ability to control their head, may lose their gag reflex, or may develop respiratory failure, requiring intubation and months of mechanical ventilation. Untreated patients usually die of mechanical upper airway obstruction or inadequate ventilation. The classic triad of botulinum toxicity is (1) descending symmetric flaccid paralysis with cranial nerve deficits, (2) afebrile, and (3) a clear sensorium. After weeks to months, patients may recover as new axon buds develop to innervate the denervated muscles.

Care for the patient with botulism is supportive, with administration of antitoxin. Early use of antitoxin will minimize further deterioration but cannot reverse existing paralysis. This antitoxin is available from the CDC.

Prehospital providers caring for victims of botulism need to be vigilant about airway compromise and inadequate ventilation. Patients may not be able to manage their secretions or maintain a patent airway. Because of diaphragm paralysis, patients may not be able to generate an adequate tidal volume. This may be exacerbated by having the patient in a supine or semirecumbent position. Patients experiencing respiratory difficulty should be intubated and adequately ventilated.

Standard Precautions are adequate for the management of patients experiencing the effects of botulinum toxicity because it is not a contagious disease. Botulism aerosols degrade readily in the environment, and it is anticipated that after delivery in a terrorist incident, substantial inactivation will occur after 2 days. Prehospital care providers responding to an overt aerosol dissemination event will require PPE suitable for a hazmat environment if working in the hot zone or warm zone. Because the aerosol can persist for approximately 2 days under average weather conditions, decontamination of victims who have been exposed to botulinum aerosol require decontamination by clothing removal and washing with soap and water. Equipment can be decontaminated using a 0.1% hypochlorite bleach solution.[28] Patients will not require isolation after arrival at the hospital, but critical care services may be needed for patients requiring mechanical ventilation.

Radiologic Disasters

Since the terrorist attacks of September 11, 2001, new consideration has been given to the likelihood of EMS systems needing to manage a radiologic emergency. Historically, planning has focused on civil service preparation for a strategic exchange of military nuclear weapons or the rare occurrence of a nuclear power plant accident. Currently, however, there is increasing awareness of the possibility that terrorists could deploy an improvised nuclear detonation device, or perhaps more likely a radiologic dispersal device, that uses conventional explosives to disseminate radioactive material into the environment.

Although radiologic accidents are rare, there have been 243 radiation accidents since 1944 in the United States with 1342 casualties that met criteria for significant exposure. Worldwide, 403 accidents have occurred, with 133,617 victims, 2965 with significant exposure, and 120 fatalities. The Chernobyl disaster was responsible for 116,500 exposed casualties and 28 deaths.[29]

Radiation disasters have the potential to generate fear and confusion in both victims and responders. Familiarization with the hazard and management principles will help to ensure an appropriate response and help to reduce panic and disorder (Box 20-4).

Exposure to ionizing radiation and radioactive contamination may result from several different scenarios: (1) detonation of a nuclear weapon, whether high grade or an improvised low-yield device; (2) detonation of a "dirty bomb" or radiation dispersion device (RDD), in which there is no nuclear detonation, but rather conventional explosives are detonated to disperse a radionuclide; (3) sabotage or accident at a nuclear reactor site; and (4) mishandled nuclear waste.

Medical Effects of Radiation Catastrophes

The injuries and risks associated with a radiologic catastrophe will be multifactorial. In the case of a nuclear detonation, casualties will be produced by the explosion, resulting in primary, secondary, and tertiary blast injuries, thermal injury, and structural collapse. Victims may be further subject to radiation injury from external irradiation; from external radioactive contamination, which can be deposited on skin and clothing; or from internal radiation through radioactive particulate contamination, which victims may inhale, ingest, or have deposited in wounds.

Accidents at nuclear reactors can generate large doses of ionizing radiation, without a nuclear detonation, especially under circumstances in which the reactor reaches a point of "criticality." Explosions, fire, and gas release can also result in radioactive gas or particulate matter, which may expose responders to risk of exposure to contamination with radioactive particles.

Radiation dispersion devices (RDDs) typically would not deliver enough radiation to cause immediate injury. However, RDDs would complicate management for prehospital care responders by distributing radioactive particulates that could contaminate victims and responders and make it difficult to manage the injuries caused by the conventional explosive. RDDs could cause confusion and panic among responders concerned about radioactivity, hindering efforts to assist victims.

Ionizing radiation causes injury to cells by interacting with atoms and depositing energy. This results in *ionization,* which can either damage the cell nucleus directly, causing cell death or malfunction, or indirectly, damaging cell components by interacting with water in the body and resulting in toxic molecules. Acute exposure to large doses of penetrating ionizing radiation (gamma rays and neutrons) in a short time can result in acute radiation illness. Types of ionizing radiation include alpha particles, beta particles, gamma rays, and neutrons.

Alpha particles are relatively large and cannot penetrate even a few layers of skin. Intact skin or a uniform offers adequate protection from external contamination emitting alpha particles. Ionizing radiation from alpha particles is a concern only if it is internalized by inhaling or ingesting alpha-particle emitters. When internalized, alpha-particle radiation can cause significant local cellular injury to adjacent cells.

Beta particles are small charged particles that can penetrate more deeply than alpha particles and can affect deeper layers of the skin, having the ability to injure the base of the skin, causing a "beta burn." Beta-particle radiation is found most frequently in nuclear fallout. Beta particles also result in local radiation injury.

Gamma rays are similar to x-rays and have the ability to easily penetrate tissue. Gamma rays are emitted with a nuclear detonation and with fallout. They can also be emitted from some radionuclides that might be present in an RDD. Gamma radiation can result in what is termed *whole-body exposure.* Whole-body exposure can result in acute radiation illness (Box 20-5).

Neutrons can penetrate tissue easily, with 20 times the destructive energy of gamma rays, disrupting the atomic structure of cells. Neutrons are released during a nuclear detonation but are not a fallout risk. Neutrons also contribute to whole-body exposure and can result in acute radiation illness. Neutrons have the ability to convert stable metals into radioactive isotopes. This has significance in patients with metal hardware or those in possession of metal objects at the time of exposure.

Whole-body exposure is measured in terms of the *gray* (Gy). The *rad* (radiation absorbed dose) was a familiar dose unit that yielded to the gray; 1 Gy equals 100 rad. The *rem* (radiation equivalent–man) describes the dose in rad multiplied by a "quality factor," which takes into account the intrinsic special deposition pattern of different types of radiation. The rem has been replaced with the *sievert* (Sv); 1 Sv equals 100 rem.

Radiation affects rapidly dividing cells most readily, resulting in injury to the bone marrow and GI tract, where high cell turnover rates occur. Higher doses can affect the CNS directly. The dose of whole-body exposure determines the medical consequences of the exposure. Patients receiving up to 1 Gy of whole-body irradiation would typically not exhibit signs of injury. At 1 to 2 Gy, less than half of

BOX 20-5   Terrorism with Ionizing Radiation: General Guide

DIAGNOSIS
Be alert to the following:

1. The acute radiation syndrome follows a predictable pattern after substantial exposure or catastrophic events (Table 20-1).
2. Individuals may become ill from contaminated sources in the community and may be identified over much longer periods based on specific syndromes (Table 20-2).
3. Specific syndromes of concern, especially with a 2- to 3-week prior history of nausea and vomiting, are:

- Thermal burn–like skin effects without documented thermal exposure
- Immunologic dysfunction with secondary infections
- Tendency to bleed (epistaxis, gingival bleeding, petechiae)
- Marrow suppression (neutropenia, lymphopenia, and thrombocytopenia)
- Epilation (hair loss)

UNDERSTANDING EXPOSURE
Exposure may be known and recognized or clandestine through:

1. Large recognized exposures, such as a nuclear bomb or damage to a nuclear power station.
2. Small radiation source emitting continuous gamma radiation, producing group or individual chronic intermittent exposures (e.g., radiologic sources from medical treatment devices, environmental water or food pollution).
3. Internal radiation from absorbed, inhaled, or ingested radioactive material (internal contamination).

Modified from Department of Veterans Affairs pocket guide produced by Employee Education System for Office of Public Health and Environmental Hazards. This information is not meant to be complete, but to be a quick guide; please consult other references and expert opinion.

patients will develop nausea and vomiting, many will subsequently develop leukopenia, and deaths will be minimal. Most victims receiving greater than 2 Gy will become ill and require hospitalization; at greater than 6 Gy, mortality becomes high. At doses greater than 30 Gy, neurologic signs are manifest, and death is most likely.[30]

Acute radiation illness manifests in a prodromal phase characterized by malaise, nausea, and vomiting. This is followed by a latent phase, in which the patient is essentially asymptomatic. The length of the latent phase depends on the total absorbed dose of radiation. The latent phase is followed by the subsequent illness, as manifested by the organ system that has been injured. Damage to the marrow occurs with total doses of 0.7 to 4.0 Gy and result in decreasing levels of white blood cells and decreased immunity over several days to weeks. Decreased platelets can result in easy bruising and bleeding. Decreased red blood cells will result in anemia. At 6 to 8 Gy the GI tract will also be affected, resulting in diarrhea, volume loss, and hematochezia. Above 30 Gy the patient will manifest symptoms of the neurovascular syndrome, experiencing the prodromal phase of nausea and vomiting, a short latent phase lasting only a few hours, followed by a rapid deterioration of mental status, coma, and death, sometimes accompanied by hemodynamic instability. Doses this high can occur after a nuclear detonation, but the victim will most likely have been killed by injuries associated with the blast. Victims could also be exposed to these high doses at a nuclear power facility where no blast has occurred, but a reactor core has reached criticality.[30]

Not all radiation accidents or terrorist events will result in high-dose radiation exposure. Low-dose radiation exposure, as would most likely occur after an RDD detonation, probably would not produce acute injury secondary to radiation. Dependent on dose, the patient may have an increased future risk of developing cancer. The acute effects of RDD detonation, besides the effects of the detonation of the conventional explosive, will likely be psychological, including stress reactions, fear, acute depression, and psychosomatic complaints, which will significantly strain the EMS agencies and medical infrastructure.

Patients can become contaminated with material that emits alpha, beta, and even gamma radiation, but the most common contaminants will emit alpha and beta radiation. Only gamma radiation contributes to whole-body irradiation, as previously described. Alpha and beta radiation have limited ability to penetrate, but still can cause local tissue injury. Patients can easily be decontaminated by clothing removal and washing. It is impossible for a patient to be so contaminated as to be a radiologic hazard to health care providers, so management of traumatic life-threatening injury is an immediate priority and should not be delayed pending decontamination.[30]

As described, radioactive particles can be inhaled, ingested, or absorbed through the skin or contaminated wounds. This type of exposure to radiation will not result in acute effects of radiation exposure but can result in delayed effects. Any victims, or responding personnel who operate in an area at risk for airborne radioactive particles, without the benefit of respiratory protection, will require subsequent evaluation to identify internal contamination, which may require medical intervention to dilute or block the effects of the radionuclide.

TABLE 20-1 Acute Radiation Syndrome

Feature	Effects of whole-body irradiation, from external radiation or internal absorption, by dose range in rad (1 rad = 1 cGy; 100 rad = 1 Gy)					
	0-100	100-200	200-600	600-800	800-3000	>3000
PRODROMAL PHASE OF SYNDROME						
Nausea, vomiting	None	5%-50%	50%-100%	75%-100%	90%-100%	100%
Time of onset		3-6 hr	2-4 hr	1-2 hr	<1 hr	Minutes
Duration		<24 hr	<24 hr	<48 hr	48 hr	N/A
Lymphocyte count	Unaffected	Minimally decreased	<1000 at 24 hr	<500 at 24 hr	Decreases within hours	Decreases within hours
Central nervous system (CNS) function	No impairment	No impairment	Routine task performance Cognitive impairment for 6-20 hr	Simple, routine task performance Cognitive impairment for >24 hr	Rapid incapacitation May have a lucid interval of several hours	
LATENT PHASE OF SYNDROME						
No symptoms	>2 wk	7-15 days	0-7 days	0-2 days	None	None
MANIFEST ILLNESS						
Signs/symptoms	None	Moderate leukopenia	Severe leukopenia, purpura, hemorrhage, pneumonia, hair loss after 300 rad		Diarrhea, fever, electrolyte disturbance	Convulsions, ataxia, tremor, lethargy
Time of onset		>2 wk	2 days-4 wk	2 days-4 wk	1-3 days	1-3 days
Critical period		None	4-6 wk; greatest potential for effective medical intervention		2-14 days	1-46 hr
Organ system	None		Hematopoietic; respiratory (mucosal) systems		GI tract Mucosal systems	CNS
Hospitalization duration	0%	<5% 45-60 days	90% 60-90 days	100% 100+ days	100% Weeks to months	100% Days to weeks
Mortality	None	Minimal	Low with aggressive therapy	High	Very high; significant neurologic symptoms indicate lethal dose	

Modified from Armed Forces Radiobiology Institute: *Medical management of radiological casualties*, Bethesda, Md, 2003.

Personal Protective Equipment

Prehospital care providers will be operating in an environment with risk of exposure to ionizing radiation after a radiologic disaster. The radiation risk will depend greatly on the type of radiologic event.

PPE available to prehospital care providers for use in chemical and biologic hazards will offer some protection from radioactive particulate contamination. It will not provide protection from high-energy radiation sources, however, such as a damaged reactor or nuclear blast at ground zero.

Radioactivity can be present in gases, aerosols, solids, or liquids. If radioactive gases are present, SCBA will offer the highest protection. If aerosols are present, an APR may be adequate to prevent internal contamination caused by

TABLE 20-2   Symptom Clusters as Delayed Effects after Radiation

1	2	3	4
Headache Fatigue Weakness	Anorexia Nausea Vomiting Diarrhea	Partial-thickness and full-thickness skin damage Epilation (hair loss) Ulceration	Lymphopenia Neutropenia Thrombocytopenia Purpura Opportunistic infections

Modified from Armed Forces Radiobiology Institute: *Medical management of radiological casualties*, Bethesda, Md, 2003.

inhalation of contaminated particles. An N-95 mask will offer some protection from inhaled particulates. Wearing a standard splash-resistant suit will protect against particulate that emits alpha radiation, will offer some protection from beta radiation, but will provide no protection from gamma radiation or neutrons. This type of barrier protection will assist in the decontamination of particulate matter from an individual, but it does not protect against the risks of acute radiation illness when the person is exposed to high-energy sources of external radiation. None of the typical PPE carried by prehospital providers protects from a high-energy point source of radiation. This type of radiation is encountered during the first minute of a nuclear detonation, in a critical reactor core, or with a high-energy radiation source such as cesium-137, which may be dispersed in an RDD. The best protection from these sources is decreased time of exposure, increased distance from the source, and shielding. Some new materials for first-responder PPE are being investigated that may offer some protection from low-level gamma radiation.

Unlike insufficient PPE for a chemical hazmat, the inhalation, ingestion, or skin absorption of radiation-emitting gas or particulate will not immediately incapacitate a prehospital care provider or victim. All prehospital providers who have operated in an environment potentially contaminated with radioactive material will have to undergo a radiation survey to determine if internal contamination has occurred and undergo active management if warranted.

Dose rate meters or alarms should be worn if available. Standards exist for acceptable doses of ionizing radiation in the occupational environment under normal and emergency conditions.[31] Dose rates of ionizing radiation can be measured to prevent responders from putting themselves at risk for acute radiation illness or an unacceptably higher incidence of cancer. The incident commander should be approached for guidance on radiation exposure readings and limits.

BOX 20-6   Treatment and Decontamination Considerations for Radiation Exposure

TREATMENT CONSIDERATIONS
- If trauma is present, treat
- If external radioactive contaminants are present, decontaminate
- If radioiodine (e.g., reactor accident) is present, consider giving prophylactic potassium iodide (Lugol's solution) within first 24 hours only (ineffective later)
- See http://www.afrri.usuhs.mil or http://www.orau.gov/reacts/guidance.htm

DECONTAMINATION CONSIDERATIONS
- Exposure without contamination requires no decontamination
- Exposure with contamination requires Standard (Universal) Precautions, removal of patient clothing, and decontamination with water
- Internal contamination will be determined at the hospital
- Treating contaminated patients before decontamination may contaminate the facility; plan for decontamination before arrival
- Patient with life-threatening condition: treat, then decontaminate
- Patient with non–life-threatening condition: decontaminate, then treat

Modified from Armed Forces Radiobiology Institute, *Medical management of radiological casualties*, Bethesda, Md, 2003.

Evaluation and Treatment

Patients who have been injured in a radiologic catastrophe should receive primary and secondary surveys as dictated by the mechanism of injury. Prehospital care providers can expect to evaluate patients who have sustained blast injury and thermal injury in the case of a nuclear detonation, or from the conventional HE detonation of an RDD (Box 20-6). Decontamination of the victim is recommended to eliminate radioactive particulate contamination but should not delay care of patients requiring immediate intervention for their injuries. If the patient does not show signs of serious injury requiring immediate intervention, the patient can be decontaminated first. If radioiodine is present in the environment, as might be encountered in a nuclear reactor or spent fuel rod accident or with detonation of a nuclear device, giving potassium iodide (KI) to responders and victims may help prevent accumulation of radioiodine in the thyroid, where it can increase the likelihood of cancer. Other blocking and decorporation therapy may be recommended by the hospital or federal assistance agencies when more information about the catastrophe is available.

Transportation Considerations

Patients should be transported to the nearest appropriate medical center that is capable of managing trauma and radiation injuries. All hospitals are required to have a plan for management of a radiologic emergency, but communities may have identified institutions that have decontamination facilities, are capable of managing trauma, and have staff trained to deal effectively with possible external or internal radioactive contamination, as well as the complications of whole-body exposure to ionizing radiation.

SUMMARY

Although weapons of mass destruction manufactured by terrorist regimes pose a significant threat to civilized society, prehospital care providers may also come in contact with explosions and chemical and radiologic material as the result of industrial mishaps. The safety of providers is paramount, and they should possess a working knowledge of levels of personal protective equipment and the fundamentals of decontamination. Explosive agents have predominated in recent terrorist attacks. High-order explosives produce primary blast injuries in survivors who are in close proximity to the blast, and secondary injuries result from flying debris.

Chemical agents may injure the skin and pulmonary system, but may also result in systemic illness, manifesting as a specific toxidrome that yields clues to the agent. Antidotes are used for some of these agents. Biologic agents can be highly virulent bacteria or viruses, or toxins produced by living organisms. The types of protective precautions used by providers vary with the specific agents. Several types of radiation exist. Exposure to these agents may result in acute radiation sickness, which is typically a function of the type of radiation and the length of exposure.

SCENARIO SOLUTION

The first priority is safety. Assess the scene. Note that a fire is still burning in the disabled train. Are there other hazards? Look for hanging debris, downed or exposed power lines, or hazmat spills. Briefly observe the crowd on the platform for evidence of a toxidrome. Is there an unusually high proportion of respiratory difficulty? Are victims vomiting and seizing? Is there evidence of agent dispersal in addition to the explosive blast? Look also for obvious evidence of a secondary device that may pose a threat to responders. Don PPE appropriate for the scenario.

Communicate with your chain of command. As the first EMS responder, the communications center will be relying on you for information. Describe pertinent details of the scene, observed hazards, numbers of victims, and likely number of resources required to manage the scene and victims. Based on your observations, the communications center and the on-duty supervisor can apprise other units and agencies of your situation and dispatch the necessary resources. A predefined disaster response plan may be activated.

Once the personal safety of the team has been assured and information has been communicated to the chain of command, prepare to serve as the incident commander until relieved by a competent authority. As soon as is feasible, approach the victims with the intention of triaging them for treatment and transport using the START algorithm. Without engaging in the medical management of victims initially, sort the victims into immediate, urgent, delayed, and expectant categories. As other assistance arrives, direct personnel to assume roles of the incident command system, until supervisory personnel arrive to assume command and control functions. ■

References

1. Hogan DE, Waeckerle JF, Dire DJ, et al: Emergency department impact of the Oklahoma City terrorist bombing, *Ann Emerg Med* 34:160, 1999.
2. Kennedy K, Aghababian R, Gans L, et al. Triage: Techniques and applications in decision making, *Ann Emerg Med* 28(2):136, 1996.
3. Garner A, Lee A, Harrison K: Comparative analysis of multiple-casualty incident triage algorithms, *Ann Emerg Med* 38:541, 2001.
4. Arnold J, Halpern P, Tsai M: Mass casualty terrorist bombings: a comparison of outcomes by bombing type, *Ann Emerg Med* 43:263, 2004.
5. Explosions and blast injuries: a primer for clinicians, http://www.bt.cdc.gov/masstrauma/explosions.asp (accessed August 2004).
6. Wightman JM, Gladish JL: Explosions and blast injuries, *Ann Emerg Med* 37:664, 2001.
7. Frykberg ER, Tepas JJ, Alexander RH: The 1983 Beirut Airport terrorist bombing: injury patterns and implications for disaster management, *Am Surg* 55:134, 1989.
8. Katz E, Ofek B, Adler J, et al: Primary blast injury after a bomb explosion in a civilian bus, *Ann Surg* 209:484, 1989.
9. Mallonee S, Shariat S, Stennies G, et al: Physical injuries and fatalities resulting from the Oklahoma City bombing, *JAMA* 276:382, 1996.
10. Peleg K, Limor A, Stein M, et al: Gunshot and explosion injuries: characteristics, outcomes, and implications for care of terror-related injuries in Israel, *Ann Surg* 239(3):311, 2004.
11. Burstein JL: CBRNE. Incendiary agents: magnesium and thermite, http://www.emedicine.com/emerg/topic917.htm less (accessed October 2004).
12. Irizarry L, Diaz-Acala J: CBRNE. Incendiary agents: white phosphorus, http://www.emedicine.com/emerg/topic918.htm (accessed October 2004).
13. Sidell FR, Takafuji ET, Franz DR, editors: *Medical aspects of chemical and biological warfare,* TMM series, Part 1, Warfare, weaponry and the casualty, Washington, DC, 1997, Office of the Surgeon General, TMM Publications.
14. Walter FG, editor: *Advanced HAZMAT life support,* ed 2, Tucson, 2000, Arizona Board of Regents.
15. Okumura T, Takasu N, Ishimatsu S, et al: Report on 640 victims of the Tokyo subway sarin attack, *Ann Emerg Med* 28(2):129, 1996.
16. US Army, Medical Research Institute of Chemical Defense: *Medical management of chemical casualties handbook,* ed 3, 2000, Aberdeen Proving Ground, Md.
17. Greenfield RA, Brown BR, Hutchins JB, et al: Microbiological, biological and chemical weapons of warfare and terrorism, *Am J Med Sci* 323(6):326, 2002.
18. US Congress, Office of Technology Assessment: *Proliferation of weapons of mass destruction,* Pub No OTA-ISC-559, Washington, DC, US Government Printing Office.
19. Ingelsby TV, Henderson DA, Bartlett JG, et al. Anthrax as a biological weapon: medical and public health management, *JAMA* 281(18):1735, 1999.
20. Bell DM, Kozarsky PE, Stephens DS: Conference summary: clinical issues in the prophylaxis, diagnosis and treatment of anthrax, *Emerg Infect Dis* 8(2):222, 2002.
21. Keim M, Kaufmann AF: Principles for emergency response to bioterrorism, *Ann Emerg Med* 34(2):177, 1999.
22. World Health Organization (WHO): *Health aspects of chemical and biological weapons,* Geneva, 1970, WHO.

23. Inglesby TV, Dennis DT, Henderson DA: Plague as a biological weapon: medical and public health management, *JAMA* 283(17):2281, 2000.

24. Henderson DA, Inglesby TV, Bartlett, JG: Smallpox as a biological weapon: medical and public health management, *JAMA* 281(22):2127, 1999.

25. Centers for Disease Control and Prevention (CDC): *Smallpox response plan and guidelines*, Version 3.0, Guide C, Part 1, Atlanta, 2002, CDC, p 13.

26. Centers for Disease Control and Prevention (CDC): *Smallpox response plan and guidelines,* Version 3.0, Guide F, Atlanta, 2003, CDC, p 1.

27. Franz DR, Jahrling PB, Friedlander AM, et al: Clinical recognition and management of patients exposed to biological warfare agents, *JAMA* 278(5):399, 1997.

28. Arnon SS, Schechter R, Inglesby TV, et al: Botulinum toxin as a biological weapon: medical and public health management, *JAMA* 285(8):1059, 2001.

29. Hogan DE, Kellison T: Nuclear terrorism, *Am J Med Sci* 323(6):341, 2002.

30. Armed Forces Radiobiology Institute: *Medical management of radiological casualties,* Bethesda, Md, 2003.

31. Department of Homeland Security Working Group on Radiological Dispersion Device Preparedness/Medical Preparedness and Response Subgroup, http://www1.va.gov/emshg/docs/Radiologic_Medical_Countermeasures_051403.pdf (accessed September 2004).

Additional Resources

http://www.bt.cdc.gov/

http://www.usamriid.army.mil/

https://ccc.apgea.army.mil/

http://hld.sbccom.army.mil/

http://wmdfirstresponders.com/

Chapter Objectives

At the completion of this chapter, the reader
will be able to do the following:

✓ Describe the components of Protective Medicine and how medical care supports each mission.

✓ Explain the benefits of a TEMS program.

✓ Discuss how emergency medical care differs in each of the three zones of care.

✓ Relate how remote assessment methodology may be used on a tactical mission.

✓ Describe the role of medical support for counterterrorism operations.

CHAPTER 21

Civilian Tactical Emergency Medical Support

SCENARIO

Your ambulance is dispatched for an injured police officer. On arrival at the scene, a police official hops on the running board of your ambulance and says, "We have an officer down inside the building. Follow me, I'll take you in to him." You rapidly recall your departmental orders prohibiting you from entering a violent crime scene until the police have secured it, and you quickly respond, "Is the scene secure?" The police official stares back at you with incredulity and says, "Didn't you hear me? A *cop* is down."

How should the prehospital care providers handle this situation? What can be done to better prepare for incidents involving injured law enforcement personnel? ∎

Increasingly, scenarios of the type just described are played out across the United States every day. To enter into an unsafe scene would violate the basic tenet of ensuring scene safety and might result in unnecessary casualties. On the other hand, an unwillingness to respond to these types of situations is also untenable. The solution has been the development of *Tactical Emergency Medical Support* as a subspecialty of prehospital emergency medicine.

Definitions

Modern Tactical Emergency Medical Support (TEMS) is the comprehensive and integrated medical care, consultation, and medical information management of law enforcement tactical operations that contribute to the safety and success of the primary law enforcement mission. It is a subspecialty of emergency medicine that involves the full spectrum of professional and paraprofessional health care providers.[1] TEMS goes far beyond the acute management of trauma, although tactical medical providers are expected to be competent in the field resuscitation of such patients. It focuses on injury control, preventive medicine, health, nutrition and fitness, and the minimization of performance decrement.[2] It is precisely because this practice is an interdisciplinary and comprehensive approach that the term tactical emergency medical *support* and not medical *services* is used. In short, TEMS is the practice of out-of-hospital medicine that focuses on enhancing the probability of tactical mission success (Figure 21-1).

The field of TEMS has grown rapidly since the late 1980s and has gained widespread acceptance in both medicine and law enforcement.[3-6] There is also considerable international acceptance of the TEMS concept for civilian law enforcement. TEMS is evolving as a more evidence-based practice.

Protective Medicine

Recently, the concept of *protective medicine* has been introduced and includes TEMS as one of its essential components. Protective medicine expands the original TEMS model beyond tactical law enforcement operations and encompasses the medical support of all law enforcement operations. The fundamental goal of protective medicine is to "protect the protectors." The specialist in protective medicine strives to be the *officer's medical advocate* to ensure that the law enforcement officer benefits from the best possible medical support infrastructure, optimal access to the medical system, accurate information and scientific support, state-of-the-art treatment, and comprehensive care. Protective medicine provides this support to the law enforcement community along the entire continuum of

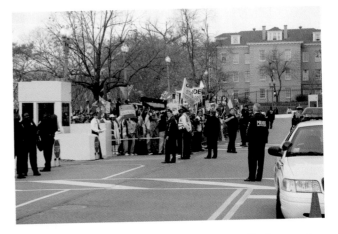

FIGURE 21-1 Special tactical emergency medical support (TEMS) skills are required to properly support crowd control and riot control law enforcement operations.

The opinions expressed in this chapter are those of the author and do not necessarily reflect the opinions or policies of the Federal Protective Service, the Department of Homeland Security, or the United States Government.

contingencies that can affect officers in the performance of their duties.

Protective medicine is extrapolated from the science of a variety of disciplines. Components under the umbrella of protective medicine include the following:

- *Medical consultation* involves the provision of timely advice and recommendations for issues pertaining to the health, safety, and performance of members of the law enforcement community and, under special circumstances, those they protect. For example, protective medicine providers can advise an individual officer regarding a medical concern, an entire agency regarding global health planning, or an operational commander regarding the medical effects of a planned enforcement operation on the occupants of a building.
- *Facility medicine* focuses on the medical, health, and safety measures that can be taken to ensure the well-being of employees and visitors to buildings during the full spectrum of law enforcement operations. Beginning with the Facility Medical Threat Assessment, protective medicine practitioners are trained to assess the medical vulnerabilities and threats associated with occupants of a structure. The provider works closely with professionals in other disciplines, such as occupational health and industrial hygiene and safety, to help the commander achieve the best possible law enforcement operations in protecting facilities.
- *Tactical emergency medicine.* As noted, TEMS focuses on the provision of medical support to law enforcement tactical teams. This support involves a constellation of measures adapted to the austere and potentially hostile special operations environment: preventive medicine, injury control, care under fire, special extraction and rescue tactics, performance decrement reduction, medical intelligence, medical threat assessment, and patient advocacy, among others.
- *Occupational health* involves workplace issues of special importance for law enforcement, such as fitness for duty determinations, immunizations, hearing protection, eye protection, and mitigating back injuries. Protective medicine providers work closely with occupational health professionals to facilitate a comprehensive, well-integrated approach.
- *Maritime medicine* involves the full spectrum of medical support in the maritime environment. The need to interdict illegal activities and other threats that use the waterways requires support for law enforcement operations on, in, and under the water. This support includes shipboard medicine, dive medicine, and rescue swimmer tactical operations.
- *Veterinary support* involves provision of preventive medicine and injury control guidance, basic medical care and resuscitation for police K-9s, as well as liaison to advanced specialized care. Coordination and

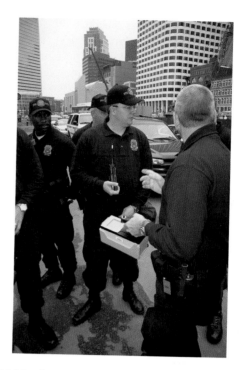

FIGURE 21-2 Support of law enforcement "hazmat" mission. Tactical medics and HazMat officers use a radiation spectrometer to determine the cause of a radiation alert. After interviewing the subject, it was determined that he had recently undergone a nuclear medicine procedure.

facilitation of veterinary care for police horse-mounted operations are also provided.

- *Hazardous materials (hazmat) emergency medicine* focuses on medical issues related to specialized teams involved in detection, assessment, and mitigation of hazardous substances and weapons of mass destruction. Medical support teams provide medical monitoring and preentry evaluation of required personnel, monitor potentially contaminated environments, support emergency rescue and extraction, provide decontamination, and treat patients exposed to toxic agents (Figure 21-2).
- *Explosive ordnance disposal* (EOD) teams, or "bomb squads," encounter some unique threats, including blast injury, exposure to toxic industrial chemicals and weaponized agents, and environmental hazards associated with the wearing of personal protective equipment. Comprehensive medical support for EOD operations includes monitoring environmental conditions and technician performance decrement, staging treatment and rescue assets, consultation on the medical and physiologic effects of blasts, treatment of blast injuries and related exposures, and clinical forensic support of postblast investigations.
- *Executive protection medicine.* Protection details are often provided for high-ranking executives and

dignitaries, persons under specific threat, and high-profile, high-target-value prisoners to ensure the safe delivery of the "protectee." Illness or injury of the protectee constitutes mission failure, regardless of the origin or cause. Executive protection medicine involves the full spectrum of medical support provided to protectees and the protection detail. This support includes planning and medical intelligence, evaluation of the protectee's medical vulnerability, special medical training for the protection detail when necessary, integration of medical response into motorcade attack countermeasures, and clinical care.

■ *Clinical forensic science* is the application of forensic principles to the living patient. This specialty service includes (1) the examination of injuries to determine their origins, nature, and mechanism; (2) evaluation of officer-involved use-of-force incidents resulting in injury; (3) scientific assessment of biologic material at potential crime scenes, such as bloodlike substances used in protests; and (4) interpretation of in-custody injuries. Physical evidence is analyzed to reconstruct the pertinent facts of an incident to corroborate or contradict other sources of information in the investigation.

Protective medicine is law enforcement medicine. Protective medicine incorporates many divergent disciplines, with the common goal of optimizing the health, safety, and welfare of the law enforcement community and those they protect. The protective medicine specialist ensures that every officer performs at his or her peak and goes home safely at the end of the day. Elements of protective medicine are shared with many other disciplines, including wilderness medicine, humanitarian assistance, disaster medicine, fireground medicine, and urban search and rescue. The common thread is the maximization of clinical outcome in a resource-poor, prolonged-transport environment while minimizing the threat to the provider.

Basic Concept and Other Considerations

In the United States, most federal and many state and local law enforcement agencies have tactical medical support programs, operating regionally, nationally, and internationally. Many other countries have also initiated TEMS efforts, including Canada and the United Kingdom.

In law enforcement, "special operations" denotes those activities that are too dangerous, complex, or technical to assign to uniformed patrol units. Special teams carry out these missions and emphasize training, coordination and speed, stealth, and violence of action to ensure success. They often use advanced technology, such as less lethal weapons systems, encrypted communications, armor, remote imaging, acoustic capture devices, and similar equipment. Special operations teams generally comprise the fittest, fastest, brightest, and most motivated personnel. The units carry a wide variety of names, including Special Weapons and Tactics (SWAT), Special Response Team (SRT), Hostage Rescue Team (HRT), Counter Assault Team (CAT), Emergency Response Team (ERT), and Special Operations Unit (SOU).

Benefits of TEMS

TEMS has additional benefits beyond improving the probability of mission success. First, a well-managed TEMS program will reduce mortality and morbidity among officers, perpetrators, and innocent parties. It is also likely to reduce line-of-duty injury and disability costs for public safety agencies. Reduction of lost work time for these officers is a significant benefit of tactical medicine because manpower is the most precious resource of any specialty team. Members have expertise, qualifications, and certifications usually acquired over long periods, and they cannot be readily replaced by lesser-trained police officers. The tactical team will often have to work short-handed if a member is injured.

Second, the impact that a TEMS program can have on the morale of the team is often underestimated. Team members are expected to take enormous risks in dangerous situations. Their willingness to engage fully in the mission, at a time when life-and-death decisions must be made in fractions of a second, is enhanced by the perception that the best possible medical care is immediately available should they be injured.

Third, the provision of far-forward medical care can dramatically enhance an agency's position in what is already a liability-prone situation. The actions of the tactical team can sometimes contribute to the creation of hazards, and some situations necessarily become temporarily less stable in the process of resolution. To create a hazard and to recognize that people might be injured, yet fail to respond to that hazard, may create liability for the law enforcement agency. The deployment of a TEMS element has proved to be an appropriate response that minimizes liability.

Fourth, the presence of a tactical medic can eliminate medically unnecessary transfer of prisoners to the hospital for evaluation. Recent court cases have asserted that law enforcement personnel who bring dangerous prisoners to hospital emergency departments and other medical facilities have a special duty to protect third parties from the prisoner.[7,8] In general, members of the public have no constitutional right to be protected by the state from harm caused by others. However, when law enforcement creates a foreseeable hazard by bringing a dangerous prisoner to a health care facility, a special obligation to protect others who may be present is incurred.

Tactical teams are specially trained and equipped to handle extraordinary law enforcement situations.[9] They take the assignments that are too dangerous or technically too complex to be handled by ordinary police procedures and, as a result, consistently push to their performance limits. Specialized medical support provided by practitioners trained and skilled in this field is one of the tools that allows special operations teams to push to that limit with reasonable safety.

Barriers to Traditional EMS Access

The scene of a law enforcement special operation represents numerous barriers to traditional emergency medical services (EMS) access. The perimeter is usually secured. Within that perimeter, it is rarely obvious which, if any, areas are safe for passage or for execution of medical activities. Furthermore, it is imperative that the medical component not become a liability by creating more problems than it resolves. Already-scarce law enforcement resources should not need to be diverted to the medical support mission. The EMS arrival-to-patient contact interval has been identified as a significant source of delay in initiation of prehospital care. In one study, police action securing the scene caused delay in 12% of all observed EMS runs and was the source of the longest EMS arrival-to-patient care delay, 39 minutes.[10] This type of delay can be much longer during SWAT missions, but can also be minimized by the implementation of TEMS, because the medical providers routinely function inside the perimeter as an integral part of the team.[11]

Some fire and rescue chiefs and EMS directors may object to their personnel practicing tactical medicine because they perceive it to be too dangerous. When asked why firefighters under their command enter burning buildings—a clearly dangerous situation—they often respond that firefighting is different from law enforcement operations because personnel are well trained and appropriately equipped against the fire threat. The same argument is true for TEMS. As noted in the opening scenario of this chapter, it is a violation of a basic prehospital trauma life support (PHTLS) principle to utilize EMS personnel who are poorly trained and inadequately equipped for this assignment to enter a secure police perimeter. However, simply waiting for the patient to be delivered outside the perimeter will result in the unnecessary loss of life, whereas far-forward medical care has been shown to reduce mortality.[12,13] The obvious solution is for the support of law enforcement special operations to be executed by well-trained and properly equipped medics who can operate safely within the perimeter.

Daily Routine Doctrine

The *daily routine doctrine* is the term coined to describe a basic axiom of disaster response. It states that the activities a provider does all the time will be performed reasonably well during a crisis, but those actions taken only in response to the crisis will be poorly executed.[14] Therefore it is best if tactical medics train on a regular basis with the elements

they support and are fully integrated into every operation. This will ensure that the medical component remains an asset to the team, not a burden or obstacle to successful mission accomplishment.

Zones of Care

Law enforcement tactical operations are usually described in terms of an "inner perimeter" and an "outer perimeter."[9] The inner perimeter is that geographic area within which police will contain the incident. It is usually represented as a circle around the crisis site and is controlled by members of the SWAT team. The outer perimeter is the area from which the public will be excluded as a safety measure. It is often represented as a larger circle surrounding the inner perimeter and is manned by law enforcement personnel other than the SWAT team, usually patrol officers. The concept of an inner and outer perimeter is useful in SWAT tactics, where decision making is focused on containing and isolating an incident, protecting the public, and controlling the threat. Tactical medics need to understand this terminology because of its use in describing tactical options.

However, the perimeter concept is not as applicable to the way in which medical decisions must be made in the tactical environment, despite its frequent reference in that context. The particular medical interventions employed, the manner of extraction, and the timing of both are highly dependent on the specific threat level present at the casualty's location. The "perimeter" construct is too broad to permit either reasonable definition of the threat at a particular location or meaningful medical decision making. Instead, a three-level characterization of the threat as hot, warm, and cold is used to describe zones of care.[2] The zones of care need not be contiguous or concentric. However, these zones may be irregularly shaped areas defined not by geography, but by variables that include (1) the available intelligence, (2) accessibility to cover and concealment (*cover* provides protection from the threat, e.g., a masonry wall through which a bullet cannot pass, whereas *concealment* merely hides one's location from the assailant), (3) weapons used, (4) terrain features, (5) threat to target distance, (6) visibility, (7) counter-sniper coverage, and (8) directed firepower. The hot, warm, and cold zones are analogous to the stages of care defined in Tactical Combat Casualty Care (TCCC) as "care under fire," "tactical field care," and "combat casualty evacuation care."

Hot Zone

The hot zone is an area where there is a direct and immediate threat. What constitutes a direct and immediate threat is determined subjectively and may vary depending on the factors previously cited. In general, however, the term *hot zone* refers to those environments where there is little protection for both patient and provider and the probability of additional injury is high. In this chapter's opening scenario, if the officer were still under fire from a gunman in the building, that area would be deemed a hot zone.

The hot zone is an extremely dangerous environment, and conventional treatment here entails enormous risk. Generally, the only appropriate care is directed fire and extraction to a safer area, although contemporaneous, momentary lifesaving interventions, such as manual airway maneuvers, may be possible. Self-care may also be possible, especially with guidance from the medic. The patient should be evaluated from appropriate cover by using Rapid and Remote Assessment Methodology (RAM) techniques[15] before a rescue or recovery is initiated (see later discussion). Because of extraordinary risk or low probability of success, the greater good may be served by delaying extraction of a viable patient until additional resources are in place. Patients who can extract themselves should do so, and body recoveries should be delayed until the scene is secure. The hot zone is the civilian law enforcement equivalent of the "care under fire" stage of TCCC.

Cold Zone

The cold zone is the area where no reasonable threat exists because of (1) distance from the crisis site, (2) employment of cover, (3) interposition of firepower, or (4) material barrier between the threat and the patient and provider. Care in the cold zone is almost identical to typical out-of-hospital care, although careful consideration should be given to the recognition and forensic preservation of evidentiary material. The cold zone is analogous to the "combat casualty evacuation care" stage of TCCC.

Warm Zone

It is in the warm zone that the difficult and defining decisions of TEMS are made. The warm zone is the area in which there is a possible threat, but the threat is not immediate or direct. For example, in the scenario at the beginning of the chapter, the perpetrator might not be actively firing at the officer, but his location within the building is still unknown and represents a significant potential threat to the patient and the caregiver. In this geographic area of uncertainty, the threat may be rapidly changing. The benefits of medical evaluation and treatment in situ must be carefully balanced against the risks of provider and patient exposure to the threat and delayed extraction to a higher echelon of care (Figure 21-3).

Multiple factors must be considered in only fractions of a second, including the relative severity of the possible threat. Not all threats are equal. Some are more severe than others for a variety of reasons, such as credibility, intelligence, type of weapon (if any), nature of injuries that

FIGURE 21-3 The defining decisions of civilian tactical emergency medical support (TEMS) are made in the warm zone, where there is a continuing threat to the safety of the patient and providers. Here, medics evaluate a patient for transport to the cold zone.

could be inflicted, and consequences of being wrong in the threat assessment. Some warm zones are simply "warmer" than others.

This environment has been insufficiently modeled, and the variables are not yet understood well enough to permit an algorithmic approach to warm zone decision making. The tactical medic must be capable of critically analyzing numerous factors and finding the right balance between risk and benefit. Traditional EMS interventions may be inappropriate. For example, spinal immobilization is of relatively little value in penetrating neck wounds, and it is time-consuming and will expose rescuers and casualty to additional danger.[16,17] Cardiopulmonary resuscitation (CPR) for cardiac arrest secondary to trauma has no place in the tactical environment.[2,18-22] (The possible exceptions are arrest caused by primary myocardial infarction, near-drowning, electrocution, hypothermia, and toxic exposure, when artificial ventilation may enable a successful resuscitation.) Interventions such as hemorrhage control, however, may be truly lifesaving. The warm zone is analogous to the "tactical field care" stage of TCCC.

Transit Risk

The health care provider not only must consider the risks associated with the particular threat zone in which the patient is located, but also must include the danger associated with extraction in the overall assessment. This is called *transit risk* and consists of three components. The first component is the amount of time it will take to move the patient to a safer area. Some areas of operation can have vast hot and warm zones because the perpetrator has a commanding field of fire, resulting in long transit times. For example, in the 1966 Texas sniper incident, a former Marine barricaded himself on the 28th-floor observation deck of the University of Texas Administration Building and killed people who were blocks away, creating a hot zone that included much of the central campus.[23] However, time can also be an inconsequential factor if it takes only a few seconds to move to a more secure area.

The second component of transit risk is route of travel. Because the zones of care are irregularly shaped, discontinuous geographic areas, there may be pockets of warm zone within seas of hot zone, and jumping from one warm zone to another can reduce the risk of traversing the hot zone. It may be necessary to cross into a "hotter" area to get to a "cooler" one, in which case the value of treating in place and deferring extraction must be considered.

The ability to deliver care during transit is the third component of transit risk. Some interventions cannot be adequately maintained during extraction, and the effect of discontinuing care on the patient's clinical condition is a factor. For example, it will be impossible to maintain a manual jaw thrust maneuver if the extraction includes a running litter carry across a hot zone. Taking the time to insert an airway adjunct may be necessary before evacuating the casualty.

The concept of transit risk can be summarized by the following formula:

$$\text{Transit Risk} = t \times R \times C$$

where t is transit time, R is the risk associated with the route of travel, and C is the risk associated with providing essential care during transit.

Differences between TEMS and EMS

Cost-Benefit Decisions

The practice of TEMS is based on the understanding of a single underlying principle: medical decisions must be made on the basis of a cost-benefit assessment that balances the cost (time, exposure, resources, etc.) of a particular intervention or approach against the potential benefit to the overall mission. With modern technology, we have the capability to bring the emergency department to the field. In this specialized and high-risk environment, however, *more* medicine is not always the *best* medicine. The costs

of implementing "more medicine" include (1) the burden of transporting more equipment and people, (2) the increased risk of physical exposure to harm while implementing additional medical procedures, (3) the increased duration of exposure, (4) the additional resources required in a resource-poor environment, and many other factors that have not yet been adequately modeled.

The physiology of injury is the same regardless of the environment in which the casualty is located; for example, hemorrhage is still controlled with direct pressure. The difference lies in the *context* in which medical decisions are made. In the example of uncontrolled hemorrhage, the tactical medic might advance more rapidly to a tourniquet if the patient had to be extracted from a warm zone where continued direct pressure could not be reliably maintained. Some prehospital procedures and practices should be modified for use in the tactical environment, whereas others are unique to this special area of practice.

Airway Management

Some have argued that cricothyrotomy instead of laryngoscopy should be the advanced airway of choice for military medics in the special operations setting.[18] In the military special operations setting, this is true because of (1) the medics' lack of experience and inability to maintain competence with laryngoscopy, (2) technical difficulty intubating in the presence of maxillofacial trauma, and (3) the undesirable light signature of the laryngoscope. These arguments support the use of alternative airways in the warm zone.

However, this proposition is not universally accepted, and significant differences exist between the military special operations environment and that of civilian law enforcement. TEMS medics are generally experienced at their respective provider level and are required by their certification or licensing programs to demonstrate skill proficiency on a periodic basis, thereby eliminating the objection to laryngoscopy based on difficulty in maintaining the skill. In regard to the light signature produced by direct laryngoscopy, digital intubation is an alternative technique taught to and practiced by TEMS providers that does not require the use of a white light, but there are few data beyond anecdotes demonstrating the technique's efficacy in this setting.[15,24,25] Digital intubation does have the advantages of a rapid technique that can be accomplished with minimal head and neck movement from a number of low-profile and protected-provider positions at the patient's side. It also requires minimal equipment and seems to be less affected by blood and secretions than visualization techniques.

In any case, airway dysfunction is a relatively infrequent problem in this population of patients, and those receiving an advanced airway are even less common. In the CONTOMS database, an airway adjunct was used in approximately 2% of all treatments rendered, and only one third of these casualties survived to arrival at the hospital.[26] In the setting of penetrating trauma, patients who are so obtunded that they cannot maintain an open airway often have serious injury to the central nervous system that decreases the likelihood of survival. Continuous monitoring of the patient may be impossible in the warm zone, and airway selection should take this into consideration. However, endotracheal intubation or cricothyrotomy should be considered if mechanical airway obstruction secondary to trauma is the primary cause of respiratory embarrassment.

Although patients may ventilate adequately on their own after a patent airway is established, an extender tube should be employed if a bag-valve device must be used. The extender tube allows more movement between the bag and the endotracheal (ET) tube without dislodging the tube during patient extraction. It is critical that the bag-valve device have the exhalation valve on the downstream side of the extender (closest to the ET tube) so that a column of exhaled gas is not moved back and forth in the tube, leading to inadequate ventilation.

Cardiac Arrest

As noted previously, CPR has little role in the tactical environment where there is an inherent risk of harm to the provider. However, several authors question the wisdom of attempted resuscitation in penetrating trauma under any circumstances. Lorenz et al[27] documented that no patients survived to discharge out of 215 victims of trauma (97 from blunt trauma and 118 from penetrating trauma) with absent signs of life on the initial assessment by paramedics. Similar findings were observed in a retrospective study in which all of the 138 trauma victims undergoing CPR at the scene or during transport died.[19] Stein and Hirshberg[28] suggest that CPR is never indicated after a terrorist mass-casualty incident, based on their experience in Israel. Also, CPR is not recommended for victims of blast or penetrating injury on the battlefield who present without pulse, respirations, or signs of life.[18] In the Oklahoma City bombing, the three patients receiving CPR did not survive.[29] However, Stratton et al[30] performed a retrospective review of outcome from 879 trauma victims (497 from penetrating trauma and 382 from blunt trauma) found pulseless and unconscious by EMS personnel. Nine (0.8%) survived to hospital discharge, including three in a vegetative state and two dependent on others for daily support. Consequently, the authors recommended attempting to resuscitate all victims. Although the very low resuscitation rate makes this approach controversial under normal circumstances, if any action is warranted in a high-risk environment, it should be limited to rapid evacuation.

A second patient group to be considered consists of non–trauma-related arrest victims. These cardiac arrests may be secondary to electrocution, toxic exposure, hypothermia, near-drowning, or an ischemic cardiac event occurring during hostilities. This latter type of cardiac arrest should be an infrequent event in a tactical setting, especially considering the relative fitness of most tactical officers. Again, the risk of resuscitative efforts needs to be evaluated against the potential benefit. In the hot and warm zones, efforts should be directed at extraction to a safer location. If extraction to a cold zone cannot be achieved, the tactical situation will mandate the approach (see later discussion on RAM).

Under no circumstances is full CPR indicated in the hot zone. In an operation with comprehensive backup from local EMS, local protocols should be followed after the victim is evacuated to the cold zone. In a remote operation with limited resources and long evacuation times, however, resuscitation efforts should be terminated in the field if there is no return of spontaneous circulation after sufficient advanced cardiac life support (ACLS) efforts or after a reasonable interval without access to ACLS. The most rigorous resuscitation efforts, including the possible acceptance of increased risk, should be considered for children, hypothermic patients, those with persistent ventricular fibrillation, and those who experience arrest after the tactical medic's arrival. This approach is based on the findings of two large studies conducted under standard field conditions. In the first study, Kellerman et al[31] retrospectively analyzed 1068 out-of-hospital cardiac arrests. Of the 758 patients without return of spontaneous circulation in the field, only three survived to discharge. All three had moderate to severe neurologic disability, and none of the three had arrested until after paramedics arrived. Similar findings were derived from a prospective study of 1461 out-of-hospital primary cardiac arrests in Houston.[32] Of the 1322 unmonitored arrests, 1252 did not achieve return of a pulse, greater than 60 beats/min for at least 5 minutes, after 25 minutes of ACLS protocol in the field. Only six of these 1252 patients survived to hospital discharge, and all six had persistent ventricular fibrillation as their field rhythm.

Spinal Immobilization

Prehospital care providers are traditionally taught to immobilize the cervical spine when there is the slightest suspicion of a spinal column injury. This is not unreasonable given the devastating effects of an occult, unstable fracture that results in cord damage. However, proper immobilization requires at least two people and approximately 5 minutes when performed by well-trained and experienced medics. This increased exposure in the warm zone is unacceptable when weighed against the low probability of an occult fracture that will benefit from immobilization of penetrating wounds.[16,17] Therefore, immobilization should generally not be considered for penetrating trauma until the patient has been removed to a cold zone. Cervical spine immobilization is more important following certain types of blunt trauma, such as high-speed vehicular crashes.

Rapid and Remote Assessment Methodology

The Rapid and Remote Assessment Methodology (RAM) was developed by the Counter Narcotics and Terrorism Operational Medical Support (CONTOMS) Program at the Uniformed Services University of the Health Sciences, the Department of Defense medical school.[15] The principal purpose of this assessment algorithm is to maximize the opportunity to extract and treat a salvageable casualty while minimizing risk to providers from attempting an unnecessary rescue. Unnecessary rescues fall into two categories: those where the casualty can extract himself and those where the casualty is already dead (more appropriately termed a "body recovery"). The RAM provides an organized approach to evaluate the totality of circumstances from a protected position before recommending a rescue attempt to the commander.

The first step in conducting a RAM is to determine if the area is secure. If it is, standard care in the cold zone is appropriate after ensuring that the patient cannot harm you. If the area is not secure, use available intelligence to determine if the patient is a perpetrator or otherwise represents a threat to you. Under such circumstances, no further medical intervention is indicated until the threat has been controlled. To do otherwise might jeopardize the safety of officers, health care providers, and innocent parties. If the patient is not a perpetrator, a remote assessment should be initiated. Attempt to evaluate the nature of the injury and the stability of the patient's condition. Remote observation is the first technique to be employed because it allows medics to gather information without revealing their position or intent to the opposing force. Technology available to SWAT teams can improve the reliability of this assessment. For example, a good pair of binoculars or night-vision goggles can often help to ascertain if the patient is breathing, the rate and quality of respiration, the presence of exsanguinating hemorrhage, and the presence of obvious wounds incompatible with life. In cold weather, a respiratory condensation plume can often be seen from the patient's mouth. Acoustic surveillance equipment can be deployed to detect speech, moans, groans, and even respiratory sounds. Thermal imaging technology has improved so much in recent years that it is currently being investigated for application in RAM.

If the patient's condition appears stable, self-care instructions and reassurance should be communicated if possible, and medical extraction should await an improvement in the tactical situation. (The commander may elect to do a tactical extraction at any time, but the tactical situation and not the patient's stable medical condition will motivate this decision.) If the patient is unstable, the risk of extraction must be weighed against the benefits of immediate access to medical care. Although this is a command decision, the team leader will rely heavily on the medic's assessment of the patient's condition and need for immediate extraction.

If the benefit/risk ratio is sufficiently high, the extraction should proceed, with only essential resuscitative procedures being performed in the "warmer" parts of the zone.

This may seem to be a relatively self-evident approach, but it is important to have a decision structure that fosters good assessment before emotion overtakes reason and a needless rescue is risked. The military experience is filled with examples of numerous casualties incurred to recover a body or attempt to rescue a casualty who eventually stood up and ran to cover without assistance.[33,34]

Noise and Light Discipline

Medical personnel as well as operators in a tactical setting need to adhere to the principles of noise and light discipline. In standard EMS, warning lights and brightly colored equipment are important because they help to identify EMS personnel at the scene of an accident and injury. Clear identification of their location will usually help protect providers from many normal hazards, such as oncoming traffic on a dark road. In a tactical situation, however, the prehospital care provider's status can change from being welcomed to being a target. The principles of noise and light discipline require rescue efforts and on-scene treatment to be conducted in a manner that eliminates the sound or light signature that an adversary could use to target the provider or the victim.

Sound discipline requires providers to approach the scene as quietly as possible. They need to whisper or use hand signals in communicating with other team members and with the victims. They need to eliminate any unnecessary noises generated by their equipment (e.g., keys dangling from belt, portable radio turned to full volume). In a similar manner, *light discipline* starts with choosing clothing and equipment that will be least detectable in the environment in which it will be used. While providing care on scene in the dark, the patient evaluation must be done primarily by touch. The use of a blue or red lens on any light used undercover will preserve the operator's night vision. The color itself is not particularly effective at preventing detection by hostile forces.

Medical Counterterrorism Operations

Many requirements for medical support of counterterrorism *crisis management* differ from those of *consequence management* and can be executed best by special operations medical providers. Law enforcement investigation and interdiction of terrorist activities are carried out in a low-profile manner that protects operators, sources of intelligence, and pending actions and that avoids unnecessary interruption of essential infrastructure or commerce. These operations are conducted under strict operational security guidelines. This is a necessary approach; a public safety response that is disproportional to the threat may result in disruption of daily living by the response itself and increase media coverage of the terrorists' cause, thus allowing terrorists to achieve their goal of instilling fear in the population. Even hoaxes can be an effective tool for the terrorist when used in this way.[28,35,36] Therefore the operational signature of the supporting medical effort, in terms of size, activity level, and equipment and logistics, must be minimized. This is best accomplished by medical providers who are accustomed to working in the law enforcement environment under circumstances in which the delivery of medical care is not the primary mission. They function regularly and effectively in a discreet or covert manner with minimal equipment and supplies.

Operational and Communications Security

Operational and communications security must be maintained. The authors of the Federal Response Plan recognized this when they wrote that only specially designated representatives of the Federal Emergency Management Agency (FEMA) would screen sensitive law enforcement reports to identify information of value to a potential consequence management effort.[37] The media will be extremely sensitive to changes in the daily operations of hospitals and EMS if these are implemented in anticipation of a counterterrorism mission. Special operations medical providers should already have the requisite background investigations and security clearances and training in security practices and needed technology (e.g., encrypted radios) to implement operational and communications security procedures.[15] The medical support package for crisis management must also be light and highly mobile to keep pace with their supported unit. The priority for mechanized transportation of supplies and equipment will be nonmedical items to support the primary mission, such as surveillance and communications electronics, weapons systems, and personal protective gear. As they regularly do for other types of missions, tactical medics will be able to select an inventory that is versatile and minimizes weight and space requirements.

Integration

Terrorism investigations are highly dynamic and frequently cross the jurisdictional boundaries of community EMS organizations, making it difficult to rely on conventional EMS systems to support crisis management operations. Furthermore, a medical unit that operates on a day-to-day basis with the police personnel involved in crisis management will be more effectively integrated into the operation. This is consistent with the Daily Routine Doctrine, as described earlier. For these reasons, a fully integrated TEMS element

that moves easily as part of the law enforcement team is usually best suited to support the crisis management component of a terrorist incident.

Forensic Science Support

Material of evidentiary value is sometimes identified and collected during the examination and treatment of a patient incidental to a terrorism investigation. This evidence can be perishable and may not survive medical treatment intact, as in the case of soot effects associated with a close-range gunshot wound. Traditionally, EMS providers have not been very good at preserving and documenting this evidence.[38-40] In contrast, TEMS providers usually have received specialized training in clinical forensic science and often carry a small evidence collection kit as part of their limited load-out. The EMT-Tactical Advanced training curriculum includes more than 8 hours of instruction in this area.[41]

Medical Intelligence

Medical support personnel need to maintain a close liaison with law enforcement intelligence components. Intelligence officers gather and receive data about potential terrorist activity but are often hesitant to share information freely, even within the law enforcement community, because of concern about compromising their sources. Some authors suggest that medical personnel are not in the intelligence business and therefore have little role before an event; they are needed only after an attack occurs.[42] However, the type of information that might be available in the intelligence community is critical to proper planning, and tactical medics must develop mechanisms that permit them to be included in the sharing of law enforcement intelligence. Furthermore, once this relationship is established, the medic can help intelligence officers by screening information for its relevance to advance notice and preparation in the traditional EMS mission.

Downey[43] noted that during the "Harbor Incident," a threatened release of sarin gas in a major U.S. amusement center, the local fire department was excluded from the information sharing and planning among federal, state, and local law enforcement. He wrote that the "fire chief was hard-pressed to institute a timely action plan to deal with the potential nerve-gas release."[43]

Medical input into the process of analyzing intelligence can be quite valuable. Medical data need to be interpreted, and it is difficult for medically naive personnel to assess the importance of medical information or even to recognize the medical value of general intelligence.

Screening for Incarceration

As noted earlier, the presence of a tactical medic can eliminate medically unnecessary transfer of prisoners and

Contents of Tactical Trauma Kit

Trauma Kit
Petroleum gauze
Bite stick
Nasopharyngeal airways
Oropharyngeal airways
Acetaminophen
Bismuth subsalicylate (Pepto-Bismol)
Ibuprofen
Moleskin
Disposable scalpel, #11 blade
Adhesive bandages
Benzoin
Trauma shears
Penlight
Forceps
Bag-valve-mask device
6-inch gauze rolls
Elastic bandages
SAM splint
ABD dressings
Stethoscope
Blood pressure cuff
Pocket mask
Tape, 2 inches wide
Chemical ice pack
Triangular bandages
4 × 4 gauze sponges
Large field dressings
Disposable gloves
60-mL syringe with tubing (for suction)
Large burn dressings
Fingertip pulse oximeter

Airway Management Kit
Endotracheal tubes (sizes 6.5, 7.0, 7.5, 8.0 mm)
Stylet
Disposable laryngoscope with light source and batteries
Large Miller blade
Large MacIntosh blade
Disposable gloves
Tape, 1 inch wide
Alcohol pads
Percutaneous cricothyrotomy kit
14-gauge angiocath needles

Intravenous (IV) Access Kit
IV administration set
Lactated Ringer's or normal saline, 250 mL
IV catheters, assorted sizes
Rubber tourniquet
Alcohol pads
Syringes, 10 mL
PRN adapters
Tape, 1 inch wide

Dental Kit
Zinc oxide power
Dental spatula and long swabs
Eugenol (oil of clove, USP)
Stomahesive
Small plate for mixing

Eye Kit
Tobramycin (0.3%) ophthalmic ointment
Ophthalmic topical anesthetic
Cobalt blue filter and penlight
Fluorescein strips
Eye patches
Tape, 1 inch wide

Example of trauma kit.

Example of pharmacology kit.

law enforcement operators to the hospital for evaluation. In everyday EMS, transport of the patient to the emergency department is sometimes seen as the ultimate "safety valve," ensuring that all patients receive adequate care by shifting the decision making from the field environment to the hospital environment. Often, this is an appropriate and effective strategy. The tactical medic always has an overriding duty to provide appropriate care under the circumstances; however, avoiding unnecessary exposure risks at a fixed medical facility makes an important contribution to overall operational security and therefore to the success of the counterterror mission. Tactical medics often have formal training and extensive experience in screening patients for incarceration.

Performance Decrement

Although the responsibilities of the tactical medic include providing field medical treatment for both trauma and illness, there are other, less obvious medical support activities that reap equal or greater benefit for the team. These include the development of appropriate physical fitness, nutrition, psychological stress prevention, and self-aid/buddy-aid programs for team personnel. Monitoring the medical effects of environmental conditions on individual and team performance is also an important function of the medical element. Problems such as sleep deprivation, heat or cold stress, rest/work cycles, and lack of opportunity for personal hygiene can degrade the performance of an entire team and should be brought to the attention of the commander.

Patient Advocacy

The primary function of a TEMS system is to bridge the gap between point of injury or illness and appropriate entry into the standing health care system. However, the medic's job does not stop when the patient is entered into the health care system. The medic continues to serve as the patient's advocate, ensuring that the appropriate care is provided in a timely manner. Done in a conscientious and diplomatic way, this function will be appreciated by a busy hospital, not resented. Success depends on establishing good working relationships with local EMS systems and receiving institutions, whether dealing with them on a regular basis or for a single mission. When the medic's jurisdiction is a well-defined geographic area, the team's tactical medicine program can be integrated with the local system so that transfer of care will be seamless.

As an insider in the medical system, the team medical officer should ensure that the needs of the patient's family and the chain of command are met. Diagnoses and treatment plans that an attending surgeon can describe to the medic in 3 minutes can be translated into lay terminology and more comfortably explained to family, unit commander, chief, or other appropriate personnel in 15 or 20 minutes.

SUMMARY

In general, the principles of medical care in the tactical environment are the same as those to which prehospital care providers are accustomed. Direct pressure still controls hemorrhage, and patients can die quickly from airway, breathing, and circulation problems. However, the austerity and danger of the operational environment require that the benefit of every medical intervention be weighed against the risks inherent in delivering that intervention. This requires a unique set of decision-making skills, and the tactical medic constantly needs to balance the benefit of a particular intervention against the special risks inherent in performing the intervention in this environment. Modification of techniques, reordering of priorities, and ongoing assessment of risk permit the tactical medic to provide the greatest good for the most people. Maximum medical intervention may actually cause the death of others and must not be attempted needlessly.

SCENARIO SOLUTION

The departmental order prohibiting you from entering a violent crime scene until secured by the police is appropriately intended to protect prehospital care providers who are not equipped or trained to operate in the law enforcement tactical environment. However, faced with this predicament, many EMS personnel would feel obligated to help their public safety brethren. You can avoid the difficult choice between violating a departmental order while jeopardizing your own safety and rescuing a downed officer by properly preparing to operate in this specialized environment.

In cooperation with your police department SWAT team, you begin a SWAT medic program. The police department provides body armor, radios, and similar equipment. EMS purchases medical gear specifically designed for tactical operations and sends selected prehospital care providers to a nationally recognized tactical medic school. The medics train with the SWAT team every month and are ready to answer the call the next time "a police officer is down." ∎

References

1. Llewellyn CH: The antecedents of tactical emergency medical support, *Top Emerg Med* 25(4): 274, 2003.

2. De Lorenzo RA, Porter RS: *Tactical emergency care,* Upper Saddle River, NJ, 1999, Prentice-Hall.

3. Carmona RH: The history and evolution of tactical emergency medical support and its impact on public safety, *Top Emerg Med* 25(4): 277, 2003.

4. Vayer JS, Schwartz RB: Developing a tactical emergency medical support program, *Top Emerg Med* 25(4):282, 2003.

5. Rooker N: The San Francisco shootings, *JEMS,* 18:74, 1993.

6. McArdle DQ, Rasumoff D, et al: Integration of emergency medical services and special weapons and tactics team: the emergence of the tactically trained medic, *Prehosp Disaster Med* 7:285, 1992.

7. *Sams v Oelrich,* 717 So2d 1044 (1998), Court of Appeal of Florida, First District.

8. *Shepherd v Washington County,* AR, 962 SW2d 779 (1998), Supreme Court of Arkansas.

9. Kolman JA: *A guide to the development of special weapons and tactics teams,* Springfield, Ill, 1982, Charles C Thomas.

10. Campbell JP, Gratton MC, Salomone JA III, et al: Ambulance arrival to patient contact: the hidden component of prehospital response time intervals, *Ann Emerg Med* 22:1254, 1993.

11. Kanable R: Peak performance: well-trained tactical medics can help the team perform at its best, *Law Enforcement Technology,* August 1999.

12. Jagoda A, Pietrzak M, Hazen S, et al: Prehospital care and the military, *Mil Med* 157:11, 1992.

13. Bellamy RF: The causes of death in conventional land warfare: implications for combat casualty care research, *Mil Med* 149:55, 1984.

14. Vayer JS, Ten Eyck RP, Cowan ML: New concepts in triage, *Ann Emerg Med* 15:927, 1986.

15. *Emergency medical technician: tactical course manual,* ed 15, Bethesda, Md, 2000, Uniformed Services University of the Health Sciences.

16. Arishita GI, Vayer JS, Bellamy RF: Cervical spine immobilization of penetrating neck wounds in a hostile environment, *J Trauma* 29:332, 1989.

17. Zajtchuk R, Jenkins DP, Bellamy RF, et al, editors: *Combat casualty care guidelines for Operation Desert Storm,* Washington, DC, 1991, Office of the Army Surgeon General.

18. Butler FK, Hagmann JH, Butler EG: Tactical combat casualty care in special operations, *Mil Med* 161(suppl 1):3, 1996.

19. Rosemurgy AS, Norris PA, Olson SM, et al: Prehospital traumatic cardiac arrest: the cost of futility, *J Trauma* 38:468, 1998.

20. Yoon RY, Harling M, Feldman JA, et al: Penetrating thoracic trauma: prehospital resuscitation for all? Minneapolis, 1993, Ninth Annual Conference and Scientific Assembly of National Association of EMS Physicians (abstract of scientific papers).

21. Hogan DE, Waeckerle JF, Dire DJ, Lillibridge SR: Emergency department impact of the Oklahoma City terrorist bombing, *Ann Emerg Med* 34:160, 1999.

22. Boehm TM, James JJ: The medical response to the La Belle Disco bombing in Berlin, 1986, *Mil Med* 153:235, 1988.

23. Lavergne GM: *A sniper in the tower,* New York, 1997, Bantam.

24. Stewart RD: Tactile orotracheal intubation, *Ann Emerg Med* 13:175, 1984.

25. Hardwick WC, Bluhm D: Digital intubation, *J Emerg Med* 1:317, 1984.

26. Counter Narcotics and Terrorism Operational Medical Support (CONTOMS) Database System, Bethesda, Md, 2004, Uniformed Services University of the Health Sciences, www.casualtycareresearchcenter.org.

27. Lorenz PH, Steinmetz B, Lieberman J, et al: Emergency thoracotomy: survival correlates with physiologic status, *J Trauma* 32:780, 1992.

28. Stein M, Hirshberg A: Trauma care in the new millennium: medical consequences of terrorism, *Surg Clin North Am* 79:1538, 1999.

29. Hogan DE, Waeckerle JF, Dire DJ, et al: Emergency department impact of the Oklahoma City terrorist bombing, *Ann Emerg Med* 34:160, 1999.

30. Stratton SJ, Brickett K, Crammer T: Prehospital pulseless, unconscious penetrating trauma victims: field assessments associated with survival, *J Trauma Injury Infect Crit Care* 45:96, 1998.

31. Kellerman AL, Hackman BB, Somes G: Predicting the outcome of unsuccessful prehospital advanced cardiac life support, *JAMA* 270:1433, 1993.

32. Bonnin MJ, Pepe PE, Kimball KT, et al: Distinct criteria for termination of resuscitation in the out-of-hospital setting, *JAMA* 270:1457, 1993.

33. Wound Data and Munitions Effectiveness Team Study, Vols I-III, Final Report, Joint Technical Coordinating Group for Munitions Effectiveness, Alexandria, Va, 1970, Defense Technical Information Center.

34. Cloonan C: In *Proceedings of the Third International Conference on Tactical Emergency Medical Support,* Bethesda, Md, 1999, Uniformed Services University of the Health Sciences, p 97.

35. US Department of Health and Human Services, Centers for Disease Control and Prevention: Bioterrorism alleging use of anthrax and interim guidelines for management—United States, 1998, *MMWR* 48(4):69, 1999.

36. MacIntyre AG, Christopher GW, Eitzen E, et al: Weapons of mass destruction events with contaminated casualties, *JAMA* 283:242, 2000.

37. Federal Response Plan, Terrorism Incident Annex, 2003, Federal Emergency Management Agency, http://www.fema.gov/rrr/frp/frpterr.shtm.

38. Carmona R, Prince K: Trauma and forensic medicine, *J Trauma* 29:1222, 1989.

39. Smialek JE: Forensic medicine in the emergency department, *Emerg Med Clin North Am* 1:693, 1983.

40. Orris KC, Lantz PE: *Interpretation of fatal multiple and exiting gunshot wounds by trauma specialists,* Boston, 1993, American Academy of Forensic Sciences.

41. US Department of Defense: *Emergency medical technician: tactical advanced student manual*, Bethesda, Md, 1998, Uniformed Services University of the Health Sciences.

42. Okumura T, Takasu N, Ishimatsu S, et al: Report on 640 victims of the Tokyo subway sarin attack, *Ann Emerg Med* 28:129, 1996.

43. Downey R: Terrorism and the fire service: preparing for today's threats, *Fire Engineering*, August 1996.

Chapter Objectives

*At the completion of this chapter, the reader
will be able to do the following:*

✓ List four factors that distinguish the "wilderness" and "street" EMS contexts.

✓ Given a particular patient situation and location, list four factors that affect the decision whether "wilderness" or "street" care is more appropriate.

✓ Describe methods used for improvised wilderness evacuation.

✓ Describe methods for dealing with elimination needs during evacuations, as well as potential medical consequences if this is not addressed.

✓ Explain the reasons for the dictum that "every wilderness patient is hypothermic, hypoglycemic, and hypovolemic until proven otherwise."

✓ Explain the meaning of the term "SPF" (sun protection factor).

✓ Describe standard ways to manage bleeding wounds in the backcountry.

✓ Describe the reasons, specific indications, and technique for wound irrigation.

✓ Explain when, in the wilderness context, an attempt at CPR is appropriate, and when it is not appropriate.

CHAPTER 22

Wilderness Trauma Care

SCENARIO

A wilderness search and rescue team is carrying a litter to a patient along a hiking trail when a member of the team, a healthy 26-year-old woman, slips and falls. She only falls 1 or 2 feet, but she "belly flops" onto a rock and has the breath knocked out of her for 1 or 2 minutes. After this, she gets up and starts carrying the litter again, insisting she feels fine. After picking up their patient, who has an ankle fracture but is otherwise well, about 2 miles from the trailhead, the team starts heading back on the trail to the road. The plan is to put the patient in a waiting ambulance and then drive him about an hour to the nearest emergency department at a small community hospital. Along the way, the woman who did the "belly flop" starts complaining about nausea and some pain in the left shoulder, then some lightheadedness. On examination, she is pale, tachycardic but with a normal blood pressure, and has some left upper quadrant tenderness.

What injuries could this rescuer have sustained? How does the team now divide their efforts to manage two patients? What additional arrangements should be made for transportation of the two patients? ■

Proper Care Depends on Context

Although our medical knowledge, understanding, and technology change from month to month, the *principles* of medical care change little over the years. "[T]he critically injured patient must be transported as quickly as possible, without detailed examination and treatment of noncritical conditions."[1] Proper care is still somewhat context dependent, however, and the definition of "detailed examination" and "noncritical conditions" may be different on an urban street than deep within a cave (Figure 22-1).

Consider a patient with a complex fracture-dislocation of the shoulder. What is the proper care in the operating room (OR)? In many cases it involves an open reduction and internal fixation (ORIF). However, proper care in the OR may not be proper care in the emergency department (ED). It would *not* be proper care to attempt an open reduction in the ED. In the ED the patient will have x-ray films taken to evaluate the fracture-dislocation, a short-acting pain medication, and a *closed* reduction of the dislocation to reduce pain and swelling, to realign the bones grossly, and to decrease pressure on nerves and blood vessels. However, the definitive ORIF will occur later, in the OR.

Furthermore, proper care in the ED may not be proper care on the street. The ambulance crew may not have the advantage of a large, warm, dry area. They may be working where it is raining or snowing, where the patient is hanging upside down inside a crushed vehicle, or where a rescue crew is using power tools to cut and crush metal all around them. On the street, the patient will have an assessment for scene safety, rescue from immediate dangers, an assessment for other injuries, a check of distal neurovascular status in the arm, immobilization of the shoulder, possibly some pain medication, and rapid transport to the ED. On the street, it would *not* be proper care to attempt an open reduction to reduce the fracture-dislocation.

Finally, proper care on the street may not be proper care in the backcountry. What if, instead of being in a crushed vehicle, the patient had fallen off a rope while a half mile into a limestone cave in the mountains, facing a multihour evacuation through the cave passages, followed by a several-hour drive to the nearest hospital? For most conditions, proper care is proper care whether it is done in the OR, in the ED, on the street, or in the backcountry, limited only by equipment and training.

For a small but significant number of common conditions, however, great differences exist between proper "street" emergency medical services (EMS) care and proper backcountry EMS care. This brings up the following important questions, as discussed later in this chapter:

- Is "street" EMS care always proper in the backcountry?
- If "street" EMS care is not proper, how do you know *what* the proper care is? Where is this written down?
- How do you deal with situations where, in the field, you are not sure precisely what the injury might be? For example, in the previous case, how do you determine a fracture-dislocation is present when you are examining the patient while you are hanging upside down, whether in a crushed vehicle or from a rope dangling down a pit deep within a cave?
- How do you decide, for a particular patient in a particular situation, which is *more* proper, street or backcountry care?
- What makes a situation "backcountry" or "street"? What about all the "in-between" cases?

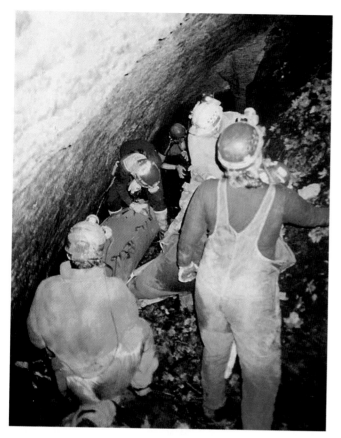

FIGURE 22-1 Trauma care in the wilderness is often hampered by adverse environmental conditions, mud, underbrush, and confined spaces.

Keep the patient with the fracture-dislocation of the shoulder and these questions in mind as you read further. Definitive answers to all the questions cannot be provided—often the answer is "it depends"—but at least good background information can be provided so that providers may, as needed and in a particular patient care situation, answer the question. The prehospital trauma life support (PHTLS) philosophy has always been that, given a good fund of knowledge and key principles, prehospital care providers such as emergency medical technicians (EMTs) are capable of making reasoned decisions regarding patient care.

This chapter considers several "backcountry" issues, chosen either because they are critical for proper backcountry patient care or because they are common backcountry problems for which management is different than on the "street."

Most importantly, this chapter provides an overview of the many issues involved in wilderness-related medical emergencies. Prehospital care providers who will be functioning in a formal capacity in the wilderness setting should obtain specific training in managing these patients. In addition, medical direction by a knowledgeable physician should be an integral component of wilderness medicine activities.

The "Wilderness EMS" Context

Many terms are used for areas far from civilization: backcountry, remote, wilderness, isolated. EMS personnel tend to lump these together under the rubric "wilderness" and to speak of "wilderness EMS." The dictionary definition of "wilderness" follows[2]:

1. a (1): a tract or region uncultivated and uninhabited by human beings;
       (2): an area essentially undisturbed by human activity together with its naturally developed life community;
    b: an empty or pathless area or region;
    c: a part of a garden devoted to wild growth;
2. wild or uncultivated state;
3. a: a confusing multitude or mass: an indefinitely great number or quantity;
    b: a bewildering situation.

Our use of "wilderness" differs from the dictionary definition, however, because we are thinking about *patient care*. Our definition is really the answer to a question: "When should we think about wilderness EMS?" That is, "When should we think and work differently from what we do on the street?"

The answer to this question goes beyond simple geography and involves the following considerations:

- Access to the scene
- Weather
- Daylight
- Terrain
- Special transport and handling needs
- Access and transport times
- Available personnel
- Communications

In a city after an earthquake, it may be very difficult to access those who are injured or trapped, there may be no road for transport, and local EMS systems may be out of action. In this situation, patients are likely to remain in their location for considerable time. They will have the same care requirements as a hiker who has fallen in the mountains and is hours—or days—away from a hospital.

A person who has fallen into a suburban landfill site, late in the evening, during an ice storm, is at risk from the same factors as in the wilderness. The patient may need a rescue team with ropes, ice axes and crampons, and medics who can anticipate and cope with issues such as hypothermia, toileting needs, prevention of pressure sores, wound management, and food and fluid requirements.

We often talk of "wilderness EMS," but in reality, *all* EMS lies on a spectrum. At one extreme is a scene half a block from a Level I trauma center, and at the other extreme are scenes such as the summit of Mount Everest or the deepest part of the Mammoth–Flint Ridge cave system in Kentucky.

Therefore, in the final analysis, where does "the street" end and "the wilderness" begin? The answer is, "It depends." It depends on the distance from the ambulance (and the ED). It depends on the weather. It depends on the terrain.

Even more importantly, it depends on the nature of the injury or illness and the capabilities of the EMS and rescue personnel on-scene. We return to this topic at the end of the chapter.

Backcountry Injury Patterns

As mentioned in Chapter 1, death from trauma has a trimodal (three-peaked) distribution. The *first peak of death* is within seconds to minutes of injury. Deaths occurring during this period are usually caused by lacerations of the brain, brainstem, high spinal cord, heart, aorta, or other large vessels and can best be managed by preventive measures such as helmets and seat belts. Only a few of the patients can be saved, and then only in large urban areas where rapid emergency transport is available. The *second death peak* occurs within minutes to a few hours after injury. **Rapid assessment and resuscitation are carried out to reduce this second peak of trauma deaths.** Deaths occurring during this period are usually caused by subdural and epidural hematomas, hemopneumothorax, ruptured spleen, lacerations of the liver, pelvic fractures, or multiple injuries associated with significant blood loss. The fundamental principles of trauma care learned in this course can best be applied to these patients. The *third death peak* occurs several days or weeks after the initial injury and is almost always caused by sepsis and organ failure.

The PHTLS course focuses mostly on saving patients from the second "peak" of the trimodal death distribution. In the backcountry, however, most of those who survive to be rescued have already weathered the first and usually most of the second "peak" of the trimodal death graph. Therefore, in the backcountry, the focus is much more on "what can we do *now* that will keep the patient from dying *tomorrow*?" We need to make sure the patient does not develop problems such as kidney failure from dehydration, overwhelming infection from poor resistance due to starvation, pulmonary embolism from deep venous thrombosis (blood clots in the legs breaking off and going to the lungs), and infections from decubiti (bedsores).

Safety

In the backcountry, even more so than on the street, scene safety is paramount. An injured or dead rescuer never did anyone any good. "Street" scene safety considerations still

apply—even in the backcountry, a civilian aircraft can offer problems similar to an automobile crash—but there are other considerations as well. In the backcountry, scene dangers are usually much less obvious than on the street; they tend to slowly "sneak up" on unwary rescuers.

The provider and patient will be exposed to the weather, and changes in weather, such as an incoming cold front with freezing rain, may complicate the operation or even injure or kill the provider and patient. If a rescue lasts for hours, the lack of food and water may cause debilitation. The terrain is often rugged, and poisonous plants and wildlife may complicate patient care (Figure 22-2). Providers need to be aware of dangers specific to the environment, such

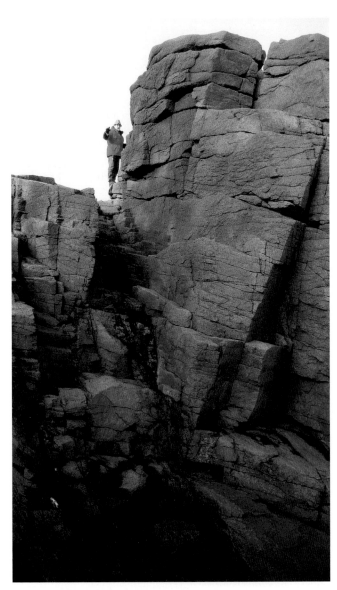

FIGURE 22-2 Steep slopes and uneven footing are a danger in wilderness rescue.

as rockfall, avalanche risk, rising water, bad air or altitude exposure, and recirculating eddies at the base of waterfalls.

The Wilderness Is Everywhere

In the rest of this chapter, we talk about "wilderness EMS" and "in the wilderness" and "wilderness patients." Remember, however, that "the wilderness" might be a short distance from the road, if it is dark and the weather is bad, or even *on* the road if a disaster has made roads impassable or made nearby hospitals unable to accept patients.

EMS Decision Making: Balancing Risks and Benefits

Experienced EMTs and medics (and even doctors and nurses) know that procedures such as airway management and wound management are the easy part of medicine. The difficult part is knowing *when* to do *what*: decision making. Even more often than on the street, in the wilderness one risk needs to be weighed carefully against another and against the potential benefits.

For *this* particular patient, in *this* particular setting, and with *these* particular resources, and with *this* particular likelihood of *this* particular help arriving at *this* particular time in the future, what are the potential risks? What are the potential benefits? Wilderness EMS is largely the art of compromise: balancing the particular risks and benefits for each patient.

To illustrate wilderness EMS decision making, we continue the discussion on management of potential spinal injury presented in Chapter 9.

"Clearing" the Cervical Spine in the Wilderness

A healthy 24-year-old woman was rock climbing along a river gorge when she fell 65 feet. All her chocks (anchors placed in cracks in the cliff) came out one by one, so she fell all the way to the ground, but was slowed by each anchor as it failed. She was wearing a helmet but hit her head and had a brief loss of consciousness. When you and your partner arrive, after an hour-long hike up the river gorge from where you parked the ambulance at the end of the road, she is alert and conscious, with no complaints, a normal neurologic examination, and a normal physical examination. It is late fall, it is getting dark, the nearest helicopter landing zone is back at the road an hour away, and the forecast is for a blizzard to start tonight. Does she need to be immobilized?

Do you have to call for a team with a Stokes litter and a long backboard? Or can you walk her out?

"Street" Cervical Spine Management History

Spinal immobilization for severely injured trauma patients became the standard of care decades ago. Even if unstable cervical spine fractures were rare in alert trauma patients, and even if no evidence indicated that spinal immobilization was effective at preventing paralysis in alert patients, being strapped to a board seemed unlikely to hurt anyone. Therefore, over the next 30 years, prehospital care providers used spinal immobilization for more and more patients. It has since been recognized that patients experience gradually increasing pain from the long backboard. Studies show moderate pain at 30 minutes and severe pain at about 45 minutes.[3]

As EMT training became more and more widely used by backcountry search and rescue teams, the practice of strapping everyone to a board after an accident did not seem to make sense, especially if the patient was on the side of a mountain in a snowstorm, and the nearest board was 10 miles away and 10,000 feet down. So search and rescue teams and the physicians working with them developed guidelines, based on the available literature, for when *not* to immobilize trauma patients in the backcountry.[4]

As described in Chapter 9, a large and important multicenter study called "NEXUS" showed that many patients can be "cleared" without x-ray films, if the following selection criteria are used:

- Absence of tenderness at the posterior midline of the cervical spine
- Absence of a focal neurologic deficit
- Normal level of alertness
- No evidence of intoxication
- Absence of clinically apparent pain that might distract the patient from the pain of a cervical spine injury

Variants of these criteria have been used by many EMS systems. A few studies suggest some problems with using these criteria in the field. The wording of some EMS "selective spinal immobilization protocols" deviate significantly from the previous wording, raising concerns about whether they really reflect the NEXUS criteria. However, it is generally accepted that the NEXUS criteria, properly applied, are a good guide to patients who do not need to be strapped to a board, whether on the street or in the backcountry.

The problem in the backcountry, however, is not as simple. What if a patient doesn't quite meet NEXUS criteria? Does that mean that the patient *has* to be immobilized?

As discussed earlier, wilderness EMS is the art of compromise, and nowhere is this more apparent than in making decisions about spinal immobilization.

What if the patient has a potential spine injury and it is a 2-hour walk from the nearest road, and no spinal immobilization equipment is at hand? Is it necessary to send someone on the 4-hour round-trip hike back to the ambulance for it?

What if the patient is in a cave, with the water level rising? Could the patient and rescuers be cut off from an escape route and drown if the team delays?

What if the patient is in the mountains, far from the ambulance, and a storm is moving in? What are the risks if the patient and rescuers are forced to spend the night on the mountain?

In each of these situations, prehospital care providers at the scene are faced with the following two options:

- Staying and waiting for the spinal immobilization to arrive.
- Starting an improvised evacuation without spinal immobilization.

Neither option is ideal, and prehospital care providers need to choose. To make this choice intelligently, the following questions must be asked and answered:

- What are the risks of an improvised evacuation without spinal immobilization, and what are the risks of waiting for spinal immobilization equipment to arrive, *for this particular patient*?
- What are the benefits of moving without waiting for spinal immobilization, and for waiting for spinal immobilization equipment to arrive, *for this particular patient*?

The benefits of spinal immobilization depend on the likelihood that this particular patient has an unstable spinal injury.

In the NEXUS study, those who did *not* meet the NEXUS criteria, and who could not be "cleared," still had a very low risk of unstable spinal fracture, as follows:

- Only 2% of those who *failed* the NEXUS "clearing" protocol had "clinically significant" fractures.
- Of that 2%, only a small fraction likely required specific treatment.
- Of *that* small fraction, only a small fraction likely had injuries that might endanger the spinal cord if not immobilized, and most of those were in patients with multiple major fractures and multiple life-threatening injuries.

Therefore, it seems likely that, for backcountry trauma patients who have survived long enough to be rescued, the incidence of unstable spine injury will be less than 1%.

Prehospital care providers at the scene need to assess these potential risks and benefits to make an informed decision.

Improvised Evacuations

When discussing spinal injury in the wilderness context, we mentioned the idea of starting an improvised evacuation rather than waiting for a litter and spinal immobilization equipment (Figure 22-3).

Carrying patients in the backcountry is an extremely difficult, time-consuming, and somewhat dangerous activity for both the patient and those doing the carrying. Those with no search and rescue (SAR) experience generally underestimate the time and difficulty of a backcountry evacuation by at least half, or sometimes up to a factor of five for more difficult evacuations, especially cave rescues.

If someone without SAR experience says, "It'll take us about 2 hours to get the patient out of here," triple this, and expect it to take 6 hours, or longer if the patient is in a cave, if the team is short on people, if the terrain is particularly difficult, or if the weather is bad. This is especially important to remember if darkness is approaching or the weather is deteriorating.

Walking a patient out, even with a couple of people helping, is almost always *much* faster. Certainly if the patient starts moving *now*, rather than waiting for a litter or spinal immobilization, the evacuation will be much, much faster. If the patient cannot walk (e.g., because of an ankle fracture), it is possible to do a piggyback carry or to make an improvised stretcher out of sticks and rope.

FIGURE 22-3 Because of uneven terrain, creativity and technical rescue skills may be needed to evacuate patients safely out of the backcountry.

Patient Care in the Wilderness

Elimination Needs

The truth described in a popular children's book called *Everyone Poops*[5] applies to backcountry patients as well. Given the relatively short transport times in an urban setting, most patients do not have an elimination need. Trauma patients almost never defecate. If you are caring for a patient who has been in the backcountry for a day, however, and it takes you several hours to get to the patient, it is *much* more likely the patient will need to urinate or defecate.

Having patient care supplies that include "blue pads" for under the patient, having some toilet paper, and even stopping to let the patient urinate or defecate are all reasonable measures (Figure 22-4).

It is possible for men and women to urinate even while immobilized in a Stokes litter with a full body vacuum splint, if packaging is planned carefully and the litter is up on an end. For women, a small funnel device commonly carried by women when backpacking will be needed.

However, people who are lying on their backsides for a long time tend to develop decubiti (bedsores). These may end up requiring surgery, resulting in a longer hospital admission. Some patients even die from infection and other complications from bedsores.

Lying in one's own urine and feces for a long time (just hours, not even days) may make bedsores more likely. If patient care is only for a few minutes during transport, urine and feces are not a major issue. However, if a provider has been taking care of a patient for several hours and then delivers the patient to the ED lying in his own feces, the nurses might (legitimately) complain about the level of care.

Food and Water Needs

Every backcountry patient is cold, hungry, and thirsty; that is, hypothermic, starved, and dehydrated, or if you prefer a good mnemonic at a slight expense of accuracy, *hypothermic, hypoglycemic,* and *hypovolemic.*

Starvation is much more than just hypoglycemia (low blood sugar), and not all starving patients are significantly hypoglycemic. Dehydration is more than just hypovolemia, which refers only to intravascular volume within the blood vascular system. Patients who are dehydrated have also lost water out of their cells and the interstitial spaces between the cells.

On the street, water or food are *not* generally given to patients. There are good reasons not to feed patients on the street. A patient will not starve or dehydrate in a few minutes. If the patient might need to go to the OR, having food or fluid in the stomach is harmful; it increases the likelihood of vomiting or, more likely, passive regurgitation when under anesthesia.

However, the stomach only needs to be empty for a few hours before anesthesia. If a patient rescued from the backcountry needs to go the OR, it will almost always take a few hours for the patient to get prepared for the OR in any event.

As noted earlier, with wilderness patients the focus is to ensure that the patient does not die *tomorrow.* Starving people is seldom good for them. Feeding the patient today will make the patient better tomorrow. Therefore, provide food and water to any reasonably alert backcountry patient.

Vomiting and aspiration are always a danger, and careful attention to the patient's airway is always important (e.g., positioning on the side for long transports, even if the patient needs spinal immobilization). However, rescuers should still attempt to provide food and water for backcountry patients, even though they have vomited once or twice, as long as their airway is protected.

Long Backboards Hurt Patients

Other important preventive measures for backcountry patients, especially those who face prolonged evacuation, include prevention of decubiti (bedsores), as follows:

- Allow (and assist) the patient to turn from side to side in the litter.
- Keep the patient's sacrum (buttocks) clean and dry.

If the patient truly needs spinal immobilization, prevention of decubiti is even more important, although correspondingly more difficult. Techniques to avoid decubiti during spinal immobilization include the following:

- Put the patient in a full-body vacuum splint rather than on a long backboard. Vacuum mattresses provide

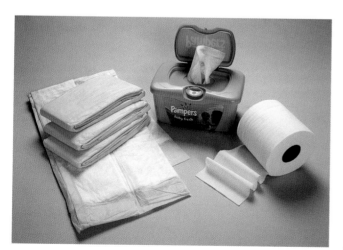

FIGURE 22-4 Elimination supplies.

excellent spinal immobilization and are much less likely to cause decubiti.[6-9]

- If no full-body vacuum splint is available, pad the long backboard well and add support under the lumbar spine, knees, and neck. Studies show that immobilization on an unpadded long backboard causes even uninjured people to experience excruciating pain in about 45 minutes and skin necrosis (cell death) in about 90 minutes.[3,10-13]
- Carry the litter first on one side, then the other, so that pressure alternates between the two hips rather than always on the sacrum.

To prevent deep venous thrombosis and pulmonary embolism, do the following:

- Package patients so that they can move their legs; do not tie them down tight.
- Consider rest stops to allow patients out of the litter to stretch their legs.

If there is mild suspicion of a cervical spine injury but not a lumbar spine injury, it might even be appropriate to allow an alert patient out of the litter, still wearing a cervical collar, and, with many trained hands to help, allow the patient to stretch the legs and urinate. Speaking with a physician conversant with wilderness EMS might be reassuring if this is contemplated.

Sun Protection

Other backcountry hazards to consider include rockfall, avalanches, and cave-stream flooding. However, one hazard worth discussing in more detail here is sun protection.

The ultraviolet (UV) rays of the sun can damage the skin, sometimes severely. Second-degree and third-degree sunburns are seen in some victims of exposure, and such severe sunburn can cause shock or death. Sunburn also makes skin cancer more likely.

Ultraviolet light comes in two frequencies, A and B (UVA and UVB). UVA was once thought to be harmless, but now we know that it works synergistically with UVB to cause sunburn. Thus, sun-blocking materials or creams must block both UVA and UVB to be effective.

Sun protection is measured by the *sun protection factor* (SPF) (Figure 22-5). The SPF is a numeric measure of how much the clothing or cream increases the minimum dose of UV light to make the skin red. For example, a sunscreen lotion with a rating of SPF 45 provides protection from sunburn for about 45 times longer than without the sunscreen.

To check clothing for SPF, hold a piece of clothing up against a light bulb. If an image of the light bulb is seen through it, the SPF is slightly below 15. If light is seen

FIGURE 22-5 Sunscreen.

through it but not the image of the light bulb, the SPF is in the range of 15 to 60 SPF.

Protective lotions with a minimum SPF of 15 should be applied to exposed skin to minimize the potential injury from sun exposure. With profuse sweating, lotion should be reapplied frequently.

Sunburn is treated as any other burn, and the care is essentially the same in the wilderness as on the street. The only major difference is that in the backcountry, the prehospital care provider needs to be aware of and treat the potential fluid loss, dehydration, or sometimes even shock, and to recognize that patients with sunburn are at higher risk for hypothermia.

Specifics of Backcountry EMS

This section reviews a few of the most important situations in which proper backcountry trauma care differs from that on the street.

Wound Management

Wound management encompasses the following:

- Hemostasis (stopping bleeding)
- Antisepsis (prevention of infection)
- Restoration of function (returning the skin to its protective function, and restoring a limb or other body part to normal function)
- Cosmesis (pleasant appearance)

In the backcountry, prevention of infection and restoration of function assume great importance.

Hemostasis

Control of bleeding is part of the primary survey. On the street, arterial bleeding can kill. In the backcountry, however, even venous bleeding can kill, if it continues for a sufficient time; every RBC counts. Therefore, bleeding control, using standard measures such as direct pressure and elevation, are as important or more important in the wilderness.

At times, however, finding a bleeding site to provide direct digital (finger) pressure over the "bleeder" (bleeding blood vessel) is not that easy. Direct digital pressure for 10 to 15 minutes is far superior to a pressure bandage at controlling bleeders.

Therefore, some wilderness EMS protocols suggest using a pressure point or a proximal blood pressure (BP) cuff as a tourniquet for 1 or 2 minutes to control the bleeding initially. Then, after letting the BP cuff down carefully, the location of the bleeder usually becomes obvious, and a gloved finger covered with a gauze pad (to prevent slipping) can be carefully placed over the bleeder for 10 to 15 minutes. If the bleeder starts bleeding again, direct digital pressure for another 10 to 15 minutes almost always stops it.

Note that we are suggesting using a BP cuff tourniquet for only a few minutes. It is important to remember to *let the BP cuff down* and not use it by itself to stop bleeding; otherwise, the limb might develop permanent damage.

Various companies market special dressings and powders and other devices to stop venous bleeding (see Chapter 7).

Prevention of Infection

After injury in the backcountry, it may be a long time until the wound receives definitive treatment in an ED. Routine wound care in the ED includes appropriate cleaning to prevent infection. Wounds contaminated by dirt or caused by penetration from a dirty object are cleaned with high-pressure irrigation. Noncontaminated wounds are cleaned with low-pressure irrigation.

High-pressure irrigation causes swelling of wounds, but in the case of contaminated wounds full of dirt and bacteria, the benefit of removing bacteria outweighs the risks from wound swelling.[14,15] Infections may set in quickly. After a wound has been open for about 8 hours, bacteria have spread from the skin deep into the wound. After 8 hours, sewing up a wound is likely to create a deep wound infection. Deep wound infections develop pressure, which keeps out white blood cells, the body's normal defense mechanism against infection.

Routine wound care on the "street" does *not* include cleansing the wound because it makes sense to delay cleansing for a few minutes until the patient reaches the ED,

which is better suited for wound cleansing and evaluating the patient. The ED can determine if the patient has a tendon or nerve laceration, an associated fracture, a spleen laceration, or a subdural hematoma in the head.

Delaying wound care does *not* make sense in the backcountry. If it will take hours to get to the ED, the wound should be cleaned. In remote areas the wound could become infected before the patient arrives at the ED several days later.

Studies have shown that early irrigation is essential to removing bacteria and reducing wound infections.[16-18] It is not necessary or practical to carry sterile solutions for wound irrigation. There is no need to add antiseptics to the water.[19] Water that is good enough to drink is good enough to irrigate a wound. Water from streams or melted snow can be treated with any standard backcountry drinking-water treatment.[14,20-24]

When cleaning an uncontaminated wound, such as a laceration sustained from banging the forehead against a teammate's helmet, it is only necessary to "slosh a bit of water through the wound." Some recommendations call for using a blue bulb syringe, usually available in the ED, but sloshing some water from a drinking-water bottle will do as well.

If the wound is contaminated, it must be irrigated with enough pressure to clean out bacteria. The original studies showed that a 35-mL syringe with an 18-gauge needle provided an appropriate amount of pressure (5-15 psi).[25-27] Squirt the water, at high pressure, throughout the wound. However, this is a major blood-borne pathogen risk; protection from the spray of blood when irrigating is necessary. Eye protection and gloves are essential.

Sometimes it is necessary to use a gauze pad or clean cloth with gloved fingers to clean out some gross dirt or foreign material. The patient's pain may need to be treated before cleaning the wound. Once done, dress and bandage the wound. Reapply a clean dressing at least daily.

If the wound is gaping open, a wet dressing will prevent tissue damage from drying out; change or at least rewet the dressing with clean water several times a day. In most cases, however, because the wound will be mostly closed by bandaging, apply a dry dressing.

Restoration of Function and Cosmesis: Closing Backcountry Wounds

Because of the lack of good lighting, x-ray films, and a warm dry place to work, it does not make sense to perform definitive wound closure in the backcountry. However, it is possible simply to cleanse the wound, dress and bandage, do good wound care for 4 days, and then do a *delayed primary closure*. Four days later, as long as the wound is not infected, it is safe to close the wound as if it had just occurred. Although bacteria move into the wound soon after injury, eventually enough of the body's defenses (e.g., white blood cells) have entered the wound and make it safe to close. This occurs about 4 days after the initial injury.

Because delayed primary closure is available, there is no pressing reason to close wounds in the backcountry. If a surgeon or someone else experienced at wound closure is present, the wound may be closed at the scene. However, it is still reasonable to only cleanse, dress, and bandage the wound and allow closure to occur later.

Closing a backcountry wound may be important in one situation: when bleeding cannot be controlled in any other way. These situations are uncommon and usually involve a scalp laceration. For this reason, some wilderness EMS personnel are trained to use disposable surgical staplers to repair scalp wounds. However, wound repair is complex and should not be attempted without sufficient training and experience.

Dislocations

A healthy 20-year-old man was kayaking along a whitewater stream when the top of his kayak paddle hit a low-hanging tree branch. Now his right shoulder is swollen and deformed and painful. He cannot bring his right arm across his chest. Distal pulses, capillary refill, sensation, and movement are intact. From the ambulance, you and your partner EMT hiked (bushwhacked) a mile through the woods to get to the stream. Should you "splint it as it lies"? Or try to reduce what looks like an anterior shoulder dislocation?

The standard of care for fractures and dislocations on the street is to "splint it as it lies" and transport for definitive treatment. The only exception is the patient whose pulse is not palpable.

Although "splint it as it lies" is a good general rule for the street, "make it look normal" is a better general rule for the wilderness context. It is certainly appropriate for both fractures and dislocations when transport is delayed.

There are many types of dislocations—finger, toe, shoulder, patella, knee, elbow, hip, ankle, and jaw—and all have been successfully reduced in the backcountry, some more easily than others. It is usually very easy to reduce dislocations of the ankle (which are almost always fracture-dislocations), patella, toe, or finger, except the proximal inter-phalangeal joint of the index finger in some cases. Elbow, knee, and hip dislocations are usually quite difficult. All are much easier with training and practice, and in particular, it takes training or experience to know, without a radiograph, *when* a joint is likely dislocated, and to attempt reduction.

EMT and paramedic courses seldom provide training in dislocation reduction. Because backcountry dislocations are so common, however, dislocation reduction is covered in almost all wilderness first-aid, wilderness first-responder, and wilderness EMT training. Those who might provide EMS in the backcountry or who regularly travel in the backcountry are advised to take one of these courses.

Cardiopulmonary Resuscitation in the Backcountry
Backcountry Traumatic Arrest

A few signs can be uniformly equated with nonsurvivability, as follows:

- Decapitation
- Transection of the torso
- Patient is frozen so hard that the chest cannot be compressed
- Patient's rectal temperature is very cold and the same as the environment
- Well-progressed decomposition (see later discussion)

The following presumptive signs of death may be of use to prehospital care providers, although no one sign by itself is reliable:

- *Rigor mortis.* Postmortem rigidity is well known but not always present, and similar rigidity is often observed in hypothermic but semiconscious patients.
- *Dependent lividity.* This is common in corpses but also is found along with pressure necrosis and frostbite in some patients exposed to the elements for a long time.
- *Decomposition.* This is usually self-evident.
- *Lack of presumptive signs of life.* Hypothermia can mimic death, in that pulses may not be palpable and respirations may be undetectable, with dilated unreactive pupils and no signs of consciousness. However, such severely hypothermic patients have occasionally been resuscitated, with full neurologic recovery.

We know that traumatic cardiac arrest "on the street," if from trauma, has a poor prognosis, even if the scene is within minutes of a Level I trauma center. No person survives more than a few minutes of cardiopulmonary resuscitation (CPR) after traumatic arrest.[28-31] This is recognized in many EMS protocols, as follows:

- For traumatic cardiac arrest, initiate CPR with cervical spine stabilization if:
  1. Cardiac arrest occurs in the presence of EMS personnel.
  2. Victim of penetrating trauma had signs of life within 15 minutes before the arrival of EMS personnel.

Therefore, in the wilderness context, CPR is inappropriate for traumatic arrest. It would be appropriate for prehospital care providers and the mountain rescue team members to examine the patient, then gently but firmly tell the companions that the victim is dead and there is no reason to initiate resuscitation. The prehospital care providers and mountain rescue team members should then deal appropriately with the expected denial and grief reactions, with a check of scene safety, especially if oncoming darkness may make exiting the area hazardous to the victim's mentally and physically exhausted companions.

Backcountry Medical Arrest

A medical arrest applies to a patient who has chest pain and then sustains a cardiac arrest. Again, in the wilderness context, the chances of survival are poor or nonexistent when the patient is more than a few minutes of CPR from defibrillation.[32-37] It is possible that a rescue team might be carrying out a patient with chest pain when the patient sustains a cardiac arrest. However, the usefulness-to-weight ratio of defibrillators is so poor that they are seldom carried by wilderness rescue teams.

There are a variety of other causes of cardiac arrest in the backcountry, and in the previous example, ventricular fibrillation (VF) cardiac arrest secondary to hypothermia or cardiac arrest secondary to pulmonary embolism is likely. For such cardiac arrests, however, survival is even less likely than with a cardiac arrest secondary to a myocardial infarction.

However, "nontraumatic" backcountry cardiac arrest might be survivable in the following situations:

- Hypothermia[38]
- Cold-water near-drowning[39-42]
- Lightning strike[43]
- Electrocution
- Drug overdose
- Avalanche burial[44]

In all these cases, a patient may appear to be in cardiac arrest but still might be resuscitated by basic CPR. For hypothermia in particular, there is a saying that "nobody's dead until they're warm and dead" (see Chapter 16). A significant minority of those who appear dead from the mechanisms listed can be resuscitated. There are special considerations for each of these situations; for example, scene safety for those who have been electrocuted and are still attached to a backcountry power line, or knowing that external cardiac compression can actually induce a VF cardiac arrest in a hypothermic patient whose heart is beating just enough to keep the patient alive.[45-48] Although appropriate in a wilderness EMT course, detailed discussion of these topics is beyond the scope of this chapter.

However, two standard wilderness CPR rules are as follows[34]:

- If the patient appears to be in cardiac arrest from causes other than trauma, attempt CPR for 15 to 30 minutes; if this does not resuscitate the patient, stop CPR and consider the patient dead.
- However, do *not* start CPR if it will put rescuers at risk and decrease their chances of retreating from the scene

safely, given concerns about daylight, terrain, weather, and available nearby shelter.

Bites and Stings

Bites and stings are common backcountry problems. The exact type of bite or sting likely in a backcountry area depends on the locale.

Bee Stings

The most widespread, common, and deadly sting is that of the common honeybee, at least to those who are allergic. Most reactions to bee stings are severe (although brief) local pain and in some cases local swelling and redness for 1 or 2 days; these latter reactions are likely directly related to injected toxins, and not an indication of allergy.

Some who are stung will progress within a few minutes to a generalized allergic reaction. This may range from urticaria to a full-blown anaphylactic reaction. Although the exact spectrum of generalized allergic reaction depends on the contents of the injected toxin (which varies among the many species of bees and wasps) and the allergic history of the patient, one or more of the following are usually seen:

- Urticaria (hives) (Figure 22-6)
- Lip swelling
- Hoarseness or stridor
- Wheezing and/or shortness of breath
- Abdominal cramping, vomiting, or diarrhea
- Tachycardia *or* bradycardia
- Low blood pressure
- Syncope
- Frank hypovolemic shock

Those with a history of a generalized allergic reaction to a sting are more likely to have another generalized reaction

FIGURE 22-6   Allergic urticaria.
(From Forbes CD, Jackson WF: *World atlas and text of clinical medicine,* ed 3, London, 1993, Mosby–Year Book Europe Limited.)

to the next sting. However, venom among different species varies enough that, despite a history of generalized allergy in the past, a patient might have no generalized reaction to the next sting.

A patient with mild urticaria after a sting probably will do well. If a patient with hives after a sting progresses to "real" anaphylaxis, however, the best early sign is hoarseness. The major cause of death after bee sting allergy is airway obstruction from hives in the airway, and hoarseness is usually the first sign of airway swelling. Any patient with a generalized reaction to a bee sting needs treatment immediately.

Basic life support (BLS) interventions involve keeping the patient flat or with the legs somewhat elevated, performing standard airway management, and providing oxygen.

One simple but useful intervention is to remove an embedded stinger properly. Although only a small fraction of bee stings still have an embedded stinger, it often requires good eyes and bright light or a magnifying glass to see the stinger, and improper removal could be deadly. Squeezing an embedded stinger with a pair of forceps, clamps, or tweezers can squeeze more venom into the skin. Instead, using a credit card or *carefully* scraping with a knife blade can remove the stinger without squeezing additional venom into the skin.

It is important to remove embedded stingers as soon as possible; the venom sac continues to squeeze in venom even after the bee has flown away.

The main medications to treat bee stings include the following:

1. Epinephrine (adrenaline). Although epinephrine only acts for a few minutes, it can be lifesaving.
2. Antihistamines (e.g., diphenhydramine [Benadryl]). Anyone who requires epinephrine for a bee sting allergy should receive an antihistamine.
3. Steroids (e.g., prednisone). Most people who require epinephrine also require steroids.

Some wilderness SAR teams carry drugs for bee sting allergy in their medical kits; the team's wilderness EMTs have special training in their use. Also, some people with a history of bee sting allergy will carry these medications in their personal first-aid kits.

The most important drug is epinephrine. Epinephrine is available as a pen-sized autoinjector (e.g., Epi-Pen), which is often prescribed to any patient who has had a generalized allergy to bee stings. These autoinjectors are found in many wilderness first-aid kits.

Snakebite

There are many species of poisonous snakes. Few are found in northern latitudes. Most occur in tropical areas, and many are deadly. Although many snakes have venom glands, in North America there are only two types of snakes with

FIGURE 22-7   Coral snake.
(From Sanders M: *Mosby's paramedic textbook,* ed 3, St Louis, 2006, Mosby.)

FIGURE 22-8   Rattlesnake
(From Sanders M: *Mosby's paramedic textbook,* ed 3, St Louis, 2006, Mosby.)

venom strong enough to cause more than minor irritation to humans.

Coral snakes are small snakes, found in the southern parts of North America, that have a venom that is neurotoxic, that is, causes paralysis (Figure 22-7). However, the snakes are small, have small fangs, cannot open their mouths very far compared to larger snakes, and have to chew to allow the venom to penetrate.

Pit vipers (Figure 22-8) are found throughout large portions of North America and include *rattlesnakes* of various types, *copperheads* (Figure 22-9), and *water moccasins,* or *cottonmouths* (Figure 22-10). The majority of pit viper bites do not occur in the backcountry, but rather occur in rural or suburban or even urban areas. A classic example is the drunk man who was kissing his pet rattlesnake when he was bitten on the tongue.

Snakebites are not as rare as one might think. This is further complicated by the variety of prehospital treat-

FIGURE 22-9 Copperhead snake.
(From Auerbach PS: *Wilderness medicine: management of wilderness and environmental emergencies,* ed 4, St Louis, 2001, Mosby.)

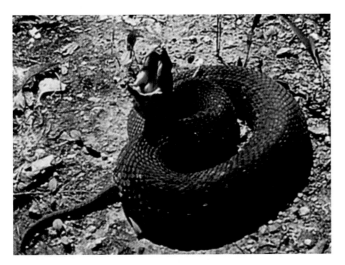

FIGURE 22-10 Water moccasin (cottonmouth) snake.
(From Auerbach PS: *Wilderness medicine: management of wilderness and environmental emergencies,* ed 4, St Louis, 2001, Mosby.)

ments attempted by patients, bystanders, or sometimes EMS personnel. The only treatment shown to be effective for envenomated pit viper bites is antivenin (antivenom), which is very expensive (thousands of dollars for a single treatment) and thus not routinely carried in first-aid kits. Indeed, the only "street" care proven to be helpful is transportation to the hospital.

1. The first thing to do to treat snakebite is to *watch for signs of envenomation.* Only a fraction of bites by pit vipers actually result in envenomation (venom was injected), and the signs of envenomation are fairly distinct. Although signs and symptoms of envenomation usually develop in a few minutes, sometimes they are delayed by 6 to 8 hours or perhaps even longer, so starting to the hospital after a suspected poisonous snakebite is appropriate. Signs of envenomation include the following:
   a. Severe local swelling, bruising and pain
   b. Continued bleeding from the bite
   c. Paresthesias in the fingers and toes (paresthesias are unusual sensations, usually caused by damage to nerves or biochemical abnormalities; a feeling of "pins and needles" is a common paresthesia)
   d. Metallic taste in the mouth
   e. Feeling of severe anxiety ("impending doom")
   f. Nausea, vomiting, and abdominal pain

The following are treatments that have been recommended but are not supported by the literature.

1. *Rest.* Some recommendations insist that those who have been bitten should always avoid exertion. Deaths from North American snakebite are very rare,[49] and it is very unlikely that the exertion of hiking out from a backcountry area will make a snakebite victim significantly more ill. If the victim can be carried out, that is ideal. However, if waiting for a carryout will delay the victim's arrival at a hospital, the victim should walk out with whatever assistance can be given.
2. *Catch the snake and bring it to the hospital.* There are numerous reports of bystanders who tried to catch a suspected poisonous snake and were bitten during the attempt. A single antivenin is used for all domestic pit viper venoms, and treatment is based on clinical degree of envenomation, relying on the previous signs and symptoms. Therefore, identifying a domestic snake is of minor importance compared with the dangers of attempting to catch the snake. A digital photograph of the snake might be useful, but identification is not worth the risk of an additional bite.
3. *Suction.* Suction, with or without cutting, has been shown to be useless for poisonous snakebite. Snakebite kits consisting of suction devices should be left out of all first-aid kits and should never be used.[50,51]
4. *Electric shock.* Electric shock, whether applied to the snake or to the snakebite, has been shown to be totally ineffective and should never be used.[52,53]
5. *Cold packs.* Cold packs have been shown to increase tissue damage from North American pit viper bites and should not be used.[54]
6. *Splinting, arterial or venous tourniquets, lymph constrictors, or elastic bandages.* Although widely recommended, none of these treatments has been shown to be effective and may worsen local damage to the bite area.[55,56]

The "Wilderness EMS" Context Revisited

At the beginning of this chapter, we asked *when* EMS is "wilderness EMS": "When should we think about wilderness

EMS; that is, when should we think and work differently from what we do on the street?"

From the bulk of the chapter, the reader can probably provide the short answer: "It depends."

Time, distance, weather, and terrain all enter into the decision. The decision that a particular patient, in a particular situation, with a particular set of injuries, needs "wilderness" care rather than "street" care is a medical decision and one best made by the prehospital care provider directly attending the patient. If the provider at the scene can contact a knowledgeable EMS physician, especially one with wilderness EMS experience or training, the advice is definitely worth seeking. Ultimately, the decision is up to the prehospital care provider at the scene.

PHTLS has always held that, given a good fund of knowledge and key principles, prehospital care providers, other EMS personnel, and EMTs are capable of making reasoned decisions regarding patient care.

SUMMARY

Wilderness EMS is the same as "street" EMS, but at the same time it is different. The principles of trauma care are the same, regardless of context. The wilderness context, which includes *much* more than designated wilderness areas, means the standard of care *changes* for certain injuries.

Clinical situations in which wilderness care is different include clearing the cervical spine, irrigating wounds, reducing dislocations, and terminating CPR. General principles for wilderness patients include dealing with elimination, prevention of decubiti, and prevention of deep venous thrombosis and pulmonary embolism. A basic principle is that all wilderness patients are hypothermic, hypoglycemic, and hypovolemic, or cold, hungry, and thirsty, and these basic bodily needs must be managed aggressively by rescuers.

Wilderness EMS involves decision making; more than anything, it is the art of compromise, the evaluation of risks and benefits for each individual patient situation. Wilderness patients seldom need more or different invasive procedures; they do usually need prehospital care providers with good thinking. A good wilderness provider carefully examines the patient, reexamines the patient on a regular basis, thinks about what is occurring, comes up with appropriate field diagnoses or perhaps a list of differential diagnoses, and uses this information to make appropriate decisions.

SCENARIO SOLUTION

The team's medic, a wilderness EMT-basic, briefly examines the patient and correctly suspects a likely hemorrhage of the spleen. The medic discusses the case with the team leader. Based on the medic's advice, the team leader details one member, another wilderness EMT-basic, to stay and bivouac with the patient with the ankle fracture. The leader calls the SAR team's base at the trailhead and arranges for a medical evacuation helicopter to meet the team at the trailhead, rather than using the ambulance for transportation. The team then uses the litter to carry the injured team member to the helicopter, which is just landing as they arrive at the trailhead. Additional team members will be dispatched along the trail, with another litter, to help evacuate the patient with the ankle fracture.

In this situation, there are no advanced techniques, only some knowledge of trauma, some knowledge of wilderness EMS, some knowledge of search and rescue, and some ability at physical examination—all applied to a difficult situation, balancing risks and benefits. In this case, the wilderness EMT's decision-making ability saves the life of the team member. She is flown to a Level I trauma center, receiving IV fluid in the helicopter when her blood pressure suddenly drops. When she arrives at the ED, she is quickly resuscitated with more fluids and blood, has a quick ultrasound of her abdomen that demonstrates free fluid, then quickly goes to the OR, where her lacerated spleen is repaired.

The goal of EMS is to "bring the hospital to the patient." The limitations of personnel and equipment, as well as the environment, place constraints on what constitutes "proper care," both on the street and in the backcountry. With their knowledge and expertise, however, and even without the use of advanced techniques, prehospital care personnel can have a major positive impact on the ultimate fate of backcountry trauma patients. ∎

References

1. Demarest JH: *Pre-hospital trauma life support,* Akron, Ohio, 1986, Emergency Training.

2. *Merriam-Webster's collegiate dictionary,* ed 10, Springfield, Mass, 1996, Merriam-Webster, Inc.

3. Chan D, Goldberg R, Tascone A, et al: The effect of spinal immobilization on healthy volunteers, *Ann Emerg Med* 23(1):48, 1994.

4. Conover K: EMTs should be able to clear the cervical spine in the wilderness, *J Wild Med* 3(4):339, 1992 (editorial).

5. Gomi T: *Everyone poops,* Brooklyn, NY, 1993, Kane/Miller Book Publishers.

6. Goldberg R, Chan D, Mason J, Chan L: Backboard versus mattress splint immobilization: a comparison of symptoms generated, *J Emerg Med,* 14(3):293, 1996.

7. Hamilton RS, Pons PT: The efficacy and comfort of full-body vacuum splints for cervical-spine immobilization, *J Emerg Med* 14(5):553, 1996.

8. Johnson DR, Hauswald M, Stockhoff C: Comparison of a vacuum splint device to a rigid backboard for spinal immobilization, *Am J Emerg Med* 14(4):369, 1996.

9. Lovell ME, Evans JH: A comparison of the spinal board and the vacuum stretcher, spinal stability and interface pressure, *Injury* 25(3):179, 1994.

10. Cordell WH, Hollingsworth JC, Olinger ML, et al: Pain and tissue-interface pressures during spine-board immobilization, *Ann Emerg Med* 26(1):31, 1995.

11. Delbridge TR, Auble TE, Garrison HG, Menengazzi JJ: Discomfort in healthy volunteers immobilized on wooden backboards and vacuum mattress splints, *Prehosp Disaster Med* 8(suppl 2), 1993.

12. Linares HA, Mawson AR, Suarez E: Association between pressure sores and immobilization in the immediate post-injury period, *Orthopedics* 10:571, 1987.

13. Mawson AR, Bundo JJ, Neville P: Risk factors for early occurring pressure ulcers following spinal cord injury, *Am J Phys Med Rehab* 67:123, 1988.

14. Edlich RF, Rodeheaver GT, Morgan RF, et al: Principles of emergency wound management, *Ann Emerg Med* 17(12):1284, 1988.

15. Edlich RF, Thacker JG, Buchanan L, Rodeheaver GT: Modern concepts of treatment of traumatic wounds, *Adv Surg* 13:169, 1979.

16. Bhandari M, Thompson K, Adili A, Shaughnessy SG: High and low pressure irrigation in contaminated wounds with exposed bone, *Int J Surg Invest* 2(3):179, 2000.

17. Bhandari M, Adili A, Lachowski RJ: High pressure pulsatile lavage of contaminated human tibiae: an in vitro study, *J Orthop Trauma* 12(7):479, 1998.

18. Bhandari M, Schemitsch EH, Adili A, et al: High and low pressure pulsatile lavage of contaminated tibial fractures: an in vitro study of bacterial adherence and bone damage, *J Orthop Trauma* 13(8):526, 1999.

19. Anglen JO: Wound irrigation in musculoskeletal injury, *J Am Acad Orthop Surg* 9(4):219, 2001.

20. Valente JH, Forti RJ, Freundlich LF, et al: Wound irrigation in children: saline solution or tap water? *Ann Emerg Med* 41(5):609, 2003.

21. Backer HD: Field water disinfection. In Auerbach PS, Geehr EC, editors: *Wilderness medicine: management of wilderness and environmental emergencies,* ed 2, St Louis, 1989, Mosby.

22. Griffiths RD, Fernandez RS, Ussia CA: Is tap water a safe alternative to normal saline for wound irrigation in the community setting? *J Wound Care* 10(10):407, 2001.

23. Moscati R, Mayrose J, Fincher L, Jehle D: Comparison of normal saline with tap water for wound irrigation, *Am J Emerg Med* 16(4):379, 1998.

24. Moscati RM, Reardon RF, Lerner EB, Mayrose J: Wound irrigation with tap water, *Acad Emerg Med* 5(11):1076, 1998.

25. Rodeheaver GT, Pettry D, Thacker JG, et al: Wound cleansing by high pressure irrigation, *Surg Gynecol Obstet* 141(3):357, 1975.

26. Edlich RF, Reddy VR: Revolutionary advances in wound repair in emergency medicine during the last three decades: a view toward the new millennium, 5th Annual David R. Boyd, MD Lecture, *J Emerg Med* 20(2):167, 2001.

27. Singer AJ, Hollander JE, Subramanian S, et al: Pressure dynamics of various irrigation techniques commonly used in the emergency department, *Ann Emerg Med* 24(1):36, 1994.

28. Fulton RL, Voigt WJ, Hilakos AS: Confusion surrounding the treatment of traumatic cardiac arrest, *J Am Coll Surg* 181:209, 1995.

29. Pasquale MD, Rhodes M, Cipolle MD, et al: Defining "dead on arrival": impact on a Level I trauma center, *J Trauma* 41:726, 1996.

30. Mattox KL, Feliciano DV: Role of external cardiac compression in truncal trauma, *J Trauma* 22:934, 1982.

31. Shimazu S, Shatney CH: Outcomes of trauma patients with no vital signs on admission, *J Trauma* 23(3):213, 1983.

32. Forgey WW, Wilderness Medical Society: *Practice guidelines for wilderness emergency care,* ed 2, Guilford, Conn, 2001, Globe Pequot Press.

33. Goth P, Garnett G, Rural Affairs Committee, National Association of EMS Physicians: Clinical guidelines for delayed/prolonged transport. I. Cardiorespiratory arrest, *Prehosp Disaster Med* 6(3):335, 1991.

34. Bowman WD: CPR and wilderness rescue: when and when not to use it, *Response,* 1987.

35. Eisenberg MS, Bergner L, Hallstrom AP: Cardiac resuscitation in the community: importance of rapid provision and implications of program planning, *JAMA* 241:1905, 1979.

36. Kellermann AL, Hackman BB, Somes G: Predicting the outcome of unsuccessful prehospital advanced cardiac life support, *JAMA* 270(12):1433, 1993.

37. Bonnin MJ, Pepe PE, Kimball KT, Clark PS: Distinct criteria for termination of resuscitation in the out-of-hospital setting, *JAMA* 270(12):1457, 1993.

38. Leavitt M, Podgorny G: Prehospital CPR and the pulseless hypothermic patient, *Ann Emerg Med* 13:492, 1984.

39. Keatinge WR: Accidental immersion hypothermia and drowning, *Practitioner* 219:183, 1977.

40. Olshaker JS: Near drowning, *Emerg Med Clin North Am* 10(2):339, 1992.

41. Bolte RG, Black PG, Bowers RS, et al: The use of extracorporeal rewarming in a child submerged for 66 minutes, *JAMA* 260(3):377, 1988.

42. Orlowski JP: Drowning, near-drowning, and ice-water drowning, *JAMA* 260(3):390, 1988 (editorial).

43. Cooper MA: Lightning injuries. In Auerbach PS, Geehr EC, editors: *Wilderness medicine: management of wilderness and environmental emergencies,* ed 2, St Louis, 1989, Mosby.

44. Durrer B, Brugger H: Recent advances in avalanche survival. Presented at the Second World Congress on Wilderness Medicine, Aspen, Colo, 1995.

45. Steinman AM: Cardiopulmonary resuscitation and hypothermia, *Circulation* 74(6, pt 2):29, 1986.

46. Zell SC: Epidemiology of wilderness-acquired diarrhea: implications for prevention and treatment, *J Wild Med* 3(3):241, 1992.

47. Lloyd EL: *Hypothermia and cold stress,* Rockville, Md, 1986, Aspen Systems.

48. Maningas PA, DeGuzman LR, Hollenbach SJ, et al: Regional blood flow during hypothermic arrest, *Ann Emerg Med* 15(4):390, 1986.

49. Curry SC, Kunkel DB: Death from a rattlesnake bite, *Am J Emerg Med* 3(3):227, 1985.

50. Bush SP: Snakebite suction devices don't remove venom: they just suck, *Ann Emerg Med* 43(2):187, 2004.

51. Alberts MB, Shalit M, LoGalbo F: Suction for venomous snakebite: a study of "mock venom" extraction in a human model, *Ann Emerg Med* 43(2):181, 2004.

52. Davis D, Branch K, Egen NB, et al: The effect of an electrical current on snake venom toxicity, *J Wild Med* 3(1):48, 1992.

53. Howe NR, Meisenheimer JL Jr: Electric shock does not save snakebitten rats, *Ann Emerg Med* 17(3):254, 1988.

54. Gill KA Jr: The evaluation of cryotherapy in the treatment of snake envenomation, *South Med J* 63:552, 1968.

55. Norris RL: A call for snakebite research, *Wilderness Environ Med* 11(3):149, 2000.

56. Stewart ME, Greenland S, Hoffman JR: First-aid treatment of poisonous snakebite: are currently recommended procedures justified? *Ann Emerg Med* 10(6):331, 1981.

Suggested Readings

Auerbach PS, editor: *Wilderness medicine: management of wilderness and environmental emergencies,* ed 4, St Louis, 2001, Mosby.

Goth P, Garnett G: Clinical guidelines for delayed or prolonged transport: II. Dislocations. Rural Affairs Committee, National Association of Emergency Medical Services Physicians, *Prehosp Disaster Med* 8(1):77, 1993.

Goth P, Garnett G: Clinical guidelines for delayed or prolonged transport: IV. Wounds. Rural Affairs Committee, Nation Association of Emergency Medical Services Physicians, *Prehosp Disaster Med* 8(3):253, 1993.

Glossary

accelerated motion   Sudden surge or increase in motion (e.g., from transference of motion in rear-impact collision); occurs as a slower-moving or stationary object is struck from behind.

acetabulum   Cup-shaped hip socket on lateral surface of the pelvis that holds head of the femur.

acidosis   Accumulation of acids and decreased pH of the blood.

acute respiratory distress syndrome (ARDS)   Respiratory insufficiency as a result of damage to the lining of the capillaries in the lung, leading to the leakage of fluid into the interstitial spaces and alveoli.

acute tubular necrosis (ATN)   Acute damage to the renal tubules, usually caused by ischemia associated with shock.

adolescent   A child with the body size and physical development normally found in children between 13 and 16 years of age. An arbitrary grouping of older children based on the similar physical characteristics common to these near-adult ages.

adult   A person (generally 16 years of age or older) whose body has reached maturity and has finished its progression through the phases of pediatric growth and development.

aerobic metabolism   Oxygen-based metabolism that is the body's principal combustion process.

afterload   The pressure against which the left ventricle must pump out (eject) blood with each beat.

air bags   Bags that automatically inflate in the event of a severe impact to cushion the impact. The bags absorb the energy slowly by increasing the body's stopping distance. These bags are designed only to cushion forward motion on the initial impact and are designed to be used in conjunction with seatbelts.

Alternate/backup airway   Airway device used when normal endotracheal intubation has failed; usually inserted blindly and provides some level of airway isolation.

alveoli   Where the respiratory system meets the circulatory system and gas exchange occurs.

Alzheimer's disease   Form of brain disease often associated with premature senile dementia.

amnesia   Loss of memory.

amputation   Severed part or part that is pathologically or surgically totally separated (removed) from the rest of the body.

anaerobic metabolism   Metabolism not using oxygen.

anatomic splinting   "Splinting" the body on a long backboard, in a supine position, and securing the patient to the board.

angina (angina pectoris)   Cramping, crushing midsternal chest pain caused by myocardial anoxia; often radiates to either arm, usually the left, and is associated with a feeling of suffocation and impending death.

anisocoria   Inequality of pupil size.

anterior cord syndrome   Condition resulting from bony fragments or pressure on spinal arteries.

anterocaudad   Forward and toward the feet.

anterograde amnesia   Amnesia for events occurring after the precipitating trauma; inability to form new memories.

anticoagulant   Substance or drug that prevents or delays coagulation or the forming of blood clots.

antihypertensive   Drug that reduces high blood pressure (hypertension). Some drugs that increase urine production (diuretics) lower the blood pressure by decreasing blood fluid volume.

aortic tear   Complete or partial tear of one or more layers of tissue of the aorta.

apnea   Absence of spontaneous breathing.

arachnoid mater (arachnoid membrane)   Spiderweb-like, transparent membrane between the dura mater and the pia mater; middle layer of the three meningeal membranes surrounding the brain.

ARDS   See *acute respiratory distress syndrome.*

ataxic breathing   Erratic breathing with no rhythm; typically associated with head injury and increased intracranial pressure.

atelectasis   Collapse of alveoli or part of the lung.

atherosclerosis   Narrowing of the blood vessels; condition in which the inner layer of the artery wall thickens while fatty deposits build up within the artery.

atlas   First cervical vertebra (C1); the skull perches on it.

avulsion   Ripping or tearing away of a part; a flap or partially separated tissue or part.

axis   Second cervical vertebra (C2); its shape allows for the wide range of rotation of the head. Also, an imaginary line that passes through the center of the body.

bag-valve-mask (BVM) device   Mechanical resuscitation device consisting of a self-inflating bag made of plastic or rubber and several one-way valves. Squeezing the bag results in positive-pressure ventilation through a mask, endotracheal tube, or alternate airway device; may be used with or without supplementary oxygen.

baroreceptor   Sensory nerve ending that is stimulated by changes in pressure. Baroreceptors are found in the walls of the atria of the heart, vena cava, aortic arch, and carotid sinus.

basilar skull fracture   Fracture to the floor of the cranium.

Battle's sign   Discoloration posterior and slightly inferior to the outer ears resulting from bleeding into the subcutaneous tissue caused by an occipital basilar skull fracture.

blunt trauma   Nonpenetrating trauma resulting from a temporary cavity in the body caused by a rapidly moving object with a small frontal projection concentrating its energy in one area.

body surface area (BSA)   Outer surface of the body covered by the skin. Percentage of the body's total surface area represented by any body part; used as one factor in determining size of a burn.

bradycardia   Pulse rate less than 60 beats per minute.

brainstem   Stemlike part of the brain that connects the cerebral hemispheres with the spinal cord.

bronchioles   The smaller divisions of the bronchial tubes.

Broselow Resuscitation Tape   Commercially available system for estimating pediatric medication dosing and equipment sizing based on patient length.

Brown-Séquard syndrome   Condition caused by penetrating injury and hemitransection of the spinal cord involving only one side of the cord.

capillaries   The smallest blood vessels; minute blood vessels that are only one cell wide, allowing for diffusion and osmosis through the capillary walls.

capnography (end-tidal carbon dioxide monitoring)   Monitoring that measures the partial pressure of carbon dioxide in a sample of gas. It can correlate very closely with the arterial partial pressure of carbon dioxide ($Paco_2$).

cardiac output   Volume of blood pumped by the heart at each contraction (reported in liters per minute).

cardioaccelerator center   Brain center that activates the sympathetic response that increases the rate of the heart.

cardiogenic shock   Shock that results from failure of the heart's pumping activity; causes can be categorized as either *intrinsic,* a result of direct damage to the heart itself, or *extrinsic,* related to a problem outside the heart.

cardioinhibitory center   Part of the medulla that slows or inhibits the heart's activity.

cardiovascular   Referring to the combination of the heart and blood vessels.

cataract   Milky lens that blocks and distorts light entering the eye and blurs vision.

catecholamines   Group of chemicals produced by the body that work as important nerve transmitters. The main catecholamines made by the body are dopamine, epinephrine (also called adrenaline), and norepinephrine. They are part of the body's sympathetic defense mechanism used in preparing the body to act.

caudad   Toward the tail (coccyx).

cavitation   Forcing tissues of the body out of their normal position and resulting in a temporary or permanent cavity (e.g., when body is struck by a bullet, acceleration of particles of tissue away from missile produces an area of injury where the large, temporary cavity occurs).

central cord syndrome   Condition that usually occurs with hyperextension of the cervical area.

central neurogenic hyperventilation   Pathologic rapid and shallow ventilatory pattern associated with head injury and increased intracranial pressure.

cephalad   Toward the head (away from the tail).

cerebellum   Portion of the brain that lies dorsal to the medulla oblongata and is concerned with coordination of movement.

cerebral perfusion pressure (CPP)   Difference between mean arterial pressure (MAP) and intracranial pressure (ICP).

cerebrospinal fluid (CSF)   Fluid found in the subarachnoid space and dural sheath; acts as a shock absorber, protecting the brain and spinal cord from jarring impact.

cerebrum   Largest part of the brain; responsible for the control of specific intellectual, sensory, and motor functions.

cervical flexion   Rotating the head forward or downward, causing bending of the neck.

cervical spine   Neck area of the spinal column containing seven vertebrae (C1-C7).

chemical burn   Burn that occurs when skin comes into contact with various caustic agents.

chemoreceptor   Sensory nerve ending that is stimulated by and reacts to certain chemical stimuli; located outside of the central nervous system. Chemoreceptors are found in the large arteries of the thorax and neck, the taste buds, and the olfactory cells of the nose.

chemoreceptor cells   Cells that stimulate nerve impulses by reacting to chemical stimuli. Certain chemoreceptor cells control the ventilatory rate.

Cheyne-Stokes breathing   Pathologic ventilatory pattern with periods of shallow, slow breathing increasing to rapid, deep breathing and then returning to shallow, slow breathing, followed by a short apneic period; often associated with traumatic brain injury and increased intracranial pressure.

chin lift   Method to open the airway of a patient with suspected cervical spine compromise; adaptation of chin lift airway maneuver that includes manual immobilization of the head in a neutral inline position.

cilia   Hairlike processes that propel foreign particles and mucus from the bronchi.

closed fracture   Fracture of a bone in which the skin is not interrupted.

coccygeal spine   Most caudad part of the spinal column; contains the three to five vertebrae that form the coccyx.

Colles' fracture Fracture of the wrist. If the victim falls forward onto outstretched hands to break a fall, this may result in a "silver fork deformity."

compartment syndrome Ischemia and compromised circulation that can occur from vascular injury; cellular edema produces increased pressure in a closed facial or bony compartment.

compensated shock Inadequate peripheral perfusion, as evidenced by signs of decreased organ perfusion but with normal blood pressure.

complete cord transection All spinal tracts are interrupted, and all cord functions distal to the site are lost.

complication Additional difficulty that occurs secondary to an injury, disease, or treatment. Also, disease or incident superimposed on another, without being specifically related, but affecting or modifying the prognosis of the original disease.

compression Type of force involved in impacts resulting in a tissue, organ, or other body part being squeezed between two or more objects or body parts.

compression injuries Injuries caused by severe crushing and squeezing forces; may occur to the external structure of the body or to the internal organs.

concussion Diagnosis made when an injured patient shows an alteration in neurologic function, most often a loss of consciousness, and no intracranial abnormality is identified by computed tomography (CT) scan.

conduction Transfer of heat between two objects in direct contact with each other.

consensual reflex Reflexive constriction of one pupil when a strong light is introduced into the other eye. A lack of consensual reflex is considered a positive sign of brain injury or eye injury.

contraindication Any sign, symptom, clinical impression, condition, or circumstance indicating that a given treatment or course of treatment is inappropriate and therefore outside of accepted medical practice. *Relative contraindication* is usually considered as a contraindication, but under special circumstances it may be overruled by a physician as an accepted medical practice on a case-by-case basis.

contralateral On the opposite side.

contrecoup injury Injury to parts of the brain located on the side opposite that of the primary injury.

contusion A bruise or bruising.

convection Heating of water or air in contact with a body, removing that air (e.g., wind) or water, then having to heat the new air or water that replaces what is left.

cord compression Pressure on the spinal cord caused by swelling, which may result in tissue ischemia and in some cases may require decompression to prevent a permanent loss of function.

cord concussion Condition resulting from the temporary disruption of the spinal cord functions distal to the injury.

cord contusion Bruising or bleeding into the spinal cord's tissue, which may also result in a temporary loss of cord functions distal to the injury.

cord laceration Injury that occurs when spinal cord tissue is torn or cut.

coup injury Injury to the brain located on the same side as the point of impact.

cranial vault The skull, or cranium.

crepitus Crackling sound made by bone ends grating together.

cyanosis Blue coloring of skin, mucous membranes, or nail beds indicating unoxygenated hemoglobin and a lack of adequate oxygen levels in the blood; usually secondary to inadequate ventilation or decreased perfusion.

decerebrate posturing Characteristic posture present in an individual with decerebrate rigidity; when a painful stimulus is introduced, the extremities are stiff and extended, and the head is retracted. One of the forms of pathologic posturing (response) typically associated with increased intracranial pressure.

decorticate posturing Characteristic pathologic posture of a patient with increased intracranial pressure; when a painful stimulus is introduced, the patient is rigidly still with the back and lower extremities extended while the arms are flexed and fists clenched.

definitive care Care that resolves the patient's illness or injury after a definitive diagnosis has been established. Clear and final care needed by the particular patient for the specific problem.

density Number of particles in each given area of tissue.

dermis Layer of skin just under the epidermis made up of a framework of connective tissues containing blood vessels, nerve endings, sebaceous glands, and sweat glands.

diaphragmatic rupture (diaphragmatic herniation) Tearing or cutting of the diaphragm so that the abdominal and thoracic cavities are no longer separated, allowing abdominal contents to enter the thoracic cavity; usually a result of increased intraabdominal pressure producing a tear in the diaphragm.

diaphyseal Part of or affecting the shaft of a long bone.

diastole Ventricular relaxation (ventricular filling).

diastolic blood pressure Resting pressure between ventricular contractions measured in millimeters of mercury (mm Hg).

diffusion Movement of solutes (substances dissolved in water) across a membrane.

distributive shock Shock that occurs when the vascular container enlarges without a proportional increase in fluid volume.

Don Juan syndrome Pattern that often occurs when victims fall or jump from a height and land on their feet. Bilateral calcaneus (heel bone) fractures are often associated with this syndrome. After the feet land and stop moving, the body is forced into flexion as the weight of the still-moving head, torso, and pelvis come to bear. This can cause compression fractures of the spinal column in the thoracic and lumbar areas.

down-and-under pathway When a vehicle ceases its forward motion, the occupant usually continues to travel downward into the seat and forward into the dashboard or steering column.

dura mater Outer membrane covering the spinal cord and brain; outer layer of the three meningeal layers; literally means "tough mother."

dural sheath Fibrous membrane that covers the brain and continues down to the second sacral vertebra.

dysarthria Difficulty speaking.

dysrhythmia (cardiac) Abnormal, disordered, or disturbed rhythm of the heart.

ecchymosis Bluish or purple, irregularly formed spot or area resulting from a hemorrhagic area below the skin.

edema Local or generalized condition in which some of the body tissues contain an excessive amount of fluid; generally includes swelling of the tissue.

edentulism Absence of teeth.

electrolytes Substances that separate into charged ions when dissolved in solution.

endotracheal intubation Insertion of a large tube into the trachea for direct ventilation from outside of the body; most desirable way of achieving definitive control of the airway in trauma casualties.

epidermis Outermost layer of the skin, made up entirely of epithelial cells with no blood vessels.

epidural hematoma Arterial bleeding that collects between the skull and dura mater.

epidural space Potential space between the dura mater surrounding the brain and the cranium; contains the meningeal arteries.

epiphyseal End of a long bone.

escharotomy Removal of sloughed tissue formed on the skin and underlying tissue of severely burned areas.

eucapnia Normal blood carbon dioxide level.

evaporation Change from liquid to vapor.

event phase Phase that begins at the time of impact between one moving object and a second object; occurrence of an incident.

evisceration Section of the intestine or other abdominal organ is displaced through an open wound and protrudes externally outside the abdominal cavity.

exsanguination Total loss of blood volume, producing death.

external respiration Transfer of oxygen molecules from the atmosphere to the blood.

fight-or-flight response Defense response produced by the sympathetic nervous system that simultaneously causes the heart to beat faster and stronger, constricts the arteries to raise blood pressure, and increases the ventilatory rate.

Fio$_2$ Fraction of oxygen in inspired air stated as a decimal; Fio$_2$ of 0.85 means that 85 hundredths or 85% of the inspired air is oxygen.

flail chest Chest with an unstable segment produced by multiple ribs fractured in two or more places, or including a fractured sternum.

flexion Bending movement around a joint that decreases the angle between the bones at the joint. In the cervical region, it is a forward bending motion of the head, bringing the chin nearer to the sternum.

foot-pounds of force Measure of mechanical force brought to bear; force equals mass times deceleration or acceleration.

foramen magnum Opening at the base of the skull.

foramina Small openings; singular, *foramen.*

fracture Broken bone. *Simple fracture* is closed without a tear or opening in the skin. In *open fracture,* initial injury or bone end has produced an open wound at or near the fracture site. *Comminuted fracture* has one or more free-floating segments of disconnected bone.

frostbite Actual freezing of body tissue as a result of exposure to freezing or below-freezing temperatures.

full-thickness (third-degree) burn Burn to the epidermis, dermis, and subcutaneous tissue (possibly deeper). Skin may look charred or leathery and may be bleeding.

G force (gravitational force) Actual force of acceleration or deceleration or of centrifugal force.

gastric ventilation Air undesirably forced down the esophagus and into the stomach rather than into the lungs.

geriatric Associated with aging and the diagnosis and treatment of injuries and diseases affecting the elderly population.

Glasgow Coma Scale (GCS) Scale for evaluating and quantifying level of consciousness or unconsciousness by determining the best responses to standardized stimuli of which the patient is capable.

global overview
Simultaneous 15- to 30-second overview of the patient's condition; focuses on patient's immediate ventilatory, circulatory, and neurologic status.

Golden Period
Time interval for patient to reach definitive care to achieve the best possible outcome.

heat cramps Acute painful spasms of the voluntary muscles after hard physical work in a hot environment, especially when patient is not acclimated to the temperature.

heat exhaustion Condition resulting from excessive fluid and electrolyte loss through sweating and lack of adequate fluid replacement when patient is exposed to high environmental temperatures for a sustained period, usually several days.

heat stress index Combination of ambient temperature and relative humidity.

heat stroke   Acute and dangerous reaction to heat exposure characterized by high body temperature.

hematocrit   Measure of the packed cell volume of red blood cells in the total blood volume.

hemianesthesia   Loss of sensation on one side of the body.

hemiparesis   Weakness limited to one side of the body.

hemiplegia   Paralysis on one side of the body.

hemoglobin   Molecule found in red blood cells that carry oxygen.

hemopericardium   Blood accumulation inside the pericardial space that can lead to pericardial tamponade.

hemorrhage   Bleeding; also, loss of a large amount of blood in a short period, either outside or inside the body.

hemothorax   Blood in the pleural space.

homeostasis   A constant, stable internal environment; balance necessary for healthy life processes.

hypercarbia   Increased level of carbon dioxide in the body.

hyperchloremia   Increase in the blood chloride level.

hyperextension
Extreme or abnormal extension; a position of maximum extension. Hyperextension of the neck is produced when the head is extended posterior to a neutral position and can result in a fracture or dislocation of the vertebrae or in spinal cord damage in patients with an unstable spine.

hyperflexion   Extreme or abnormal flexion; a position of maximum flexion. Increased flexion of the neck can result in a fracture or dislocation of the vertebrae or in spinal cord damage in patients with an unstable spine.

hyperkalemia   Increased blood potassium.

hypertension   Blood pressure greater than the upper limits of the normal range; generally considered to exist if patient's systolic pressure is greater than 150 mm Hg.

hypertensive crisis   Sudden, severe increase in blood pressure exceeding 200/120 mm Hg.

hyperthermia   Body temperature much higher than the normal range.

hypertonic   Greater osmotic pressure than normal serum or plasma.

hypoglycemia   Decreased blood glucose.

hypoperfusion   Inadequate perfusion (bathing) of cells with properly oxygenated blood.

hypopharynx   Lower portion of the pharynx that opens into the larynx anteriorly and the esophagus posteriorly.

hypotension   Blood pressure below the normal acceptable range.

hypothenar eminence   Fleshy part of the palm along the ulnar margin.

hypothermia   Subnormal core body temperature below the normal range, usually between 78° and 90° F (26° and 32° C).

hypotonic   Solution of lower osmotic pressure than another. Also, lower osmotic pressure than normal serum or plasma.

hypovolemia   Inadequate fluid volume of blood (below the normal range).

hypovolemic shock   Shock caused by loss of blood.

hypoxia (hypoxemia)   Deficiency of oxygen; inadequate available oxygen. Lack of adequate oxygenation of the lungs caused by inadequate minute volume (air exchange in the lungs) or a decreased concentration of oxygen in the inspired air. *Cellular hypoxia* is inadequate oxygen available to the cells.

immune system   Related group of responses of various body organs that protects the body from disease organisms, other foreign bodies, and cancers. The main components of the immune response system are the bone marrow, thymus, lymphoid tissues, spleen, and liver.

incisura (tentorial incisura)   Opening in the tentorium cerebelli at the junction of the midbrain and the cerebrum; the brainstem is inferior to the incisura.

incomplete cord transection   Transection of the spinal cord in which some tracts and motor/sensory functions remain intact.

infant   A child between 7 weeks and 1 year of age.

injury   Harmful event that arises from the release of specific forms of physical energy or barriers to normal flow of energy.

internal respiration   Movement or diffusion of oxygen molecules from the red blood cells into the tissue cells.

interstitial fluid   Extracellular fluid located between the cell wall and the capillary wall.

intervertebral disc   Cartilage-like discs that lie between the body of each vertebra and act as shock absorbers.

intervertebral foramen   Notch through which nerves pass in the inferior lateral side of the vertebra.

intracellular fluid   Fluid within the cells.

intracranial hypertension   Increased intracranial pressure.

intraosseous   Within the bone substance.

intubation   Passing a tube into a body aperture. *Endotracheal intubation* is the insertion of a breathing tube through the mouth or nose into the trachea to provide an airway for oxygen or an anesthetic gas.

ipsilateral   On the same side.

ischemia   Local and temporary deficiency of blood supply caused by obstruction of circulation to a body part or tissue.

ischemic sensitivity   Sensitivity of tissue cells to the lack of oxygen; usefulness of anaerobic metabolism before cell death occurs.

jaw thrust   Maneuver that enables the airway of a trauma patient to be opened while the head and cervical spine are manually maintained in a neutral inline position.

jugular vein distention (JVD)   Backup of pressure on the right side of the heart resulting in venous pooling and neck vein distention (engorgement) caused by decreased filling of the left side of the heart and reduced left-sided heart output.

kinematics   Process of examining the mechanism of injury of an incident to determine what injuries likely resulted from the forces and motion and changes in motion involved; the science of motion.

kinetic energy (KE)   Energy available from movement; function of the weight of an item and its speed: KE equals one-half the mass times the velocity squared.

kyphosis   Forward, humplike curvature of the spine often associated with the aging process; also may be caused by rickets or tuberculosis of the spine.

Laryngeal mask airway (LMA)   Alternative airway device used to provide airway support when endotracheal intubation is unsuccessful or not available; consists of an inflatable silicone mask and rubber connecting tube; is inserted blindly into the pharynx, forming a low-pressure seal around the laryngeal inlet.

laws of motion   Scientific laws relating to motion. *Newton's first law of motion:* A body at rest will remain at rest and a body in motion will remain in motion unless acted on by some outside force.

ligament   Band of tough, fibrous tissue connecting bone to bone.

ligamentum arteriosum   Remnant of fetal circulation and point of fixation at the arch of the aorta.

logroll   Method to turn patients with possible spine injury from one side to the other or completely over while manually protecting the spine from excessive, dangerous movement. Used to place patients with a suspected unstable spine onto a longboard.

lucid interval   Period of normal mental functioning between periods of disorientation, unconsciousness, or mental illness.

lumbar spine   Part of the spinal column found at the lower back inferior to the thoracic spine, containing the five lumbar vertebrae (L1-L5).

mass   A patient's weight.

mass-casualty (multiple-casualty) incident (MCI)   Event (e.g., plane crash, building collapse, fire) that produces a large number of patients from one mechanism, at one place, and at the same time.

mean arterial pressure   Average pressure in the vascular system; estimated by adding one-third the pulse pressure to the diastolic pressure.

mechanical energy   Form of energy dealing with movement.

mediastinum   Middle of the thoracic cavity containing the heart, great vessels, trachea, mainstem bronchi, and esophagus.

medulla (medulla oblongata)   Part of the brainstem; primary regulatory center of autonomic control of the cardiovascular system.

meninges   Three membranes that cover the brain tissue and the spinal cord.

metabolic acidosis   Acidosis resulting from an increase in acids other than carbonic acid.

metabolism   Sum of all physical and chemical changes that take place within an organism; all energy and material transformations that occur within living cells.

minute volume   Amount of air exchanged each minute; calculated by multiplying the volume of each breath (tidal volume) by the number of breaths per minute (rate).

myocardial contusion   Bruising of the heart or the heart muscle.

myocardium   Middle and thickest layer of the heart wall; composed of cardiac muscle.

nares   Openings in the nose that allow passage of the air from the outside to the throat (singular, *naris*). Anterior nares are the nostrils. Posterior nares are a pair of openings in the back of the nasal cavity where it connects with the upper throat.

nasopharyngeal airway   Airway that is placed in the nostril and follows the floor of the nasal cavity directly posterior to the nasopharynx. This airway is usually well tolerated by patients with a gag reflex.

nasopharynx   Upper portion of the airway, situated above the soft palate.

neural arches   Two curved sides of the vertebrae.

neurogenic shock   Shock that occurs when a cervical spine injury damages the spinal cord above where the nerves of the sympathetic nervous system exit.

newborn   A child from birth to 6 weeks of age.

nonpatent airway   An obstructed airway.

nonrebreather reservoir mask (NRB)   Oxygen mask with reservoir bag and nonrebreather valves that allow exhaled air to exit. It delivers high oxygen concentrations (85%-100%) to patients when attached to a high-liter-flow oxygen source.

obtundation   Sensory dullness.

occipital condyles   Two rounded, knuckle-like bumps at the end of the occipital bone at the back of the head.

oculomotor nerve   Third cranial nerve (CN III); controls pupillary constriction.

odontoid process   Toothlike protrusion on upper surface of the second vertebra (axis) around which the first cervical vertebra (atlas) turns, allowing the head to rotate through approximately 180 degrees.

offline medical direction   Written protocols that can direct most prehospital care.

oncotic pressure   Pressure that determines the amount of fluid within the vascular space.

online medical direction   Medical direction that allows the prehospital care provider to discuss patient care over the radio or phone while in the field.

open fracture   Fracture of a bone in which the skin is broken.

open pneumothorax   Penetrating wound to the chest causes the chest wall to open, producing a preferential pathway for air moving from the outside environment into the thorax; also called "sucking chest wound."

oropharyngeal airway   Airway that, when placed in the oropharynx superior to the tongue, holds the tongue forward to assist in maintaining an open airway. It is only used in patients with no gag reflex.

oropharynx   Central portion of the pharynx lying between the soft palate and upper portion of the epiglottis.

osmosis   Movement of water (or other solvent) across a membrane from an area that is hypotonic to an area that is hypertonic.

osteoporosis   Loss of normal bone density, with thinning of bone tissue and growth of small holes in the bone; may cause pain (especially in lower back), frequent broken bones, loss of body height, and various poorly formed parts of the body; often part of the normal aging process.

overtriage   Problem resulting when minimally injured or noninjured patients are taken to trauma centers.

oxygen consumption   Volume of oxygen consumed by the body in 1 minute.

palpation   Process of examination performed by applying the hands or fingers to the external surface of the body to detect evidence of disease, abnormalities, or underlying injury.

para-anesthesia   Loss of sensation in the lower extremities.

paradoxical motion   Motion caused by the combination of lower pressure in the chest and higher atmospheric pressure outside the chest that causes a flail segment to move inward, rather than outward, during inspiration.

paradoxical pulse   Condition in which patient's systolic blood pressure drops more than 10 to 15 mm Hg during each inspiration, usually caused by increased intrathoracic pressure.

paraplegia   Paralysis of the lower extremities.

parasympathetic acute stress reaction   Response that slows bodily functions and may result in syncope.

parasympathetic nervous system   Division of the nervous system that maintains normal body functions.

paresis   Undue localized weakness or partial (less than total) paralysis that may be related to nerve inflammation or injury.

parietal pleura   Thin membrane that lines the inner side of the thoracic cavity.

Parkland formula   Formula for fluid replacement of the burn patient.

partial-thickness (second-degree) burn   Burn to both epidermis and dermis; skin presents with reddened areas, blisters, or open, weeping wounds.

patent airway   Open, unobstructed airway of sufficient size to allow for normal volumes of air exchange.

pathophysiology   The study of how normal physiologic processes are altered by disease or injury.

PEARRL   Pupils equal and round, reactive to light; used when checking patient's eyes to determine if they are round, appear normal, and appropriately react to light by constricting, or abnormal and unresponsive; generally includes the presence of consensual reflex.

pediatric   Dealing with children; dealing with injuries and diseases affecting children (birth to 16 years of age).

pediatric trauma score (PTS)   Clinical scoring system based on clinical information known to be predictive of severity of injury; can be used for triage decision making.

penetrating trauma   Trauma when an object penetrates the skin; generally produces both permanent and temporary cavities.

percutaneous transtracheal ventilation (PTV)   Procedure for patient ventilation in which 16-gauge or larger needle is inserted directly into lumen of the trachea through the cricothyroid membrane or directly through the tracheal wall.

perfusion   Fluid passing through an organ or a part of the body. Also, the surrounding and bathing of a tissue or cell with blood or fluid parts of the blood.

pericardial space   Potential space existing between the heart muscle (myocardium) and the pericardium.

pericardial tamponade   Compression of the heart by blood collecting in the pericardial sac, which surrounds the heart muscle (myocardium); also called *cardiac tamponade.*

pericardiocentesis   Procedure to remove accumulated blood inside the pericardial space.

pericardium   Tough, fibrous, flexible but inelastic membrane that surrounds the heart.

peristalsis   Propulsive muscular movements of the intestines.

peritoneal space   Space in the anterior abdominal cavity that contains the bowel, spleen, liver, stomach, and gallbladder; lined with the peritoneum.

peritoneum   Lining of the abdominal cavity.

peritonitis   Inflammation of the peritoneum.

phantom pain   The experience of sensation in the missing part or limb after amputation.

pharynx   The throat; a tubelike structure that is a passage for both breathing and digestive tract. *Oropharynx* is area of pharynx posterior to the mouth; *nasopharynx* is area of pharynx beyond the posterior nares.

pia mater   Thin, vascular membrane closely adhering to the brain and spinal cord and proximal portions of the nerves; innermost layer of the three meningeal membranes that cover the brain.

pleura   Thin membrane that lines the inner side of the thoracic cavity and the lungs. The part that lines the thoracic cavity is called the *parietal pleura;* the fold covering the lung is called the *visceral pleura.*

pleural fluid   Fluid that creates surface tension between the two pleural membranes and causes them to cling together.

pneumatic antishock garment (PASG)   Garment designed to put pressure on the lower portion of the body and prevent pooling of blood in the abdomen and pelvis; also called *military* or *medical antishock trousers* (MAST).

pneumothorax   Injury that produces air in the pleural space; often associated with a collapsed lung. A pneumothorax can be *open,* with an opening through the chest wall to the outside, or *closed,* resulting from blunt trauma or a spontaneous collapse.

postevent phase   Phase that begins as soon as energy from the crash is absorbed and patient is traumatized. The phase of prehospital care that includes response time, "golden period," and critique of a call.

preevent phase   Phase that includes all the events that precede the incident (e.g., ingestion of drugs and alcohol) and conditions that predate the incident (e.g., acute or preexisting medical conditions). This phase includes injury prevention and preparedness.

preload   Volume and pressure of the blood coming into the heart from the systemic circulatory system (venous return); the process outside of the heart in the vena cava.

premature ventricular contraction   Irregular, extra contraction of the ventricles resulting from an ectopic stimulus, causing a contraction rather than the normal stimuli from the normal pacing node. Second most common abnormal rhythm of the heart.

presbycusis   Gradual decline in hearing.

presbyopia   Farsightedness.

preschooler   A child with the body size and physical development normally found in children between 2 and 6 years of age. An arbitrary grouping of children based on the similar physical characteristics common to these ages.

priapism   Penis remains erect, usually for a prolonged period; may be caused by a urinary stone or an injury to the lower spinal column.

primary brain injury   Direct trauma to the brain and associated vascular injuries.

primary injuries of blasts   Injuries caused by the pressure wave of the blast (e.g., pulmonary bleeding, pneumothorax, perforation of gastrointestinal tract).

primary survey   Initial assessment of airway, breathing, circulation, disability, and expose/environment to identify and manage any life-threatening injuries.

psychogenic shock   Temporary neurogenic shock as a result of psychological stress (fainting).

pulmonary contusion   Bruising of the lungs; can be secondary to blunt or penetrating trauma.

pulmonary diffusion   Movement of oxygen from the alveoli across the alveolar capillary membrane and into the red blood cells or the plasma.

pulmonary function   Controlled patent airway, ventilation, diffusion, and perfusion, resulting in arterial blood that contains adequate oxygen for aerobic metabolism and a proper level of carbon dioxide to maintain tissue acid-base balance.

pulse oximeter   Device that measures arterial oxyhemoglobin saturation, by determining the absorption ratio of red and infrared light passed through the tissue.

pulse pressure   Increase in pressure (surge) created as each new bolus of blood leaves the left ventricle. Also, the difference between the systolic and diastolic blood pressures (systolic pressure minus diastolic pressure equals pulse pressure).

quadriplegia   Paralysis of all four extremities.

raccoon eyes (periorbital ecchymosis)   Distinct bruised (ecchymotic) area around each eye, limited by the orbital margins.

radiation   Direct transfer of energy from a warm object to a cooler one by infrared radiation.

rapid deceleration mechanism   A series of three collisions that occur when a vehicle suddenly ceases forward motion: (1) vehicle, (2) occupant inside vehicle, and (3) occupant's internal organs.

rapid-sequence intubation (RSI)   Method of patient preparation for intubation that includes pharmacologic adjuncts for sedation and muscle relaxation.

residual volume   Air that remains trapped in the alveoli and bronchi that cannot be forcibly exhaled.

respiration   Total ventilatory and circulatory steps involved in the exchange of oxygen and carbon dioxide between the outside atmosphere and the cells of the body; in medicine, may be limited to breathing and the steps in ventilation.

respiratory tract   Pathway for air movement between the outside air and the alveoli; includes the nasal cavity, oral cavity, pharynx, larynx, trachea, bronchi, and lungs.

response time   From the time an incident occurs until arrival of emergency medical services (EMS) on scene.

retrograde amnesia   Loss of memory for events and situations just preceding the time (immediate preinsult period) of patient's injury or illness. Also, loss of memory for past events.

retroperitoneal space   Space in the posterior abdominal cavity that contains the kidneys, ureters, bladder, reproductive organs, inferior vena cava, abdominal aorta, pancreas, a portion of the duodenum, colon, and rectum.

revised trauma score   Method for scoring and quantifying the severity of trauma in pediatric patients.

rotational impact   When one vehicle strikes the front or rear side of another, causing it to rotate away from the point of impact. Also, when one corner of the vehicle strikes an immovable object or one moving slower or in the opposite direction of the vehicle, resulting in it rotating.

rule of nines   Topographic breakdown (mostly of 9% and 18% portions) of the body to estimate the amount of body surface covered by burns.

sacral spine   Part of the spinal column below the lumbar spine containing the five sacral vertebrae (S1-S5), which are connected by immovable joints to form the *sacrum,* the weight-bearing base of the spinal column and part of the pelvic girdle.

safety   Evaluation of all possible dangers and ensuring that no unreasonable threats or risks still exist.

SAR   Search and rescue.

scalp   Outermost covering of the head.

scene   Environment to be evaluated in which injury occurred. In a motor vehicle crash, this includes evaluation of the number of vehicles, the forces that acted on each, and the degree and type of damage to each.

school-age child   A child with the body size and physical development normally found in children between about 6 and 12 years of age. An arbitrary grouping of children based on the similar physical characteristics common to these ages.

secondary brain injury   Extension of the magnitude of the primary brain injury by factors that result in a larger, more permanent neurologic deficit.

secondary injuries of blasts   Injuries that occur when the victim is struck by flying glass, falling mortar, or other debris from the blast.

secondary survey   Head-to-toe evaluation of the trauma patient. This assessment is done only after the primary survey is complete and there are no immediate life-threatening problems; usually done en route in urgent patients.

semipermeable membrane   Membrane that will allow fluids (solvents), but not the dissolved substance, to pass through it.

senescence   The process of aging.

sensory examination   Gross examination of sensory capability and response to determine the presence or absence of loss of sensation in each of the four extremities.

sepsis   Infection.

septic shock   Shock caused by widespread systemic infection, resulting in release of locally active hormones and causing damage to the walls of blood vessels, producing both peripheral vasodilation and leakage of fluid from the capillaries into the interstitial space.

shear   Change-of-speed force resulting in a cutting or tearing of body parts.

shock   Widespread lack of tissue perfusion with oxygenated red blood cells that leads to anaerobic metabolism and decreased energy production.

sinoatrial node   Node at junction of superior vena cava with right cardiac atrium; regarded as the pacing or starting point of the heartbeat. In healthy patients, pacing from this node causes atrial contraction, is slowed, and then produces ensuing contraction of the ventricles.

situation   Events, relationships, and roles of those parties who, with the patient, were involved in a call. The situation (e.g., domestic dispute, single-vehicle crash without apparent cause, elderly person living alone, a shooting) is important in scene assessment.

skull (cranium)   Several bones that fuse into a single structure during childhood.

sniffing position   Slightly superior and anterior position of the midface.

spinal shock   Injury to the spinal cord that results in a temporary loss of sensory and motor function.

spinal stenosis   Narrowing of the spinal canal.

spinous process   Tail-like structure on the posterior region of the vertebrae.

sprain   Injury in which ligaments are stretched or even partially torn.

strain   Soft tissue injury or muscle spasm that occurs around a joint anywhere in the musculature.

stroke volume   Volume of blood pumped out by each contraction (stroke) of the left ventricle.

subarachnoid hemorrhage   Bleeding into the cerebrospinal fluid-filled space.

subarachnoid space   Space between pia mater proper and arachnoid membrane; contains cerebrospinal fluid and meningeal veins. The subarachnoid space is a common site of subdural hematomas.

subcutaneous layer   Layer of skin just under the dermis that is a combination of elastic and fibrous tissue as well as fat deposits.

subdural hematoma   Collection of blood between dura mater and arachnoid membrane.

superficial (first-degree) burn   Burn to the epidermis only; red, inflamed, and painful skin.

supine hypotension syndrome   Decrease in blood pressure caused by compression of the vena cava by the uterus.

surgical cricothyrotomy   Procedure to open a patient's airway that should be considered a "last resort"; accomplished by cutting a slit into the cricoid cartilage in the neck to open the airway into the trachea; also *cricothyroidotomy.*

sympathetic acute stress reaction   "Fight-or-flight" response in which bodily functions increase and pain masking occurs.

sympathetic nervous system   Division of the nervous system that produces the fight-or-flight response.

synovial fluid   Fluid found inside joints.

systemic vascular resistance (SVR)   Amount of resistance to the flow of blood through the vessels. SVR increases as the vessel constricts. Any change in lumen diameter or vessel elasticity can influence the amount of SVR.

systole   Ventricular contraction.

systolic blood pressure   Peak blood pressure produced by the force of the contraction (systole) of the ventricles of the heart.

tachycardia   Abnormally fast rate of heartbeats; defined as greater than 100 beats per minute in an adult.

tachypnea   Increased breathing rate.

tendon   Band of tough, inelastic, fibrous tissue that connects a muscle to bone.

tension pneumothorax   Condition occurring when the air pressure in the pleural space exceeds the outside atmospheric pressure and cannot escape. The affected side becomes hyperinflated, compressing the lung on the involved side and shifting the mediastinum to partially collapse the other lung. A tension pneumothorax is usually progressive and is an imminently life-threatening condition.

tentorial herniation   Normally the cerebrum (brain) is supratentorial. When part of the brain is pushed down through the incisura as a result of increased intracranial pressure, tentorial herniation occurs.

tentorium cerebelli (tentorium)   An infolding of the dura that forms a covering over the cerebellum. The tentorium is a part of the floor of the upper skull just below the brain (cerebrum).

tertiary injuries of blasts   Third group of injuries sustained in a sequence (or pattern) of injury-producing events (e.g., explosions); occur when the victim becomes a missile and is thrown against some object. These injuries are similar to those sustained in ejections from vehicles, in falls from significant heights, or when the victim is thrown against an object by the force wave resulting from an explosion. Tertiary injuries are usually obvious injuries.

thoracic spine   Part of the spinal column between the cervical spine (superiorly) and the lumbar spine (inferiorly) containing the 12 thoracic vertebrae (T1-T12). The 12 pairs of ribs connect to the thoracic vertebrae.

thorax (thoracic cavity)   Hollow cylinder supported by 12 pairs of ribs that articulate posteriorly with the thoracic spine and 10 pairs that articulate anteriorly with the sternum. The two lowest pairs are only fastened posteriorly (to the vertebrae) and are called *floating ribs.* The thoracic cavity is defined and separated inferiorly by the diaphragm.

tidal volume   Normal volume of air exchanged with each ventilation. About 500 mL of air is exchanged between the lungs and the atmosphere with each breath in a healthy adult at rest.

toddler   A child with the body size and physical development normally found in children between about 1 and 2 years of age.

tonsil-tip catheter   Rigid suction catheter designed for rapid removal of large amounts of fluid, vomitus, blood, and debris from the mouth and pharynx to avoid aspiration.

total lung capacity   Total volume of air in the lungs after a forced inhalation.

toxemia   Distribution throughout the body of poisonous products of bacteria (toxins) growing in a focal or local site.

trauma chin lift   Maneuver ideally used to relieve a variety of anatomic airway obstructions in patients who are breathing spontaneously; accomplished by grasping the chin and lower incisors, then lifting to pull the mandible forward.

trauma jaw thrust   Maneuver that allows an open airway with little or no movement of the head and cervical spine. The mandible is thrust forward by placing the thumbs on each zygomatic arch and placing the index and long fingers under the mandible and at the same angle, thrusting the mandible forward.

traumatic aneurysm   Abnormal dilation, bursting, or tearing of a major blood vessel (usually an artery) caused by or related to an injury.

traumatic asphyxia   Blunt and crushing injuries to the chest and abdomen with marked increase of intravascular pressure, producing rupture of the capillaries.

Trendelenburg position   Simultaneous lowering of patient's head while elevating patient's legs. Usually done by raising foot end of a flat bed or longboard higher than head end. In this position (with abdomen higher than thorax), weight of the abdominal contents presses on the diaphragm, producing some ventilatory difficulty. A modified Trendelenburg position, with the head and torso horizontal and only the legs elevated, will minimize ventilatory problems.

triage   French word meaning "to sort"; a process in which a group of patients is categorized according to their priority of need for care. When only several patients are involved, triage involves alternating from patient to patient, meeting all the patients' highest-priority needs first, then moving to lower-priority items. In a mass-casualty incident, triage is done by determining both urgency and potential for survival.

tumble   End-over-end motion. Bullets usually tumble when resistance is met by the leading edge of the missile.

undertriage   Problem that arises when seriously injured patients are not recognized as such and are mistakenly taken to nontrauma centers.

up-and-over pathway   Body's forward motion carries it up and over steering wheel; chest or abdomen typically impacts steering wheel, and head strikes windshield. In semisitting position common in passenger vehicles, once the down-and-under motion has ended, as the knees are stopped by the dashboard, the body then continues in an up-and-over movement. In some trucks, where the driver is sitting fully upright with feet stopped by the pedals, the up-and-over movement may occur initially.

vagal Dealing with stimulation of the vagus (tenth cranial) nerve; parasympathetic system's response that slows the heart rate and reduces the force of contractions, keeping the body within workable limits. This response can normally override the sympathetic nervous system's chemical release, keeping the heart rate in an acceptable range. Accidental vagal stimulation, however, can produce an undesirable bradycardia, further reducing the patient's cardiac output and circulation.

vagus nerve Tenth cranial nerve (CN X); when stimulated, slows the heart rate, regardless of catecholamine levels. It contains motor and sensory functions and a wider distribution than the other cranial nerves.

velocity Quickness of motion; speed, as in the speed of a moving mass.

ventilation Movement of air into and out of the lungs through the normal breathing process. The mechanical process by which air moves from the atmosphere outside the body through the mouth, nose, pharynx, trachea, bronchi, and bronchioles, and into and out of the alveoli. To ventilate a patient is to provide positive-pressure inspirations with a ventilating device, such as a bag-valve-mask device, and then alternately allowing time for passive exhalation to occur; used in patients who are apneic or who cannot provide adequate ventilation for themselves.

vertebra Any of the 33 bony segments of the spinal column; plural, *vertebrae*.

vertebral body Area of the vertebrae that bears most of the weight of the spine.

vertebral foramen Opening in the vertebral body; plural, *foramina*.

visceral pleura Thin membrane that covers the outer surface of each lung.

whistle-stop catheter (whistle-tip catheter) Soft catheter used for suctioning the nasal passage, deep oropharynx, or endotracheal tube; allows for controlled intermittent suction. Its name is derived from the opening (whistle-stop) found in the side of the proximal end of the catheter. Suction is not produced at the distal tip until this hole or port is covered with one of the operator's fingers, producing a closed system to the opening at the distal tip.

zygomatic arches Bones that form superior area of the cheeks of the face. Laterally, superior to the molars, these extend more anteriorly than the maxilla, giving the individual some of his or her unique facial structure; commonly called the "cheekbones."

Index

Page numbers followed by b indicate boxes; f, figures; t, tables.

Mannitol, 216, 369

Manual clearing of airway, 95, 124, 126f, 140-141

Manual inline stabilization of head, 138-139, 237, 247-248, 486-487

Manually triggered ventilatory devices, 134

MAP. *See* Mean arterial pressure (MAP).

Maritime medicine, 531

Mark-1 kit, 514

Mask squeeze, 461, 462t

Masks
  donning and removing, 515b, 516b
  face or pocket, 134
  guidelines for, 75, 516

Mass, kinetic energy and, 34

Mass effect, 201-203, 204

Mass-casualty incidents (MCIs). *See also* Disasters; Weapons of mass destruction (WMD).
  cardiopulmonary resuscitation in, 536
  management of, 492, 493-494
  pediatric triage for, 373-377
  priorities for, 70, 93
  triage for, 83-86, 87b-88b

Mean arterial pressure (MAP), 166, 199-200

Mechanical energy, 18, 34

Mechanical principles
  of pressure, 459-461
  of trauma, 32, 38-64

Mechanisms of injury. *See also* Kinematics.
  for drowning, 448-449
  for explosives, 509
  for geriatric trauma, 391-392
  for lightning, 454-455
  for musculoskeletal trauma, 317
  for spinal trauma, 224-225, 231-232, 233-234

Media, partnering with, 495

Mediastinal emphysema, 463

Mediastinal shift, 281f

Mediastinum, 273

Medical and surgical history, past, 104. *See also* History.

Medical assistance teams, 498

Medical consultation for law enforcement, 531

Medical counterterrorism operations, 537-538, 540

Medical evaluation
  for fitness to dive, 458, 467, 469b
  for heat stress, 423b

Medical intelligence, 538

Medical response to disasters, 493, 495-499

Medications. *See also* Pain management.
  AMPLE history for, 104
  for bee sting allergy, 556
  for brain injury, 216, 369-370
  for cyanide poisoning, 344-345, 513
  elderly use of, 212, 394-395

Medications—*cont'd*
  heat illness and, 407-408
  for high-altitude illness, 472t, 473-474, 475
  high-altitude illness and, 470
  for hypothermia, 434
  for intubation, 129, 130b, 131t
  for nerve agents, 513-514
  postexposure prophylactic, 77b
  for scuba-related injuries, 474
  shock and, 178-179
  storage of, 421, 424
  topical burn, 340
  vital sign changes and, 392

Medline, 9b

Medulla
  function of, 198b, 199
  injury to, 203

Meninges, 196, 197f, 198

Mental health, disasters and, 499-500

Mental status
  altered, immobilization for, 234
  in elderly, 389, 392-393, 394
  in heat stroke, 412

Meperidine, 326

Metabolic acidosis, 169

Metabolism
  aerobic, 118, 121, 122
  anaerobic, 94, 118, 169
  energy production in, 482
  heat production in, 405-406

Methemoglobin, 344-345

Methylprednisolone, 242

Metropolitan Medical Response System (MMRS), 495, 498

Microcirculatory changes in shock, 169, 170f

Midazolam (Versed), 131t

Midbrain, 198b

Middle ear squeeze, 461, 462t

Midface fractures, 209

Miliaria rubra, 407, 409

Minor triage category, 86, 87b, 88b

Minute ventilation (V_E), 275b

Minute volume
  calculation of, 121
  decreased, 123

Miosis, 513

Missile injuries. *See* Gunshot wounds; Penetrating trauma.

Monitoring and reassessment, 110
  for brain injury, 207
  terminology for, 93t

Monro-Kellie doctrine, 201-202

Morgan lens, 347, 348f

Morphine, 112
  for frostbite pain, 438
  for musculoskeletal trauma, 325
  for pediatric trauma, 372

Mortality. *See* Death.

Motion, laws of, 33-35

Motor function, assessment of, 317, 318

Motor nerves, spinal, 229

Motor vehicle crashes (MVC), 38-45
  abdominal trauma in, 302
  air bags and, 45

Motor vehicle crashes (MVC)—*cont'd*
  among elderly, 384, 391-392
  deaths from, 5f, 15f, 16b, 32
  energy in, 33-35
  impact and injury patterns in, 38-43, 44f
  pediatric trauma in, 46, 356, 357t, 358b
  phases of, 20, 21t, 32-33
  prevention of, 5
  scene assessment for, 33
  scene safety for, 71-72, 73f
  seat belts and, 44-45
  spinal injuries in, 234
  terminology for, 20
  vehicle incompatibility in, 43-44

Motorcycle crashes, 5f, 45-47

Motorcycle helmet laws, 5, 46

Mountain sickness, acute. *See* Acute mountain sickness (AMS).

Mouth-to-mouth/mask ventilation, 134t

Moyer's solution, 347

MTWHF mnemonic for nerve agent poisoning, 513

Mucocutaneous exposure to blood, 74, 76, 77b

Multiple organ failure, 174, 482, 483

Multiple-patient incidents, 70, 93. *See also* Mass-casualty incidents (MCIs).

Multisystem trauma patient, 93, 94b
  hypothermia in, 429
  principles of care for, 483-489

Muscarinic effects of nerve agents, 513

Muscle cramps, 409-410

Muscles, 315, 316f
  aging of, 390, 394
  of breathing, 272, 273f, 274f

Musculoskeletal system
  aging of, 389-390, 394
  anatomy and physiology of, 314-315, 316f

Musculoskeletal trauma
  algorithm for, 329
  assessment of, 316-318
  fractures and dislocations in, 319-324
  hemorrhage in, 178, 318-319
  management of, 314, 330, 486
  pediatric, 371
  prolonged transport for, 330
  special considerations for, 325-328

Mustard agents, 514

Myocardial hypertrophy, 388

Myocardial infarction, 387

Myocardial injuries, 61-62, 173, 283-284

Myoglobin, release of, 327-328, 343

Myoglobinuria, 343

N

N-95 mask, 524

Narcotics, 112
  for frostbite pain, 438
  intubation using, 129, 131t